9899

MORECAMBE BAY HOSPITALS NHS TRUST

D1388122

Farquharson's textbook of operative general surgery

Farquharson's textbook of operative general surgery

Ninth edition

Margaret Farquharson FRCSEd

and

Brendan Moran FRCSI

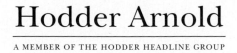

General Surgeons, North Hampshire Hospital, Basingstoke, UK

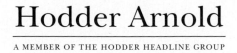

Hodder Arnold

A MEMBER OF THE HODDER HEADLINE GROUP

First published in 1954 by E&S Livingstone
Second edition published in 1962
Third edition published in 1966
Fourth edition published in 1969
Fifth edition published in 1972
Sixth edition published in 1978
Seventh edition published in 1986
Eighth edition published in 1995

This edition published in Great Britain in 2005 by
Hodder Education, a member of the Hodder Headline Group,
338 Euston Road, London NW1 3BH

http://www.hoddereducation.com

Distributed in the United States of America by
Oxford University Press Inc.,
198 Madison Avenue, New York, NY10016
Oxford is a registered trademark of Oxford University Press

Whilst the advice and information in this book are believed to be true and
accurate at the date of going to press, neither the author[s] nor the publisher
can accept any legal responsibility or liability for any errors or omissions
that may be made. In particular, (but without limiting the generality of the
preceding disclaimer) every effort has been made to check drug dosages;
however it is still possible that errors have been missed. Furthermore,
dosage schedules are constantly being revised and new side-effects
recognized. For these reasons the reader is strongly urged to consult the
drug companies' printed instructions before administering any of the drugs
recommended in this book.

British Library Cataloguing in Publication Data
A catalogue record for this book is available from the British Library

Library of Congress Cataloging-in-Publication Data
A catalog record for this book is available from the Library of Congress

ISBN-10: 0 340 81498 5
ISBN-13: 978 0 340 81498 7
ISBN-10: 0 340 81496 9 (International Students' Edition, restricted territorial availability)
ISBN-13: 978 0 340 81496 3

1 2 3 4 5 6 7 8 9 10

Commissioning Editor: Joanna Koster
Development Editor: Sarah Burrows
Production Controller: Lindsay Smith
Cover Design: Sarah Rees
Artwork: Gillian Lee Illustrations

Typeset in 10 on 12pt Minion by Phoenix Photosetting, Chatham, Lordswood, Kent
Printed and bound in India.

617.91
FAR

What do you think about this book? Or any other Hodder Arnold title?
Please visit our website at www.hoddereducation.com

Contents

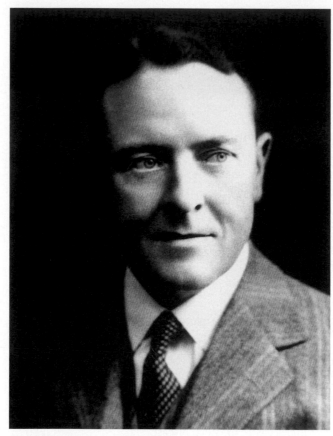

Eric L Farquharson 1905–1970.
This photograph was taken around the time of the publication of the 1st edition.

Foreword to the Ninth Edition

Eric Farquharson was a surgeon ahead of his time. As one who was taught by him and who worked for him, it is easy to remember the many innovations which he introduced, the many ideas which he had and his ability to look beyond conventional wisdom. He was heavily involved both with the Royal College of Surgeons of Edinburgh and the Royal College of Surgeons of England, a position which is commendable even today.

Although he championed single authorship, I believe that he would have been one of the first to recognise how essential it is for operative surgery to be taught by surgeons operating within their individual speciality. In this ninth edition of his textbook, the areas covered are comprehensive but, more importantly, they have been covered by authors who clearly speak from experience and with authority. It is therefore inevitable that both surgical trainees and trained surgeons will benefit from this important new text.

JAR Smith PhD PRCSEd FRCSEng
President of The Royal College of Surgeons of Edinburgh
2005

Preface to the Ninth Edition

Eric Farquharson wrote the 1st edition of *Operative Surgery* in 1954. He was a general surgeon in an era when general surgery still included orthopaedics and urology, and most surgeons regularly operated on a wide range of problems. He intended the book to be of value to the surgeon in training, and he described the common operations within the boundaries of general surgery in the early 1950s. However, half a century later, surgical practice has expanded and changed. Urology and orthopaedics are now separate surgical disciplines. General surgery itself is subdividing, and the more advanced procedures in each subspecialty are not performed by those in other subspecialties, and only rarely by generalists. Special expertise and the availability of advanced technology have encouraged development of centres of excellence for specific conditions, and referral between surgical colleagues has increased.

For this edition to continue to be a valuable companion for the practising surgeon, it also has had to evolve. The kernel of the book remains the description of operations within the present narrower boundaries of general surgery, with discussion of the possible surgical options. Non-operative surgical topics are, of necessity, condensed although it is acknowledged that the practice of surgery increasingly encompasses preoperative investigation, the planning of optimal management in conjunction with non-surgical colleagues, and the care of the critically ill surgical patient.

Operative surgery in specialities other than general surgery has now in general been omitted. However, in an emergency, even those surgeons practising in well-equipped hospitals in the developed world must occasionally operate outside their specialty. In addition, previous editions have proved to be of value to the surgeon working in parts of the world where general surgery has to be a more all-encompassing surgical discipline. For these reasons, selective operations have been retained, including some older techniques, which may still be of value in certain circumstances.

Eric Farquharson believed in single authorship to give balance and continuity of style. Specialization, however, was starting in the 1950s and he sought advice from colleagues whose practice concentrated on orthopaedics, neurosurgery and urology. This philosophy has been followed for much of this new edition. In some chapters advice from several specialists was obtained, and in the chapters which cover other surgical disciplines the approach has been from the viewpoint of the general surgeon. However, in some chapters a separate general surgical subspeciality author has been more appropriate. In each chapter a few references, including some to historic papers, have been selected by the authors. The choice has been personal, and there has been no attempt to provide a comprehensive list which can be obtained from other sources.

This edition is intended for the surgical trainee in general surgery and should be of value throughout training. It should also continue to serve more experienced general surgeons when faced with an operative surgical challenge outside their chosen area of expertise. Despite subspecialization, there will always be a need for general surgical knowledge and skills, and we hope that this book fulfils this purpose.

Acknowledgements

A textbook entering its 9th edition, some 50 years after its first publication, is inevitably a hybrid text which has been modified with each successive edition. Much has changed in surgery during this period, and some sections have had to be extensively rewritten.

However, there are passages originally written by Eric Farquharson which are still valid today and these have been retained, along with some of the original illustrations. Eric Farquharson died in 1970, and entrusted his book to Forbes Rintoul who has edited it until his own recent retirement. Much of the work of Forbes Rintoul, and of the contributors and artists to the editions during his editorship, has been retained. The legacy to the Ninth Edition from all of these sources is gratefully acknowledged. We have been privileged to receive letters of encouragement from many of the former contributors, and in addition they have almost without exception been happy for any of their text that is still relevant to be used in this new edition. They have made offers to proof-read, or to try and find replacement contributors when they have been no longer able to contribute themselves due to retirement or increasing commitments. Their continuing interest in the book has been an enormous encouragement, but our particular thanks must go to Forbes Rintoul who, after his retirement, has so generously handed the future of the book back to Eric Farquharson's family, and has given us his full support.

This edition has only been possible as a result of the help we have received from so many people. We are extremely grateful to them all. The list of contributors to this edition includes all those who have written sections for this edition, and all who have acted as advisors in their field of expertise. Where a contributor has written the greater part of a chapter his or her name is given as the author of that chapter. Some contributors who have written their own chapters have, in addition, advised in other sections of the book which pertain to their specialty. Other contributors, who are not authors of chapters, have also advised in their area of expertise throughout the book, as outlined below.

Anatomy	Chummy Sinnantamby
Breast and Endocrine	Robert Carpenter
Cardiothoracic	David Wheatley
Colorectal	David Bartolo
Head and Neck	Simon Keightley (Ophthalmology)
	Cyrus Kerawala (Maxillofacial)
	Robert Sanderson (Otolaryngology)
Gynaecology	David Farquharson
	Colin Jardine-Brown
Neurosurgery	Carl Meyer
Orthopaedics	Geoffrey Hooper
Paediatric surgery	John Orr
Peri-operative care	Alsion Milne (Haematology)
	Piers Wilson (Aneasthetics)
Plastic surgery	Kenneth Stewart
Urology	Timothy Hargreave
	Anthony Richards

In addition, there are many un-named colleagues whom we wish to thank. Trainees have read chapters, and advised on content and whether explanations are clear. Surgeons who have worked in isolated hospitals have suggested what operations should be included, and local colleagues have provided many unofficial answers to questions.

We would like to thank our immediate families for all their support, and in particular our long-suffering spouses. All the time spent on preparation is time when we have been unavailable for them. In the preface to the 1st Edition, Eric Farquharson expresses his gratitude to his wife for her active interest and support. She proof-read the first and every subsequent edition including this one, and has been an invaluable source of help and encouragement.

Contributors

David CC Bartolo MS FRCS FRCSE
Consultant Colorectal Surgeon
Western General Hospital
Edinburgh, UK

Robert Carpenter MB BS MS FRCS
Consultant Breast and Endocrine Surgeon
Breast and Endocrine Unit
St Bartholomew's Hospital
London, UK

David IM Farquharson FRCOG FRCS(Ed)
Consultant Gynaecologist
Simpson Centre for Reproductive Health
Royal Infirmary of Edinburgh
Edinburgh, UK

Timothy B Hargreave MS FRCS FRCS(Ed) FRCP(Ed) FEB(Urol)
Senior Fellow
Department of Oncology
Edinburgh University
Western General Hospital
Edinburgh, UK

Geoffrey Hooper MB ChB MMSc FRCS(Eng) FRCS(Ed)(Orth)
Consultant Orthopaedic and Hand Surgeon
St John's Hospital
Livingston
West Lothian, UK

Colin P Jardine Brown MBBS FRCS FRCS(Ed) FRCOG
Consultant Obstretrician and Gynaecologist
The North Hampshire Hospital
Basingstoke
Hampshire, UK
(1979–2002; Retired)
Internal Professional Adviser & Parliamentary and Health Service
Ombudsman
(2002 onwards)

Myles Joyce MB BCH BAO MD
Specialist Registrar in General Surgery
Department of Academic Surgery
University College Hospital
Galway, Ireland

Simon Keightley BSc DO FRCS FRCOphth
Consultant Ophthalmic Surgeon
The North Hampshire Hospital
Basingstoke
Hampshire, UK

Cyrus J Kerawala BDS FDSRCS MBBS FRCS(Ed) FRCS(Max-Fac)
Consultant in Oral and Maxillofacial Surgery
The North Hampshire Hospital
Basingstoke
Hampshire, UK

Oliver McAnena MCh FRCSI
Consultant Surgeon
Lecturer in Surgery
Department of Academic Surgery
University College Hospital
Galway, Ireland

Carl HA Meyer FRACS
Consultant Neurosurgeon
Queen Elizabeth Hospital
Birmingham, UK

Alison Milne MB BS FRCP FRCPath
Consultant Haematologist
Department of Haematology
The North Hampshire Hospital
Basingstoke
Hampshire, UK

John D Orr MBChB MBA FRCS(Ed)
Consultant Paediatric Surgeon
Department of Paediatric Surgery
The Royal Hospital for Sick Children
Edinburgh, UK

Rowan W Parks MD FRCSI FRCS(Ed)
Senior Lecturer in Surgery and Honorary Consultant Surgeon
Royal Infirmary of Edinburgh
Edinburgh, UK

James Powell BSc MD FRCSEd
Clinical Lecturer in Surgery
Department of Clinical and Surgical Sciences
University of Edinburgh
Royal Infirmary of Edinburgh
Edinburgh, UK

Myrddin Rees MS FRCS FRCS(Ed)
Consultant Hepatobiliary Surgeon
The North Hampshire Hospital
Basingstoke
Hampshire, UK

Anthony B Richards MChir FRCS
Consultant Urologist
The North Hampshire Hospital
Basingstoke
Hampshire, UK

Robert J Sanderson MBChB FRCS(Eng) FRCS(Ed) FRCS(ORL-HNS)
Consultant Otolaryngologist / Head and Neck Surgeon
Department of Otolaryngology
Western General Hospital
Edinburgh, UK

Chummy S Sinnatamby FRCS
Surgical Anatomy Tutor
The Royal College of Surgeons of England
Lincoln's Inn Fields
London, UK

Kenneth J Stewart MD FRCS(Ed) Plast
Consultant Plastic and Reconstructive Surgeon
Royal Hospital for Sick Children
Edinburgh, UK

Wesley Stuart MD FRCS(Ed) (Gen Surg)
Consultant Vascular Surgeon
Southern General Hospital
Glasgow, UK

Fenella Welsh MA MD FRCS(GenSurg)
Clinical Fellow in HPB and Transplant Surgery
Royal Infirmary of Edinburgh
Edinburgh, UK

David J Wheatley MD ChM FRCS(Eng) FRCS(Ed) FRCS(Glas) FMedSci FECTS
BHF Professor of Cardiac Surgery
Division of Cardiovascular and Medical Sciences
Glasgow Royal Infirmary
Glasgow, UK

Piers TJ Wilson MBBS FRCA
Consultant Anaesthetist
The North Hampshire Hospital
Basingstoke
Hampshire, UK

SURGERY OF THE SKIN AND SUBCUTANEOUS TISSUE

1

The skin is one of the largest organs of the human body. It serves a multitude of purposes: a barrier to infection; a controller of heat and fluid loss; and a sensory interface with the world. Its aesthetic qualities are of the utmost importance to the individual. The mobility and elasticity of the skin are necessary for joint movement, and its strength essential in areas where it is subjected to repeated minor trauma, especially in the hands and feet. The skin of each part of the body is modified to suit specific purposes; for example, the thick-ridged, sensitive and moist skin of the finger tip is ideal for gripping tiny objects, whilst the thin, compliant skin of the eyelid provides ideal mobility and protection of the globe.

Every skin incision heals with a scar which has the potential to cause disturbance of function or appearance. Scars are to a certain extent unpredictable. However, certain parts of the body are notorious for their propensity to form hard, red, elevated hypertrophic scars. Furthermore, the position of a scar has a great bearing on its visibility and its connotations; the pre-auricular face lift scar is, for example, a barely apparent trade-off for the aesthetic enhancement, whereas a scar of equivalent length only a few centimetres further forward in the mid cheek can be socially and economically devastating.

Skin incisions and suturing are often the first surgical skills acquired by a trainee. Very few operations can be performed without cutting through the skin. It may be incised to gain access to deeper structures, or the surgery may be primarily on the skin itself whether for the repair of trauma or for the excision of a skin lesion. An understanding of the surgical challenges of the integument is therefore fundamental to all surgeons, even if certain techniques are the preserve of those specializing in cutaneous surgery.

Many basic surgical techniques of dissection, tissue handling and repair are encountered first in the skin and subcutaneous tissue, and are therefore discussed in this chapter.

The general preoperative preparation of a patient, the perioperative environment and the postoperative care are summarized in Appendices I–III.

GENERAL TECHNIQUE

Incisions and tissue handling

Skin incisions must be carefully planned, not only to excise a skin lesion or to give good access to underlying structures but, wherever possible, they should lie in – or parallel to – the natural crease lines of the skin (Fig. 1.1). Alternatively, they may sometimes be placed at a more remote site to disguise their existence. Scars should not be placed across the flexor aspect of a joint, and ideal skin incisions on the palm of the hand are shown in Figure 1.2. Surgeons will, however, encounter situations where they are forced to compromise upon this counsel of perfection.

Incisions through the skin must be made cleanly with a sharp knife held at right-angles to the surface. If the skin is

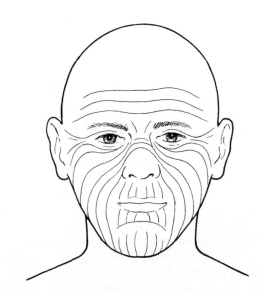

Figure 1.1 *Natural crease lines on the face.*

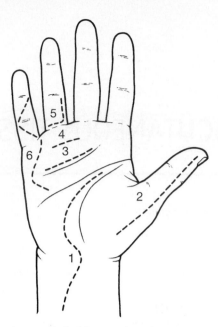

Figure 1.2 *Acceptable incisions on the palmar aspect of the hand.*

loose and wrinkled it should be held gently stretched or it will not cut cleanly. Diathermy incision of the skin is preferred by some surgeons as it reduces bleeding. However, there is a risk of thermal injury to the skin to the detriment of wound healing and scar quality. Therefore, although diathermy is often used for the skin incision of, for example, a laparotomy, it cannot be recommended in cosmetically sensitive areas except when used by very experienced surgeons. If diathermy is utilized for the skin, the 'cut' rather than the 'coagulation' setting must be selected to minimize thermal damage. Fine-toothed forceps and fine skin hooks are recommended when operating on the skin. Although all living tissue must be handled gently, the effects of rough handling of the skin are more visible than that of deep tissue.

Arrest of haemorrhage

Small bleeding points appear as the dermis is cut. If necessary, these may be coagulated with fine bipolar forceps. However, again there is a risk of thermal injury. In most circumstances, patience in tolerating this early bleeding will be rewarded by haemostasis. As the incision continues into the subcutaneous fat, larger bleeding vessels are encountered. When a vessel has already been divided it can either be picked up in diathermy forceps and coagulated, or it can be secured first with artery forceps, after which it is either ligated or sealed with coagulation diathermy. A vessel in the subcutaneous fat which is identified before it is divided, can be coagulated by diathermy before division, but larger vessels should be divided between artery forceps and ligated. Diathermy can be used for the dissection deep to the skin and has the advantage that it prevents multiple small bleeding points, but larger vessels still require individual attention.

The vessel should be held without a mass of surrounding tissue. Extra tissue in diathermy forceps leads to less effective coagulation and greater tissue damage, and extra tissue held in artery forceps makes the secure ligation of a vessel more difficult. Bleeding from vessels which 'perforate' the deep fascia from underlying muscles can be troublesome. It is essential to control these bleeding vessels promptly before they retract. Coagulation diathermy or ligation is appropriate if they can be isolated. Alternatively a suture, or a custom-made metallic clip, may be employed.

Most vessels clamped in an artery forceps should be ligated. A small vessel, however, may be coagulated by applying diathermy to the artery forceps. If no diathermy is available, the pressure of the artery forceps left on for a minute or two and then released may be sufficient, but there is a danger of bleeding restarting. For the 'tying off' or ligation of bleeding points close cooperation between surgeon and assistant is required. The surgeon passes the ligature material around the forceps; the assistant holds the forceps, depressing the handle and elevating the point as much as possible, so that the tissue which is clamped is encircled by the ligature (Fig. 1.3). Just as the surgeon is tightening the first hitch of the knot, the assistant slowly releases the forceps. Sudden release of the forceps should be avoided as the blood vessel is liable to slip out of the grasp of the ligature. Every time a vessel is ligated, two 'foreign bodies' are introduced – the ligature itself and the strangulated tissue beyond it. It is therefore important to include as little adjacent tissue as possible in the clamp, to use the finest material consistent with security, and not to leave the cut ends longer than necessary. An absorbable material in the subcutaneous tissue is preferable.

If an artery forceps has been applied to a bleeding point in such a way that it is difficult for the assistant to elevate the point, simple ligation is unlikely to be secure. Transfixion ligation is then safer (Fig. 1.4). The surgeon passes the suture needle under the forceps through the middle portion of the grasped tissue. The first throw of a knot is then formed and this loop is settled deep to the points of the artery forceps to encircle half of the tissue. The ligature is then passed round, under the handle of the forceps, to encircle the other half of the tissue and the first hitch of the knot tied. As the surgeon tightens this first hitch, and therefore the whole figure-of-eight ligature, the assistant slowly releases the artery forceps. An even safer transfixion suture favoured by some surgeons

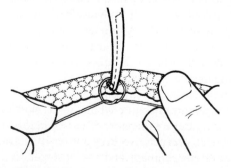

Figure 1.3 *Method of 'tying-off' a bleeding point.*

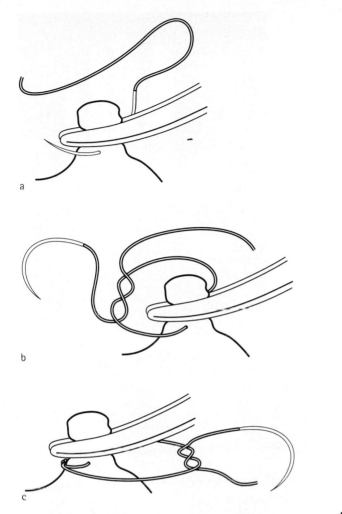

Figure 1.4 *A transfixion suture. The figure-of-eight ligature is prevented from slipping off by its anchorage through the tissue.*

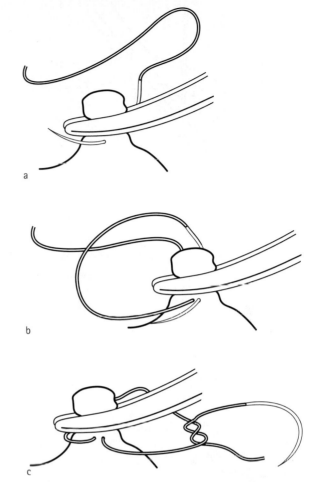

Figure 1.5 *An alternative transfixion suture which passes twice through the tissue.*

is shown in Figure 1.5. In this, the needle is passed a second time through the tissue held in the artery forceps with the loop of suture material passing under the tips of the forceps. The figure-of-eight is then completed by the tie under the handles. These transfixion sutures have greater application in securing major vessels.

Sometimes a thin-walled wide vein can be dealt with more safely by passing a ligature above and below the point of intended division and only dividing the vessel after both ligatures are tied (Fig. 1.6). An artery forceps is first passed carefully under the vessel and the jaws opened sufficiently to grasp the ligature material, which is carried to the open jaws by a second artery forceps – 'a *mounted* tie' (Fig. 1.6a). The ligature is then drawn round under the vessel.

There is increasing use of clips and staples for securing vessels, and these devices have proved invaluable, both in minimal access surgery, and in situations where access is difficult. Small linear cutting stapling devices have been of particular benefit in the safe division of large veins, where the length of the vein is too short to accommodate ligatures. The

right renal vein and the hepatic veins are examples. It is a faster and more secure technique than that of oversewing the vein. The angled head of these stapling devices allows access into restricted surgical fields. Another relatively recent development has been that of heat bonding with 'Ligasure'. A vessel, often with surrounding fat, is held in the instrument until it is sealed by heat. The device alerts the surgeon with a small 'beeping' sound when the process is complete. This has proved a useful device for dividing the mesentery of the bowel, and gives a secure seal even for vessels up to the size of the inferior mesenteric artery.

Tourniquets

Tourniquets can be used to obtain a bloodless field, and should be used for most fine procedures on the distal limbs. A finger or toe tourniquet made from the finger of a rubber glove can also exsanguinate the digit as it is rolled down into position (Fig. 1.7a). It is useful for minor surgery on the distal portion of a digit, but for any more major procedure a pneumatic tourniquet (Fig. 1.7b) is preferable. The tourni-

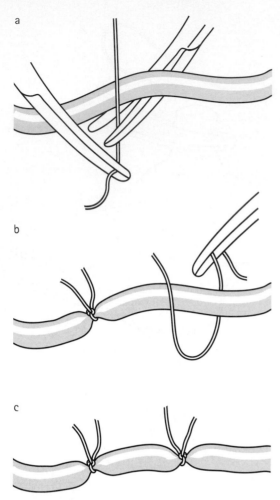

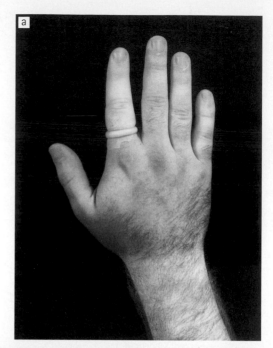

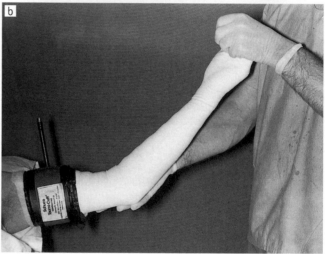

Figure 1.6   *(a) A 'mounted tie' is used to carry a ligature to the open jaws of an artery forceps passed beneath a vessel. (b) After ligation the procedure is repeated. (c) An isolated section for division is obtained.*

Figure 1.7   *(a) A finger tourniquet, fashioned from a surgical glove finger, with the tip cut off, is placed on the finger and rolled to the base. A size should be chosen which is a firm fit before it is rolled. (b) A pneumatic tourniquet. After applying the tourniquet around the upper arm, the arm is exsanguinated by elevating it and wrapping a rubber bandage around it, starting distally. The tourniquet is then inflated and the bandage removed*

quet is applied and, before inflation, the limb is emptied by elevation alone, or by elevation combined with the firm application of a rubber bandage from the digits up to the tourniquet. The tourniquet is then inflated to 50 mm of mercury above systolic pressure and the bandage removed. The pressure is maintained at this level until surgery is completed, and in a fit young patient may be left inflated for up to 90 minutes. Alcohol-based antiseptic skin preparation should be avoided as seepage of the solution under the tourniquet may result in iatrogenic chemical burns.

Knots

The simple and reliable reef knot is well known, and is universally advocated for surgical purposes. It is essential that it is kept 'square' by being tightened in the correct directions, for an insecure slip-knot results if this precaution is not observed (Fig. 1.8). A *triple* knot is the modification of the reef knot commonly used, and at least three throws are

required for security. With slippery monofilament material, multiple throws are required to provide a safe knot, and the ends should not be cut too short. Extra turns in all, or just the first throw, can give added security especially to a knot of thicker monofilament material.

Knots may be tied using the needle holder to grasp the end of the suture material which must be wound around the instrument in the opposite direction on the second throw to achieve a reef knot (Fig. 1.9). This method is suitable for tying the knots of skin sutures, and is also used for the knots

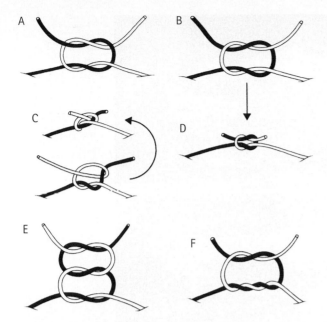

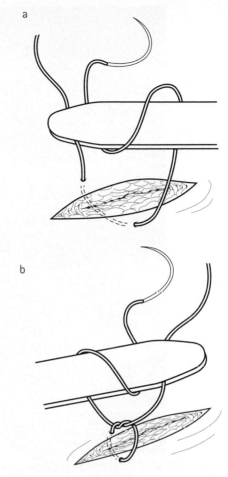

Figure 1.8 *Different types of knots. (A) A* granny knot*: this is an unsafe knot, which should never be used. (B) A* reef knot*: this must be kept 'square' by tightening in the correct directions and with equal tension on the ends. (C) A* reef knot *which has been spoiled by careless tightening, so that an insecure knot results. The white strand has been pulled to the left. (D) The white strand has been correctly pulled to the right, the black to the left; see (B). (E) A* triple knot. *(F) A* surgeon's knot *with an extra turn on the first loop.*

Figure 1.9 *An instrument tie. Note that the suture material is wound in the opposite direction in the second throw to achieve a reef knot. The direction of pull on the suture ends must also be reversed for each throw to keep the knot square.*

in laparoscopic surgery which have to be executed entirely by instrument. In open surgery, a hand technique is preferred for tying the knot of a ligature, or of a deep suture, as it is felt to be more secure. The left-hand technique is shown in Figure 1.10. It is important to remember that whichever technique is used, if a reef knot is not kept 'square' a 'slip-knot' results. In a deep wound the index finger of the left hand is used after each throw to settle the new throw onto the previous throw and to tighten the knot.

At the end of a continuous suture the surgeon is left to tie a 'loop' to an 'end' which is not ideal, especially in slippery monofilament material. The Aberdeen knot is useful in this situation and is shown in Figure 1.11.

Closure of superficial wounds

Healing by first intention is a realistic expectation after most surgical and traumatic breaches to the skin, and the skin edges are approximated. Grossly contaminated wounds presenting late, with possible concern over viability of deeper tissue, are obviously unsuitable for primary closure, and their management is considered in more detail in Chapter 3. More minor contamination is not a contraindication to primary closure if surgical debridement is radical. Any dirt or foreign material must be removed.

Wounds of the hand require particular attention. Blunt injuries, which have produced a bursting injury with gross oedema, should not be sutured as the tension will be too great. Wounds of the wrist and hand are easy to underestimate. There is little subcutaneous fat and tendons and nerves are vulnerable. Often, an apparently simple skin laceration has been repaired, and only later does it become apparent that a superficial tendon or nerve has also been severed. In every hand and wrist laceration the surgeon must, before exploring the wound, check for distal function of any structure which could have been injured. Exploration for deep damage requires good operative and anaesthetic conditions, and is discussed further in Chapter 3.

Failure of primary healing in a sutured skin wound is usually due to a collection of serosanginous fluid or blood in the subcutaneous fat. This has collected due to failure to obliterate a dead space, combined with suboptimal haemostasis. Rough handling of tissue may have caused devitalized areas and any minor contamination then results in an infected collection. The potential dead space in the subcutaneous fat may be obliterated by the skin suture (Fig. 1.12), or a sepa-

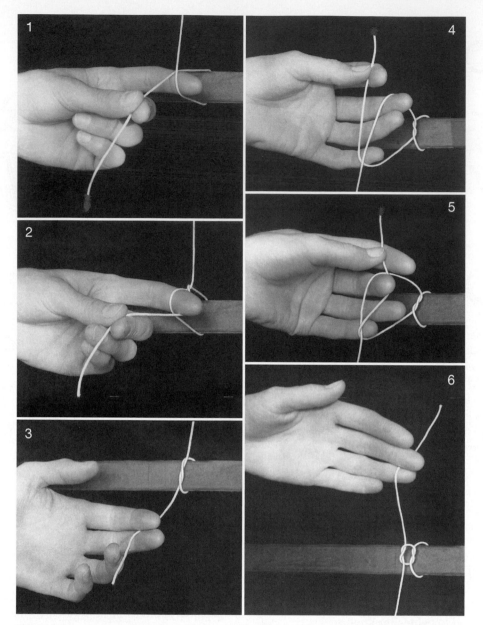

Figure 1.10   *Method of tying a reef knot with the left hand. Note how the knot is kept 'square' by tightening in the correct directions (the end of suture material passing off the edge of each photograph is held in the right hand). This is an original illustration from the 1954 edition. The photographs were taken by Eric Farquharson himself of knot tying by his wife, Elizabeth Farquharson, who is also a doctor.*

rate absorbable suture can be used to appose the fat. The latter is more successful in areas where there is a membranous layer to the superficial fascia as in the groin. In many instances the subcutaneous fat, although thick, lies in apposition and no further action is needed other than careful haemostasis. The routine use of surgical drains in the subcutaneous fat is being challenged in many areas of surgery. However, there are situations where most surgeons would recommend vacuum drainage of the subcutaneous fat for 24–48 hours, or for longer if drainage is significant. A potentially large dead space, as after the removal of a large lipoma,

is one instance. A drain may also be beneficial when bacterial contamination of the wound has occurred in colonic surgery, as even a small collection of blood in the subcutaneous fat is likely to become infected.

After dealing with the subcutaneous fat, the skin edges must be held in accurate apposition and supported for as long as it takes for the scar to develop the tensile strength necessary to protect against distraction.

Interrupted skin sutures may cause scarring, especially if the sutures are too tight and postoperative tissue swelling causes them to cut into the skin. Vertical 'mattress sutures'

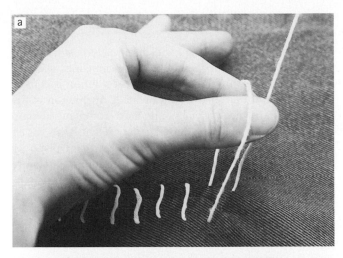

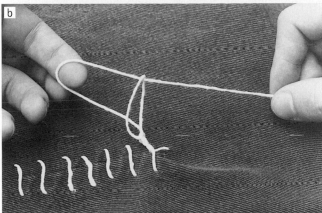

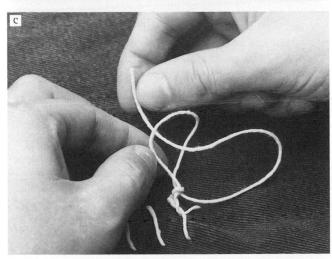

Figure 1.11 *The Aberdeen knot. (a) After the last suture has been inserted, it is drawn through until there is only a small loop. The surgeon passes his or her index finger and thumb through the loop to grasp the suture and pull it through to form the next loop. (b) As each new loop is formed, the previous loop is allowed to close to form the next layer of the knot. (c) Finally, the end of the suture – rather than a loop of it – is passed through the loop and the knot tightened.*

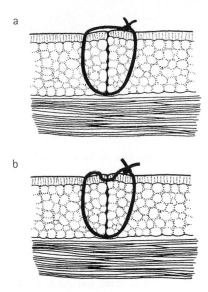

Figure 1.12 *(a) A simple suture securing apposition of skin and underlying fat. (b) A vertical mattress suture.*

used to evert the skin edges have even greater potential to scar the skin if they are drawn too tight (Fig. 1.12b). Interrupted skin sutures should be of a fine smooth non-absorbable material such as nylon or polypropylene (Prolene), which causes less tissue reaction than silk. Cutting needles are required for skin. The needle should be passed perpendicularly through the skin and the stitches tied with only sufficient tightness to bring the skin edges together without constriction. Knots should be placed laterally away from the wound. Tight sutures cause ischaemia, delay healing, and increase scarring. The intrusive cross-hatched scars, associated with interrupted sutures, are a result of suture-induced ischaemic necrosis. An interrupted suture closure can give excellent cosmetic results on the face where sutures should be removed at around 5 days. Epidermal downgrowth of spurs occurs around suture material *in situ* for over a week and results in small punctate scars. As the skin in most areas of the body requires the support of sutures for the healing wound for at least 7 days, these little punctate scars may be unavoidable. Below the knee, and on the back, sutures are needed to prevent skin dehiscence for around 2 weeks.

A continuous subcuticular suture to appose the dermal layers of the skin is a fast and cosmetically satisfactory method of skin closure (Fig. 1.13). The additional scarring from sutures is avoided, but it should be noted that a subcuticular suture gives no support to the underlying tissue. Synthetic absorbable materials are frequently used by general surgeons to close incisions. However, these can cause a tissue reaction and may in some cases be blamed for poor scars. Any knots of absorbable suture should be placed deep and well away from the wound edge. The tissue reaction induced by catgut was sufficiently severe to preclude its use as a subcuticular suture. A non-absorbable nylon or Prolene subcuticular suture avoids the tissue reaction associated with

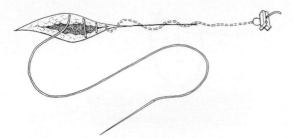

Figure 1.13 *A subcuticular non-absorbable suture should be of a smooth material such as Prolene for easy removal, and the ends are brought out beyond the wound. If an absorbable suture is used the ends are secured by buried knots.*

absorbable sutures, and is removed after 10–14 days. The needle is introduced beyond one end of the wound and after completion is brought out beyond the other end. Steristrips can be used to provide support and to secure the suture. A crushed bead on the suture will also secure it, but has the disadvantage that such beads prevent any suture material being drawn into the closure as the wound swells postoperatively, and thus the beads are pulled into the skin causing discomfort, and occasionally additional scarring.

Skin clips, steristrips and tissue glue can also be used for skin closure in certain circumstances. If clips are used, they should be removed early as they can be associated with cosmetically unacceptable cross-hatching of the scar.

SURGERY OF SKIN LESIONS

Surgical removal of benign tumours and other skin lesions is often requested purely on cosmetic grounds. Alternatively, there may be recurrent infection, bleeding or pain making removal desirable. The patient or the surgeon may be concerned about malignancy. Before embarking on cosmetic excisions the surgeon must be confident that the scar will be less conspicuous than the original blemish. He or she should also consider the natural history of the lesions, for example the disfiguring cavernous haemangiomata, which may enlarge dramatically in late infancy, are self-limiting, and the results of surgical intervention are usually worse than the results of natural regression. The differential diagnosis of skin lesions is beyond the scope of this chapter, but many simple excisions can be avoided if the patient can be confidently reassured that a lesion is benign. Accurate clinical diagnosis is therefore important.[1] Cooperation with a dermatologist is invaluable for this, and for the management of those skin lesions better treated by curettage, cryotherapy or topical applications.[2] Lasers also have a valuable role in the management of certain skin lesions such as capillary malformations and *café-au-lait* macules.

Anaesthesia

Local infiltrative anaesthesia with lignocaine is suitable for most minor superficial operations. Lignocaine is available as 1 or 2 per cent solutions. A 0.5 per cent solution is equally effective and, if unavailable, can be made by dilution of the above strengths with normal saline. The recommended maximum dose of lignocaine is 3 mg/kg bodyweight. Thus, for an average 70-kg man the surgeon may use only 10 mL of a 2 per cent solution but 40 mL of a 0.5 per cent solution. The more dilute solutions therefore have advantages when more extensive surgery is planned. Lignocaine with adrenaline is suitable for local infiltrative anaesthesia, except in the vicinity of end arteries where arterial spasm could endanger blood supply and, in particular, should be avoided in a finger or toe. An adrenaline-containing local anaesthetic agent has several benefits. The arteriolar constriction reduces small vessel ooze during surgery, and also slows the absorption of local anaesthetic agent into the circulation. This gives both a longer period of anaesthesia and allows a higher dose to be used before there is concern over systemic toxicity. Proprietary solutions contain 1 part adrenaline in 200 000. Local anaesthetic agents are introduced into the subcutaneous fat as shown in Figure 1.14. If the injection is close to the skin the delay before anaesthesia is minimized, but if it is injected intradermally, although effective, the initial injection is more painful. It should be remembered that the skin will require to be anaesthetized wide of the incision to include the skin through which the sutures are to be placed. As the solution is injected the point of the needle is slowly moved, thus minimizing any risk of significant intravenous injection. Aspiration before injection is only necessary when a large volume of local anaesthetic agent is injected at one site. To anaesthetize a large area of skin, the needle may have to be introduced at multiple points.

Bupivicaine (0.5% and 0.25% solutions with, and without, adrenaline) is a longer-acting local anaesthetic agent. Its onset is slower than lignocaine, but its effectiveness for up to 8 hours is useful for postoperative pain relief.

A local anaesthetic agent may be used around a nerve to give anaesthesia in the area which it serves. A digital nerve block (Fig. 1.15) is commonly used for surgery on a digit. Lignocaine *without adrenaline* is injected into the web spaces on either side of the finger around the dorsal and palmar digital nerves. Other common nerve blocks include brachial, intercostal, ilio-inguinal and femoral.

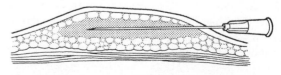

Figure 1.14 *Subcutaneous infiltration of a local anaesthetic agent.*

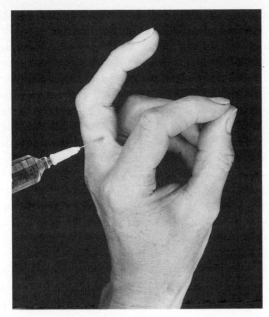

Figure 1.15   *Digital nerve block anaesthesia.*

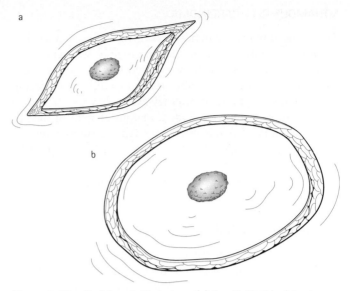

Figure 1.16   *Excision of skin lesions. (a) An elliptical incision is most suitable if a linear closure is planned. (b) A circular or oval incision is more appropriate if a skin graft is planned.*

Subcutaneous fat has very few nerve endings, and a large subcutaneous lipoma can often be removed painlessly with local anaesthesia only infiltrated just beneath the overlying skin. However, if a cutaneous nerve which has not been anaesthetized is encountered severe pain may ensue.

Infiltration of local anaesthesia is painful. The pain can be minimized by warming the solution, adding bicarbonate to render it less acidic, injecting slowly with a fine-gauge needle, prior topical application of local anaesthetic creams such as EMLA (a combination of lignocaine and prilocaine), infiltrating areas of looser tissue first, and by performing local nerve blocks prior to more extensive infiltration. However, pain is always worse in an anxious patient and gentle reassurance can also minimize distress.

Excision of a benign skin lesion

An ellipse of skin is excised so that a linear closure can be effected (Fig. 1.16a), and the long axis of the ellipse should ideally be in, or parallel to, the natural skin creases. The width of the ellipse should be such that the lesion is fully excised plus a small margin of macroscopically normal skin. The resultant scar is thus seldom shorter than three times the diameter of the original lesion. Underlying subcutaneous fat may have to be included in the ellipse if the lesion extends into it. In other instances, fat underlying the excised skin ellipse must be excised to allow the skin edges to be brought together without tension. Haemostasis and closure of the defect are performed as discussed above.

Excision of a malignant skin lesion

The three most common skin cancers have different behaviour patterns and thus pose different challenges for the surgeon.

BASAL CELL CARCINOMA (RODENT ULCER)

This is the most common malignant skin tumour. It is slow-growing and metastases are extremely rare, but if left untreated it may penetrate deeply and erode into soft tissue, and even into bone. The excision should be planned to include at least 3 mm of normal tissue on all aspects, including the deep surface. The microscopic edge of the tumour may be wide of the clinical edge, and the histology is important to check the completeness of excision, especially at the deep margin. Complete excision is associated with a recurrence rate of less than 2 per cent. A technique of excision in layers, with horizontal frozen section control, has been described by Mohs. Its use is not widely accepted for primary basal cell carcinomas but it may have advantages for recurrent lesions in ensuring complete tumour ablation.[3] It is not a technique that can be recommended for general surgical practice. Penetrating tumours around the eyes, nose, mouth and ears can pose major surgical problems, requiring skilled reconstruction following excision. This is considered in more detail both later in this chapter and in Chapter 10. Radiotherapy can also be used to treat these difficult lesions, but scarring still occurs and cosmesis may be no better. In addition, radiotherapy is contraindicated in certain areas, for example the pinna and close to the lacrimal canaliculi.

SQUAMOUS CELL CARCINOMA

This tumour may arise in normal skin, but areas damaged by chronic traumatic or venous ulceration, or by solar exposure, are at increased risk. The tumour is sensitive to radiotherapy, which may be used as an alternative to surgical excision in some sites. Carcinoma in situ may extend beyond the visible lesion, and excision to include a margin of 1 cm of macroscopically normal skin is recommended. Advanced tumours metastasize to regional nodes. The multiple superficial tumours of sun-damaged skin appear to be a less aggressive subgroup. Surgery for squamous cell carcinoma of the lip and pinna are discussed further in Chapter 10.

MALIGNANT MELANOMA

This is the most aggressive of the skin cancers. Tumour thickness and depth of penetration are major determinants of survival,[4,5] as metastatic spread is increasingly likely with thicker tumours. A wider excision is recommended than for other skin malignancies as there is a real risk of local recurrence in the skin and subcutaneous tissue adjacent to the scar. This risk is also related to tumour thickness, and recommended clearance margins for excision are based on the thickness of the melanoma.[6] The very wide excisions previously performed have, however, been shown to be unnecessary, and a 1-cm margin of normal skin around tumours of less than 1 mm in depth has been demonstrated to be sufficient. Between 1 and 2 mm the evidence is open to interpretation, and a margin of between 1 and 2 cm is normally accepted. A 2-cm clearance is recommended for lesions between 2 and 4 mm in depth. Thus, a 3 mm-thick tumour requires a margin of 2 cm of normal skin. Assuming that the tumour itself is 1 cm in diameter, the width of the ellipse needs to be 5 cm. The excision should be carried down to, but not through, deep fascia to achieve optimum clearance margins in the deep plane. The excision of the underlying subcutaneous fat has the additional advantage that it may reduce the tension on a primary closure, but in many areas of the body simple closure is not possible and skin grafting or flap reconstruction is required. Reconstruction with a flap may be cosmetically preferable. The limb proximal to a melanoma is avoided as a donor site for a skin graft for fear of encouraging the development of recurrent skin nodules within it.

Preoperative decisions in malignant melanomata are difficult, especially as clinical diagnosis is far from infallible. Lesions which appear benign clinically are excised and the diagnosis of malignant melanoma is only made at histological examination. Conversely, many surgeons have experience of a patient who has had a wide excision with the inevitable challenge of skin closure and scarring, only to find that the confident clinical diagnosis is not confirmed histologically. Malignant melanomata may arise in normal skin, from within a pre-existing benign naevus, or from a single area of an *in-situ* lentigo maligna. The tumours vary in appearance and although dark pigmentation is usual, amelanotic lesions also occur. Even if a confident diagnosis is made preoperatively the estimation of thickness is uncertain, especially if it has arisen from the edge of a pre-existing benign naevus. Fortunately, an initial excision followed by a wider clearance is not detrimental and is thus the surgical management of choice for most suspicious lesions. If a suspicious lesion is excised under local anaesthesia with a 2-mm clearance, urgent paraffin section histology will give a firm diagnosis and an accurate measurement of the thickness of the lesion. This will allow definitive further surgery, if indicated, to be planned a few days later. Incision biopsies or frozen-section histology are seldom helpful. A minimal excision biopsy margin ensures tension-free healing and also maintains the local lymphatic drainage patterns. This is important if a subsequent sentinel node biopsy technique is to be employed.

When grafting or flap reconstruction is planned, rather than linear closure, a more rounded ellipse, or circle, of tissue is excised (Fig. 1.16b). Malignant melanomata around, or under a nail, often require at least partial amputation of the digit to achieve the necessary local clearance and skin cover.

The spread of malignant melanoma occurs by both lymphatic and haematogenous pathways, and there has been much debate over the years regarding the potential benefit of *prophylactic* radical excision of the drainage lymph nodes.[7] If the nodes are tumour-free the operation has been unnecessary and carries significant morbidity. If nodes are positive, it may still have been unnecessary if haematogenous spread has already occurred, as death from distant metastases may precede symptoms from the regional nodes. Theoretically, however, there may be a few patients in which the surgery might prevent further spread. The most accurate method of identifying nodal metastases, prior to a full nodal dissection, is by a sentinel node biopsy.

Sentinel node biopsy

Sentinel node biopsy is based on the premise that if there is no metastasis in the first drainage node (sentinel node), then the risk of any further nodal metastases is so low as to make a radical lymphadenectomy unjustified. The technique is employed in both malignant melanoma and in breast cancer. Two methods of identification of the sentinel node have been developed, but most surgeons now favour a combination of the two. Radiolabelled colloid or vital dye is injected into tissue adjacent to a primary tumour, on the premise that the lymphatic drainage of this tissue will be identical to that of the tumour itself. The sentinel node is then identified by the concentration of the isotope, as shown by scintigraphic images or hand-held gamma ray probes, and also by the concentration of blue dye, as seen at operation. Timing is of great importance, as the clearance of the two substances differs. Radiolabelled colloid is slow to reach the regional nodes, but once there remains concentrated in the sentinel node. Vital dye, in contrast, reaches the sentinel node within 5–10 minutes, and then rapidly drains on into further nodes.

In melanoma surgery, radiolabelled colloid is injected

around the biopsy site the day before surgery, and a subsequent preoperative scintigraphic scan will identify the position of the sentinel node. This is of particular help in planning surgery when it is not immediately apparent to which nodal group the lymphatics of the tumour drain. Nodal dissection can be guided by a hand-held gamma ray detector, but accuracy is increased if blue dye is also injected intraoperatively. At around 10 minutes after injection there should be one intensely stained node which is excised for histology. Lymph node clearance is then performed only in those patients with a positive sentinel node. This technique, although undoubtedly logical, has not to date been demonstrated to produce a survival benefit.[8] The surgery of lymph nodes is discussed further in Chapters 2, 9 and 24.

Radiotherapy has no place in the treatment of primary melanoma but can be valuable for the treatment of intracranial or spinal metastases. Systemic chemotherapy has been disappointing and isolated limb perfusion, although controlling local disease, does not significantly alter survival.[9]

Excision of a sebaceous cyst

Excision of sebaceous cysts is recommended as they enlarge, often become infected, and seldom regress spontaneously. It is important to excise them completely in order to prevent recurrence. They arise from the deep layers of the skin and are most satisfactorily excised in a similar manner to that used for other skin lesions, through an elliptical incision. The punctum, where the overlying skin is tethered to the cyst, should be in the centre of an ellipse. The length of the ellipse approximates the diameter of the cyst. The width of the ellipse is determined by planning the skin closure, and will vary with the degree of skin stretching that has occurred. For example, a sebaceous cyst on the scalp is protuberant with stretched overlying skin and a wide ellipse is removed. Sebaceous cysts on the back lie mainly in the subcutaneous tissue with minimal stretching of the overlying skin, and only a narrow ellipse of skin need be removed.

First the skin ellipse is incised, and care must be taken not to enter the cyst with this initial incision. The plane is then developed immediately outside the cyst wall. This plane can be difficult to enter, especially where stretched skin is closely applied to the cyst wall. It is often easier to dissect initially at the two ends of the ellipse ensuring that the skin incision is full thickness into subcutaneous fat. Artery forceps, applied to the freed ends of the ellipse, and a skin hook placed under the lateral skin edge, can be used to retract and counter-retract to identify the plane (Fig. 1.17). In all dissections natural planes between structures can be found and developed by a blunt or a sharp method of dissection. In *blunt dissection*, reliance is placed on the assumption that natural cleavage occurs between structures. If however there is inflammatory scarring, the line of least resistance to separation may be through the cyst wall or out into the fat, and there is tearing of tissue. In all areas of surgery *sharp dissec-*

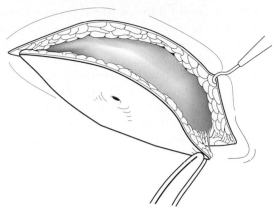

Figure 1.17 *Excision of a sebaceous cyst. The artery forceps on the freed corner is useful for retraction as the lateral skin edge is lifted initially with a skin hook.*

tion allows far more accurate dissection, and has the potential for more complete removal of pathology with preservation of delicate adjacent structures. This principle is discussed further in the chapters on abdominal surgery. Forceps or scissors can be used to develop a plane by blunt dissection. For sharp dissection the areolar tissue of the plane must be held on stretch and divided under direct vision with scissors, scalpel or diathermy.

An alternative method of cyst excision can be utilized to minimize cutaneous scarring. Instead of excising the cyst unruptured, the cyst is deliberately punctured by driving a 3–4-mm punch through the overlying skin and superficial cyst wall. The contents are expressed and the cyst wall is then teased out through the skin opening. The resultant wound is relatively small and can be closed primarily or left open to heal by secondary intention with a pleasing cosmetic outcome.

If any inflammation is present, removal of the cyst should be deferred until this has subsided. A frankly infected sebaceous cyst should be simply incised and the contents drained. No attempt should be made to excise it as wound complications and disappointing scars are often the result. In addition, the infection frequently destroys the lining of the cyst and no further treatment may be necessary. If the cyst does recur, excision can be planned at a later date.

SURGERY OF FINGER AND TOE NAILS

If a finger or toenail is avulsed the nail regrows from the nail bed. Avulsion can therefore only be a good surgical option for a self-limiting condition. For example, trauma to a digit – with the associated soft tissue swelling – can result in a previously trouble-free nail growing into the oedematous tissue of the nail fold and causing further damage and infection. The curved nails which cause 'in-growing toenails' are really only a chronic variant of this as the condition is almost unknown in bare-foot people. An avulsion to allow the infection to settle may be successful if the patient is prepared to adapt their nailcutting and footcare when the new nail regrows. A nail may also be avulsed to examine – and even biopsy – a dark stain under a nail when there is doubt as to whether this is a haematoma or a malignant melanoma. If, however, there have been recurrent problems with an ingrowing nail, or a nail is thickened with onychogryphosis, the nail bed must be removed, or destroyed, otherwise the problem will simply recur as the nail regrows. The nail bed may be excised using a Zadek's operation (Fig. 1.18), or it can be destroyed with phenol.

Either a general anaesthetic or a digital block is suitable for toenail surgery, and a toe tourniquet will give a bloodless field. Bleeding can obscure the anatomy in a Zadek dissection and it will displace the phenol during phenolization. The nail is first avulsed. One blade of a heavy artery forceps is introduced under the nail, either in the medial or the lateral third. Rotation of the closed forceps lifts the medial or lateral nail edge out of the basal corner and the nail fold (Fig. 1.18a). The manoeuvre is repeated on the other side and the whole nail avulsed. The tissue overgrowth and proud granulations are curetted or excised from the nail folds. The raw nail bed is dressed with tulle gras, absorbent dressings and a crepe bandage. The distal pulp skin should be visible beyond the dressing so that adequate perfusion can be confirmed.

To excise the nail bed two incisions are made out from the basal corners, and the flap of skin overlying the base of the nail is elevated (Fig. 1.18c). The germinal area of the nail bed is dissected out, paying particular attention to the medial and lateral extensions, which are loosely attached to the bony expansions at the base of the proximal phalanx. This is not, therefore, a suitable operation if there is sepsis as there is a risk of spreading the infection into the bone or joint. An infected ingrowing nail should be avulsed and the excision of the nail bed postponed for around 6 weeks, by which time all infection should have settled. For the same reason, excision *combined* with phenolization should be condemned as the phenol damages the joint capsule if the excision is already complete. At the end of a Zadek excision the medial and lateral corner extensions of the germinal matrix should be checked for completeness (Fig. 1.18d). An artery forceps, inserted into the excised lateral corner, will only pass out through it if excision has been incomplete. Regrowth from germinal matrix left *in situ* can result in recurrent nail spicules. The incisions **WX** and **YZ** are closed with a suture, and the raw tissue of the nail bed is dressed with tulle gras and absorbent dressings.

Immediate phenolization after avulsion is safe in the presence of infection and avoids the necessity of a second procedure. Phenolization must be carried out with great care in order to avoid burns to surrounding tissue. Aqueous phenol crystals are used and melted over hot water. After 3–5 minutes of contact with the germinal nail bed the phenol is neutralized with alcohol. The nail bed is then dressed in the standard fashion. Healing is slow as this is a chemical burn.

Recurrent nail growth may be a problem with either

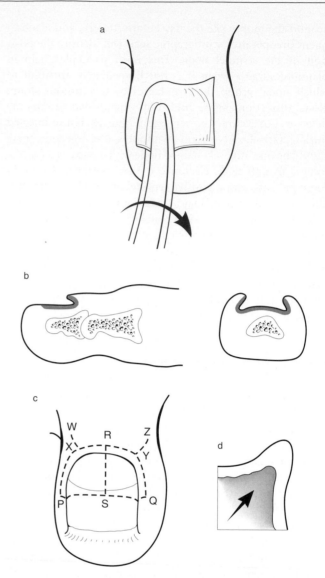

Figure 1.18 *Zadek's nailbed excision. (a) The medial edge of the nail has been avulsed and the forceps are in place to avulse the lateral edge. (b) The germinal matrix of the nail is in the proximal third of the nailbed. It extends under the skin fold at the base of the nail and laterally under the skin at the edge. In the basal corners there is often a significant extension (d). (c) The incision **WXYZ** is made and the flap elevated to expose the basal germinal matrix. The incisions **XP** and **YQ** then allow retraction of the lateral skin folds. The incision **PQ** is distal to the half moon on the nail bed which indicates the end of the germinal portion. The whole area of germinal matrix is then excised but this is easier after it has been divided into two lateral halves by the incision **RS**. Both **PQ** and **RS** are incisions through the whole thickness of the germinal matrix. In the corners the germinal matrix extends further than is often appreciated (as far as **Z**). (d) A complete specimen of germinal matrix. An artery forceps inserted into the corner should not protrude out through a defect.*

method but can be largely avoided by meticulous technique. Some patients with in-growing toenails are anxious to retain a toenail. It is possible to avulse only a lateral or a medial third of the nail, and then to excise or destroy only that area of germinal matrix. Unfortunately, the original problem may recur at the new edge of the nail, and many of these patients will finally need a full nail bed ablation.

EXCISION OF A LIPOMA

Lipomata are the commonest tumours of the subcutaneous tissue, and excision is only indicated if they are painful, or large and unsightly. A rapid increase in size occasionally causes concern that the tumour might be a sarcoma. A linear incision through the overlying skin is deepened through the overlying fat until the surface of the lipoma is reached. It can be distinguished from the surrounding fat by a slightly different colour, and the fatty lobules are larger. In addition, there is a suggestion of a fine transparent 'capsule'. A lipoma can be shelled out using *blunt dissection*, and this is often the most appropriate method. Alternatively, a *sharp dissection* can be used to cut the fine areolar tissue put on stretch between the lipoma and the surrounding fat (Fig. 1.19). Even a large lipoma can be easily excised under local anaesthesia unless it is clinically adherent to the underlying muscle. The plane on the edge of a lipoma will be clear of subcutaneous vessels and nerves, and very little in the way of either enter the lipoma. A lipoma which is clinically adherent to underlying muscles has extensions tracking deep between muscle bellies, often around small vessels and nerves entering the lipoma. This is a particular problem in lipomata on the back of the neck, and not only explains the aching and shooting pains sometimes associated with these lesions, but can also make their removal under local anaesthesia very challenging. The closure of the subcutaneous tissue and skin is discussed above.

If histology shows the presence of a liposarcoma, a re-excision should be undertaken to include the scar and a margin of the surrounding tissue in order to prevent local recurrence.

The use of liposuction to treat lipomata is controversial. Although often effacious, the small risk of misdiagnosis, and inadvertent liposuction of a malignancy, is cause for concern.

SURGERY FOR SKIN LOSS OR DESTRUCTION

Skin may be lost by direct mechanical trauma or irretrievably damaged by pressure, ischaemia, heat, chemicals or infection. The final pathway of treatment in all of these situations is the subsequent restoration of skin cover by surgical means.[10] Early excision of obviously dead skin reduces the risk of secondary infection and, in conditions such as extensive burns, is associated with improved survival and outcome. It is therefore no longer regarded as advisable to watch and wait as skin sloughs. In an appropriate setting, early excision is more often the treatment of choice. However, in the

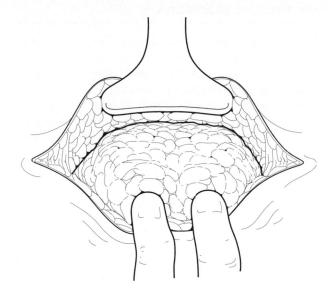

Figure 1.19   *Retraction, with counter-traction, demonstrates the fine strands of areolar tissue which are all that cross the plane between a lipoma and the surrounding fat.*

two situations below, early surgery to dead skin is mandatory.

Constricting eschars

Thermal and chemical burns may cause full-thickness destruction so that the skin is replaced by a hard, constricting eschar. If this is circumferential on a limb or the chest it may threaten the distal circulation or prevent adequate respiratory movement. Such eschars require early linear incision down to live tissue to allow release of the constriction.

Necrotizing skin infections

Here, the progressive skin destruction is often only arrested by surgery. Although bacterial in aetiology, antibiotics alone are ineffective as tissue death is occurring ahead of bacterial colonization, by the combined effects of cytotoxic bacterial toxins and ischaemia secondary to small vessel damage. Antibiotics do not penetrate dead tissue. *Fournier's gangrene* and *necrotizing fasciitis* are examples of this process. As soon as the diagnosis is suspected, the extent of the damage must be explored under general anaesthetic, and the patient forewarned of the extensive nature of the surgery which may be required. In necrotizing fasciitis an apparently localized abscess, which may have been explored locally a few hours before, is associated with extensive death of fascia, subcutaneous fat and overlying skin. The patient may be extremely unwell and require intensive care support in addition to antibiotics, but the only chance of cure is complete excision of all the dead tissue.[11] Fortunately, tissue deep to the deep fascia is normally spared. Extensive reconstruction is postponed until the infection is under control and the patient's general state has improved.

Necrotizing infections of muscle are discussed in Chapter 3.

Reconstructive procedures

Not every wound can be closed directly, especially after skin has been lost by trauma or surgical excision. If direct suture without tension is impossible, then a range of choices is available. The simplest effective measure is usually the best, but the long-term cosmetic result should be considered. Many of these procedures are suitable for general surgeons, but some will yield poor results to an occasional operator. If extensive reconstruction is anticipated, and especially on the face, the help of a plastic surgeon is essential if at all possible.

SIMPLE UNDERMINING AND ADVANCEMENT

Careful undermining of the adjacent tissues away from the edge of a wound may permit primary closure without tension. The level at which this undermining should be carried out is important. In the face, undercutting must be close to the skin to avoid branches of the facial nerve. In the limbs and trunk, the most suitable plane is on the deep fascia, while on the scalp the best plane is between the galea and the pericranium (Fig. 1.20). Carefully placed parallel incisions to the under surface of the galea may allow further advancement without tension. If skin closure is not possible even after undermining, skin grafting should be considered, along with any possible benefit in opting for a flap technique instead.

SKIN GRAFTS

Grafts are completely detached from their origin and, to survive, must obtain adequate nourishment from the bed on which they are placed.

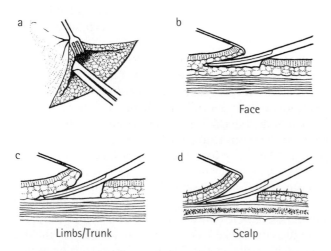

Figure 1.20 *Undermining of skin edges can reduce tension on a suture line. The general technique is shown in (a). The optimum depth for this undermining varies in different parts of the body (b–d).*

Split skin grafts

These are the general-purpose grafts most frequently used. They can be taken from any part of the body, but the commonest donor site is the lateral surface of the thigh. The grafts may be cut at different depths. Thin grafts, consisting of little more than epidermis, are used mainly to cover granulating areas where the urgent need is for wound healing. They 'take' well, even in the presence of infection, but their inability to withstand wear and tear, and their tendency to contract relegates them to the category of temporary grafts that will need later replacement by thicker grafts or flaps. Thicker grafts contain more dermis and are far more durable and pleasing in appearance. Indeed, the thicker *split-skin grafts* are almost indistinguishable from a full-thickness graft. However, the surgeon must be careful to select an unobtrusive donor site, as the thicker the skin graft the more unsatisfactory may be the healed donor area.

PREPARATION OF THE RECIPIENT AREA

A clean, freshly made 'tidy' wound (whether surgical or traumatic) presents no problems, provided that complete haemostasis is secured, preferably with bipolar diathermy coagulation. The base of the wound should be as even as possible, and any spaces between muscle bellies obliterated by a few interrupted fine sutures. If ideal conditions are not met it is possible to store skin grafts for a limited period of time (see below) and apply them to the wound at a later date.

By contrast, 'untidy' wounds and granulating areas may require careful preparation. Adherent slough must be excised, and any crevices in the granulating area removed by scraping away the exuberant soft granulations. Regular wet dressings, soaked in saline or an antimicrobial solution, can be applied until a healthy, pink, flat granulating surface is produced. The process of establishing a healthy granulating bed can be accelerated by the use of the KCI mediscus VAC system, which comprises a foam dressing placed under negative pressure by a suction device. The fitness of the wound for grafting is probably best judged by the clinical appearance, as the information obtained by bacterial investigation is not always helpful and may be misleading. Complete sterility is usually unobtainable, and is not essential. However, the presence of β-haemolytic streptococci group A is a contraindication to grafting and must be treated first with systemic antibiotic therapy. A heavy growth of any pathogenic organism can interfere with the graft 'take', and frequent dressings – possibly containing an antibacterial agent such as povidone iodine – may first be required to reduce bacterial colonization. The indiscriminate local application of antibiotic powders, solutions and creams or various desloughing agents (enzymatic, chemical or hydrophilic) is an extremely expensive and largely worthless substitute for a good dressing technique.

In the operating theatre a healthy granulating area requires little extra preparation other than cleansing with povidone iodine or Hibitane, followed by saline. If some of the granulations are still exuberant and unhealthy in appearance, they should be scraped away and bleeding controlled with moist warm packs.

CUTTING AND PREPARING THE GRAFT

The donor site, which should have been shaved if hairy, is simply prepared like any other operation site. Grafts can be harvested with a hand-held knife, but more consistent results are achieved with a powered dermatome device. The blade of the knife and the donor site are smeared with a lubricant such as liquid paraffin. The limb should be held firmly by the assistant whose hands provide counterpressure from behind to present the surgeon with a flat surface from which to cut the graft. The surgeon creates tension on the donor site just in front of the skin-grafting knife, either with a swab or a wooden board (Fig. 1.21). A hand-held skin-grafting knife is pressed firmly against the skin and, with a steady to-and-fro sawing motion, the knife and skin grafting board move steadily forwards (Fig. 1.21b).

Although the blade in the knife has been set at a predetermined depth, the thickness of the graft is also influenced by the pressure applied to the skin and the angle of the blade. The surgeon must check the thickness of the graft as he or she cuts it. This can be judged by the translucency of the graft and the pattern of bleeding and appearance of the donor site. A very thin graft is translucent so that the knife blade will appear bluish grey in colour through it, and the bleeding points on the donor surface will be closely packed and confluent. A thicker graft will appear white in colour, and the

bleeding points on the donor surface are few and far apart (Fig. 1.21c). If the skin graft has been cut at too deep a level and subcutaneous fat appears, the surgeon has two choices: (i) to resuture the graft in place and take a thinner graft elsewhere; or (ii) to use the thick graft as a full-thickness graft and place a thin split-skin graft on the unintentionally deep donor site. The donor site should be dressed as soon as the grafts have been cut. A variety of dressings may be used, but these should be adhesive in order to avoid slide, and semipermeable to avoid collection of exudate. Inner dressings should be covered by absorbent dressings and crepe bandaging, and should be left undisturbed for at least 10 days.

The use of a graft in its unmeshed state provides the most acceptable cosmesis. However, if extensive grafting is required – as after major burns – the graft may be *meshed* to expand it and make the most economical use of the available skin. It may be passed through a meshing device (Fig. 1.22) in which the mesh size is related to the degree of expansion of the skin graft, and is determined either by the plastic board utilized as a carrier for the meshing machine or by the offset of the blades within the machine. A ratio of 1.5:1 expansion of the graft provides minimal expansion, but improves the ability of the graft to conform to an irregular bed, and allows serum or blood to exude. Ratios of 3:1 or even 6:1 can be used for more extensive burns. If a mesher is unavailable, the graft can be 'fenestrated' by cutting slits in it with a knife while it is lying on a wooden preparation board. In extensive burns, stored cadaveric graft can be utilized to provide temporary wound cover. Strips may be alternated with autograft. As the allograft is rejected, the patient's own epithelial cells

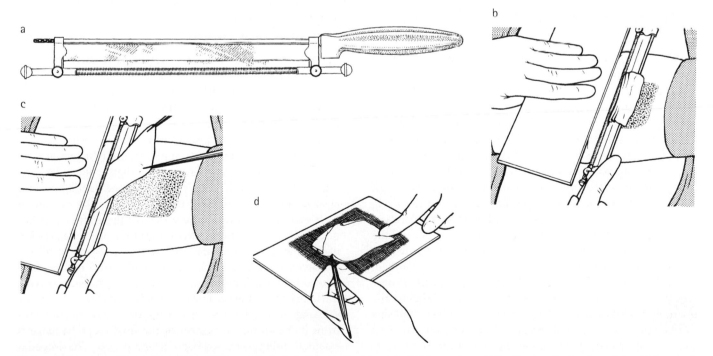

Figure 1.21 (a) A skin-grafting knife. (b) The method of cutting a split-skin graft. (c) The pattern of bleeding is an indication of the thickness of the graft which has been taken. (d) The graft is spread out on tulle gras.

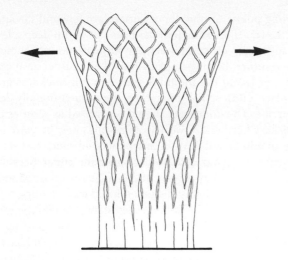

Figure 1.22   *Expansion of meshed skin.*

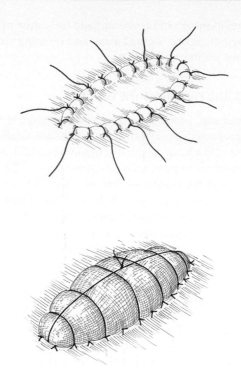

Figure 1.23   *Tie-over dressing.*

grow out to replace them. All of these methods result in parts of the wound healing by secondary intention with more resultant scarring and contracture.

Skin grafts may be *stored* for up to 2 weeks in a refrigerator at 4°C. Microbiological counts in the stored graft increase with time, and its use beyond 14 days is undesirable. After spreading the graft on tulle gras, the raw surfaces should be folded together, the graft rolled up and lightly wrapped in a gauze swab wrung out in normal saline, and placed in a sterile container.

GRAFT APPLICATION AND FIXATION

The graft is placed over the recipient site and adjusted so that it conforms to any irregularity of the bed. Any portion of the graft not in contact with underlying tissue will die. The graft is tacked to the edges of the defect with a few well-spaced sutures which can be left long, and used to fix a 'tie-over' dressing (Fig. 1.23). The graft can be either placed directly on the recipient site or first prepared on a sheet of paraffin gauze spread on a wooden board. The sheets of graft skin are laid with their superficial surface in contact with the paraffin gauze (see Fig. 1.21d). If the gauze has been cut to the size of the recipient site – remembering that uneven contours will increase the size necessary – this can often make preparation easier. Any wrinkles or curled edges are attended to, and the graft is trimmed as required. If several sheets of graft are necessary the best configuration of the pieces can be planned. When no meshing device is available, and expansion is necessary, the graft can be meshed using a scalpel as it lies on the board as described above. Alternatively, just a few small slits can be cut to give the graft greater ability to conform. This will also allow exudate to escape and prevent it from lifting the graft off its new bed. The graft can then be transferred to its new site on the tulle gras.

CARE OF GRAFTS: DRESSINGS OR EXPOSURE

Failure of the split skin graft to 'take' completely is due to:

- a collection of serum or blood beneath the graft;
- infection; and/or
- dislodgement of the graft.

Exposure of skin grafts allows exudate or haematoma to be expressed in the first few hours and prevents shearing by a dressing. The graft is however exposed to other potential trauma, and patient cooperation and expert nursing are essential.

A dressing protects the graft from outside interference, but great care is needed over its application. Light pressure on the surface of the graft will reduce the chance of exudate lifting it from the underlying tissue. A crepe bandage over a layer of absorbent dressing is suitable for a flat or convex graft surface. However, if the surface of the graft is irregular or concave – for example, after the grafting of a wide excision of a malignant melanoma – a 'tie-over' dressing to fill the concavity is needed. This can be made from cotton wool soaked in sterile liquid paraffin and is held in place by tying the long ends of the sutures together over it (Fig. 1.23). If the dressing slips or rotates, a shearing force may tear the graft from its position, so fixation of the final crepe bandage is essential, either by elastoplast or a light plaster. The dressings should be left undisturbed for 5–8 days unless pain, pyrexia or smell indicate the presence of infection.

Excision and grafting of burns

The extensive restoration of skin cover after major burns is rightly the domain of the specialist plastic surgeon. Every surgeon should be familiar with the immediate management of the burned patient before transfer to a specialist unit. Isolated general surgeons may have to continue the management themselves, and it must be remembered that tissue damage may extend deep to the skin[12] and that the operative reconstruction is only a small but important part of the management of the severely burned patient.[13]

Split skin grafts are used to cover the raw areas produced by full-thickness burns. The ideal management of a full-thickness burn is early excision of the dead skin, followed by immediate or delayed skin grafting. However, a general surgeon managing a severely burned patient, with limited resources and no available blood for transfusion, may still be better to opt for the traditional delay until the dead skin has separated spontaneously with the help of dressings. In deep dermal burns tangential excision (using a skin-grafting knife) down to the zone of punctate bleeding with immediate cover using thin split grafts gives the best results.[14]

Full–thickness skin grafts (Wolfe grafts)

These grafts, which are composed of the full thickness of the skin, are unsuitable for use on granulating areas, but are ideal for resurfacing clean surgical wounds produced by excision of scars or tumours. They are particularly useful where texture, colour or durability are important. For this reason, they are widely used to correct facial deformities such as ectropion, scars and growths of the eyelids, nose and cheek, and also in the hand to correct deformities, burn contractures of the fingers, finger tip injuries and in the treatment of syndactyly.

The recipient site must have absolute haemostasis. An exact pattern of the defect is made in paper or foil, and a suitable donor site chosen which has skin of similar colour and texture. It should also be in an area where the resultant defect can be easily closed and a scar inconspicuous. The postauricular sulcus (Fig. 1.24), the supraclavicular and infraclavicular regions are good donor sites. So, too, is the inframammary crease in the woman and the lateral groin in either sex, provided that care is taken not to transplant hairy skin. The pattern is used on the donor site to ensure the correct size and shape is cut. The skin is dissected off the subcutaneous fat and any remaining fat trimmed from the under surface of the graft before it is placed in the defect and secured in a similar fashion to a split skin graft. The donor defect can usually be closed as a linear wound.

New technologies

A variety of new technologies are currently being explored to improve the quantity and quality of skin grafting. Intgra is a

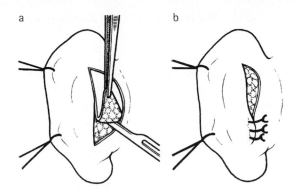

Figure 1.24   *A post-auricular full-thickness skin graft. (a) The exact size and shape required is cut from the post-auricular sulcus. (b) Linear closure of the defect is usually possible.*

dermal substitute with a silicone cover. Grafting this onto a clean wound 3–4 weeks prior to split-skin grafting may enhance the quality of the replaced skin. However, this is an expensive product with significant risks, and its use should be confined to specialist centres. Likewise, the use of cultured epithelial autografts as an adjunct to the resurfacing of extensive burns should only be considered in specialist centres in the context of research.

TISSUE FLAPS

A flap differs from a graft in that it carries its own blood supply and is therefore not reliant on obtaining a blood supply from its bed. In certain circumstances, a flap may be mandatory as the bed of a defect is not suitable for skin grafting – as may be the case when there is exposed bone, tendon or joint. At other times, a flap may be chosen as a more aesthetic – or indeed a 'safer' – reconstruction. Great care must be taken in planning a flap, as in inexperienced hands the decision to use a flap may result in an escalation of the original problem.

The classification of flaps can be simplified by understanding that there are a number of methods of classification. Cars can be classified according to engine size, colour, body, shape or fuel requirements. Flaps can be classified according to congruity, configuration, components, circulation or conditioning (the 'five Cs'). A description of the vast array of flaps available is beyond the scope of this chapter. Flap surgery is mainly in the domain of the reconstructive specialist, but general surgeons should understand the principles on which they are based.[15] Surgeons should also be aware of the potential role of flaps in their subspecialty, and may wish to master some simple flap techniques that are relevant to their surgical practice. For example, a colorectal surgeon may wish to use a gluteal musculocutaneous rotation flap to close a perineal wound at the end of an abdominoperineal resection, and a fasciocutaneous rhomboid Limberg flap is commonly employed in the treatment of pilonidal disease (see Chapter 23).

Congruity

Flaps may be described as *local* when they lie immediately adjacent to the soft tissue defect. Alternatively, flaps may be regarded as *regional* when they are moved from an adjacent anatomical area, or *distant* when they are moved from a remote anatomical site. A flap may be referred to as *pedicled* when it is moved with an intact tissue bridge to support it, or *islanded* when there is no intact skin bridge, but an island of skin is moved under a bridge to fill a non-contiguous defect. Local skin flaps have the advantage that they provide skin of similar colour and texture to that which is lost.

Configuration

Local skin flaps can be moved to an adjacent area by one of three methods. They may be either advanced (Fig. 1.25), rotated (Fig. 1.26), or transposed (Fig. 1.27). The amount of movement possible is dependent on the skin laxity. In general, *advancement flaps* give only limited mobility but are of great value in certain situations such as the finger tip. Their mobility may be enhanced by carefully 'islanding' them on a vascular pedicle. The geometry of *rotation flaps* requires a large flap to fill a relatively small defect. A rotation flap of buttock skin and muscle is widely used in the reconstruction of sacral pressure sores, and a rotation flap of cheek skin in facial reconstruction. The mobility of the rotation can be enhanced by a back cut at the point furthest from the defect (see Fig. 1.27). *Transposition* of a flap results in the greatest degree of flexibility. However, flexibility is dependent on adequate mobilization, which is in turn limited by blood supply. The rich blood supply of the face allows a flap with a relatively long length-to-breadth ratio to be raised. The donor site from flap transposition may be closed directly if there is sufficient laxity, but a skin graft is sometimes required.

Z-*plasties* are a manoeuvre in which two interdigitated triangular flaps are transposed to cover a defect. It is a particularly useful method of closure after the excision of linear contracted scars restricting movement in the neck, axilla and hand. From the extremities of the primary incision, incisions are made at an angle of 60 degrees so that the full incision resembles the letter 'Z' (Fig. 1.28).

Components

Flaps may contain one or more tissue types. Local flaps of skin alone are commonly used to fill small cutaneous defects. Sometimes, a flap may consist purely of another anatomical component such as fascia, muscle, bone or even bowel. Flaps containing more than one variety of tissue are described in terms such as 'musculocutaneous' or 'fasciocutaneous'. The addition of muscle to a flap can provide the extra bulk required to fill a deep defect such as a sacral pressure sore. Even when extra bulk is not required, muscle or fascia within the pedicle and base of a flap may enhance its circulation.

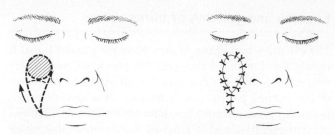

Figure 1.25   V–Y *advancement flap on a subcutaneous pedicle.*

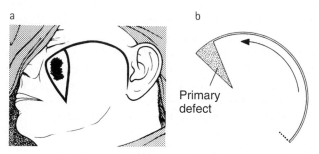

Figure 1.26   *A cheek rotation flap. (a) A large flap is necessary even when the defect is small. (b) A 'back cut' can be used to reduce tension.*

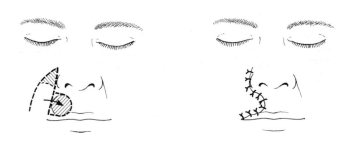

Figure 1.27   *Transposition flap from naso-labial fold to defect in upper lip.*

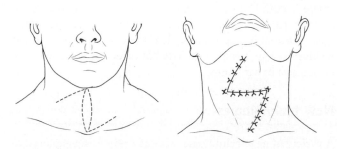

Figure 1.28   Z-*plasty to release a contracture on the neck.*

Circulation

The raising of a flap deprives it of any circulation except that which arrives through its pedicle. Even in experienced hands, partial or complete flap necrosis may occur. Flaps may be regarded as having a random pattern circulation when they are raised without respect to the prevailing underlying circulation. In reality, because of incremental knowledge and experience, very few truly *random pattern flaps* are elevated. If they were, then theoretically the length-to-breadth ratio may be more limited in areas of poor vascularity (e.g., the lower leg) than in the richly supplied face. It has long been appreciated that flaps may be made longer and narrower when a vessel courses along their long axis. Examples of these *axial pattern flaps* include the groin flap (supplied by the superficial circumflex iliac artery) and the deltopectoral flap (supplied by perforating branches of the internal mammary artery). The long groin skin flap in particular was exploited for many years by plastic surgeons on the basis of experience, rather than anatomical knowledge. There is now a much greater understanding of cutaneous blood supply, to the extent that every body area has been mapped in detail. Skin may be supplied either by vessels running directly under the skin, or by vessels which perforate through or between muscles. Thus, a large island of skin can be raised and moved to a distant site for reconstruction by utilizing muscle as its pedicle. The latissimus dorsi flap, which is used in breast reconstruction, is an example and is described in Chapter 2. The rectus abdominis flap, used to reconstruct sternal, or perineal defects, is described in Chapter 12. The pectoralis flap, used in head and neck reconstruction, is described in Chapter 10, page 187, and the gastrocnemius flap, which is a standard flap technique for the reconstruction of defects in the upper third of the leg, is described in Chapter 3, page 37.

The addition of anatomical components to a flap may enhance its circulation. For example, by incorporating deep fascia within a flap on the lower leg, a longer flap can be raised safely (see Fig. 1.30). This is partly so because vessels perforate in the intermuscular septi, and then arborize upon the fascia. However, perhaps the greatest revolution in plastic surgery in recent years has been the greater understanding of the location of these 'perforating' vessels and their exploitation to raise 'perforator' flaps in a variety of anatomical locations.

Conditioning

The safety of a flap may be improved by enhancing its 'axiality', classically by cutting down either side of a flap as a prelude to raising it off the body, some days or weeks later. This is done to encourage the blood supply of the flap to run parallel along its long axis. Such a manoeuvre opens up 'choke' vessels which connect adjacent areas of skin, and thus allows the capture of territories which would not, under most circumstances, be supplied by the vessel within the pedicle of the flap. This phenomenon is known as 'delay'. It should not be confused with the period of delay between inserting a flap into its recipient site and dividing its pedicle. In the simple

flaps, shown in Figures 1.29 to 1.32, the pedicle is only divided when the flap has established a blood supply from its new site – a process which normally takes around 3 weeks. Some of these older techniques are now used less frequently in specialist practice as the variety of reconstructive flaps has increased. Further reading is recommended for those general surgeons with a particular interest.[15]

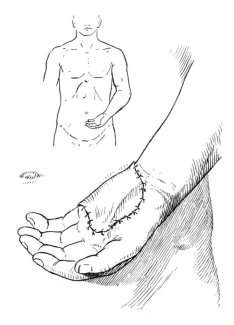

Figure 1.29 *Full-thickness skin cover is essential for the palm of the hand. A simple direct flap technique which may still be of value when more sophisticated reconstruction is not available.*

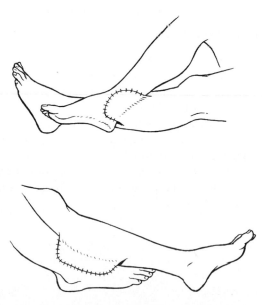

Figure 1.30 *Direct pedicle grafts from one leg to another. The disadvantages of several weeks of immobilization were not insignificant, and these flaps have been virtually replaced by more advanced reconstructive procedures.*

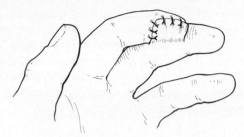

Figure 1.31 *Cross-finger flap. The flap has been raised from the dorsum of the middle phalanx of the middle finger to cover a defect on the tip of the index finger. (A split-skin graft will have adequate durability on the donor site.) After 3 weeks the pedicle of the flap is divided.*

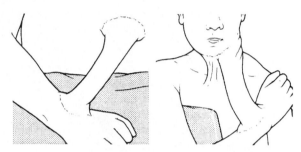

Figure 1.32 *An historical illustration. The long abdominal or groin skin flap was raised and its pedicle 'tubed' to protect the raw surfaces. The end of the flap was implanted into the wrist. Once safely established on the wrist, the pedicle was divided and it was carried on its new blood supply to cover a defect on the face or neck. More sophisticated reconstructive procedures have replaced this ingenious technique.*

FREE TISSUE TRANSFER

Many of the composite flaps described above can be raised on their vascular pedicle, which is then divided to allow the tissue to be transposed as a free flap to almost any recipient site where there are suitable vessels to allow revascularization of the free flap by microvascular anastomosis. This is a technique for the surgeon specializing in reconstructive surgery. One of many examples of free tissue transfer is the use of the radial forearm (Chinese) flap which can be moved with the underlying radial artery and associated veins to a wide variety of locations for countless purposes.

TISSUE EXPANSION

This is a technique of gaining extra skin by the subcutaneous insertion of a silicone bag which can be gradually expanded by the injection of normal saline over a period of several weeks. The expanded skin may be used to provide a local flap, and has particular application in expanding the area of hairy skin available to cover large scalp defects. The technique is also used to provide a pocket for a breast implant.

REFERENCES

1. *Atlas of Clinical Dermatology*, 3rd edn. A du Vivier, Edinburgh: Elsevier Churchill Livingstone, 2002.
2. *ABC of Dermatology*, 4th edn. PK Buxton, London: BMJ Publishing Group, BMJ Books, 1998.
3. Rowe DE, Carroll RJ, Day CL. Mohs surgery is the treatment of choice for recurrent (previously treated) basal cell carcinoma. *J Dermatol Surg Oncol* 1989; **15**: 424–31.
4. Breslow A. Thickness, cross-sectional areas and depth of invasion in the prognosis of cutaneous melanoma. *Ann Surg* 1970; **172**: 902–8.
5. Clark WH, From L, Bernadino EA, *et al.* The histogenesis and biological behavior of primary human malignant melonomas of the skin. *Cancer Res* 1969; **29**: 705–15.
6. Ng AKT, Jones WO, Shaw JHF. Analysis of local recurrence and optimizing excision margins for cutaneous melanoma. *Br J Surg* 2001; **88**: 137–42.
7. Stone CA, Goodacre TEE. Surgical management of regional lymph nodes in primary cutaneous malignant melanoma. Review. *Br J Surg* 1995; **82**: 1015–22.
8. Thomas JM, Patocskai EJ. The argument against sentinel node biopsy for malignant melanoma. Editorial. *Br Med J* 2000; **321**: 3–4.
9. Vrouenraets BC, Nieweg OE, Kroon BBR. Thirty-five years of isolated limb perfusion for melanoma: indications and results. Review. *Br J Surg* 1996; **83**: 1319–28.
10. *Fundamental Techniques of Plastic Surgery and their Surgical Application*, 10th edn. AD McGregor, Edinburgh: Elsevier Churchill Livingstone, 2000.
11. Elliot DC, Kufera JA, Myers RAM. Necrotizing soft tissue infections. *Ann Surg* 1996; **224**: 672–83.
12. *A Colour Atlas of Burn Injuries*. JA Clarke, London: Hodder Arnold, 1992.
13. *Burn Care and Therapy*. GJ Carrougher, London: Mosby, 1998.
14. Janžekovič Z. A new concept in the early excision and immediate grafting of burns. *J Trauma* 1970; **10**: 1103–8.
15. *Reconstructive Surgery; Principles, Anatomy and Techniques*. SJ Mathes, F Nahai, Edinburgh: Quality Medical Publishing, 1996.

2

SURGERY OF THE BREAST AND AXILLA

SURGICAL ANATOMY

The breast

The breast is a skin appendage which develops from modified sweat glands deep to the nipple. Accessory breast tissue may occur along a line from groin to axilla. The development of the rudimentary breast is stimulated by hormones, and commences as a nodule or *breast bud* deep to the areola in early puberty. The adult breast lies predominantly on the deep fascia of pectoralis major and extends from the second to the sixth costal cartilages. Medially, it extends almost to the midline and laterally it continues as the *axillary tail* of the breast over the lateral edge of pectoralis major into the axilla. Superficially, it is separated from the skin by subcutaneous fat, except over the areola and the nipple. The breast substance consists of glandular tissue and surrounding fat. Alterations in hormonal levels cause structural and functional changes in the breast during pregnancy, lactation and, to a lesser extent, throughout the menstrual cycle.

The blood supply of the breast is mainly from branches of the internal thoracic (mammary) artery and the intercostal arteries which pierce the intercostal muscles, and laterally from branches of the lateral thoracic artery. The lymphatic drainage of the breast follows all these routes, but the predominant drainage is to the axillary lymph nodes. There is significant drainage to the internal thoracic nodes from the medial breast (Fig. 2.1).

The axilla

The *axillary contents* are the fat and lymph nodes bounded by the axillary walls. The medial wall is bounded by the chest wall covered with serratus anterior. The anterior wall of the axilla is formed by the pectoral muscles and the clavipectoral fascia. The posterior wall comprises latissimus dorsi, teres

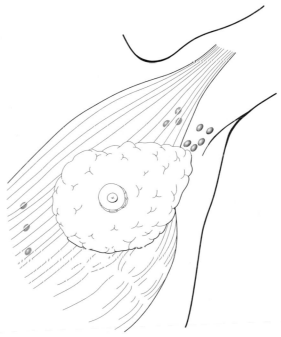

Figure 2.1 *Diagram of the left breast. The breast lies on the fascia of pectoralis major except for the axillary tail which extends beyond the lateral edge of the muscle into the axilla. The lymphatic drainage is to the axillary and internal thoracic (mammary) nodes.*

major and subscapularis. The axillary vessels and the brachial plexus lie along the narrow superolateral wall of the axilla. The axillary vein is the superolateral boundary of an axillary dissection. The axillary artery, with the brachial plexus around it, is superolateral to the vein and is thus safe and out of sight during an axillary dissection. Some branches of the plexus, however, will be encountered (Fig. 2.2). The thoracodorsal nerve (the nerve to latissimus dorsi) and the thoracodorsal artery (a terminal branch of the subscapular artery) lie on the surface of the posterior wall, and the nerve to ser-

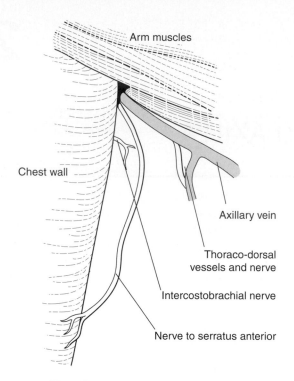

Figure 2.2   *The axillary vein is the superolateral limit of an axillary dissection. The thoracodorsal vessels and nerve are preserved on the posterior wall. The intercostobrachial nerve (shown divided) and the nerve to serratus anterior are encountered on the medial wall. The medial and lateral pectoral nerves which cross the apex of the axilla and the medial cutaneous nerve of the arm, running below and parallel to the vein, are not shown.*

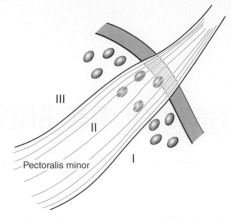

Figure 2.3   *Pectoralis minor is the landmark used to divide the lymph nodes into level I (below and lateral), level II (behind) and level III (above and medial) to the muscle.*

TREATMENT MODALITIES IN BREAST CANCER

Surgery of the breast is dominated by the surgery of breast cancer, which affects up to 1 in 12 women at some time during their lifetime. Cancer of the male breast is an uncommon tumour, but the principles of treatment are similar. A comprehensive discussion of the management of breast cancer is beyond the scope of a general operative textbook, but operative decisions cannot be taken in isolation and a brief summary of the issues therefore follows, although further reading on general management is essential.[1,2]

Radical surgery for breast cancer traditionally involved the excision of the whole breast and the axillary lymph nodes. The original radical operation of *Halstead radical mastectomy*[3] included removal of the whole breast, the axillary contents and the pectoral muscles. *Extended radical mastectomy* was a logical extension to a Halstead radical mastectomy which achieved more radical lymphatic clearance by excision of the internal thoracic and supraclavicular nodes. However, morbidity was increased without significant advantages in survival or local control, and these extensive procedures were for the most part abandoned.

Pectoralis major was excised in a radical mastectomy as it was believed that the lymphatic drainage was mainly through the muscle; in addition, removal improved access to the axilla. Adequate access to the axilla is obtained by pectoral muscle retraction, however, and it is now known that there is no oncological benefit in removing the pectoral muscles unless they are invaded by tumour. Even if the pectoral muscles are invaded, other treatment modalities may be more appropriate than surgery. The radical surgical option is therefore now the *Patey modified radical mastectomy,* or more simply described as a *total mastectomy and axillary clearance,* in which pectoralis major is retained.

Conservative excision of a malignant breast lump with no

ratus anterior on the medial wall; they should be identified and preserved. The nerves to the pectoral muscles cross the apex of the axilla, and the medial cutaneous nerve of the arm runs parallel and inferomedial to the axillary vein. The intercostobrachial nerves cross the axilla from medial to lateral.

The axillary lymph nodes lie in the fat of the axilla and receive lymphatic drainage from the upper limb and the superficial tissue of the chest wall in addition to the breast. Lymphatic channels from the breast drain predominantly first to the nodes lowest in the axilla, and then subsequently to the higher nodes, and finally through the apex of the axilla to the supraclavicular nodes. The axillary nodes are arbitrarily divided into levels I, II and III dependent upon their relationship to the pectoralis minor muscle (Fig. 2.3). *Level I nodes* are lateral and below the muscle, *level II nodes* are behind it, and *level III nodes* are above and medial.

As in malignant melanoma (see Chapter 1), there is increasing appreciation that the lymph node drainage of the breast is first to one or more specific nodes called sentinel nodes. These are usually in the axilla but they can be in the internal thoracic chain or, more rarely, within the breast itself. Axillary sentinel node biopsy is discussed later in this chapter.

other treatment often resulted in a recurrence within the breast. Similarly, performing a *simple total mastectomy* without treatment to the axilla was often followed by axillary recurrence. Large trials confirmed these clinical observations.[4,5] However, some women were cured without disfiguring surgery and others died of distant metastases before the development of symptomatic local recurrence. Patients who fall into either of these two groups are now easier to identify, and unnecessarily radical therapy to breast or axilla may be avoided.

Radiotherapy is effective in the treatment of breast cancer and can be used as an alternative treatment to surgery both for the breast and the axilla. Combining more conservative surgery with radiotherapy gives results comparable to radical surgery. This was first reported by McWhirter[6] and confirmed by many subsequent studies.[4,5] The principle remains, however, that radical treatment includes treatment of the whole breast and axilla by one or other modality unless it can be shown that the individual patient does not require it. Safe avoidance of radical treatment of the axillary nodes in selected patients relies on the axillary staging operations described later in the chapter.

Breast cancer responds both to *hormonal manipulation* and to *cytotoxic chemotherapy*. These approaches are useful not only in the control of metastatic disease but, if used as *adjuvant treatment*, they also increase survival. Decisions on the use of adjuvant chemotherapy are based on predictions of tumour behaviour such as the Nottingham Prognostic Index.[7] Tumour size, histological grade and node status have been found to be important. Patient age and menopausal status, and the tumour receptor status to hormones, are all taken into consideration when considering options of hormonal manipulation and chemotherapy.

The practice of optimal breast cancer surgery therefore requires cooperation between surgeon, radiotherapist and oncologist. Surgeons specializing in breast cancer have been shown to have better results than generalists.[8] This is primarily the result of the appropriate treatment modality being chosen for the individual patient, and is dependent on a high standard of histological, cytological and radiological diagnostic services. Surgeons practising in areas of the world where these diagnostic services are suboptimal, or where access to radiotherapy or chemotherapy is limited, can still obtain excellent results although they may have to rely more on the use of radical surgery.

A prophylactic bilateral mastectomy may be requested by patients at high genetic risk of breast cancer. A *subcutaneous mastectomy* is performed in which the whole breast except for areola and nipple are removed via an inframammary incision. No ellipse of skin is excised, and an immediate reconstruction with a silicone implant can be undertaken with good cosmetic result. Unfortunately, the operation does not totally eliminate the risk of death from breast cancer as not all breast tissue is removed.[9]

SURGERY FOR CARCINOMA OF THE BREAST

Diagnostic surgery

The first role of the surgeon is the confirmation or exclusion of the tentative diagnosis. *Triple assessment* is the combined evidence of the clinical, mammographic and cytological examinations, and results in a confident preoperative diagnosis in almost all patients. If these assessments all suggest malignancy, excision with a margin of normal tissue (*wide local excision*) is usually the most appropriate next surgical step. This will not only give final confirmatory histology but also is often sufficient surgical treatment of the primary lesion within the breast. When the results of the initial assessment are contradictory, more information may be gained by a *core biopsy* being taken for histology. The patient may have presented with a palpable mass, or a suspicious area may have been detected by screening mammography. If the lesion is palpable, the surgeon can take the core biopsy with a specially designed needle passed through a small stab incision in the overlying skin which has been infiltrated with local anaesthetic. Core biopsy of an impalpable lesion detected on imaging requires sophisticated stereotactic localization devices, or guidance by ultrasound. A preoperative definitive diagnosis can usually be made, but *excision biopsy* may have to be the final diagnostic procedure.

Surgical treatment of the breast primary tumour

EARLY BREAST CANCER

Radical treatment is undertaken with an intention to cure. After local excision alone, recurrence may occur within the remaining breast tissue.[4] It is, therefore, generally accepted that the majority of patients should be advised to have more radical treatment; either radiotherapy to the affected breast after conservative surgery, or a mastectomy. Most patients prefer to avoid mastectomy, and in most instances the two treatment options are comparable in terms of both local control and long-term survival. However, a mastectomy is known to offer superior local control when there is extensive carcinoma in situ, or multifocal invasion. A mastectomy may also be a better option in some medial or centrally placed tumours when local excision is expected to give a disappointing cosmetic result. Mastectomy may also be indicated if radiotherapy is contraindicated or unavailable.

LOCALLY ADVANCED BREAST CANCER

Primary surgery is contraindicated if there is evidence of extensive skin involvement by tumour or features of advanced disease such as inflammation or cutaneous oedema (peau d'orange). Similarly, when tumour or involved axillary nodes are fixed to muscle, primary surgery is best avoided. In these circumstances primary systemic therapy with chemotherapy or endocrine manipulation – or both – can bring advanced locoregional disease under control. This approach is also clearly indicated when distant disease is found at presentation. Locoregional radiotherapy can also achieve useful locoregional control. Since survival under these circumstances is likely to be poor, surgery can often be avoided, and is reserved for those cases where chemotherapy, endocrine manipulation and radiotherapy have failed to achieve useful local palliation. These operations follow the standard pattern of wide excision of highly symptomatic malignant infiltration followed by reconstruction onto healthy surrounding tissue.[10] The indications for such operations are, fortunately, rare.

PHYLLODES TUMOUR

This tumour is usually initially excised as a suspected fibroadenoma. Phyllodes tumours require adequate wide local excision. Although malignant potential varies, local recurrence and rarely blood-borne dissemination may occur. Lymph node metastases are not a feature.[11] Wide local excision, or on rare occasions mastectomy without axillary sampling or clearance, is thus the standard management.

Wide local excision

This is indicated for a proven malignancy or for a lesion that is suspected to be malignant after full assessment. The lesion is removed with a margin of macroscopically normal breast tissue. If a subsequent mastectomy is likely, the scar should be within the ellipse of skin which would be excised at mastectomy. Invasion, or carcinoma in situ, beyond the primary tumour may extend to the margins of the excision and necessitate a later, more radical local excision or mastectomy. Segmentectomy, and breast disc repair, can have oncological and aesthetic advantages over a wide local excision.

If the lesion is impalpable, some method of marking the area to be excised must first be undertaken. Similar stereotactic and ultrasound methods can be used as for core biopsy and a fine wire marker introduced into the lesion. This can be done in the breast imaging suite under local anaesthesia prior to surgery. After the excision, the excised tissue should be X-rayed to check that the radiologically suspicious area is within it.

Simple mastectomy

An appreciation of the development of the breast as a skin appendage is fundamental to the concept of a mastectomy. The whole breast is excised with an overlying ellipse of skin which includes the nipple and areola. General anaesthesia is routine, but the operation can be undertaken with infiltration of large volumes of dilute local anaesthetic agent. The patient is placed supine with the arm abducted and

supported on an arm board. In order to prevent shoulder capsular strain and nerve damage, abduction should be less than 90 degrees and the elbow should not be at a lower level than the shoulder.

The skin ellipse is marked. A horizontal ellipse lies in the natural skin creases, but some obliquity affords better access to the axilla and also the medial end of the scar will be lower and below the area of visible 'cleavage' (Fig. 2.4a). The width of the ellipse is decided by issues of skin closure. Tension should be avoided, but excess skin may give an ugly folded scar and haematoma formation is also more likely.

The skin is incised as planned and the incisions deepened through the subcutaneous fat. The ideal plane of dissection is between the subcutaneous fat and the breast tissue, but it is not an easy plane to follow. Skin flaps that are too thick leave residual breast tissue in situ, whilst if they are cut too thin the skin is in danger of losing its blood supply or even being 'button-holed'. The upper flap and then the lower flap are raised until, at the edge of the breast, the plane comes down onto the deep fascia (Fig. 2.4b). The breast is then dissected off the deep fascia from above downwards and multiple bleeding vessels secured (Fig. 2.4c). If an area is encountered where the tumour has breached this plane, a disc of pectoralis fascia and muscle should be excised with the specimen. The lateral end of the dissection is the most difficult as the plane between axillary tail of breast and the axillary fat is indistinct and the deep plane is also less obvious beyond the lateral border of pectoralis major. After careful haemostasis, the skin is closed over vacuum drainage. Avoidance of drains by meticulous haemostasis and obliteration of the dead space with sutures has proved possible without increase in morbidity in a specialist centre.[12]

Subcutaneous mastectomy

This is usually the preferred option for a prophylactic mastectomy. The operation can be performed through a submammary incision, but the same mastectomy planes are followed both between breast tissue and skin, and between the breast and the deep fascia. The only difference is that all the breast skin, the nipple and the areola are preserved. An immediate reconstruction is then undertaken which can give excellent cosmesis. When a mastectomy is indicated in malignant disease, preservation of the nipple and areola will usually be contraindicated.

Skin-sparing mastectomy

This alternative to a simple total mastectomy for breast cancer can be used when immediate reconstruction is planned, and usually results in a better cosmetic appearance. A total mastectomy is performed through a circumareolar incision. The nipple and areola are excised with the rest of the breast, but the breast skin is preserved as an envelope which receives an immediate reconstruction.[13]

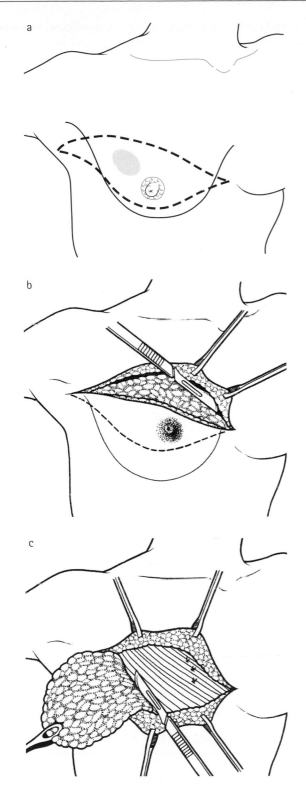

Figure 2.4 *A right simple mastectomy. (a) A slightly oblique ellipse keeps the medial end of the scar low and less conspicuous while also giving good access laterally to the axilla. (b) Dissection of the upper skin flap. The natural plane between subcutaneous fat and breast tissue is followed. (c) The breast is then dissected off the deep fascia from above downwards. When the lateral edge of pectoralis major is reached the dissection of the axillary tail is continued into the axilla.*

BREAST RECONSTRUCTION AFTER CANCER SURGERY

As a greater proportion of women are now able to be treated for breast cancer without mastectomy, those who are advised to have a mastectomy are increasingly interested in the possibility of breast reconstruction. This may be undertaken at the initial mastectomy or even several years later. For late reconstruction, a silicone implant can be used, after prior tissue expansion (see Chapter 1, page 20). Permanent tissue expander-implants with a surrounding silicone compartment are available. However, the original mastectomy scar traverses the summit of the new breast mound, and the final appearance may be poor. The use of tissue expansion is contraindicated in areas which have been subjected to radiotherapy. A superior cosmetic result can be achieved with a flap which transfers skin and fatty bulk to create a breast replacement. A pedicled flap of latissimus dorsi or rectus abdominis with overlying skin can be used, and free flaps are an alternative in skilled hands.

Latissimus dorsi musculocutaneous flap

This is the most widely used method of breast reconstruction following mastectomy. After completion of the mastectomy and any axillary clearance, the patient is turned on her side and a suitably sized ellipse of skin marked overlying the latissimus dorsi muscle. The long axis of the skin ellipse or 'paddle', can be made in a variety of directions. It may be made transverse to hide the scar under the bra strap, or it may be made perpendicular to the muscle fibres as this is the line of maximum skin laxity. The paddle is placed sufficiently posteriorly to afford adequate length to the flap (Fig. 2.5a). The skin is incised, leaving it attached to the underlying muscle. The skin and fascia are dissected off the muscle proximal and distal to the skin ellipse, and the muscle freed on its deep surface, prior to dividing its posterior attachment. It may then be elevated as a flap based on the branches of the subscapular vessels. Dissection is carried along the flap pedicle until it can be rotated and passed subcutaneously round to fill the breast defect (Fig. 2.5b). The vessels, on which the viability of the flap depend, lie in the flap pedicle separate from the muscle and on its deep surface. Care must be taken not to divide the vessels. The anterior muscle attachment may be divided for extra length but it is often left intact. The flap is then rotated through the axilla to the anterior defect. Ideally, the muscle should be denervated to avoid future painful contractions. The donor site is closed over suction drains and the patient returned to the supine position. The latissimus dorsi muscle forms the tissue replacement for the excised breast, and its overlying ellipse of skin is sutured to the upper and lower mastectomy flaps. A latissimus dorsi flap is often used in reconstruction in conjunction with a submuscular silicone implant to provide adequate volume.

a

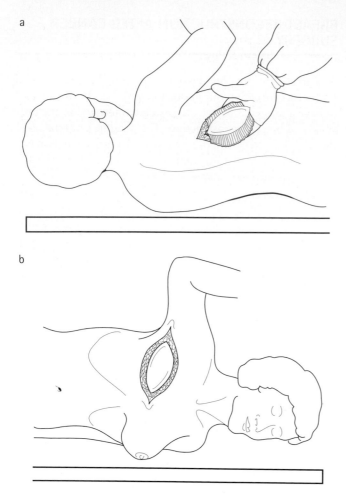

b

Figure 2.5   *A right latissimus dorsi reconstruction. (a) An ellipse of skin is circumcised just below the scapula and raised with its underlying portion of latissimus dorsi. The posterior origin of these muscle fibres is divided to create a compound flap on a pivot point close to the origin of the subscapular artery. (b) The myocutaneous flap is rotated and tunnelled subcutaneously into the mastectomy wound defect. The donor site is closed as a linear scar.*

Alternative flaps

Reconstructive plastic surgery of the breast after excisions for cancer has become increasingly sophisticated, and excellent cosmetic results can be obtained. Although pedicled transverse rectus abdominis myocutaneous (TRAM) flaps based on the internal thoracic artery have a somewhat perilous blood supply, free TRAM flaps, or free deep inferior epigastric artery perforator (DIEP) flaps, based on the inferior epigastric artery are increasingly employed where microsurgical skills are available (see Chapters 1 and 12). These are preferred by some surgeons to latissimus dorsi flaps. A free superior gluteal artery perforator flap is another alternative. These flap techniques are suitable both for immediate and for late reconstruction.

Wide local excision of a medial or centrally placed tumour can give a poor cosmetic result, especially if the tumour is large and the breast is small. Latissimus dorsi mini-flaps have proved useful as 'fillers' after large local excisions. A single long incision down the lateral edge of the breast allows the breast with the pectoral fascia to be reflected off pectoralis major. A wide local excision of the tumour is performed through the deep aspect of the breast. The limited latissimus dorsi flap is then harvested from within the axilla through the same incision, and is rotated into the breast defect to replace the bulk of tissue excised.[14]

Oncoplastic surgery

There is a growing appreciation that both oncological and aesthetic principles should be applied when planning and executing breast cancer surgery. Safe margins around a breast cancer are essential to minimize the risk of local recurrence, but this can result in an unacceptable appearance to the breast following surgery. With an understanding of plastic surgical techniques this risk can be reduced. For example, after segmental excision the breast disc can be mobilized from the overlying skin and the defect repaired. The skin is then re-draped over a smaller breast mound. When appropriate, excess skin can also be removed as in a standard breast reduction operation (see Fig. 2.11), although the underlying excision of breast tissue will differ as it has been planned around the excision of the malignancy. To achieve symmetry, contralateral breast reduction surgery might be necessary, and this is usually undertaken at a separate and later operation. Alternatively, new tissue can be used to fill the defect as in the limited latissimus dorsi flap technique described above.

Similar considerations apply when a mastectomy is indicated and breast reconstruction is requested. Is immediate or delayed reconstruction more appropriate? If immediate reconstruction is selected, should a skin-sparing approach be undertaken? Breast surgeons need to appreciate all of these possibilities to achieve the best result for their patients.

This approach might be termed 'oncoplastic' surgery, and this sort of surgery can be undertaken with collaboration between breast and plastic surgeon where the plastic surgeon is involved in planning the approach and repairing the defect. Alternatively, and with appropriate training, breast surgeons can acquire plastic surgical skills.

AXILLARY SURGERY FOR CANCER

Surgical staging in the axilla

Breast cancer can spread early in the course of the disease to the axilla, and radical treatment of the axilla by surgery or radiotherapy at initial presentation reduces symptomatic axillary recurrence.[5] Surgical clearance and radiotherapy have similar success and morbidity. However, if the axillae of all patients are treated, about 60 per cent of patients have unnecessary axillary treatment as they have no nodal secondaries. This group is difficult to identify, however. Clinical staging of the axilla has little to offer, as shown beautifully in the simple classic study by McNair and Dudley in 1954.[15] Imaging of lymph nodes for staging has been used mainly to detect enlargement, and altered signal on imaging, of inaccessible intra-abdominal and intra-thoracic nodes. Imaging techniques, however, have little to add in the assessment of these relatively superficial axillary nodes in the staging of breast cancer. Benign axillary nodal enlargement is common, and normal-sized nodes containing small metastases within them will elicit a normal signal. Surgical removal of nodes for histology is the only accurate staging modality for the axilla. The three operations which are commonly used to stage the axilla are a level I dissection, lymph node sampling,[16] and sentinel node biopsy.[17]

A concern over all lymph node staging procedures is that the more thorough the examination, the greater the chance of detecting a small nodal metastasis. If a pathologist has only one node to examine and takes multiple sections, the chance of detecting a microscopic focus within it is obviously higher than if the node is one of fifteen apparently normal nodes. A further dimension has been added to this debate with the advent of histocytochemistry techniques which can identify single or small clumps of malignant cells in a lymph node. It is impossible to know whether such cells are merely awaiting their death by the action of the immune defences, or are in the process of establishing their own microcirculation to become a viable metastasis.[18] In all staging surgery the advantages of immediate frozen section histology have to be balanced against a more thorough and accurate delayed histological examination, but with the possibility of a second operation being indicated.

AXILLARY SAMPLING

This is an operation in which the axilla is explored, and the four most obvious nodes are removed for histology. It only requires entry into the axillary fat to remove the most easily palpable nodes. These are commonly in the lower axilla, and a formal dissection of the axillary vein is seldom necessary. When this procedure is combined with a mastectomy or the excision of a lateral tumour, access from the breast wound is often adequate, otherwise a small transverse incision will suffice.

LEVEL I AXILLARY DISSECTION

A level I axillary dissection removes the lower axillary nodes (below the lateral border of pectoralis minor). The operation follows the same principles of dissection as the level III operation described below, but the dissection is only taken to the level of the lower border of pectoralis minor.

SENTINEL NODE BIOPSY

This technique is similar to that used for malignant melanoma as described in Chapter 1, page 10. Basically, the first node in the axilla to receive lymphatic drainage from the breast is the relatively constant sentinel node. This node is identified, after injecting either a radiotracer or blue dye (or both) into the breast, and is removed for pathological evaluation. If negative for metastases, no further axillary surgery is undertaken – that is, axillary clearance surgery is reserved for those with proven metastatic disease. There has been debate regarding the validity of this technique,[19] and this resolves into two basic issues. First, identification of the node can be difficult; and second, there is a false-negative rate in terms of predicting axillary involvement. Both of these problems can be minimized to acceptable levels by appropriate selection of cases suitable for the technique, and by perfecting the localizing procedures and the pathological evaluation of the sentinel node. There is a learning curve – as with all new techniques – and audit of outcomes is an essential part of introducing the procedure. Some feel that results from randomized prospective trials will be necessary before sentinel node biopsy is introduced into routine clinical practice. Others have undertaken their own evaluation and have already introduced the procedure.

Surgical treatment or clearance of the axilla

The staging procedures discussed above are not surgical treatment. A *level III clearance* (the removal of all three groups of axillary glands) is a radical surgical treatment of an axilla. Radiotherapy is an alternative and can be used after axillary staging surgery. A surgeon may opt for surgical clearance in those patients with a high predicted risk of nodal involvement, but perform nodal sampling in those with a low risk. If metastases are detected in the sampled nodes, radiotherapy can then be given to the axilla, or an axillary clearance undertaken. Radiotherapy combined with a level III dissection increases morbidity, and should, if possible, be avoided.

LEVEL II AND LEVEL III AXILLARY CLEARANCE

A level II and level III axillary clearance may be performed in conjunction with a simple mastectomy or a wide local excision of a lump in any part of the breast. It may also be undertaken as an isolated procedure when earlier axillary node sampling has shown tumour, and surgery is felt to be preferable to radiotherapy. It may very occasionally be indicated for obvious recurrent axillary disease in a patient who has already had radiotherapy, but should be avoided if at all possible due to the almost inevitable subsequent lymphoedema. Surgery after previous axillary surgery or radiotherapy is often more difficult, but the operation is essentially the same.

The patient is placed supine with the arm abducted in a similar position as for a simple mastectomy. It is important during the preparation of the skin with antiseptic that the arm is lifted forwards so that the skin over the posterior axillary wall is included, and a sterile drape is placed beneath it.

Some surgeons then suspend the forearm, with the elbow flexed, above the patient in preference to placing it on an armboard. This produces less tension in pectoralis major which can be retracted more easily.

The axilla is most often explored through a transverse lower axillary incision. It may be the lateral end of a mastectomy incision, or an extension of the incision for the wide local excision of a laterally placed breast tumour. The axilla can also be explored through the vertical oblique incision at the lateral edge of the breast if this incision has already been used for the breast surgery. When an axillary dissection is undertaken as part of a mastectomy, the breast and axillary contents are excised as a single specimen. The mastectomy dissection can be completed, except for the axillary tail, before entering the axilla. Other surgeons prefer to dissect up the upper flap only and then dissect the axilla, leaving the final freeing of the breast from the chest wall until later.

The lateral border of pectoralis major is defined and the fascia incised along its length (Fig. 2.6a) to allow entry into the axilla. The axillary contents are retracted downwards and the fat is carefully incised over and parallel to the axillary vein until the vein is visible (Fig. 2.6b). This is the superolateral border of the dissection. Tributaries entering the vein from the axillary fat are secured, divided and ligated with absorbable sutures. The clearing of the vein continues until the vessels lying on the muscles of the posterior wall of the axilla come into view. The most obvious are the thoracodorsal vessels. (This artery is the branch of the subscapular artery on which a latissimus dorsi flap depends.) The thoracodorsal nerve to latissimus dorsi emerges from behind the axillary vein just medial to the thoracodorsal vessels and then runs obliquely towards the vessels forming an easily identifiable triangle on the posterior wall muscles (see Fig. 2.2). Both the vessels and the nerve are preserved, but all of the fat and nodes should be dissected off them. The lateral border of latissimus dorsi is identified and marks the inferolateral limit of the dissection. The vein is then cleared up towards the apex of the axilla, behind pectoralis minor which will have to be firmly retracted. To obtain sufficient access to perform a level III clearance, the division of the tendon of insertion of pectoralis minor into the coracoid process may be essential. The pectoral nerves and accompanying vessels will be encountered, crossing the upper axilla to the anterior axillary wall. The lateral pectoral nerve may have to be sacrificed. The medial should be preserved if at all possible. Before completing the apical dissection it is easier to turn attention first to the medial wall and dissect the axillary contents off serratus anterior.

On the medial axillary wall, the large lateral branch of the 2nd intercostal nerve (the intercostobrachial nerve) is almost immediately encountered entering the axillary fat. Most surgeons sacrifice it, although some try to dissect it out and preserve it. Further posteriorly, the nerve to serratus anterior tends to be lifted off the muscle with the axillary contents and needs to be carefully freed and allowed to drop back. Once this dissection joins the posterior wall dissection the remaining apical fat and lymphatics are divided (Fig. 2.6c).

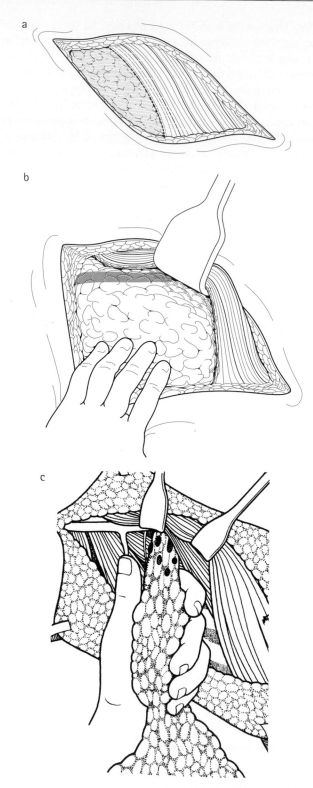

Figure 2.6   *A right axillary clearance. (a) The lateral border of pectoralis major is defined and the fascia incised along its length to gain access into the axilla. (b) The axillary contents are retracted downwards and the fat over the axillary vein is carefully incised until it can be identified. (c) The apical division of fat and lymphatics is easier after the medial and posterior wall dissection has been completed. (In this illustration the axillary dissection has been combined with a mastectomy which has been completed first.)*

Finally, the fat which still attaches the specimen to the lateral end of the lower flap is divided. Haemostasis should be meticulous, but lymphatic drainage will continue and vacuum drainage of the axilla is favoured by most surgeons despite recent evidence that drains can be avoided.[12] This drain may have to remain *in situ* for 2 weeks or more to prevent collection of lymph. Reducing arm movement decreases lymph production but increases the longer-term problem of a reduction in the range of shoulder movement. Early shoulder movement is therefore encouraged.

SURGERY OF BENIGN BREAST DISEASE

Breast lumps

Improvements in diagnostic facilities, combined with a greater understanding of the normal cyclical changes within the breast, have reduced the number of benign breast lump excisions. Palpable cysts can be aspirated and many nodular areas can be safely left *in situ*. A solid, discrete breast lump which is believed to be benign on all assessment criteria may also be left, but some patients and surgeons prefer the excision of such lumps because of the small risk of a missed malignancy. Surgeons who do not have access to reliable mammographic or cytological diagnostic facilities will inevitably have to excise more benign lumps to avoid a missed malignancy.

Children in early puberty are sometimes referred to a surgeon with a tender lump deep to one nipple. This is a normal developing breast bud, and one breast frequently starts developing a few months ahead of the other. Excision biopsy of this 'lump' is a disaster in a girl as she loses all potential breast tissue on that side.

LOCAL EXCISION OF A BREAST LUMP

Only the lump itself is excised, without a surrounding margin of normal breast tissue. This is, therefore, a suitable technique for the removal of lumps which are expected to be benign on histological examination. A good cosmetic result should be sought, and circumferential scars are better than radial. A scar may sometimes be hidden in the inframammary crease. This scar may, however, pose difficulties if the lesion proves to be malignant as it does not lie naturally within the ellipse of skin to be excised if a mastectomy is indicated. Scars in the superomedial quadrant of the breast often become hypertrophic and can sometimes be avoided by an incision hidden at the areolar edge.

Haemostasis is important, and vacuum drainage should be considered after large excisions. Absorbable sutures may be used to reconstitute the breast tissue, and a subcuticular suture is suitable for skin closure. A breast in pregnancy is significantly more vascular but otherwise poses no difficulties. A lactating breast continues to secrete milk at the operation site. A vacuum drain may compound the problem and establish a milk fistula, and the situation may be better managed by repeat aspiration of the milk cyst as it recollects.

Breast infections

Infection occurs most commonly – but not exclusively – in a lactating breast. In the early stage of inflammation the appropriate antibiotic may be all that is required. Once pus has formed drainage is required. Deep pus in the breast is difficult to assess clinically, but may be confirmed by ultrasound. Good results have been obtained by ultrasound-guided aspiration combined with aggressive antibiotic therapy,[20] and this treatment has been shown to be effective even if ultrasound is not available.[21] However, open surgical drainage is still sometimes required. Whichever treatment is undertaken, there appears to be no contraindication to continuing breast feeding, and this should be encouraged – especially in areas of the world where it is crucial to the survival of the baby.

A recurrent or chronic abscess at the areolar edge is most often the result of an underlying *mammillary fistula*. Recurrence will continue until the fistula is laid open by deroofing of the track. Recurrent infections deep to the nipple – often associated with nipple retraction and nipple discharge – are usually secondary to *periductal mastitis*. A major duct excision eradicates the source of the infection and, if eversion of the nipple can be achieved, then cosmesis is also improved.

Neonatal swelling of breast tissue in either sex is a physiological response to maternal hormones. Occasionally there is associated infection and a neonatal breast abscess. In a female child care should be taken in draining this to cause minimal damage to the rudimentary breast bud.

DRAINAGE OF A BREAST ABSCESS

General anaesthesia is preferable as the loculi of a deep abscess must be broken down with a finger to obtain good drainage; surface local anaesthesia is inadequate here. A linear incision should be made in a position where it will allow dependent drainage, but cosmetic implications should also be considered. An abscess in the upper breast may be drained satisfactorily through an incision on the areolar edge. A corrugated or similar drain should be left in situ to allow continuing drainage of the depths of the cavity and to prevent premature skin closure (Fig. 2.7). This can also be achieved by a more radical deroofing of an abscess, but it gives a less satisfactory final scar.

LAYING OPEN OF A MAMMILLARY FISTULA

A probe is introduced into the chronic abscess cavity at the areolar edge and the track gently sought with the probe towards the apex of the nipple. The track is then laid open by incision onto the probe and the wound left to heal by granu-

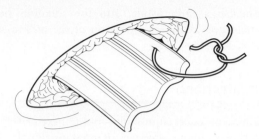

Figure 2.7 *A corrugated drain prevents premature skin closure.*

lation from beneath (Fig. 2.8). These patients usually have an underlying periductal mastitis, and recurrence is common. They may be better served by a formal major duct excision with the removal of all the diseased tissue.

Nipple discharge

The discharge from multiple ducts which occurs in galactorrhoea requires medical rather than surgical management. Discharge from multiple ducts can also occur in duct ectasia, and in association with periductal mastitis. When symptoms cannot be controlled by other measures a formal major duct excision is indicated. Discharge from a single duct is commonly secondary to a duct ectasia. However, if the discharge is bloodstained there is the possibility that the underlying pathology is an intraduct papilloma or carcinoma. A microdochectomy (the excision of a single major duct) may be performed for discharge from a single duct, either to alleviate distressing symptoms or to obtain a specimen for histological examination and exclusion of an underlying neoplasm.

MICRODOCHECTOMY

Local anaesthesia is satisfactory, but most patients prefer a general anaesthesia for nipple and areolar surgery. The nipple is squeezed to identify the appropriate duct into which a fine blunt probe is introduced. A sawn-off needle has the extra advantage of an eye which can be used to secure the probe in place with a fine suture for the duration of the operation. The probe is then used to guide the surgeon in the removal of 3–5 cm of the appropriate duct. This can be approached by a radial incision in the areola, or alternatively by an areolar edge incision which may be cosmetically superior (Fig. 2.9). After removal of the duct, which is sent for histology, the wound is closed with fine sutures.

MAJOR DUCT EXCISION

Antibiotic cover is recommended if there is chronic infection. All the ducts under the nipple and areola are excised and it is, therefore, obviously contraindicated if future breastfeeding is anticipated. The approach is via an incision at the inferior areolar edge. A deep purse-string suture, to encourage nipple eversion before the skin suture is inserted, can improve the final cosmetic result.

BREAST REDUCTION AND AUGMENTATION SURGERY

Although much of this work is cosmetic, there are often sound medical or psychological indications for intervention. Gynaecomastia in pubertal boys is so common as to be considered a variant of normal. Excision of the tender nodule deep to the nipple is straightforward but seldom justified as the condition usually settles spontaneously. However, occasionally this breast disc spreads to form a noticeable 'breast'

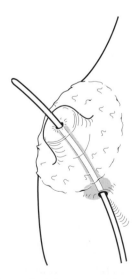

Figure 2.8 *The fine probe is in a mammillary fistula which extends from a chronic areolar edge abscess to the opening of a duct onto the nipple.*

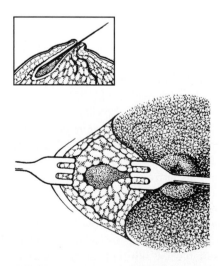

Figure 2.9 *A blunt probe, or sawn-off needle, is introduced into the discharging duct. Excision of this duct can be through either a radial areolar incision or an incision at the areolar edge.*

which can cause great distress, and surgical intervention is justified. Liposuction is an alternative to excision if the breast tissue is fatty rather than fibrous.

Reconstruction after mastectomy is offered routinely in many centres, and the reconstructive options have been described above. Symmetry may not be possible without the augmentation of a silicone implant, or a reduction mammaplasty on the remaining breast. The patient may also request the creation of a nipple (by local flaps) and areola (by skin grafting or tattooing) on the reconstructed breast. Complete or partial failure of breast development – either bilaterally or unilaterally – causes major distress to a young woman, and is another indication for reconstructive surgery. Excessive breast development can cause a woman both discomfort from the weight of tissue to be supported and embarrassment at her appearance. General surgeons who have not subspecialized in breast surgery should not undertake these more complex operations. Even breast surgeons often refer this work to a plastic surgeon unless they have a special interest and further training in plastic surgery. Patient expectations are high, and good cosmetic results will only be obtained by those specializing in the field.

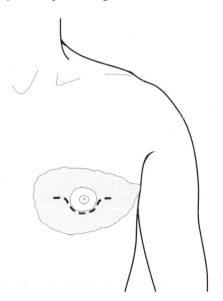

Figure 2.10 *Excision for gynaecomastia can involve the removal of breast tissue extending out over the whole shaded area. Lateral and medial extensions to the initial areolar edge incision may be necessary, but should be avoided if possible.*

Excision of gynaecomastia

An inframammary scar is distressing as it is a continuing source of embarrassment. It is usually possible to excise even a broad-based breast through an inferior circum-areolar incision. Dissection is commenced by lifting the areola and nipple from the underlying breast. A little breast tissue should be left attached to the undersurface of the nipple and

areola to safeguard the blood supply, and also to prevent a hollow in this region due to a lack of subcutaneous fat. The skin is then undermined circumferentially to the edge of the breast tissue, where the plane of dissection comes onto the pectoral fascia. The breast is then dissected off the pectoral fascia and delivered out through the wound. Access is restricted, and much of the dissection can not be under direct vision; moreover, haemostasis is difficult until the whole breast has been excised. If difficulty is encountered, the breast can be transected and removed a quadrant at a time. A small extension at either end of the incision improves access but should be avoided, if possible, as the scar will be more apparent (Fig. 2.10). Even if haemostasis is good, a

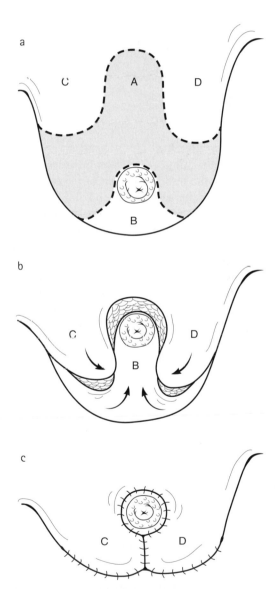

Figure 2.11 *A breast reduction operation. (a) The shaded area of breast tissue is excised. The 'keyhole' area 'A' is to accommodate the nipple and areola when elevated to the new position. They are retained on a pedicle of inframammary skin and breast tissue. (b) The nipple is now elevated to its new position 'A'. (c) The skin on 'B' is shaved off and 'C' and 'D' are rotated over for skin closure.*

vacuum drain is recommended as haematoma formation under the flaps is a common complication.

Breast augmentation

This can be achieved by a silicone implant. The commonest approach is through an incision in the inframammary fold of the breast, where it will be least conspicuous. The implant is placed either deep to the pectoral fascia, or deep to the pectoralis muscle. Early complications include haematoma formation and infection. Complications can also occur years later. Capsular contracture around the implant is not uncommon with a worsening cosmetic result. Leakage of the silicone into the tissues may occur and implants may rupture. The safety of silicone gel implants has been extensively studied following major public concern. Several government-commissioned reports have affirmed that there is no association with connective tissue diseases or breast cancer.

Breast reduction

There are several techniques in which breast tissue and skin are excised from the inferior portion of the breast, which is then reconstructed by mobilizing and drawing round the breast tissue from either side. Careful planning of the incisions is mandatory to achieve good results. Symmetry of both breast size and shape is important, and also the projection of the breast and the final position of the nipple and areola, which must be moved cranially. The nipple and the areola can be moved to their new position as a full-thickness graft, but it is more satisfactory to move them with their blood supply preserved by adjacent tissue. This can be with a strip of de-epithelialized inferior breast skin (Fig. 2.11) or with a cone of underlying breast tissue.[22] Early complications include nipple necrosis. Careful preoperative counselling is important or patients may be disappointed with the final result. They should be warned of possible asymmetry, reduced nipple sensation, and that subsequent lactation is seldom an option.

REFERENCES

1. *ABC of Breast Diseases*, 2nd edn. JM Dixon, BMJ Books, 2002.
2. *Breast Surgery: A Companion to Specialist Surgical Practice*, 2nd edn. JR Farndon, Philadelphia: Elsevier Saunders, 2001.
3. Halstead WS. The results of operations for the cure of cancer of the breast performed at the John Hopkins Hospital from June 1889 to January 1894. *Ann Surg* 1894: **20**: 497–555.
4. Fisher B, Redmond C, Poisson R, *et al*. Eight-year results of a randomized clinical trial comparing total mastectomy and lumpectomy with or without radiation in the treatment of breast cancer. *N Engl J Med* 1989; **320**: 822–8.
5. Fisher B, Redmond C, Fisher ER, *et al*. Ten-year results of a randomized clinical trial comparing radical mastectomy and total mastectomy with or without radiation. *N Engl J Med* 1985; **312**: 674–81.
6. McWhirter R. The value of simple mastectomy and radiotherapy in the treatment of cancer of the breast. *Br J Radiol* 1948; **21**: 599–610.
7. Galea MH, Blamey RW, Elston CE, *et al*. The Nottingham Prognostic Index in primary breast cancer. *Breast Cancer Res Treat* 1992; **22**: 207–19.
8. Gillis CR, Hole DJ. Survival outcome of care by specialist surgeons in breast cancer: a study of 3786 patients in the west of Scotland. *Br Med J* 1996; **312**: 145–8.
9. Hartmann LC, Schaid DJ, Woods JE, *et al*. Efficacy of bilateral prophylactic mastectomy in women with a family history of breast cancer. *N Engl J Med* 1999; **340**: 77–84.
10. Hathaway CL, Rand RP, Moe R, *et al*. Salvage surgery for locally advanced and locally recurrent breast cancer. *Arch Surg* 1994; **129**: 582–6.
11. Mangi AA, *et al*. Surgical management of Phyllodes tumors. *Arch Surg* 1999; **134**: 487–92.
12. Purushotham AD, McLatchie E, Young D, *et al*. Randomized clinical trial of no wound drains and early discharge in the treatment of women with breast cancer. *Br J Surg* 2002; **89**: 286–92.
13. Peyser PM, Abel JA, Straker VF, *et al*. Ultra-conservative skin-sparing 'keyhole' mastectomy and immediate breast and areola reconstruction. *Ann R Coll Surg Engl* 2000; **82**: 227–35.
14. Raja MAK, Straker VF, Rainsbury RM. Extending the role of breast-conserving surgery by immediate volume replacement. *Br J Surg* 1997; **84**: 101–5.
15. McNair TJ, Dudley HAF. Axillary lymph nodes in patients without breast carcinoma. *Lancet* 1960; **i**: 713–15.
16. Steele RJC, Forrest APM, Gibson T, *et al*. The efficacy of lower axillary sampling in obtaining lymph node status in breast cancer: a controlled randomized trial. *Br J Surg* 1985; **72**: 368–9.
17. McIntosh SA, Purushotham AD. Lymphatic mapping and sentinel node biopsy in breast cancer. Review. *Br J Surg* 1998; **85**: 1347–56.
18. Page DL, Anderson TJ, Carter BA. Minimal solid tumour involvement of regional and distant sites – when is a metastasis not a metastasis? Editorial. *Cancer* 1999; **86**: 2589–92.
19. Carpenter R. Sentinel node biopsy should be introduced into routine clinical practice before results of randomized trials are available. Invited article. *Breast* 2001; **10**: 281–4.
20. O'Hara RJ, Dexter SP, Fox JN. Conservative management of infective mastitis and breast abscesses after ultrasonographic assessment. *Br J Surg* 1996; **83**: 1413–14.
21. Schwarz RJ, Shrestha R. Needle aspiration of breast abscesses. *Am J Surg* 2001; **182**: 117–9.
22. Bolger WE, Seyfer AE, Jackson SM. Reduction mammaplasty using the inferior glandular 'pyramid' pedicle: experience with 300 patients. *Plast Reconstruct Surg* 1987; **80**: 75–84.

3

SOFT TISSUE SURGERY: MUSCLES, TENDONS, LIGAMENTS AND NERVES

Although it is the orthopaedic surgeon who operates most frequently on these tissues, an understanding of the surgical principles is still essential to the general surgeon. Trauma and infection occur in the soft tissue of both the trunk and the limbs, and there is significant overlap between surgical specialties. This chapter may also be of some value to the general surgeon who is unable to obtain specialist help and has to operate in unfamiliar 'orthopaedic territory'. However, the true surgical generalist may find that a large proportion of his or her surgical practice is in this mainly orthopaedic area, and will wish to supplement this chapter with further operative texts.[1]

SURGERY OF SOFT TISSUE TRAUMA

The severity of damage both to muscle, and to other tissue, is often underestimated as attention is focused on the more obvious skin wound, or the fractured bone visible on X-ray. For example, a high-velocity bullet which has passed through the upper calf may have inflicted a small entry and exit wound and a tibial fracture. The fracture appears to be the most significant injury, and initially it may not be appreciated that almost the entire calf musculature is necrotic, that there is nerve and arterial damage, and that the viability of the distal limb is under threat. Soft tissue trauma inflicts three separate insults: direct tissue injury; tissue ischaemia; and the introduction of infection.

DIRECT TRAUMATIC DAMAGE

A knowledge of the mode of injury is a useful predictor of the likely damage. A stab wound with a sharp knife causes minimal damage except to the tissue which is severed. A blunt impact may cause a small wound but a large surrounding area of damaged, or even non-viable tissue. A high-velocity missile imparts kinetic energy to the surrounding tissue, a temporary cavity forms with traction forces on the tissue, and disruption of small vessels. The cavity sucks in contaminants and then collapses. The final result is extensive contaminated tissue death surrounding an apparently small-calibre track (Fig. 3.1).

DAMAGE TO THE BLOOD SUPPLY

An injury may sever a major vessel. However, the damage to an artery may be more subtle with only a partial tear. In this situation the distal circulation may initially be preserved but deteriorate later. This is discussed more fully in Chapter 5.

Injury to a major vessel in the vicinity of a penetrating wound must always be suspected, and evidence of associated nerve damage should heighten suspicion further.

More commonly, the swelling of injured soft tissue within

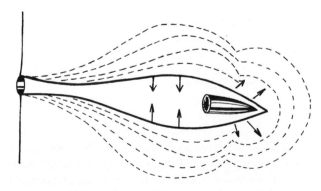

Figure 3.1 *A high-velocity missile causes extensive damage to the tissue around the track.*

a closed fascial compartment allows the tissue pressure to exceed perfusion pressure. This causes ischaemic muscle damage (*compartment syndrome*), and finally muscle death ensues some hours after the injury.

INFECTION

Any traumatic damage associated with breach of the skin, or mucosa, has the potential to introduce infection. However, a sharp injury inflicted with a non-sterile knife seldom results in significant infection. In contrast, penetrating injuries with blunt objects are associated with a high risk of infection, as virulent organisms may be carried into tissue which has also been contused, or rendered ischaemic, by the injury. Thus, animal bites were always treated by delayed suture in the pre-antibiotic era. Infection of damaged tissue leads to further tissue necrosis. Gross contamination, with soil or clothing carried into necrotic tissue, almost inevitably results in severe limb- and life-threatening infection as the necrotic debris and haematoma are an ideal culture medium.

Surgical removal of dead tissue and contaminants

The nature of the injury gives a good preoperative indication of the likelihood of extensive soft tissue necrosis, or gross contamination. All dead tissue must be excised and all vegetable debris removed, or severe complications are inevitable. A small skin wound may have to be extensively enlarged in order to achieve adequate access. Any doubtfully viable tissue can be left for a second inspection after 24–48 hours (see *Delayed repair* below). Metallic foreign bodies, such as bullets, shotgun pellets and pieces of shrapnel, may remain quiescent for a lifetime and should not be removed unless the surgery will be straightforward, otherwise the surgeon is at risk of causing more damage than the original weapon.[2] An exception is a lead-containing foreign body which, if left *in situ*, may cause lead poisoning.

Surgical preservation of tissue perfusion

If a major vessel has been severed and there is distal ischaemia, arterial repair is of the utmost urgency if amputation is to be avoided (see Chapter 5).

Oedema and **swelling** occurs with any injury, and is more marked in blunt injuries with significant tissue contusion. Elevation of the affected part (Fig. 3.2) reduces oedema, but this can be counterproductive in a patient with peripheral arterial occlusive disease, as it reduces further an already low arterial pressure. *Compartment syndrome,* as outlined above, leads to a loss of perfusion to the muscle. It is the result of swelling within a restricted space leading to excessive interstitial pressure. It can be caused not only by blunt trauma but also by other insults. An acutely ischaemic limb, which has been revascularized after a delay of some hours, will have

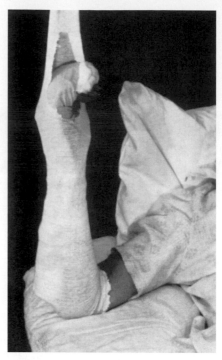

Figure 3.2   *Elevation of an injured hand. The photograph was taken by Eric Farquharson using a member of his family as the model.*

muscles which have suffered an ischaemic insult and will later swell. Even severe unaccustomed exercise can cause a compartment syndrome. Urgent decompression by fasciotomy, before irreversible ischaemic muscle damage occurs, is important. Minor compartment syndromes will settle spontaneously with elevation and rest, and the decision whether to operate is sometimes difficult. More is lost, however, by failure to act than by an unnecessary operation. Severe muscle tenderness, and pain exacerbated by any contraction of the muscle, should at least alert the surgeon to consider fasciotomy.

FASCIOTOMY

Fasciotomy is the treatment of a compartment syndrome.[3] The fascia must be opened along the length of the muscle belly. This can be achieved by a subcutaneous fasciotomy but it is easier – and much safer – to incise the whole length of overlying skin. This has the additional advantage of releasing any associated skin constriction. Closure by secondary suture is appropriate when the swelling subsides after a few days, but skin grafts may be needed. Occasionally only one fascial compartment is at risk. More often all compartments need release.

In the *leg* an incision behind the medial border of the tibia can be used to release the deep and superficial posterior compartments. A second incision, 4 cm lateral to the tibia, is required if release of the anterior and peroneal compartments is also indicated (Fig. 3.3). Alternatively, if flaps are

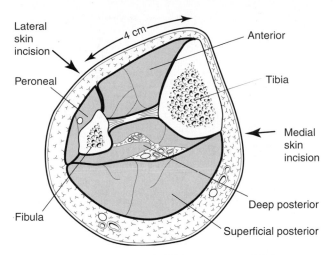

Figure 3.3 *An incision behind the medial border of the tibia affords access to both posterior compartments of the calf. A second incision 4 cm lateral to the anterior border of the tibia is required for access to the anterior and peroneal compartments.*

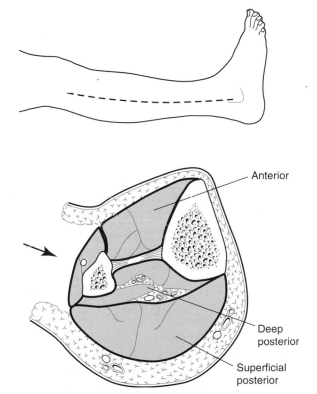

Figure 3.4 *A single incision over the fibula with elevation of flaps allows access to all four compartments.*

raised at the level of the deep fascia, a single lateral incision will provide access to all four compartments (Fig. 3.4). When the peroneal compartment needs to be released, the level of the fibular head should be identified, and used as a landmark to avoid damage to the common peroneal nerve as it winds around the neck of the fibula. Although the leg is the commonest site for a compartment syndrome, it can also occur

in the thigh and upper limb, but these less frequently require decompression.

Surgical repair of soft tissue injury

Primary suture

Primary suture of deep tissues and skin is suitable in clean wounds. It may also be appropriate management in selected contaminated wounds, but thorough wound toilet combined with excision of devitalised tissue is essential prior to closure. Antibiotic cover should be considered for any potentially contaminated wound which has been closed primarily.

Delayed repair

This is always the safer option. Before the advent of antibiotics it was considered mandatory for any potentially contaminated wound, and for any wound in which wound toilet had been delayed. Antibiotics have merely moved the dividing line between those wounds which can be treated by primary closure and those which cannot. If there is established infection, and tissue of doubtful viability has been left *in situ*, then primary closure is still potentially disastrous. The wound is cleaned, dead tissue excised and the cavity lightly packed with saline-soaked gauze. Some 48 hours later the wound is re-explored. If there is no infection, and the doubtfully viable tissue is now healthy, the deep tissues can be repaired and the wound closed. If, however, there is now further necrosis and infection the wound is again debrided and left open.

MUSCLE REPAIR

Longitudinal clean incisions of muscle do not require suture. A loose suture is at best harmless, whilst a tighter suture strangulates muscle fibres. However, the overlying fascia may be sutured if there is no significant muscle swelling, and closure of the deep fascia prevents a potential *muscle hernia*. A transverse incision of a muscle may, however, warrant repair. Divided muscle fibres retract and finally heal with a fibrous scar. The divided fibres atrophy and there is compensatory hypertrophy of the remaining intact fibres. A surgical repair is therefore usually only indicated for a laceration, or tear, which has divided a significant proportion of the muscle. When the fascia has also been divided, sutures to appose the fascia may be sufficient to hold the muscle fibres in apposition. It is on this principle that the closure of a Kocher subcostal incision is based (see Chapter 12). If a muscle belly repair is indicated, a figure-of-eight suture will be the least likely to cut out (Fig. 3.5). An absorbable suture which loses its tensile strength relatively slowly (e.g. vicryl) is suitable. Splintage for about 6 weeks after repair is recommended.

Closed trauma in the form of a severe force may disrupt

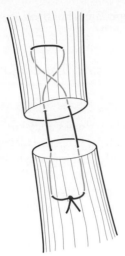

Figure 3.5   *A figure-of-eight suture is less likely to cut through muscle.*

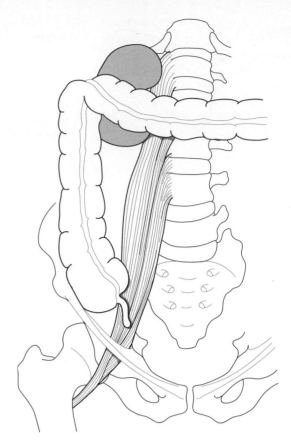

Figure 3.6   *Colon, appendix, kidney and vertebral bodies are all closely related to the psoas muscle. Infection originating from them may present as a psoas abscess tracking to the groin insertion.*

the *muscle tendon unit*. In children and adolescents the epiphysis into which the tendon is inserted may be pulled away from the bone, in the young adult a transverse muscle belly tear occurs, in the older adult the tendon itself ruptures and in old age the tendon may avulse a fragment of osteoporotic bone. A partial muscle belly tear causes a 'tumour' proximal to the injury when the muscle contracts. No treatment other than reassurance is required unless a major portion of a muscle has disrupted.

RECONSTRUCTION AND TISSUE COVER

This should normally be delayed until both the patient and the wound have entered a healing phase, and there is no longer any concern over non-viable tissue or infection. However, sometimes there is an urgency to establish tissue cover to allow healing, and so a compromise has to be struck. A muscle flap (see below) may be utilized to cover exposed bone.

INFECTION OF MUSCLE

Pyogenic muscle infection

This most commonly occurs secondary to penetrating trauma, even if this is only in the form of a minor puncture wound. Occasionally pus tracks into a muscle from an adjacent deep abscess. The commonest example is a psoas abscess which is pointing in the groin, but is caused by an underlying retroperitoneal infection which has tracked into the psoas muscle. The original pathology may be vertebral, renal or colonic (Fig. 3.6). In malnourished or immunocompromised individuals, a primary pyomyositis of large muscles may occur, and this is a common condition in some tropical countries. Whatever the aetiology, adequate drainage of pus, and the excision of any necrotic tissue, is indicated. A drain should be left into the depths of the abscess to prevent premature closure of the track. A corrugated drain, sutured to the skin, as used for a deep breast abscess (see Fig. 2.7, page 30), is satisfactory for this purpose.

Anaerobic muscle infection

Clostridium welchii, the causative organism of gas gangrene, and *Clostridium tetani*, the causative organism of tetanus, are found in soil and faeces, and these anaerobic organisms thrive in necrotic and ischaemic muscle. Gas gangrene was a common – and much feared – complication in the battlefields of the First World War.[4] Amputation was thus often considered a safer option than attempting to save a severely damaged limb which was already potentially contaminated with bacterial spores.

GAS GANGRENE

Clostridium welchii multiplies in ischaemic damaged tissue. The toxins produced by the bacteria damage previously healthy tissue which is then colonized, and the infection spreads longitudinally within muscle sheaths. The patient is usually profoundly unwell, and crepitus may be apparent from small bubbles of gas.

Prevention consists of thorough early wound toilet with removal of all necrotic tissue. A high-risk wound is then left open as described above. Although the organism is sensitive to penicillin, the use of the antibiotic for prophylaxis or treatment may be disappointing as the high blood levels do not reach the dead tissue in which the organism is multiplying.

Treatment of gas gangrene is primarily surgical for the same reason. All infected tissue must be excised as soon as the patient's general condition allows. The patient may be extremely ill with signs of multiple organ failure and require general resuscitation, but a surgical delay of more than a few hours will be counterproductive. This situation can pose a similar dilemma regarding the optimum timing of surgery to that encountered in patients with peritonitis, and this is discussed in Chapter 14. If gas gangrene in a wound is suspected, it must be opened and explored. In the early stages of anaerobic infection the affected muscle fibres are paler than normal, a lustreless pinkish grey shade being described: later they become deeply congested, slate blue or frankly gangrenous. Bubbles of gas are apparent. All unhealthy and potentially infected tissue must be excised, as leaving traumatized, or ischaemic, tissue in the vicinity is an unacceptable risk. The possibility of saving a limb should always be considered, but unfortunately amputation is often the only safe option. Parenteral penicillin is administered at high dosage and hyperbaric oxygen therapy, if available, may be beneficial.

Tissue gas is not pathognomonic of gas gangrene as saprophytic, non-pathogenic, gas-forming anaerobes may multiply in necrotic tissue. This scenario is occasionally encountered around a retroperitoneal colonic perforation. The excision of the necrotic tissue alone is adequate in this situation.

TETANUS

Tetanus is the other feared anaerobic infection of contaminated wounds. The incidence shows great regional variation, possibly related to soil acidity, and infection can occur after a very minor puncture wound. Immunization, antibiotics and anti-serum are all effective in its prevention. In established infection, there is no local tissue destruction, and excision of the wound has no great therapeutic merit unless indicated for other reasons. Penicillin is effective in destroying residual organisms, and antiserum will neutralize any unfixed toxin. However, by the time of presentation, much of the toxin is already fixed within the central nervous system, and clinical deterioration will continue for some days despite the administration of antibiotics and antiserum. The mainstay of treatment is the control of spasms, and general intensive support.

Necrotizing fasciitis and Fournier's gangrene

These are discussed in Chapter 1.

MUSCLE FLAPS

Healthy muscle has an excellent blood supply, and the overlying skin derives a significant proportion of its blood supply from the muscles, by vessels passing through the deep fascia. Many muscles have only one or two nutrient arteries supplying the whole muscle. These enter near either the muscle origin or insertion, and this anatomical arrangement allows for the isolation of a muscle, with the overlying skin if appropriate, as a 'flap'. A vascular pedicle at one end of the muscle is carefully preserved, and the other end of the muscle is separated from its origin or its insertion. This allows the musculocutaneous flap to be rotated around a vascular pedicle, to cover a tissue defect in an adjacent area.[5] The principles underlying flap surgery are discussed in more detail in Chapter 1. Numerous adaptations of this principle have been developed in reconstructive surgery.

In sites to which no suitable flap can reach, a free flap of tissue – such as muscle, or muscle and skin – is achieved by detaching the tissue completely and dividing the nutrient artery. The artery and its accompanying vein are then anastomosed to suitable vessels in the recipient site using microvascular techniques.

The latissimus dorsi flap is described in Chapter 2 in relation to breast reconstruction surgery, the rectus abdominis flap in Chapter 12, the gracilis flap in Chapter 23, and the pectoralis flap in Chapters 9 and 10. Reconstructive flap surgery is the province of the plastic surgeon, but many general surgeons are experienced with the technique for the one or two flaps that are useful in their area of interest.

The gastrocnemius flap is useful in lower-limb trauma. Tissue loss over a compound fracture of the tibia is an injury which is slow to heal, and prone to complications. The rotation of a musculocutaneous flap to cover the fracture site has proved very beneficial in this situation. For example, the medial head of gastrocnemius has a neurovascular bundle close to its origin. The muscle can be divided distally at the musculotendinous junction, and swung medially to cover an exposed fracture of the upper tibia. The functional defect is compensated for by the other muscles in the flexor compartment. If a muscle flap is used without overlying skin, a split-skin graft can then be used to cover the muscle.

SOFT TISSUE MALIGNANCY

These malignant tumours are sarcomata which metastasize by the bloodstream, and not via the lymphatics. Treatment of the primary lesion must be adequate, or local recurrence is common, but no benefit is gained by lymph node dissection.

The apparent 'capsule' of these sarcomata is merely a layer of compressed tumour cells and, therefore, excision in the natural plane just outside this capsule inevitably leaves a tumour bed which is contaminated with malignant cells. Surgical excision should therefore include a circumferential margin of normal tissue. When a sarcoma arises within a muscle the excision usually includes the whole muscle, or fascial compartment. Frequently, an initial excision has been undertaken for what was believed to be a benign lump, and a second more radical operation is indicated once there is confirmatory histology of malignancy. Limb amputation can usually be avoided. Radiotherapy may be an alternative to radical surgery in those tumours which are highly radiosensitive. Patients with these relatively rare tumours should have the benefit of referral to centres with a special interest.[6]

Pulmonary metastases are usually the first indication of metastatic spread, and occasionally surgical removal of isolated metastases in liver or lung can still offer the chance of cure. Chemotherapy and radiotherapy may both have a role, in adjuvant and in palliative therapy.

TENDON REPAIR

A tendon is a condensation of fibrous tissue in continuity with a muscle. The origin of a muscle is commonly fleshy from a wide area of bony cortex, but if it arises from a localized area it may be tendinous. The common extensor tendon, arising from the lateral epicondyle of the humerus, is an example of this. The insertion of most muscles is tendinous, as the muscle is commonly only inserted into a localized area of bone. The tendon may be short in proportion to the muscle belly (e.g. the patella tendon) or long, as in the tendons of the finger flexors and extensors.

A tendon may be severed by a laceration, and the long flexor and extensor tendons to the fingers are particularly vulnerable, due to their superficial position. Tendon rupture can also be caused by a blunt force. This may represent excessive force on a normal tendon or a minor strain on a degenerative tendon. A tendon may also disrupt at its attachment to bone or it may avulse the fragment of bony cortex to which it is attached.

If no action is taken after tendon disruption, the muscle tone pulls the tendon ends apart and any healing will be with lengthening, and resultant diminution of function. On occasion the ends can be approximated by extension, or flexion, of the relevant joint, but results are better with a formal repair. The suture material must be of adequate strength to overcome the forces channelled through the tendon. In practice, the tendency for the suture to cut through the fibres of the tendon is more often the limiting factor than the strength of the material used, and sutures should be placed so as to minimize this risk (Fig. 3.7). Catgut loses tensile strength too rapidly, while silk causes excessive tissue reaction. In the past, wire was extensively used but this has been generally super-

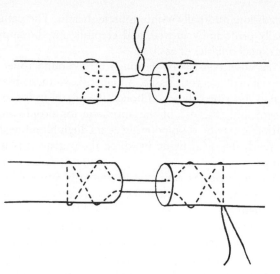

Figure 3.7 *The propensity of a suture to cut through a tendon can be minimized by the suturing techniques illustrated. An additional finer continuous suture can then be inserted circumferentially in the paratendon.*

seded by polypropylene (Prolene). Techniques using strips of fascia as suture material have been tried for the large tendons. If the tendon has severed at its bony attachment, then tendon to bone fixation is required. This can be achieved by drilling a hole through the bone and passing the Prolene (or wire) suture through the hole. Two other methods are shown in Figure 3.8. A spontaneous rupture of a degenerative tendon can seldom be satisfactorily repaired, and the choice lies between acceptance of the disability, attempted repair – with a high chance of failure – or a tendon transfer operation.

Even after a tendon repair, splintage of the joint is then used to reduce tension during healing. For example, an Achilles tendon rupture treated surgically may still require splintage of the ankle in plantar flexion for 6 weeks.

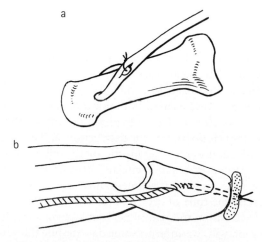

Figure 3.8 *(a) The tendon has been passed through a hole drilled in the bone and sutured to itself. (b) A suture passed through the tendon and out through the terminal phalanx to the skin is tied over a button. After 3–4 weeks the suture and the button are removed.*

EXTENSOR TENDONS IN THE HAND

These heal well, and may be repaired primarily by simple apposition. Some surgeons favour an absorbable suture as it is impractical to bury a knot in these flat tendons. Avulsion of the extensor tendon from the base of the terminal, or less commonly the middle, phalanx of a finger can be successfully treated conservatively by splinting the affected joint in extension for 4–6 weeks.

EXTENSOR POLLICIS LONGUS

The repair of a spontaneous rupture of this tendon is seldom practical. It may be ignored, or a tendon transfer performed (see below). Eric Farquharson had a spontaneous rupture of his extensor pollicis longus a few years before retirement. He was advised to postpone a decision regarding a tendon transfer repair until he had ascertained the severity of the disability. Within 2 weeks he had adapted sufficiently to return to operative surgery – much earlier than would have been possible after a tendon transfer.

FLEXOR TENDON INJURY IN THE HAND

Surgical repair can give disappointing results, even when undertaken by specialist surgeons. Referral is therefore indicated, if at all possible. In Zone 2 the tendons and their synovial sheaths are within the fibrous flexor sheath (Fig. 3.9). In this zone – and also in Zone 4, behind the flexor retinaculum – dense and permanent adhesions commonly form during healing.[7] It is recommended that no repair is attempted when there is an isolated division of a superficial tendon within Zone 2. If both flexor tendons are divided, only the profundus tendon should be repaired and, except in very experienced hands, primary repair is best not attempted. Instead, a secondary repair is undertaken with a tendon graft of palmaris longus, or plantaris. At operation the fibrous flexor sheath is excised except for three intact pulleys which are left *in situ* to prevent bow stringing of the tendon graft. The superficial tendon is excised, and the profundus tendon excised from Zone 2. The tendon graft is then carefully drawn through the pulleys. The two tendon suture lines, to the distal profundus stump and to the proximal tendon in the palm, are thus outside this area which is particularly prone to fibrosis. After finger tendon repair splintage to protect against excess force is required for 6–8 weeks.

INFECTIONS IN THE HANDS AND FEET

Hand infections

Treatment is dominated by the need to prevent stiffness and the subsequent loss of function.[8] The hand – whether injured by infection or trauma – is at high risk of a poor long-term functional outcome if restoration of mobility is prolonged. Correct splintage during the early phase, followed by inten-

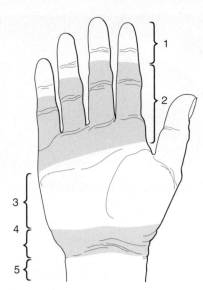

Figure 3.9 *Primary repair of flexor tendons in Zones 1, 3 and 5 is satisfactory, whereas repair in Zones 2 and 4 is often disappointing due to the formation of dense adhesions.*

sive physiotherapy, is essential (Figs 3.10–3.12). Early treatment of an infected hand with an appropriate antibiotic is often successful but, if rapid resolution does not occur, trapped pus must be suspected and released. It is not always immediately apparent in which compartment the pus is trapped as the whole digit or hand will swell. Even the eventual 'pointing' may mislead if the anatomy is not appreciated (Figs 3.13 and 3.14).

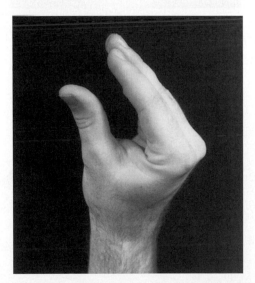

Figure 3.10 *The 'position of immobilization' for the hand. Relevant capsular structures are held at maximum length to prevent joint contractures. The wrist is slightly dorsiflexed, the interphalangeal joints are extended and the metacarpophalangeal joints are flexed. The thumb lies parallel to the fingers.*

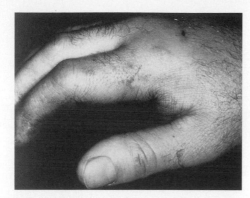

Figure 3.11   *Injured joints seldom lie naturally in either the 'position of immobilization' or the 'position of function'. Injured hips and knees lie flexed, and the injured hand adopts this position (cf. Fig. 3.10). The hand must be elevated to reduce swelling, and splinted in the correct position to prevent secondary contractures.*

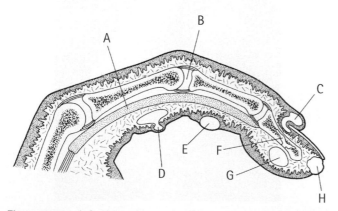

Figure 3.12   *The 'position of function'. A hand fixed in this position is still of functional use. This is not the correct position for immobilization unless loss of joint movement is inevitable.*

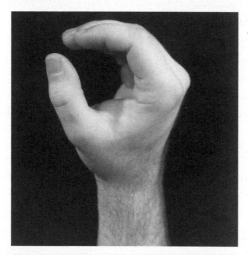

Figure 3.13   *Infections which may affect a digit. A Tendon sheath infection; B Septic arthritis; C Paronychia; D Subcutaneous infection with a subcuticular 'collar stud' extension; E Subcuticular abscess; F Osteomyelitis; G Pulp space infection; H Apical pulp space infection.*

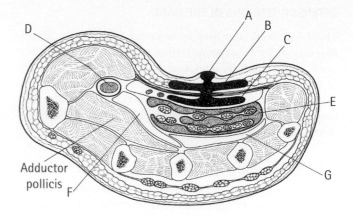

Figure 3.14   *The anatomy of hand infections, shown on transverse section. A Subcuticular palmar abscess; B Subcutaneous palmar abscess; C Subaponeurotic palmar abscess; D Tendon sheath infection (radial bursa); E Tendon sheath infection (ulnar bursa); F Thenar space; G Deep mid palmar space.*

SYNOVIAL SHEATH INFECTIONS

Infection within the synovial sheaths of the flexor tendons (Fig. 3.15) can result in fibrous adhesions within the sheath, or even sloughing of the tendon. The sheath should therefore be explored if pus is suspected, or if complete resolution has not occurred within 48 hours of antibiotic treatment. Surgical exploration is carried out through two skin crease incisions – one placed over the proximal sheath, and the other in the distal skin crease of the finger over the distal sheath. The sheath is drained and then irrigated with saline via a fine catheter which can be left *in situ* for further irrigation over the ensuing 24–48 hours.

OTHER SOFT TISSUE INFECTIONS IN THE HAND

Early diagnosis and antibiotic therapy has reduced the need for surgical intervention, but once pus has formed it should be drained. It should be remembered that deep pus may be difficult to diagnose if it fails to point superficially, and that pus pointing superficially may be associated with a deeper collection which also requires drainage. For example, a *paronychia* may extend under the nail necessitating nail avulsion for adequate drainage, while a *superficial septic blister* may connect with a deeper subcutaneous or pulp space collection. Between the palmar aponeurosis and the flexor tendons is the *superficial middle palmar space*. An infection of this space is usually caused by a penetrating wound of the palm; this presents as a 'collar stud' abscess in the palm (see Fig. 3.14) and should be drained anteriorly. Behind the flexor tendons are the *deep mid palmar space* and the *thenar space*. Infection within these spaces is less common, and initially presents with a generally swollen hand, this often being more noticeable on the dorsum. Drainage is undertaken from the web space, which is also where the pus will eventually point after tracking via the lumbrical canals (Fig. 3.16).

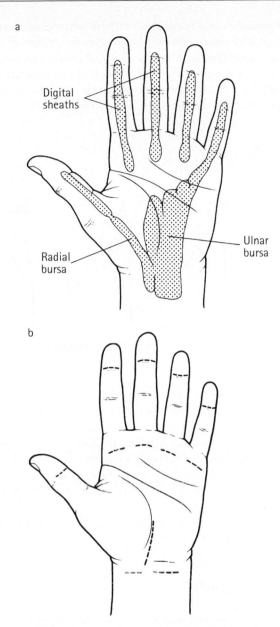

Figure 3.15   *(a) The flexor tendon sheaths. (b) The incisions for drainage of tendon sheath infections.*

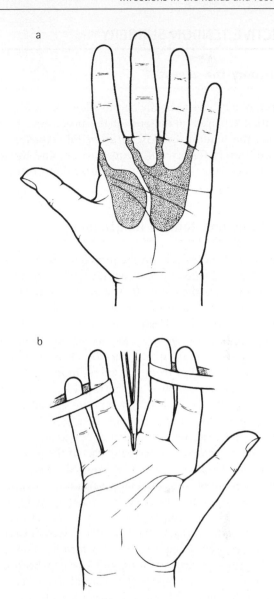

Figure 3.16   *(a) The thenar and deep mid palmar spaces communicate with the web spaces via the lumbrical canals. (b) Drainage is via the web space.*

Foot infections

In contrast to infections in the hand, where the predominant concern is regarding stiffness and loss of function, infections in the feet carry a significant risk of loss of a limb. Penetrating trauma is common in the barefoot farm worker in the developing world. The wound is contaminated by soil and then often neglected until there is established deep infection, and even infected gangrene. Treatment follows the general principles in the management of soft tissue infections. Adequate drainage of pus is essential, combined with removal of dead tissue and contaminants. Systemic antibiotics, and repeated local treatment, are continued until the infection has settled and healing has commenced. Only then should secondary

suture, or reconstruction, be considered. Amputation in the presence of infected gangrene is discussed in Chapter 4. In the developed world most foot infections follow very minor trauma in diabetic patients. Diabetic neuropathy may have rendered the patient oblivious both to the trauma, and to the early stages of infection. Impaired circulation, from both large vessel atheroma and diabetic microangiopathy, reduces the tissue resistance, and the raised blood glucose provides an excellent environment for bacteria. Underlying pus must be considered if prompt resolution on antibiotics does not occur. Associated osteomyelitis of phalanges and metatarsal heads, and septic arthritis may also occur early. Pus can be drained from a web space but often a ray amputation is required, either for a gangrenous toe or when additional bone or joint infection has become established (see also Chapter 4).

ELECTIVE TENDON SURGERY

Tenotomy for access

A tendon may have to be divided to allow access for surgery. It is then repaired at the end of the procedure. Examples include the tendon division to allow full exposure of the popliteal artery for arterial reconstruction, and the tendon division necessary to enable the transposition of the ulnar nerve to the flexor aspect of the elbow.

Tenotomy and tendon lengthening

Here, the techniques rely on the principle that natural healing of a divided tendon occurs with lengthening as the muscle tone distracts the cut ends. Whereas a simple tenotomy may be satisfactory in some circumstances, a formal tendon lengthening procedure is superior when the muscle is functionally important (Fig. 3.17). *Sternomastoid* tenotomy may be used to correct congenital torticollis. Division of the common extensor tendon from the lateral humeral epicondyle may be undertaken for an intractable 'tennis elbow'. *Adductor*, *hamstring* and *Achilles* tendons can all be divided or lengthened to allow correction of a flexion deformity. Unfortunately, the tendon which is felt as the tight band restricting movement is often only part of the problem, and a further soft tissue release may be required. This is seen both in the treatment of congenital talipes equinovarus, and in the *late contractures* after neglected trauma and paralysis which are so often encountered in areas with poor access to medical care. In the latter situation there is often a fixed flexion of the hip and knee with an equinus ankle deformity. The surgeon is aiming for a plantigrade foot, and a weight-bearing limb with possible caliper support. Very careful assessment before surgery is essential. Shortened major vessels and nerves crossing the flexor aspect of the joint may still prevent extension. In addition, the correction of an equinus deformity may be counterproductive if it is compensating for a shortened limb.

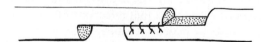

Figure 3.17   *A tendon-lengthening technique suitable for a short Achilles tendon.*

Tendon transfers

Tendon transfers are used to restore active movement where it has been lost as a result of damage to muscles or tendons. The muscle must be strong enough for its new role, with adequate amplitude of motion in a similar direction. It is also essential that it can be spared from its original function.

Extensor indicis fulfils these criteria when used to replace a ruptured *extensor pollicis longus*. Tendon transfers can also be undertaken to correct imbalance from neurological disease. Thorough assessment is essential before embarking on surgery, and any fixed deformity must have been corrected. Tendons may be joined as shown in Figure 3.18.

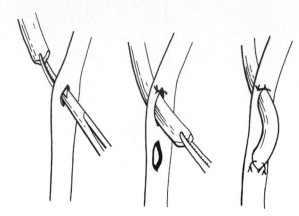

Figure 3.18   *A technique for joining two tendons.*

The *tibialis posterior* tendon may be transferred to correct the drop foot of paralysed peroneal muscles. The distal muscle and proximal tendon are mobilized above and behind the medial malleolus. The tendon insertion into the navicula is divided through a separate incision. The tendon is transferred anteriorly and, through a separate incision over the base of the fifth metatarsal, it is attached to the paralysed peroneus brevis. This is a useful technique for surgeons practising in countries with a high incidence of polio or leprosy.

Tendon grafts

The non-essential tendons of palmaris longus and plantaris can be used as grafts to bridge gaps in essential finger flexor tendons, as discussed above.

Tendon release

Stenosing tenosynovitis prevents free movement of a tendon within its sheath. In *trigger finger or thumb* there is a nodular swelling on the flexor tendon which catches as it is pulled under the proximal end of the fibrous flexor sheath during extension of the digit. Surgical release is indicated if steroid injection fails, and is performed through a short transverse, or longitudinal, incision just distal to the distal transverse palmar skin crease. Extensor pollicis brevis and abductor pollicis longus may be trapped in the first compartment of the extensor retinaculum at the wrist. If steroid injection fails to relieve pain and swelling, surgical release can be undertaken. Care must be taken of the terminal branches of the radial nerve as intractable pain can occur if they are damaged. Sometimes the compartment contains subdivisions of the nerve which must be sought and released.

SURGERY OF LIGAMENTS AND JOINTS

Consideration must always be given to the position of any injured or inflamed joint, as even a healthy immobilized joint stiffens. If a joint requires splintage, it should be immobilized in a position which holds the relevant capsular structures at their maximum length, rendering contractures less likely (see Fig. 3.10). This is often a different position from that which the injured joint assumes naturally (see Fig. 3.11). If long-term loss of movement, and even bony ankylosis, are inevitable it is important that the joint is in the best position for any subsequent use of the damaged limb (Fig. 3.19; see also Fig. 3.12). Ligaments are condensations of fibrous tissue on which the stability of a joint depends. Some – such as the cruciate ligaments of the knee and the ligament to the femoral head – are within the joint, and the latter also carries an important nutrient artery. More often they are outside the joint, and are closely associated with the joint capsule. In traumatic rupture the ligament itself may tear, or it may avulse a fragment of bone from its insertion. Disruption of a ligament should be suspected if there is a haemarthrosis, or if a small fragment of bone is seen on X-ray in the vicinity of a

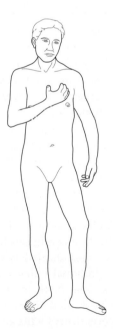

Figure 3.19 *The 'position of function' in the lower limb is with the hip extended, the knee flexed to 10° only, and the ankle dorsiflexed to 90°. Elbows fixed in acute flexion allow patients to feed themselves; extended elbows allow them to attend to toilet needs. When joint destruction is anticipated after an advanced septic arthritis or injury, splintage to obtain a joint position consistent with a functional limb is essential.*

ligamentous insertion. Ligament disruption and instability of a joint is confirmed on stress X-rays, taken under general anaesthesia to overcome the stability being maintained by the surrounding muscles.

Repair of ligaments and joints

Immediate repair using similar techniques to tendon repair may be performed. However, as there is no muscle distraction of the cut ends of a ligament, a plaster cast to prevent any 'opening' of the joint while healing takes place may be sufficient in some circumstances. Unfortunately, some patients present long after the initial injury with unstable joints, and delayed reconstructive repair of ligaments must then be considered. Good results can be obtained in ligament reconstruction for unstable joints and, in particular, cruciate reconstruction with a portion of the patella tendon has proved very successful. However, these are operations for experts in the field, and an occasional surgeon would expect results worse than with conservative management.

Pyogenic arthritis

The management of joint infections forms only a small part of the practice of a specialized orthopaedic surgeon, but in some areas of the world they are common and a major cause of long-term disability.[9] Urgent action is required to save the joint. Differential diagnosis from traumatic haemarthrosis and gouty arthritis may be obvious clinically, but if pus or blood are suspected in a joint then aspiration is essential to establish the diagnosis and facilitate appropriate treatment. A needle is introduced through an area of locally anaesthetized skin. If pus or blood are encountered, a wide-bore needle is required to ensure adequate drainage. There are several routes for aspiration of most joints, and a grossly swollen joint normally poses little difficulty in access with a needle. Anatomical consideration must be given to avoid overlying vessels and nerves. The hip joint however can be more difficult as it is deep, and a joint effusion does not produce obvious swelling. A satisfactory method is to introduce the needle just above the tip of the greater trochanter, and to pass it upwards and medially, in the line of the femoral neck, until the joint is reached.

When all blood or pus has been evacuated the joint is irrigated with normal saline. A septic arthritis requires high doses of antibiotics – preferably given intravenously – and repeat aspirations and irrigation should be performed daily until inflammation has settled. If the pus is thick and cannot be aspirated the joint requires formal exploration for drainage. Consideration should be given to the best position for splintage (see above).

In a young child, if there is as yet no epiphyseal barrier to infection, a septic arthritis may be associated with an osteomyelitis. Failure to recognize and treat the additional pathology may have serious consequences (see Chapter 4).

Elective surgery of joints

Ganglia

These arise most commonly from the wrist and interphalangeal joints. Often, no surgery is indicated, and some will disappear spontaneously as a result of rupture. This can be attempted therapeutically by aspiration of the contents with a wide-bore needle under local anaesthesia, followed by further disruption of the wall of the ganglion by multiple punctures with the same needle. If a ganglion is to be excised, it must be traced down to the joint capsule where, if there is a connection, it should be transected but left open. Adequate anaesthesia, and a bloodless field, are mandatory. Even if the excision is complete recurrences are common.

Surgery within joints

This includes reconstructive ligament surgery, the trimming of meniscal tears, the removal of loose bodies and synovectomies. Many open surgical procedures have been virtually replaced by minimally invasive techniques with the arthroscope. This is not surgery in which a general surgeon should be involved without additional orthopaedic training.

Arthrodesis and excision arthroplasty

Ankylosis, or spontaneous bony union, may develop across a joint which has been severely injured by trauma or infection. Ankylosis may give a good functional result if fusion occurs in the position of function. *Arthrodesis,* in which a joint is surgically obliterated, inducing bony union, is based on the same principle. A severely diseased, painful joint may be excised as an *excision arthroplasty,* in which the aim is to obtain a fibrous rather than a bony union. These procedures are discussed briefly in Chapter 4 as they may be of value to the isolated generalist.

Joint replacement

This is now a standard technique for hip and knee joints badly damaged by degenerative and other pathologies. Other joint replacements are performed less frequently. Orthopaedic operative texts cover this enlarging field.[1]

NERVE INJURIES

A major peripheral nerve is made up of a large number of fibres – for example, there may be as many as 50 000 in the median nerve in the forearm. Each fibre consists of an *axon* surrounded by its Schwann cell sheath. The axon is the process of a nerve cell, the main body of which lies within a ganglion or within the central nervous system. The peripheral nerves carry, to a varying degree, fibres concerned with motor, sensory and autonomic functions. Groups of nerve fibres are aggregated into bundles, or fascicles, which are surrounded by a thin layer of connective tissue. There is a strong and distinct layer of connective tissue, the *epineurium,* which surrounds the fascicles which make up a nerve trunk (Fig. 3.20). The connective tissues of a peripheral nerve are surprisingly strong so that it is not uncommon to find the major nerves as the only intact structures in a severely injured limb. The peripheral nerves are supplied by many small arteries which communicate freely within the nerve. It is possible, therefore, to mobilize quite long lengths of nerve without damaging the blood supply.

Nerve injuries may be divided into three degrees of severity:

- In *neurapraxia* the axons are not disrupted, but nerve conductivity is temporarily lost. Recovery occurs spontaneously within hours or days of the injury.
- In *axonotmesis* the axon is disrupted but the supportive connective tissues of the nerve remain in continuity. The axon has to regrow along the intact sheath, and there is no functional recovery until it reaches the end organ. The growth rate is around 1 mm a day.
- In *neurotmesis* the nerve is completely divided. No recovery occurs unless surgical repair is undertaken as the ends retract, the axonal outgrowths fail to find an axonal sheath, and scar tissue forms.

Surgical repair is an attempt to convert a neurotmesis into a situation similar to an axonotmesis, but the result is never as good as many axons still fail to grow down a sheath. In addition, sensory regrowth towards a motor endplate, and vice versa, is of no functional benefit.

Nerve repair

A loss of nerve function in a *closed injury* is usually either a neurapraxia or an axonotmesis, and the initial management can be conservative. If recovery does not occur within a few days, the injury is probably an axonotmesis, and there will be a long wait as the axons regrow. However, the possibility that the nerve is divided should be considered, even in a blunt injury. If doubt continues, surgical exploration should be considered. The integrity of a nerve in the vicinity of any *open injury* should be checked and a loss of nerve function, distal to a wound, always suggests a divided nerve. When the wound is explored the severed nerve ends are identified and a decision is then made as to whether to proceed with a primary nerve repair. A bloodless field with a tourniquet (see Chapter 1) provides the best conditions for nerve repair, but a tourniquet may be contraindicated in an extensively damaged limb in which additional ischaemic insult should be avoided. Primary repair may be the best option, but only in clean, incised wounds of limited extent where surgeons have the necessary experience, instruments and time at their disposal. Most general surgeons will wish therefore to enlist the help of an orthopaedic or plastic surgical colleague with special expertise and, if not available, to opt for secondary repair. An isolated general surgeon may have limited experience, combined with a lack of fine equipment but, if referral is impractical, will have to proceed with either primary or secondary repair.

If repair is to be delayed, the nerve ends should be prevented from retraction. If the ends reach with ease they can be apposed with two or three inert sutures and await a more formal repair. Correct orientation at this stage may be easier than subsequently, and should be attempted and documented. If the severed ends cannot be apposed, they should be fixed to surrounding tissue to prevent further retraction. Attempts have been made to isolate the nerve ends with silastic to prevent the formation of adhesions which can make the secondary repair more difficult.

Nerve repair, if at all possible, should be performed with the help of some form of magnification, either loupes or operating microscope, to prevent further damage to the nerve by clumsy dissection, and to ensure accurate orientation of the nerve and placement of sutures. Sutures should be of a relatively inert material, such as nylon or Prolene and very fine (8/0 or finer). Silk and absorbable sutures provoke an inflammatory response and should not be used.

PRIMARY REPAIR

For primary suture only minimal trimming of the nerve ends is required. It is carried out with a sharp razor blade with the nerve resting on a firm surface. Correct orientation of the nerve is facilitated by noting the arrangement of the fasicular bundles within the nerve (Fig. 3.20) and the presence of any blood vessels on the surface. The repair is then by epineural suture. The first two sutures may be held as stay sutures to steady and rotate the nerve (Fig. 3.21). Excessive suturing should be avoided. For example, six to eight sutures are sufficient for the median nerve, and two to three for a digital nerve.

SECONDARY REPAIR

At a secondary repair, it is safer first to identify the nerve, both proximal and distal to the scar tissue, and only then to dissect the injured site. If the ends have been aligned at the original exploration, guide sutures placed before excising the bridge of neuroma and scar tissue will facilitate maintaining correct alignment, and in addition these sutures can be used to draw the ends together. The neuroma must be excised, and both ends must be cut back to undamaged nerve beyond the scar tissue (Fig. 3.21b). This is recognized when the nerve bundles pout separately from the cut surface and may

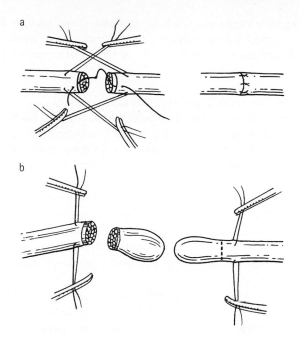

Figure 3.21 *Nerve repair is by epineural sutures, and correct orientation of nerve bundles is essential. (a) The initial guide sutures hold the orientation and prevent inadvertent subsequent rotation of one end. They can also be used to rotate both ends of the nerve together so that the posterior sutures can be inserted. (b) In secondary repair the neuroma must first be excised.*

require up to 1 cm of excision. Orientation, alignment and suturing are carried out as for a primary repair. The epineurium is thicker than in a primary repair, and suturing is easier. Mobilization of the ends will be required to achieve apposition without tension, but if the defect is greater than 2–3 cm direct suture is not possible without shortening the course of the nerve by transposition, or by flexion of a joint. Alternatively, a nerve which can be spared – such as the sural or saphenous – is used as a graft to bridge the gap. Techniques for nerve grafting, and for the repair of partially severed nerves, are for specialists with expertise in the field, and will give disappointing results when used by generalists.

After any nerve repair, immobilization is indicated for 3 weeks to protect the suture line from tension. Flexion of a joint may be required to prevent initial tension on a shortened nerve, but marked flexion should be avoided by the use of nerve grafts. Subsequent extension of the joint must be a controlled slow increase over several weeks to prevent disruption of the repair. While awaiting axonal regrowth – whether after axonotmesis or nerve repair – the patient must be advised of the need to protect anaesthetic skin from accidental injury. The patient must also be shown how to retain, by passive movement, the mobility of joints for which the muscles are paralysed. It may be necessary to provide some form of splintage to maintain function, and prevent contractures, during the recovery period.

Good functional recovery is dependent not only on the technical success of the repair but also on the distance the

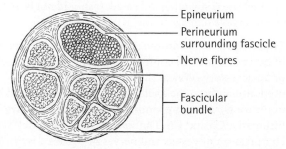

Figure 3.20 *Diagrammatic cross-section of a peripheral nerve.*

Epineurium
Perineurium surrounding fascicle
Nerve fibres
Fascicular bundle

axons have to grow to reach the end plates, and whether the nerve is mixed, or mainly either sensory or motor. The technical challenges, and the functional results of repair, of different nerves therefore vary.

- Facial nerve: this nerve may be damaged, or intentionally sacrificed for oncological reasons, during parotid surgery. Direct apposition is seldom possible, but good results can be achieved with nerve grafts. If this is unsuccessful, management can be with dynamic muscle transfer. Neurapraxia after a superficial parotidectomy is not uncommon, but if the surgeon is confident that all branches of the nerve were identified and preserved, there can be reasonable confidence that function will recover, commonly within a day or two if there has been no axonal disruption (see also Chapters 9 and 10).
- Recurrent laryngeal nerve: this nerve may be injured in thyroid surgery (see also Chapter 9). Neurapraxia will recover but a severed nerve causes permanent cord paralysis, with a resultant deepening, and reduced force to the voice. A bilateral injury results in both cords drifting medially. A tracheotomy may have to be performed to maintain the airway. Any form of nerve reconstruction is very difficult.
- Brachial plexus: injury to the brachial plexus is most often seen after motor cycle accidents and is caused by a severe traction force which may also have damaged the proximal subclavian artery. The injury is often of mixed severity, with some portions of the brachial plexus suffering only neurapraxia, whilst other portions have axonal disruption or are completely severed. The prognosis is therefore very varied. Surgical repair of a severed nerve is seldom practical as the commonest site of damage is an avulsion of the roots from the spinal cord. Some surgeons advocate early exploration, but as access is difficult and often little can be achieved in the way of a repair, this is unlikely to appeal to the generalist who, with limited experience of the problem, is in danger of causing more harm than good.
- Radial nerve: this nerve is vulnerable to damage from the bone ends in a humeral shaft fracture. Repair of the nerve may produce good results as it is mainly a motor nerve. The distance to the end plates, however, delays recovery for a year or more and a splint for wrist drop is required. If the nerve repair is unsuccessful the wrist drop can be treated by tendon transfer.
- Median nerve: this nerve is most often divided in a laceration of the wrist or forearm. The radial or ulnar artery may also have been divided, and additional tendon damage is also common. At the wrist the median nerve is flattened and easily mistaken for a tendon. It is therefore important that exploration, as well as repair, is undertaken under optimum conditions; this requires a bloodless field with a tourniquet. Postoperative flexion of the elbow reduces tension on a median nerve repair at the wrist, and is preferable to palmar flexion of the wrist. If the wrist is held in acute flexion during healing, the adherence of the nerve at the site of injury to adjacent tissues can cause traction problems when the wrist is mobilized.
- Ulnar nerve: this nerve may be divided at the wrist, where the challenges in diagnosis and successful repair are similar to those encountered in median nerve damage. If the ulnar nerve is severed at the elbow, it is advisable to bring the divided ends anteriorly for a tension free-repair. Anterior translocation of an intact ulnar nerve is described below.
- Sciatic nerve: repair of this nerve, although technically straightforward, gives poor functional results.
- Autonomic nerve repair is not a surgical option, as these are non-myelinated nerve fibres; effective axonal regrowth is not possible in the absence of axonal sheaths, even if the ends are approximated. Pelvic surgery endangers both the sympathetic and parasympathetic nerves to the bladder and sexual organs and great care must be taken to cause the minimum of damage.

Nerve infections

In the early stages of a *herpes zoster* infection (shingles) the dermatome pain precedes the skin rash and can cause major diagnostic confusion. Renal colic or cholecystitis are frequently suspected at this stage. *Poliomyelitis* presents to the surgeon with limb paralysis and deformity. The nerve infections in *leprosy* also lead to paralysis and deformity, but in addition the loss of sensation results in distal soft tissue damage. The surgical implications of polio and leprosy are substantial but the surgery is not on the nerves themselves.

ELECTIVE SURGERY OF NERVES

Nerve release

This is indicated if a nerve is suffering repeated trauma or constriction resulting in an 'entrapment' neuropathy. The neuropathy may take the form of pain, altered sensation or muscle weakness and wasting. Conservative measures include rest and/or local steroid injection to reduce local oedema, but surgical release is still often indicated. It should not be delayed until irreversible damage to the nerve has occurred.

- **Thoracic outlet syndrome** presents with a mixed pattern of nerve and arterial compression. A prominent 1st rib, or an accessory cervical rib, causes trauma predominantly to the axillary artery and the C8 and T1 nerve roots, whereas prominent scalene bands may traumatise C5 and C6. The surgery to release the compression of vessels and nerves in this area is described in Chapter 6.

- **Intercostal nerves** may be trapped as they emerge from under the costal margin, but more commonly the entrapment occurs as they enter the rectus sheath. Surgical release is seldom indicated as symptoms usually settle with steroid injections, but they can present diagnostic problems.
- **Carpal tunnel release** is indicated when conservative management has failed to relieve median nerve compression. The operation is performed under regional or general anaesthetic with a tourniquet. The incision (Fig. 3.22) is deepened through the palmar fascia to expose the flexor retinaculum. The flexor retinaculum must be divided completely to release the median nerve and the proximal edge sought under the skin, if the skin incision stops short of the wrist crease. An incision to the ulnar side of the nerve is safer than directly over it. Only the skin is sutured. The operation may be performed as a minimal access technique through a small proximal incision, and this has advantages in avoidance of a potentially troublesome scar. A surgeon inexperienced in the operation would, however, be at greater risk of performing an inadequate release or damaging the nerve.
- **Ulnar nerve transposition** to the front of the elbow shortens the course of the nerve, and reduces tension. Through an incision over the medial epicondyle, the common flexor tendon is divided, the ulnar nerve is transposed anteriorly, and the tendon repaired. To ensure sound healing of the tendon, the elbow should be immobilized for 3 weeks.
- The **lateral cutaneous nerve of the thigh** may be trapped under the inguinal ligament, and symptoms usually settle with steroid injections.

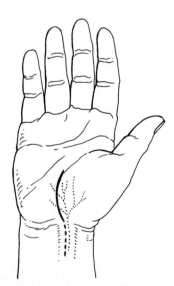

Figure 3.22   *The incision for carpal tunnel decompression is placed slightly towards the ulnar side of the midline to avoid palmar cutaneous branches of the median nerve. The skin incision can stop short of the wrist crease.*

Nerve division

Intentional surgical division of nerves is now restricted to vagotomies and sympathectomies. Historically, *phrenic nerve*-crushing techniques were used to cause an axonotemesis. The diaphragm was paralysed, and 'rest' of the tuberculous lung was believed to encourage healing. As the axons regrew the function recovered.

- **Truncal**, **selective** and **highly selective vagotomies** are discussed in the section on the upper gastrointestinal tract (see Chapters 16 and 17).
- **Cervical sympathectomy** is the somewhat misleading misnomer for the operation performed to obliterate the sympathetic innervation to the upper limb. (The inferior cervical ganglion, which may be fused to the first thoracic ganglion as the composite *stellate ganglion*, is in fact carefully preserved to prevent a *Horner's syndrome*.) The operation has a declining role in the management of vasospastic disorders, but has proved valuable in the treatment of hyperhidrosis. The upper thoracic sympathetic chain lies on the necks of the ribs (Fig. 3.23), and the outflow to the upper limb is from the 2nd to the 5th thoracic ganglia. One traditional surgical approach was through a limited lateral thoracotomy in the axilla, but this operation is now almost exclusively performed by a transthoracic endoscopic approach (this is described in Chapter 7). The alternative anterior cervical approach, which is also now rarely performed, is described in Chapter 9. Whichever approach is employed, the operation on the sympathetic chain is similar. A T2 sympathectomy consists of division of the sympathetic chain below the neck of the 2nd rib, and destruction of the 2nd thoracic ganglion. This is the standard operation for palmar hyperhidrosis. If repeat surgery is indicated after initial failure of this operation a T3 sympathectomy is performed, and the lower half of the stellate ganglion on the neck of the first rib may also be sacrificed. Any damage to the upper portion of this

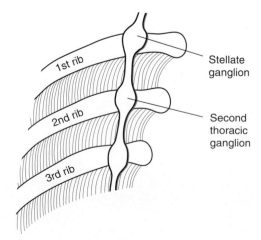

Figure 3.23   *The sympathetic chain lies on the neck of the ribs.*

ganglion will result in a Horner's syndrome. Control of axillary hyperhidrosis requires a T2/T3 sympathectomy, whilst extension to a T4 sympathectomy may be indicated if repeat surgery is required. However, more extensive destruction of sympathetic innervation often results in troublesome compensatory sweating.[10]

- **Lumbar sympathectomy** has a limited role in increasing skin perfusion in an ischaemic lower limb. It is now most often achieved with a chemical ablation of the sympathetic chain, by a paravertebral injection under radiological control. The alternative surgical sympathectomy is performed through a retroperitoneal approach via an oblique loin incision. The sympathetic chain is found lying in the groove between the vertebral bodies and the psoas muscle. On the right it is behind the inferior vena cava (Fig. 3.24), and on the left it is beside the left margin of the aorta. The 1st lumbar

ganglion is high up under the crus of the diaphragm, and the 4th may be obscured by the common iliac vessels. Removal of the 2nd and 3rd ganglia obliterates the sympathetic innervation distal to the mid thigh and is normally sufficient. If the 1st lumbar ganglion is destroyed bilaterally, ejaculatory failure will be inevitable.

- **Splanchnectomy:** bilateral thoracoscopic splanchnectomy has been employed for relief of pain in chronic pancreatitis. The sympathetic chains are exposed from the level of T5–T12 ganglia, and their splanchnic branches divided.[11]

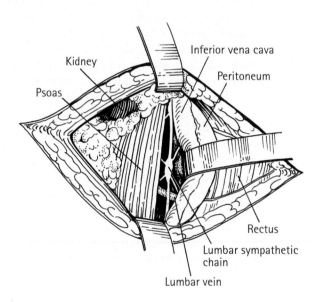

Figure 3.24   *The lumbar sympathetic trunk lies in the groove between the psoas muscle and the vertebral bodies. On the right, the inferior vena cava may overlap it and must be gently retracted.*

REFERENCES

1. *Campbell's Operative Orthopaedics*, 10th edn. T Canale. St. Louis: Elsevier Mosby, 2003.
2. *Surgery of Modern Warfare*. Hamilton Bailey. Edinburgh: Livingstone, 1941.
3. Tiwari A, Haq AI, Myint F, *et al*. Acute compartment syndromes. Review. *Br J Surg* 2002; **89**: 397–412.
4. Haycraft JB. On the treatment of acute emphysematous gangrene during the present war: experience in a clearing hospital. *Lancet* 1915; **1**; 592–5.
5. *An Atlas of Flaps in Limb Reconstruction*. AC Masquelek. Philadelphia: AG Dunnitz, 1995.
6. Brennan MF. Management of soft tissue sarcoma. Leading article. *Br J Surg* 1996; **83**: 577–9.
7. *Green's Operative Hand Surgery*. DP Green, R Hotchkiss, R Lampert (eds). Edinburgh: Churchill Livingstone, 1998.
8. *Hand Therapy*. L Cheshire, M Slater (eds). Oxford: Elsevier Butterworth Heinemann, 2000.
9. *Primary Surgery*, Volume 1. M King. Oxford University Press, 1990.
10. Andrews BT, Rennie JA. Predicting changes in the distribution of sweating following thoracoscopic sympathectomy. *Br J Surg* 1997; **84**: 1702–4.
11. Buscher HCJL, Jansen JJMB, van Goor H. Bilateral thoracoscopic splanchnicectomy in patients with chronic pancreatitis. *Scand J Gastroenterol* 1999; **34** (Suppl. 230): 29–34.

SURGERY OF BONE AND AMPUTATIONS

4

Although skeletal surgery is perceived to be almost exclusively within the province of the orthopaedic surgeon, all surgeons must have an understanding of the principles of surgery on bone. Rib resection, and division of the sternum or clavicle, may be required for access to intrathoracic structures, and access through bone is required for surgery to the brain and spinal cord. A general surgical operation may include the excision of bone en bloc with the main specimen, ranging from the central portion of the hyoid bone with a thyroglossal sinus, to part of the sacrum with an advanced intra-pelvic malignancy.

Trauma to bone – and the resulting fractures – do not occur in isolation, and general and orthopaedic surgeons, caring jointly for a patient with multiple injuries, must understand the challenges in the other specialty. Vascular and orthopaedic surgeons may have to work in parallel to save a limb with an unstable compound fracture and a severed major artery (see Chapter 5). Unstable pelvic ring fractures with massive pelvic haemorrhage, and abdominal organ trauma, require close interdisciplinary cooperation. Many cranial, sternal and rib fractures are of little significance in themselves, and healing will occur without treatment, but they are indicators of major impact and signify the possibility of injury to underlying organs. Conversely, a surgeon caring for a patient with severe intra-abdominal, chest or head injuries must understand the priorities – and principles – of the management of the associated orthopaedic trauma.

Amputations in the developed world are most commonly performed for peripheral arterial occlusive disease. These amputations are routinely undertaken by general or vascular surgeons, whereas the amputations for trauma are the province of the orthopaedic surgeon.

For these reasons – and as many isolated general surgeons may feel the need to offer a limited orthopaedic service – some basic orthopaedic techniques, the principles of stabilization of fractures, and the treatment of osteomyelitis are discussed. A true surgical generalist who has the necessary facilities and resources to offer a more comprehensive orthopaedic service however will find this chapter lacking in detail, and further orthopaedic training and reading will be essential.[1,2]

INFECTION IN BONE

Most elective orthopaedic surgery is 'clean' surgery, in as much as the bone is approached through prepared skin, and the risk of contamination from respiratory, urinary or gut organisms is minimal. If infection is introduced into bone the consequences can be disastrous, especially if foreign material (e.g. an internal fixation device or a prosthesis) is to be left *in situ*. Meticulous aseptic technique is mandatory and, for joint replacement work, a dedicated theatre and additional methods to maintain extra clean air are needed if infective complications are to be avoided. Elective surgery should be postponed if the patient has any septic focus. The surgery is routinely covered with prophylactic antibiotics (see Appendix II), but general methods of preventing the conditions predisposing to infection, as discussed in Chapter 1, are equally important. Surgical trauma can be minimized by gentle tissue handling and haematoma formation can be reduced by meticulous haemostasis, with postoperative vacuum drainage when appropriate.

A *compound fracture* is already contaminated, and early wound toilet is mandatory to prevent infection becoming established. Risk of infection in compound fractures varies. The fracture may be compound merely because the fractured sharp end of a superficial bone has punctured the skin from within. Alternatively, there may be extensive soft tissue damage from a direct blow from without, which has also carried soil and clothing into the shattered bone and damaged soft tissues. The management of the associated soft tissue and vascular damage is discussed in Chapters 3 and 5.

Osteomyelitis

ACUTE OSTEOMYELITIS

This condition requires urgent treatment with antibiotics, which are most effective when administered intravenously to guarantee high blood levels. The commonest organism is *Staphylococcus aureus*, and an appropriate antibiotic for this organism is chosen, while results of blood cultures are awaited. *Salmonella* infections are common in patients who have sickle cell disease. If there is not a dramatic improvement within 24 hours, trapped pus must be suspected and drained. With late presentation pus may already have formed, and delaying surgical drainage further for a trial of antibiotics is contraindicated. In the developed world osteomyelitis is no longer common; when it does occur it usually presents early, settles on antibiotic therapy, and surgical drainage is seldom required.

The increased pressure from the inflammatory swelling and trapped pus, compromises bone perfusion. In addition, subperiosteal pus strips the periosteum with the nutrient arteries off the underlying bony cortex. Thus, untreated osteomyelitis rapidly progresses to ischaemic necrosis of bone. A state of chronic osteomyelitis is then established which can last a lifetime. In the child, damage to the adjacent growth plate may cause long-term sequelae and, in the very young, metaphyseal osteomyelitis may spread into a neighbouring joint with resultant septic arthritis.

Surgical drainage consists of an incision down to bone at the level of maximum tenderness and swelling. Any subperiosteal abscess is evacuated, and several drill holes are then made through the cortex of the metaphysis to allow the release of an intra-osseous abscess. The skin incision may be closed over a vacuum drain, but the wound should remain visible for inspection. A plaster cast should be applied if there is any danger of a pathological fracture developing, but a window must be cut for wound inspection.

CHRONIC OSTEOMYELITIS

This condition is characterized by chronic bony sepsis associated with necrotic bone. The dead bone forms a 'foreign body', and any organisms which persist within it are safe from high blood levels of antibiotics. Eradication of infection, and finally healing, is only possible after the removal of any sequestra of dead bone. At operation, abscess cavities within the bone are deroofed, and any sequestra – which are recognized by their white appearance – are lifted out. This is usually easy if all overhanging bone has been removed, and sequestra are lying free within the pus. Involucrum (new bone) laid down around a sequestrum may make the surgery more difficult. All the dead bone must be removed and, if encased within involucrum, much of this healthy new bone may have to be sacrificed. However, if the need for major bony reconstruction is to be avoided, the retention of some involucrum may be essential to maintain the integrity of the

bone. The dead space can then be filled with viable soft tissue such as a muscle flap (see Chapter 3).

SURGERY OF BONE: BASIC SURGICAL TECHNIQUE

Most surgery on soft tissue consists of dissection, following an anatomical plane, and the approximation of tissues with sutures. The skills required for surgery on bone are very different.[2] Bone cutters will cut a thin bone, and small pieces of bone can be removed with bone nibblers. Larger bones may be cut with a classical hand saw, while the soft tissues are retracted so that they are not damaged. Retraction is difficult in some circumstances. A Gigli saw is useful where access is difficult (Fig. 4.1), and a combination of techniques may solve a difficult problem. Hand-held electric saws with an oscillating circular blade have overcome many of the problems, both of access and of potential soft tissue injury. Bone may also be cut using an osteotome and hammer. Drill holes in bone can be made by a hand-held brace and bit but, now more commonly, by an electric drill. Drills have many further uses in the surgery of bone. They are used to introduce Kirschner wires and guide wires, and the pins for skeletal traction. They may be used to drill a hole through the bone

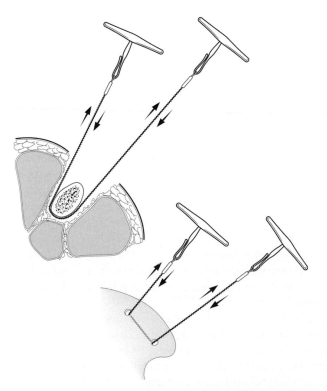

Figure 4.1 *Access to bone with a classical saw may be obstructed by soft tissue. A Gigli saw overcomes this problem. It can also be used to divide a flat bone (e.g. ilium or cranium) between two drill holes. Modern electric circular saws are now preferred in most situations.*

for a screw, or to make a shallow hole which can be gripped by the tongs used for skull traction. A hole may also be required for a ligature for soft tissue re-attachment, or for a wire to fix two pieces of bone.

Bone cannot be sutured directly, and alternative methods of attaching soft tissue to bone have been devised (see Chapter 3). If bone-to-bone apposition requires stabilization, this may be achieved by placing a screw (Fig. 4.2a), an intramedullary rod (see Fig. 4.10) or a Kirschner wire (see Fig. 4.5) from one piece of bone into the other. This may require open apposition of bone ends or, in some techniques, the apposition can be achieved by a closed method, and the wire or pin inserted percutaneously at a distance from the fracture site. Bone can also be wired together around pins inserted into the bone (see Fig. 4.6), or a plate may be laid over the fracture, and the plate fixed to both segments with screws (Fig. 4.2b). A bone staple is another method of fixation (Fig. 4.3a). An alternative to fixation within the tissues is a rigid external 'fixator' outside the limb, to which pins are fixed which have been drilled into the bony fragments (see Fig. 4.12).

BONE HEALING IN FRACTURES AND IN ELECTIVE ORTHOPAEDIC SURGERY

Bone ends in apposition normally heal. Initially there is a haematoma between the ends, and fibroblasts and capillary

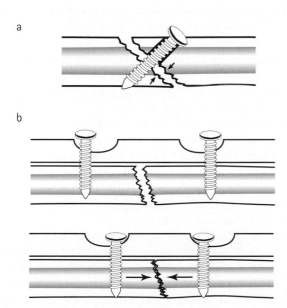

Figure 4.2 *(a) Screw fixation across a fracture. The screw should cross the fracture at right-angles. 'Overdrilling' of the proximal cortex results in compression of the fracture as the thread 'bites' in the distal cortex. (b) Internal fixation of a fracture with a plate must hold the bone ends in apposition. Additional compression of the fracture can be achieved by a variety of techniques. The simplest is a plate with obliquely bevelled oval screw holes. As the sloping shoulder of the screw is tightened against the plate the small lateral movement compresses the fracture.*

loops grow into the haematoma. As the first bone is laid down the *callus* between the bone ends becomes visible on X-ray. Organization within the callus results in increasing strength. Finally, remodelling of the bone occurs which compensates for minor mal-alignment of the fracture. This process occurs spontaneously after most fractures, and many heal satisfactorily without any intervention. Skull, rib, minor vertebral, pubic, clavicular, humeral, metacarpal and digital fractures are all examples. Some form of splintage may reduce pain, but is not essential for healing.

MAL-UNION

If a grossly displaced fracture is allowed to heal without reduction into a satisfactory alignment, the fracture is described as 'mal-united'. Compensatory remodelling will be insufficient to restore normal anatomy. The deformity may be from overlap of bone ends and subsequent limb shortening, from angulation, or from rotation at the fracture site. Even after an initial satisfactory reduction, significant mal-alignment recurs if the forces across the fracture displace the alignment of the bone ends. In these situations stabilization of the fracture site is essential for satisfactory healing. In some instances traction is suitable, whilst in other fractures either external or internal fixation of the fracture may be more appropriate.

Fractures into a joint form a subgroup in which even minor degrees of malalignment are unacceptable. Accurate apposition of articular surfaces is essential to avoid post-traumatic arthritic changes in the joint.

NON-UNION

A non-united fracture is one in which no rigid bony bridge has formed between the bone ends. Instead, there is a bridge of fibrous tissue. A few fractures are notorious for problems with non-union. The distal tibia, the scaphoid and the femoral neck are probably the three most common, and in the latter two cases the underlying problem is, at least in part, a poor blood supply to one fragment of bone. Rigid immobilization of the fracture site improves the chances of satisfactory healing.

Fracture immobilization

EXTERNAL SUPPORT

If a fracture requires immobilization, the simplest method is an *external plaster of Paris splint*, after reduction of the fracture if necessary.[3] In order to immobilize the fracture of the shaft of a long bone, the plaster must extend to include the joint both proximal and distal to the fracture. However, fractures in the vicinity of a joint can normally be satisfactorily immobilized by a cast which includes that joint, but which stops short of the second joint. For example, a fracture of the tibial shaft requires a plaster of Paris splint which

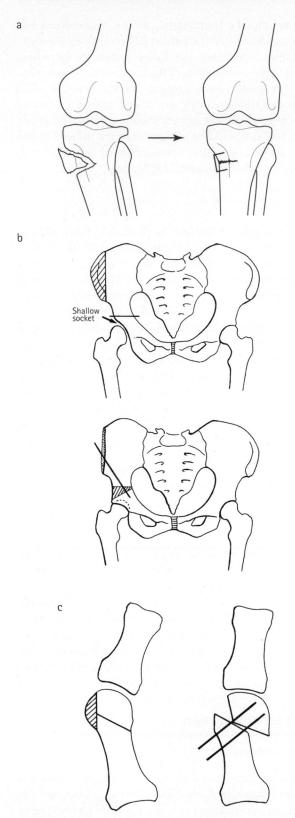

a

b

Shallow socket

c

Figure 4.3 *Osteotomy. (a) Osteotomy of the proximal tibia to correct a varus deformity. A wedge of bone has been excised and the new position held with a bone staple. (b) An innominate osteotomy which alters the angle of the shallow acetabulum of a congenital dislocated hip. The wedge opening is packed with cancellous bone chips. (c) Wilson's osteotomy for hallux valgus.*

includes the knee and ankle, whereas a malleolar fracture only needs a below-knee cast, and a tibial platform fracture requires a plaster cylinder extending from the upper thigh to above the ankle. The disadvantages of an external rigid cast are immediately apparent. One or two joints are to be held immobilized for 6–12 weeks, with resultant stiffness (see Chapter 3) and the plaster may be very heavy and make nursing difficult. (This is a particular problem when a hip spica is applied for a fractured femur.) The injured limb is hidden from view, and if there is an associated soft tissue injury which needs attention, windows have to be cut in the plaster. In addition, an external plaster cannot hold accurate bone apposition, as is ideal for an intra-articular fracture.

OPEN FIXATION

Open fixation of a fracture overcomes many of these problems.[4] Fracture apposition, which is so important in an intra-articular fracture, can be more accurate. The healing phase is generally more efficient and precise, without the need to lay down a large mass of callus followed by remodelling. The fractured bone is stabilized but the joints are kept mobile, and soft tissue wounds are more accessible. There is, however, the disadvantage of a skin wound. Healing of this wound, which is often through tissues that are already traumatised, may be troublesome and there is the possibility of introducing infection. Compound fractures may be grossly contaminated, and the introduction of an internal fixation device in this situation can increase the danger of osteomyelitis. The cosmetic implications of the scar may be distressing to some patients. The later removal of the plate or screw may be indicated, and this will require a second operation. (If a plate is left *in situ* the natural stress lines within the bone are distorted, and it is at increased risk of further fracture, usually at the ends of the plate.) In addition, a bone is at increased risk of a fracture for a period after the plate is removed. Internal fixation also has the potential for increasing the chance of non-union by holding the bone ends apart. Most plates and screws are now designed so that they compress the fracture to reduce this problem (see Fig. 4.2a and b).

If a pathological fracture occurs through a bony metastasis healing will not occur spontaneously. Local radiotherapy may allow the fracture to heal and is often all that is required in, for example, a fracture of the pubic ramus or vertebral body. If, however, the fracture itself requires prolonged immobilization or traction, open fixation – in addition to radiotherapy – will improve the quality of the patient's remaining life.

Elective surgery on bone

Principles of bone healing are used by orthopaedic surgeons in some simple elective procedures:

- Osteotomy. A bone may be cut, and realigned, to correct a deformity. Three variants are shown in Figure 4.3.
- Arthrodesis. If the articular cartilage of a joint is destroyed by inflammation, spontaneous bony union (*ankylosis*) may occur. This can produce a rigid, but stable and pain-free, joint. It is therefore most important that the joint is immobilized in the optimum position for function (see Chapter 3). A similar situation can be achieved surgically by arthrodesis. The articular cartilage and underlying cortical bone are excised, and the two denuded bone ends are then fixed in apposition (see Fig. 4.14). The addition of a bone graft across the joint is also sometimes employed.
- Excision arthroplasty. If fractured bone ends are not in apposition, a non-union or loose fibrous union may result. This principle is used in *excision arthroplasty*. It gives good results in non-weight-bearing joints such as an interphalangeal joint, where it can be useful for a claw toe deformity (Fig. 4.4). Despite the fact that the hip is a major weight-bearing joint an excision arthroplasty (Girdlestone's operation) is a valuable operation for a severely damaged hip, if a joint replacement is not possible (see Fig. 4.11).
- Joint replacements. Artificial joint replacements (*arthroplasties*) are now possible for many damaged joints. The fixation of the prosthesis to the bone, to maintain a long-term rigid bond, was one of the most difficult early challenges for this surgery. This specialist orthopaedic surgery cannot be covered in a general surgical operative text.
- Bone grafting. This may be performed with either cancellous or cortical bone. Bone grafts do not survive, but act as a trellis for the formation of new bone. Bone allografts, if available, are as satisfactory as the patient's own bone; both are absorbed and replaced, and therefore immunological rejection is not an issue. Small grafts are more rapidly replaced than large, and the least possible amount of bone should be used. Cancellous bone is more easily vascularized, and offers less volume of bone to be re-absorbed. It is therefore preferred unless there is an overriding mechanical requirement which demands the denser, stronger cortical bone. A cortical bone graft can be used as a 'strut', or as a stabilizing 'pin' or 'plate'.

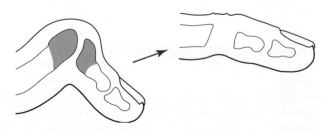

Figure 4.4 *Excision athroplasty is a satisfactory operation for a painful non-weight-bearing joint.*

The fibula, or a portion of rib, make an ideal strut or pin, and a rectangle of cortical bone can be cut from the tibia and used as an on-lay plate. A cortical strut of bone can be used in reconstructive surgery; for example, to bridge a mandibular defect after a radical excision for cancer of the floor of the mouth. The iliac crest is the favoured site for harvesting the more useful cancellous bone. Bone grafting techniques are of value in arthrodesis of some joints, and may also be used across a fracture which has formed an unstable fibrous union. They are, however, used less frequently with the development of more sophisticated internal fixation devices.

A general surgeon, whose practice also includes orthopaedics, may wish to undertake some of the simpler elective orthopaedic procedures. Unfortunately, space does not permit their inclusion in a general surgical operative textbook, and orthopaedic texts should be consulted. However, individual fractures and the surgical approaches to the long bones are discussed briefly, along with a few selected orthopaedic procedures. It is hoped that this, combined with the general principles outlined above, may be of some value to a general surgeon who finds him or herself forced by circumstance to stray into orthopaedic territory.

SURGICAL EXPOSURE AND THE MANAGEMENT OF SPECIFIC FRACTURES

Cranial bones

Fractures of the skull and access to the brain are discussed in Chapter 8.

Faciomaxillary skeleton

Fractures of the zygoma, maxilla and mandible are discussed in Chapter 10.

Vertebral column

Minor stable fractures may need little treatment other than pain relief. In unstable fractures the major concern is protection of the spinal cord, and this can often be achieved by the external support of special beds or plaster shells or, in the case of cervical fractures, with traction. Operative fixation has many advantages in allowing early mobilization, but these are not operations for a surgeon unfamiliar in this territory, as the potential for secondary spinal cord damage should not be underestimated. Internal fixation between vertebral bodies requires an anterior approach which can be technically demanding and, in the thoracic spine, will necessitate a thoracotomy. A posterior approach is directly onto the more superficially placed veterbral arches, but the patient must be turned, and additional spinal cord insult can occur from this manoeuvre alone. Additionally, in general, anterior fixation between vertebral bodies gives greater skeletal stability than posterior fixation between vertebral arches. Conservative management will often be the safer option for a general surgeon.

The position of an unstable cervical spine fracture can be maintained in cervical traction, which can also be used for the reduction of a cervical dislocation. Traction is attached to skull callipers, which grip the outer table of the skull, and the patient is nursed on his or her back in a 10-degree head-up tilt. The patient's weight in this position provides the counter-traction. Alternatively, a four-point skull fixation to an external halo attached to a body jacket will allow the patient to be ambulant. When there is an unstable cervical fracture, the drill holes for the pins of the skull callipers are safer established under local, rather than general, anaesthesia. The anaesthetic agent must be infiltrated deeply to include the pericranium. A 2- to 3-cm incision is made a few centimetres above the external auditory meatus on both sides. The pericranium is incised and a small area of bone bared. The outer table of the skull is then drilled, with the guard preventing the drill from penetrating too deeply.

Surgery to decompress a spinal cord, perhaps threatened by a disc prolapse or an abscess, is an emergency, but one which should be transferred if at all possible to specialist services. Occasionally an isolated surgeon may have to proceed and, if pus causing the compression can be drained, there is a good chance of success. This is discussed further in Chapter 8.

Elective surgery of the vertebral column is highly specialized, and is unsuitable territory for the occasional operator in this field.

Ribs, sternum, scapula and clavicle

Surgical stabilization of these fractures is seldom required. The injuries are important, not in terms of their damage to the skeletal system but as an indicator of likely damage to underlying organs. A fractured sternum may be associated with contusion to the heart. A severely displaced fracture or dislocation of the clavicle can be associated with trauma to the major vessels of the superior mediastinum, or with compression of the trachea. A fractured rib may tear an intercostal vessel, or the underlying lung, with subsequent haemothorax or pneumothorax, and there will also inevitably be underlying lung contusion. Multiple rib fractures may cause mechanical difficulties with breathing. The management, however, is mainly of the underlying organ trauma and is discussed further in Chapter 7.

Clavicular fractures, even when displaced, seldom require formal fixation. However, in a severe avulsion-type upper-limb injury there may be a partial brachial plexus injury and associated concern over major vessel damage in a severely injured patient. A fractured clavicle may be the only apparent skeletal injury in the region, even though there is often significant tearing of scapular musculature and the whole shoulder girdle is 'floating'. These patients may have severe head and chest injuries, and it is easy to ignore an apparently minor clavicular fracture. However, in this situation, internal fixation of the clavicle is indicated to stabilize the shoulder girdle. A simple plate across the fracture site is suitable. Sternal division, rib resection and clavicular division are all employed to gain access to the heart, great vessels and lungs. The techniques are discussed in Chapter 7.

Humerus

Many humeral neck and shaft fractures heal with minimal intervention. External stabilization with a plaster cast is unsatisfactory and, if rigid fixation is deemed necessary, an intramedullary nail is the usual choice. For example, rigid fixation of any fracture is normally mandatory in circumstances when there has been associated damage, and subsequent repair, to an artery or nerve. The radial nerve is occasionally torn by a mid-shaft fracture and, if division is suspected, surgical exploration is indicated (see Chapter 3).

Supracondylar fractures are common in childhood. The elbow, with the distal humoral fragment, is displaced posteriorly; this causes the brachial artery to be stretched over the deformity and to be endangered by the sharp bone ends. If the artery is undamaged, closed reduction of the fracture usually restores the radial pulse, and the elbow is then held in acute flexion in a high collar and cuff sling. If the pulse is again lost, it may be only due to compression from swelling, and straightening the elbow may restore it. The fracture can then be managed temporarily by skin traction, while resting the limb on a splint until any swelling has subsided. If any concern remains over the artery, it should be explored as described in Chapter 5. The surgeon should be alert for a developing compartment syndrome (see Chapter 3), which is a not uncommon complication of this injury. Increasing pain, exacerbated by passive extension of the fingers, is an indication for fasciotomy of the flexor compartment of the forearm. Supracondylar fractures, and fractures of the medial and lateral epicondyle, can also be managed by open reduction and fixation with a Kirschner wire (Fig. 4.5). The wire is drilled into the distal fragment, the fracture reduced, and the wire advanced across the fracture into the main portion of the humerus.

The shaft of the humerus can be approached anteriorly or posteriorly. The anterior approach to the proximal shaft is between deltoid and pectoralis major, and a cephalad extension of this incision is used for anterior access to the shoulder joint. More distally, the anterior approach is through an incision placed just lateral to the lateral border of biceps. The cephalic vein and biceps are retracted medially to expose brachialis, which is then split in the direction of its fibres. The

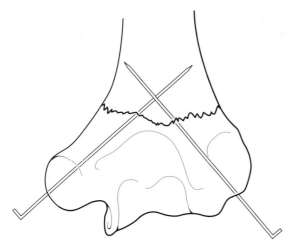

Figure 4.5 *The reduction of an unstable supracondylar fracture may be held with Kirschner wires.*

posterior approach to the shaft of the humerus is between the long and lateral heads of triceps. The radial nerve must be identified and preserved. The humeral condyles are superficial and access is straightforward through a medial, lateral or posterior longitudinal incision, depending upon the position of the fracture. The ulnar nerve, lying posteriorly on the medial side, must be safeguarded.

Radius and ulna

Olecranon fractures cross an articular surface, and the triceps pulls the fragments apart. Open fixation is therefore indicated, and tension wiring may be employed. Two Kirschner wires are introduced across the reduced fracture, via a posterior approach. A drill hole in the ulna allows a wire figure-of-eight to be formed around the Kirschner wires and through the hole and then tightened (Fig. 4.6). Radial head fractures may be treated conservatively but, if comminuted and displaced, the radial head is better excised. A dislocated radial head requires surgery for accurate reduction, and repair of the annular ligament. The radial head can be approached posteriorly in both these situations. The associated ulnar fracture

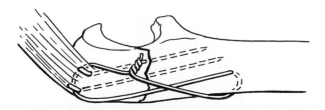

Figure 4.6 *A hole is drilled in the ulna and Kirschner wires are inserted across the fracture from the olecranon fragment. Tension wiring compresses and further stabilizes the fracture.*

then requires open fixation. Mid-shaft combined radial and ulnar fractures cannot be held satisfactorily by external splintage. Open fixation with plates is performed through two separate incisions. The ulna is easily approached posteriorly, where it can be felt subcutaneously. The radius is approached anteriorly by an incision along the medial border of brachioradialis. The muscle is then retracted laterally, together with extensor carpi radialis longus and brevis. The radial nerve is on the deep surface of brachioradialis and is displaced laterally. The radial vessels are retracted medially with the anterior muscles. Distal radial fractures seldom require operative intervention. If reduction cannot be maintained, a Kirschner wire across the fracture site may be helpful.

Hand

Most fractures of the hand heal without intervention. A scaphoid fracture requires rigid immobilization, but closed treatment is usually satisfactory. Metacarpal and phalangeal fractures often require little treatment. Displaced unstable fractures may be held with Kirschner wires, and this is more often indicated in fractures of the thumb and first metacarpal. Compound fractures, associated with tendon and digital vessel trauma, require very careful assessment as early amputation may be the best option (see later). If it is possible to save useful digits, any flexor tendon repair required should probably be delayed. Preservation of function in a severely damaged hand by splintage and physiotherapy is most important (see Chapter 3).

Pelvis

Many minor fractures of the pubic rami, or blade of the ilium, without disruption to the pelvic ring, require no intervention. Displaced anterior fractures may be associated with bladder or urethral injuries (see Chapters 24 and 25). An unstable anterior fracture can be stabilized by using a simple plate. Fractures through the acetabulum often lead to later arthritis of the hip. They may be treated with skeletal traction, as discussed below, but more accurate open reduction of the bone, and internal fixation, allows earlier mobilization and may give a better final outcome. These injuries are sometimes associated with pelvic organ, or vascular damage, and cooperation in management is needed between specialist surgeons.

Major **pelvic ring disruption** may be a life-threatening injury. It most often takes the form of an anterior fracture which opens on a 'hinge' formed by a disrupted sacro-iliac joint, or a fracture in the vicinity of this joint. Major force has caused this injury and there may also be damage to bladder, urethra and rectum. The initial life-threatening problem, however, is haemorrhage from torn pelvic veins. The retroperitoneal pelvic haematoma further opens the pelvic ring, and the increasing distortion of normal anatomy results in additional venous disruption. The patient may also have severe injuries in the upper abdomen and chest, and the correct decisions over surgical priorities are essential for a successful outcome. The pelvis must be stabilized urgently in the accident department to prevent further opening of the pelvic ring with subsequent venous tearing (Fig. 4.7). Stabilization also compresses the haematoma and reduces the venous haemorrhage.[5] Laparotomy, unless mandatory for some other intra-abdominal injury, is not indicated. Exploration of the haematoma will obviously remove all tamponade effect, and venous bleeding will again increase.

If the haematoma is still increasing after pelvic fixation –

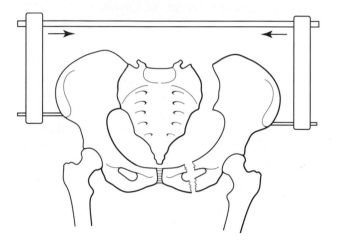

Figure 4.7 *External stabilization of a pelvic fracture is the most effective manoeuvre to reduce venous bleeding from torn posterior pelvic veins. The lateral pins are inserted percutaneously into the lateral surface of the ilium and the two side arms pulled inwards to close the opened pelvic ring. Rotation of the device allows access for a laparotomy.*

and especially if additional arterial bleeding is suspected – then interventional radiology, if available, is the best management option. Angiography, and embolization of bleeding vessels, can be very successful.[6] The alternative of surgical exploration is difficult. The bleeding site itself, of torn veins within a haematoma, is relatively inaccessible, and veins which have torn where they emerge from the ilium may not be amenable to surgical suture. Ligation of the internal iliac artery or vein on the affected side is less effective than selective embolization as the ligation is some distance from the bleeding point, and the extensive cross-circulation within the pelvis maintains blood flow through the damaged vessels.

ILIAC BONE GRAFTS

Cancellous bone may be harvested from the iliac crest for use as a bone graft. An incision is made parallel to, and just below, the crest extending from the anterior superior spine posteriorly as far as required. The lateral surface of the ilium is exposed subperiosteally, the crest with its attached muscles

is detached with an osteotome and reflected medially, care being taken to leave the anterior spine undisturbed. The medial aspect of the ilium is then exposed. Thin slivers of cancellous bone are cut from the exposed margin of the ilium, with five or six slivers, each 6–10 cm in length, being sufficient for most purposes. The detached crest is then sutured back to the periosteum and muscles on the outer face of the ilium.

Femur and hip joint

Intertrochanteric fractures, and fractures of the femoral neck, are mainly fractures of the elderly. Although the former may heal with traction they are better treated by internal fixation. Femoral neck fractures heal poorly. They require rigid intramedullary fixation across the fracture line, or prosthetic replacement of the femoral head. Stabilization must be of sufficient strength to allow immediate weight bearing and avoid prolonged immobilization of an elderly patient (Fig. 4.8). The treatment of these common fractures involves skills which the true surgical generalist may wish to acquire if his or her practice is to include orthopaedics. The operations are not included here as, unless a general surgeon has planned a relatively comprehensive orthopaedic service, he or she will not have the equipment and skills necessary to undertake these operations. In addition, the technique varies with the equipment available. The operative management of congenital dislocation of the hip, and the surgery for hip replacement, are excluded for the same reasons.

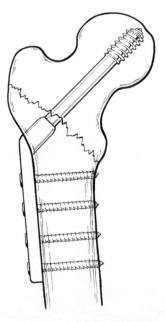

Figure 4.8 *Internal fixation of a hip fracture should be sufficiently robust to allow early weight-bearing. Intraoperative X-rays are necessary for the accurate placement of the pin or screw along the femoral neck into the proximal fragment.*

Fractures of the femoral shaft may be treated with a plaster of Paris cast, but the method is seldom used except in childhood. The plaster is very heavy as it extends both up around the pelvis and down to below the knee. It does however allow a child to be nursed at home. Accurate apposition, and rigid immobilization, are not essential for the healing of these fractures, but overlap and shortening must be avoided. The simplest form of treatment is therefore traction, with the limb supported on a Thomas splint (Fig. 4.9a). The alternative 'gallows' traction is suitable for a baby or toddler (Fig. 4.9b). Skin traction is very satisfactory in children as the skin is relatively strong, the traction required is less, and the duration of traction required is approximately half that required for an adult. Skeletal traction is usually preferred in

an adult and, with balanced traction, allows flexion of the knee to maintain the range of movement. A Steinmann or Denham pin is introduced, under general or local anaesthesia, through the upper tibia just posterior to the tibial tubercle. The weight required is around 10 kg in an adult. Alternatively, intramedullary nailing of the fracture can be used to avoid the long period in traction (Fig. 4.10). Fractures of the femoral condyles, and supracondylar fractures, are often better treated with a pin to stabilize the reduction. The possibility of associated popliteal vessel damage must be considered.

The upper femoral shaft is most satisfactorily approached through a posterolateral incision. The vertical skin incision is continued through tensor fascia lata, and then deepened to bone at the posterior border of vastus lateralis. Distally, the femoral shaft is more easily approached anterolaterally between vastus lateralis and rectus femoris.

The optimal treatment of a severely damaged hip joint is a prosthetic replacement, and this is now one of the commonest elective orthopaedic operations in the developed world. Many patients are elderly, and the commonest underlying pathology is osteoarthritis. In areas of the world with a poor standard of living and limited health facilities, severely damaged hip joints are common and the patients are often young. The original underlying pathology may be a tuberculous or pyogenic arthritis, or a premature osteoarthritis in a joint damaged by untreated trauma. Prosthetic hip replacement is often unavailable to these patients, but a **Girdlestone excision arthroplasty** can restore a pain-free weight-bearing limb with a good range of hip movement. No specialist equipment or skills are needed and, as it may be of value to the isolated generalist, this now almost historic operation is described.

The patient is placed on his or her side. The incision is from the posterior superior iliac spine, over the greater trochanter, and then distally in line with the femur. Gluteus maximus is divided in line with the skin incision, exposing

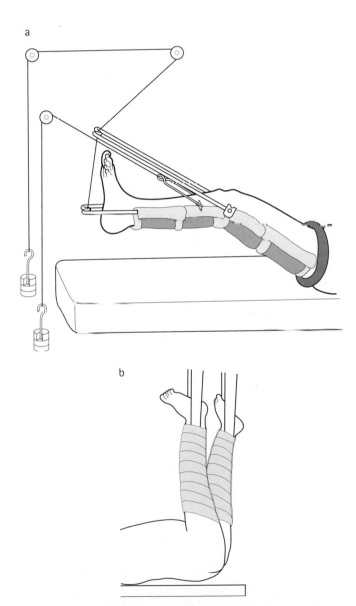

a

b

Figure 4.9 *Accurate apposition and rigid immobilization are not essential for femoral shaft fractures, but traction is required to prevent overlap. (a) Skeletal traction in a Thomas's splint. (b) 'Gallows' skin traction in a baby.*

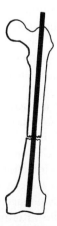

Figure 4.10 *An intra-medullary nail in* situ *after an open insertion. More sophisticated closed locked intramedullary nails are now widely used.*

the short rotator muscles of the hip joint. Figure 4.11 shows the portion of bone which is excised. Postoperatively, traction for 4–6 weeks allows firm scarring and prevents flexion deformity, telescoping and limb shortening.

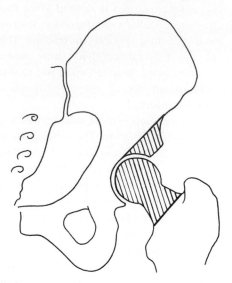

Figure 4.11 *Extent of the bone resection in a Girdlestone pseudarthrosis. This old operation still has a role when a joint replacement is not possible.*

Tibia and fibula: the knee and ankle joint

The possibility of damage to the popliteal vessels must be considered in any severe skeletal injury around the knee. Angiography should be employed if there is any concern over distal pulses, and if this does not exclude arterial injury the vessel should be explored. The surgeon must remember that an intimal tear in an intact artery can progress to a thrombotic occlusion which can easily be overlooked in a patient whose limb is encased in plaster of Paris (see Chapter 5). Fractures of the tibial plateau that cross the articular surface of the knee joint require accurate reduction to reduce the risk of later osteoarthritic changes. The reduction often has to be held with a pin. Small bony fragments separated from the upper tibia should alert the surgeon to a possible avulsed ligament. A patella fracture which is not reduced will cause underlying arthritis. The reduction must then be held by a screw, or tension wiring, but if comminuted, the patella is better excised.

Tibial shaft fractures can often be treated satisfactorily by closed reduction and immobilization in a full-length plaster of Paris cast. Open fixation with a plate (Fig. 4.2b) may be preferred, but a plate which does not compress the fracture site – or which introduces infection – will cause major problems. Severe injuries, with associated vascular and soft tissue damage, require interdisciplinary cooperation to save the limb (see Chapters 3 and 5). Restoration of blood supply is crucial but the vascular surgeon requires limb stability to proceed with fine vascular anastomoses. Rigid external fixation is ideal in this situation (Fig. 4.12).

Fibular fractures are of little significance except in the distal quarter where they may compromise the alignment, or stability, of the ankle joint. Fractures of the medial and lateral malleoli are important if there is disruption of the ankle mortis. Minor fractures may be reduced and held in plaster of Paris. More major fractures should be stabilized by internal fixation (Fig. 4.13).

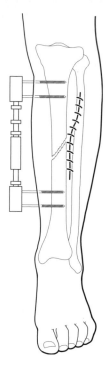

Figure 4.12 *A tibial fracture can be reduced and then stabilized with an external fixator. This can be a temporary solution while a vascular repair is undertaken, or it can be the chosen method of stabilization during bony healing. It is of particular value when extensive soft tissue trauma and contamination makes the use of internal fixation unwise.*

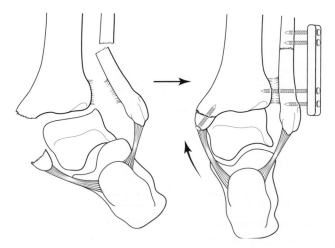

Figure 4.13 *Accurate apposition is necessary when a fracture involves a joint.*

A patient with an unstable knee may benefit from reconstructive ligament surgery, whilst one with a painful arthritic knee may benefit from a joint replacement. These are both specialist orthopaedic operations. **Arthrodesis** of a knee can give a sound weight-bearing limb and may still have a place when a joint replacement is not available (Fig. 4.14). Through an anterior transverse incision, the knee joint is entered by division of the patella tendon. The knee is flexed to expose the cruciate and collateral ligaments which are divided. The joint surfaces are then resected, and the cancellous bone ends held in compression apposition as shown. Correct alignment, and 15 degrees of flexion, are important for good function.

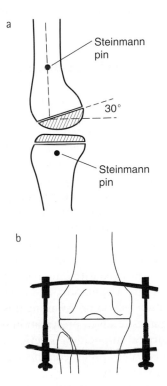

Figure 4.14 *Arthrodesis of a severely damaged knee is an option when a joint replacement is not possible. The articular surfaces are resected and Steinmann pins inserted to which the Charnley compression apparatus is fixed.*

Feet

Most fractures of the feet need no intervention other than support for pain relief. A crush fracture of the calcaneum, however, distorts the subtalar joint making subsequent degenerative change inevitable. The articular surface can be levered back into position with an instrument inserted into the body of the calcaneum from a posterolateral approach. Severe degeneration can be managed with a triple arthrodesis of the subtalar and midtarsal joints. Much of the elective orthopaedic surgery of the feet follows the general principles of osteotomies to correct malalignment, and excision arthroplasties of damaged joints.[2]

AMPUTATIONS: INDICATIONS AND GENERAL CONSIDERATIONS

The amputation of a limb – or part of a limb – is required when the vitality of the part is destroyed by injury or disease, or when the life of the patient is threatened by infective or malignant pathology in the extremity. Amputation may also be indicated for a deformed or paralysed limb, which is of little functional use to the patient, particularly in those instances where an artificial limb would be of greater value.

Trauma

In severe trauma the decision of whether to amputate or persevere with limb salvage is not always straightforward. Vessels and nerves can be repaired, and it may even be possible to re-attach a totally severed limb if the injury has been a sharp amputation rather than an avulsion. However, in general, if a limb has received a blunt injury which has severed the bone, in addition to causing vascular and nerve damage, the final result from salvage surgery is likely to be disappointing. The division of bone is often already completed and can be accepted as the level for amputation, if adequate soft tissue cover is possible (Fig. 4.15). In other situations, the considerations of soft tissue cover dictate the level of bone division (Fig. 4.16). In some instances, the stump length will have to be shortened to make it suitable for a future prosthesis, but in general extra length is beneficial. If the trauma is recent and relatively clean, it may be possible after careful wound toilet and with antibiotic cover, to appose the soft tissue definitively with a few loose sutures over a drain. This may also be appropriate when a patient presents early with an injury such as that sustained from a landmine explosion, provided that wound toilet is meticulous.[7] However, when a patient presents late with such a wound, it is unwise initially to do anything other than excise

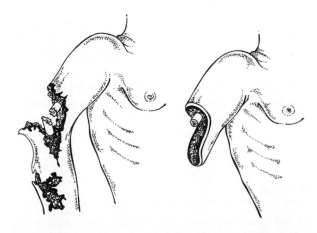

Figure 4.15 *In severe trauma bone division is often complete and dictates the level of amputation if soft tissue cover is possible. A single flap may make the best use of viable soft tissue.*

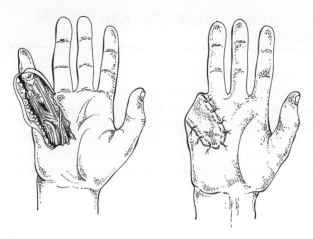

Figure 4.16 *Severe soft tissue loss of palmar skin and tendons necessitates a proximal amputation despite intact bone.*

non-viable tissue, and proceed to the fashioning of the definitive stump several days later. Occasionally, amputation is necessary when trauma has caused little damage except that it has severed a major vessel, and vascular reconstruction has been impossible or unsuccessful. The considerations are then more ischaemic than traumatic, but with the advantage that the patient does not have the generalized advanced atherosclerosis which complicates most amputations for limb ischaemia.

Deformity and paralysis

In considering the indications for amputation it is necessary to make a clear distinction between the upper and lower extremities. It is important to preserve length and stability in the lower limb. Stability of a paralysed limb, without associated deformity, can usually be achieved with external calliper support. A deformed, shortened, unstable lower limb may be the result of a congenital malformation, or the end result of severe trauma, septic arthritis or osteomyelitis, especially if it occurred in early childhood and the growth of the bone was arrested. Whatever the initial pathology, if corrective surgery cannot achieve a weight-bearing limb, the patient will be better served by an amputation to allow the fitting of a prosthesis.

Stability and length are not crucial to useful function in the upper limb, and a grossly deformed, or shortened, limb is often of more use than a prosthesis. However, the retention of a paralysed upper limb is of little benefit to the patient who may request an amputation.

Malignancy

In most soft tissue sarcomata, the excision of a compartment of soft tissue is adequate local treatment. In bone sarcomata, advanced reconstructive techniques have allowed radical excision of the bone primary with preservation of the limb.

However, a limb amputation is still occasionally the only surgical option. In subungual melanoma a distal digital amputation is necessary to achieve a radical tissue margin.

Infection

Amputation is indicated as an urgent life-saving intervention in infective gangrene. Gas gangrene is the most serious form of this, and is discussed in Chapter 3. Gangrene was traditionally divided into 'wet' and 'dry' gangrene. An infective gangrene is always a 'wet' gangrene. There is a rapid deterioration of the patient due to absorption into the systemic circulation of chemicals released from dead tissue, and delay in amputation inevitably leads to death from multiple organ failure.

Peripheral arterial occlusive disease

This accounts for over 90 per cent of amputations in the Western world. Unless there is already irreversible ischaemic damage, restoration of tissue perfusion by arterial reconstruction (or angioplasty) must be considered initially in an effort to avoid amputation. Amputation is reserved for situations where this has failed, or has been shown to be impractical. An amputation may be carried out at the stage of severe intractable ischaemic rest pain and incipient gangrene, or for established gangrene. An ischaemic gangrene may be either a 'wet' or a 'dry' gangrene. Urgent amputation is mandatory for wet gangrene. The 'dry' variety, with black desiccated digits or distal foot, is associated with minimal systemic toxicity. There is no urgency for amputation, and eventually demarcation and separation will occur. Awaiting this natural resolution may sometimes result in preservation of more tissue than if an early surgical amputation is performed, but a surgical amputation is usually preferred. This form of dry gangrene is also seen in frostbite.

In general, in peripheral arterial occlusive disease the amputation is performed at the most distal level consistent with healing. Many of these patients have widespread disease of the vascular tree with major vessel involvement, and surgery for gangrene of the toes usually necessitates an amputation at mid calf, or even above the knee, unless perfusion of the limb can be improved by arterial reconstruction, or angioplasty. It must be remembered when planning an amputation that the tissue perfusion necessary to heal an amputation wound is much greater than that merely required to sustain tissue viability. A relatively small number of patients, particularly those with diabetes, have predominately small vessel disease and consequently relatively localized peripheral ischaemic changes. In these circumstances it is possible to consider one of the more conservative amputations. In diabetic patients the gangrene is often of mixed aetiology. Neuropathic trauma occurs in a foot with poor perfusion from both major and small vessel disease and infection then adds the final insult. However, many diabetic patients unfortunately still require major amputations as the overriding pathology is often one of accelerated atheroma formation in major vessels.

Many patients are elderly, with poor general mobility and cardiorespiratory reserve. They may manage to walk again with a below-knee amputation, but only a minority manage after an above-knee amputation. If, however, there is no prospect of future walking, an above-knee amputation, which results in faster and more secure stump healing, may allow an earlier return to mobility in a wheelchair. It must be remembered that patients with peripheral vascular disease have similar pathology in their coronary and carotid vasculature. Perioperative mortality, and poor late survival after amputation, reflects this.

Stump length

Consideration must be given to the function desired of the stump. Even the most fragmentary portion of a hand is of great value to the patient, and should be preserved (Fig. 4.17). Overzealous attempts to preserve a foot may be misguided, although the preservation of a weight-bearing heel is of value. Above the wrist or ankle the stump should be fashioned with the aim of fitting a prosthesis. In the upper

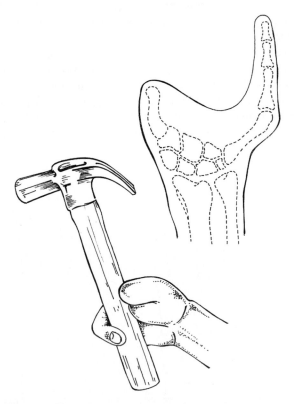

Figure 4.17 *Even a fragmentary portion of a hand is of great value. The drawing is taken from the X-ray and photograph of a man injured in the 1914–18 war. He retained sufficient strength of grip between the 5th finger and the 1st metacarpal to return to manual employment.*

arm and forearm, a 20-cm stump is recommended. For the lower leg a 14-cm tibial stump is ideal, and a stump of less than 8 cm is difficult to secure in a prosthesis. In an above-knee amputation a 25–30 cm stump measured from the tip of the trochanter is optimum. Amputations through joints are often difficult to fit to a satisfactory prosthesis. These general guidelines should be modified to adapt to local circumstances and the available prostheses (see Figs 4.24 and 4.27).

Stump length in childhood is difficult to judge as the divided bone loses its distal growing epiphysis, and proportional amputation is therefore not appropriate. Bony overgrowth in the immature stump does not significantly increase the length of the stump, but periosteal spikes of new bone cause discomfort and frequently require revisional surgery. In an above-knee amputation in childhood, the major growing epiphysis of the femur is lost and thus very little increase in length occurs. It is therefore essential that as much length as possible is preserved and, if at all possible, a through-knee amputation is to be preferred. Growth in length of the stump is also diminished after a below-knee amputation as the proximal tibial epiphysis fails to contribute its full expected growth. When feasible, a Syme's amputation – which retains the distal growing epiphysis of the tibia – is therefore a good alternative in childhood. Alternatively, a proportionally long 13-cm tibial stump is recommended.

Division of skin and muscle

A stump, to which a prosthesis is to be fitted, should be firm and smoothly rounded, and it should be conical in shape, tapering distally. A bony stump has inadequate muscle cover, while a bulbous floppy stump has the retention of excessive muscle and skin, distal to the division of bone. The skin and soft tissue division must therefore be carefully planned. A *racquet incision*, in which a straight incision is carried proximally from a circular or elliptical incision, is used for disarticulation at the metacarpo- or metatarso-phalangeal joint (see Fig. 4.19), and is applicable for amputation at the shoulder or hip (see Figs 4.21 and 4.30). Amputation using *flaps* is the most widely used method of amputation. Either two flaps cut from opposite sides of a limb, or a single longer flap, may be used. In order that the bone may be adequately covered, it is essential that the combined length of the two flaps, or the total length of a single flap, should be equal to 1.5 times the diameter of the limb at the level that the bone is divided. Each flap should be cut to a semicircular, rather than rectangular, shape since a conical, and not a cylindrical, stump is desired. Unequal flaps may be indicated because of tissue loss, or to maximize the use of tissue with good perfusion. This also avoids a terminal scar. When unequal flaps are used, the shorter flap should be rather broader than the longer flap so that the skin edges to be sutured are of equal length. A good blood supply to the skin of the flap must be assured, and is a particularly important consideration in amputation for peripheral arterial occlusive disease. As the blood supply of the skin is often partly from the underlying muscle, by vessels which pierce the deep fascia, there are obvious advantages in a combined myocutaneous flap. The muscle, however, may need to be thinned distally to avoid a bulky stump (see Fig. 4.26). The alternative is to plan separate flaps, and this is more suitable for some amputations. The initial flaps are of skin and subcutaneous fat alone, and the muscle flaps are raised separately.

NERVES

Nerves are divided cleanly with a knife and allowed to retract into the soft tissues, thus avoiding a troublesome neuroma. Ligation of a major nerve with a fine ligature prevents bleeding from accompanying vessels, but the ligature may be implicated in neuroma formation. Ligation of the sciatic nerve may be necessary if the small accompanying artery has become enlarged as a significant collateral vessel. Phantom pain after amputation may be significantly reduced by perioperative epidural anaesthesia.

BLOOD VESSELS

Blood vessels require ligation. Large superficial veins will be encountered in the subcutaneous fat, and can be simply ligated. The major vessels of a limb require careful ligation, with ligatures of a gauge and strength appropriate to their size. Double ligation, or a transfixion technique as described in Chapter 1, is recommended. A tourniquet should not be used in amputations for peripheral arterial occlusive disease as any reduction in the perfusion of the flaps may be critical for healing.

BONE

Bone is divided by any of the methods discussed above, and rough edges removed with a rasp or file. Care must be taken to avoid soft tissue damage while dividing the bone.

CLOSURE

Opposing muscle groups are sutured together over the bone ends, both to cover the divided bone and to balance the muscle action on the stump. Younger patients may benefit from a more formal *myodesis* in which the muscle is secured to the bone ends by sutures passed through drill holes in the bone. Tension-free skin closure is important and, in a major amputation, vacuum drainage is recommended. Postoperatively the first priority is healing, but care must be taken to maintain the mobility of proximal joints. A stiff hand, or a flexion deformity at the hip, is easier prevented than treated. In major lower-limb amputations there are some advantages in early bandaging of stumps to improve the shape for a prosthesis, and in the application of a plaster to allow early weight-bearing through a prosthetic extension. However, these manoeuvres carry some risk of compromising healing in vulnerable stumps with marginally adequate perfusion.

UPPER–LIMB AMPUTATIONS

Hand

The amputation of fingers is most commonly undertaken for severe trauma in which there is skin loss combined with additional bone, vessel or tendon damage. The advantages of alternative lengthy reconstruction procedures must be considered, and the correct decision may depend on the patient's occupation and preference, as much as on the extent of the injury. The type of amputation is often determined by the availability of skin and soft tissue, rather than by following formal procedures (see Fig. 4.16). It is, however, always preferable to cover the bony stump with volar skin and soft tissue. Every effort must be made to preserve as much of the thumb as circumstances will allow, as it is of pre-eminent importance in the hand. Even a stump composed of the metacarpal alone, or part of the metacarpal, is of great value (see Fig. 4.17). A stiff or deformed finger from previous infection, or trauma, may hinder the use of the hand and the patient may request amputation. Occasionally a finger must be amputated for adequate local treatment of a malignancy.

In general, amputation through the base of a phalanx is preferable to disarticulation at the joint immediately proximal, as this preserves the attachments of tendons and intrinsic muscles and results in a stronger grip. An amputation through the base of the proximal phalanx, or through the metacarpo-phalangeal joint, of the index or little finger leaves a somewhat conspicuous deformity. The hand has a better cosmetic appearance if the metacarpal head is sectioned obliquely, preserving the attachment of the metacarpal ligament, and the metacarpal arch (Fig. 4.18). After oblique removal of the metacarpal head, the stump of the metacarpal should be covered by interosseous muscle.

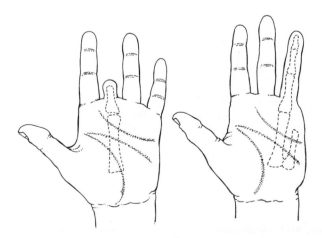

Figure 4.18 *Amputation through the base of a proximal phalanx gives a strong grip. An oblique metacarpal amputation results in a more satisfactory appearance if the index or little finger has to be sacrificed.*

Distal amputations of the fingers are best covered by a single volar flap, whereas an equal lateral flap technique is suitable for more proximal amputations. A racquet extension to the incision allows the transection of the metacarpal head (Fig. 4.19). Difficulty is encountered in digital amputations if the flaps are too short. This will occur if the surgeon is not aware of the surface marking of the joints when planning the flaps. The joints are more distal than is immediately apparent (Fig. 4.20).

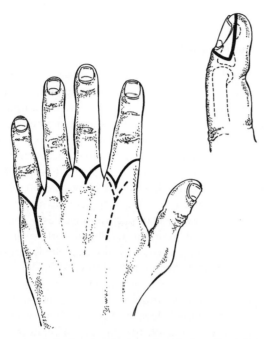

Figure 4.19 *A single volar flap is preferable for a distal digital amputation. Equal lateral flaps are suitable for more proximal amputations. A racquet extension affords access to the metacarpal head.*

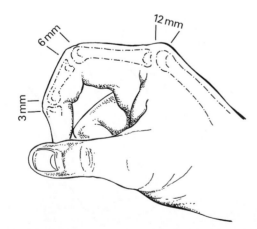

Figure 4.20 *A surgeon unfamiliar with the surface markings of the joints will have difficulty in planning satisfactory flaps. The measurements given indicate the distance of each joint distal to the angle of the knuckle.*

Arm and forearm

These amputations are not commonly indicated except for major trauma, and follow the general rules of amputation discussed previously. Bilateral amputations often deprive a patient of independence, although sophisticated functional prostheses have greatly improved in recent years. Occasionally after a clean traumatic amputation, a limb has been successfully reattached with microsurgical techniques. Unfortunately many of these injuries occur during periods of war and its aftermath in areas of the world with limited resources. The *Krukenberg amputation* may have a place when a bilateral forearm amputation is inevitable in these circumstances. The operation separates radius and ulna, thus providing a crude pincer grasp.[8]

Shoulder

These major amputations are seldom indicated. Amputation through the humoral neck preserves the normal contours of the shoulder and is preferable to the more proximal amputations unless they are specifically indicated. For *disarticulation through the shoulder joint* a racquet incision is used (Fig. 4.21a). The incision commences at the tip of the coracoid and extends distally in line with the humerus to the axillary folds where it splits to encircle the arm. The vertical part of the incision is deepened to bone, by the division of clavicular fibres of the deltoid and pectoralis. The posterolateral part of the circular incision is then deepened to bone, by the division of the deltoid muscle close to its insertion. The deltoid muscle is retained in the large lateral flap. The joint capsule and capsular muscles are then divided to allow dislocation of the humeral head. The brachial vessels are secured, and the nerves and remaining muscle divided. A *forequarter amputation* is an even more radical procedure, and the loss of the normal shoulder contour is a significant deformity. The

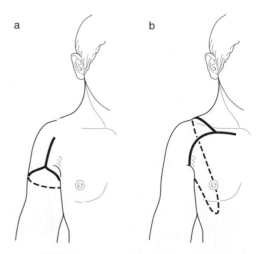

Figure 4.21 *(a) The incision for disarticulation of the shoulder. (b) The incision for a forequarter amputation.*

linear portion of the racquet incision is along the clavicle, the lateral two-thirds of which is excised (Fig. 4.21b). The clavicular excision affords access to the subclavian vessels and the brachial plexus, both of which require division. The pectoral muscles are divided. Posteriorly the scapula is excised after division of all muscles attaching the scapula to the trunk.

LOWER–LIMB AMPUTATIONS

Foot and ankle

These amputations may be for infective gangrene, trauma or frostbite. Ischaemic gangrene of the toes, or forefoot, from peripheral arterial occlusive disease nearly always indicates that tissue perfusion will be inadequate to sustain the increased requirements of a healing amputation wound at any site below mid calf. A more proximal amputation is thus indicated unless tissue perfusion can be improved by arterial reconstruction, or angioplasty.

A **distal amputation** is sometimes appropriate in diabetes. A patient with diabetic neuropathy may be unaware of minor trauma and subsequent infection, and present with localized infective gangrene. Even if there is an ischaemic element to the gangrene, it may only be due to diabetic microangiopathy, and a distal amputation wound may still heal. However, many diabetic patients also have major vessel disease and this should be carefully assessed before recommending a limited amputation. Furthermore, the spread of web space infection can be particularly rapid in diabetic patients.

RAY AMPUTATION

The most common amputation in the foot is a ray amputation of the affected toe with the distal half of the associated metatarsal (Fig. 4.22). This also allows good drainage of infected deep spaces of the foot, and the wound is left open.

The advisability of a first or fifth ray local amputation should be carefully considered, as healing is more likely to be troublesome.

TRANSMETATARSAL, TARSOMETATARSAL AND MIDTARSAL AMPUTATIONS

These are also satisfactory amputations for distal gangrene with adequate perfusion of the hindfoot, and leave a patient with a weight-bearing heel. The amputation is undertaken using a long plantar flap which covers the end of the stump, and the dorsal incision is at the level of bone division (Fig. 4.23).

SYME'S AMPUTATION

This classical ankle amputation, first described by Syme in 1842, produces a durable weight-bearing stump, which is often superior in the long term to the forefoot amputations described above. It is particularly suitable in young patients who have sustained a crushing injury to the foot, and is of special value to patients who do not have access to modern artificial limbs. The end of the stump is at a height of about 6–8 cm from the ground, and may be walked on without a prosthesis. Alternatively, a simple appliance which raises the stump is inexpensive to manufacture (Fig. 4.24). The amputation fell into disfavour in the developed world as there were difficulties in fitting a cosmetically acceptable prosthesis. There has, however, been renewed interest in this amputation.[9] Syme's amputation may have a place in diabetics but if there is significant large vessel atheroma it is not suitable.

The incision starts below the tip of the lateral malleolus and is drawn across the sole to a point 2 cm below the medial

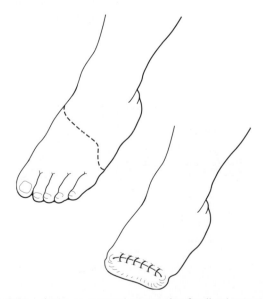

Figure 4.23 *A transmetatarsal amputation for distal gangrene is only satisfactory if the hindfoot perfusion is good. A single plantar flap has the optimum blood supply and also covers the stump with the skin which is most suitable to withstand trauma.*

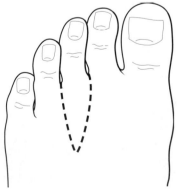

Figure 4.22 *A ray amputation of a toe with the distal half of the metatarsal will often suffice if distal gangrene is of infective origin.*

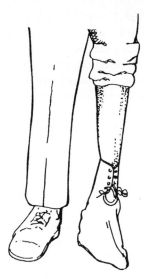

Figure 4.24   *A primitive 'elephant boot' prosthesis that can be used after a Syme's amputation.*

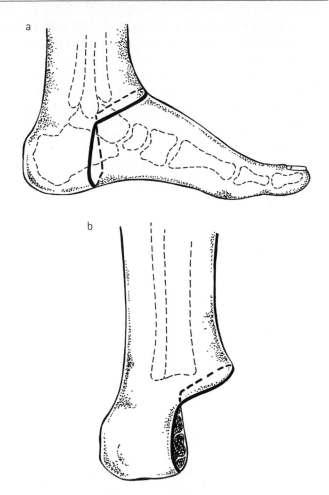

Figure 4.25   *Syme's amputation. (a) The incision. (b) The calcaneum has been dissected out of the heel flap. The malleoli and the distal articular surface of the tibia have been excised.*

malleolus (Fig. 4.25). The two ends of the incision are then joined by the shortest route across the front of the ankle joint. Throughout the incision, all structures are divided down to bone. Extensor, flexor and peroneal tendons are divided, as are the anterior tibial and plantar vessels and nerves. Vessels are ligated and nerves cut short as discussed previously. The ankle joint is then entered anteriorly and the lateral ligament divided. The foot is then dislocated in a plantar direction to expose the back of the joint.

The next part of the operation is the most important and the most difficult. It consists of the division of the posterior ligaments of the joint, the detachment of the insertion of the Achilles tendon and the dissection of the calcaneum out of the heel flap. There is great danger in injuring the posterior tibial and peroneal arteries, as both arteries are closely applied to the back of the posterior ligament. Their branches, which supply the skin of the heel, are also in danger when the calcaneum is dissected out of the flap. The knife is kept closely applied to the bone to prevent damage at this stage. The malleoli and a thin slice of tibia are then removed. The saw is applied exactly at right-angles to the long axis of the tibia. The heel flap is folded over the bone ends and sutured in position over a vacuum drain.

Modifications

Modifications have been sought to increase the length of the stump. The distal articular surface of the tibia may be left *in situ*, and a larger heel flap fashioned by siting the incision more distally, starting 1 cm in front of the medial malleolus. In *Pirogoff's* modification, the posterior part of the calcaneum is retained in the heel flap, and is opposed to the sawn surface of the tibia. It is fixed in place by periosteal sutures, or fixed internally with a pin. However, the advantages of a full-length, weight-bearing stump is offset by the delay in mobility while awaiting bony union, and this can be a major consideration in the elderly.

Below–knee amputations

These operations are most commonly performed for peripheral arterial occlusive disease, and the standard techniques are designed to maximize the use of well-perfused tissue. It is not always possible to retain the ideal 15 cm of tibia, but if less than 8 cm can be retained there will be difficulty in fitting a satisfactory prosthesis. The long posterior flap is marked out, and should be of a length 1.5 times the diameter of the leg. The anterior flap, which has the poorer blood supply, is cut down to bone at the level of bone division. Elevation of the anterior flap of skin and muscle off the underlying bone is kept to a minimum, and 1 cm is adequate. The tibia is then divided and bevelled anteriorly. The fibula is divided 1 cm more proximally. The posterior flap should retain deep fascia, and some underlying muscle, throughout its length to safeguard skin perfusion. However, the muscle bulk must be reduced to obtain a tapered stump. The posterior muscles are divided obliquely so that virtually all of the deep muscle is removed and, distally, only a thin remnant of the superficial gastrocnemius remains (Fig. 4.26). Arteries are ligated as they are encountered, and nerves divided so that they can retract. The muscles of the flaps are opposed over the bone with sutures through deep fascia, and the skin is closed over suction drainage.

Variations

Variations of the standard method are numerous:

- A 'skew' flap technique is favoured by some surgeons.[10] Skin and muscle flaps are fashioned separately. Equal skin flaps are based on the blood supply of the skin, which in this site is anatomically related to the venous drainage of the long and short saphenous veins, and relies on collateral vessels running with the sural and saphenous nerves. A single posterior muscle flap is still used.
- If the patient does not have peripheral arterial occlusive disease, two rather than one musculocutaneous flaps may be preferred. Unequal length of these flaps has the advantage that the scar is away from the end of the stump. Periosteum may be raised from the tibia distal to the level of bone resection, preserved and swung over to the fibula to form a periosteal bridge between the bones. This may form a better stump for a young active amputee.
- A very short stump, although generally unsatisfactory, may be ideal for a primitive prosthesis (Fig. 4.27).

Disarticulation through the knee

This amputation produces a stump which is functionally satisfactory and which can sustain end weight-bearing. As discussed previously, a through-knee amputation has advantages in children in order to preserve final femoral length. However, the bulbous end, and the external hinge usually required in the prosthesis, can make it cosmetically inferior to other alternatives. In peripheral arterial occlusive disease, if the tissue perfusion will not sustain the healing of a below-knee amputation, a through-knee amputation will probably also be problematic, and an above-knee amputation becomes a better option.

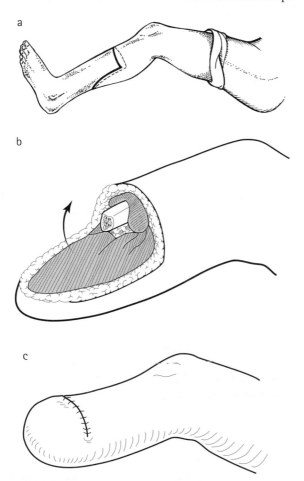

Figure 4.26 *Below-knee amputation. (a) The single long posterior flap utilizes the superior blood supply to the calf skin which is critical for successful healing in peripheral vascular disease. (b) The posterior muscle groups are divided obliquely from the tibia to the skin to reduce the bulk of the flap. (c) The scar is away from the weight-bearing end.*

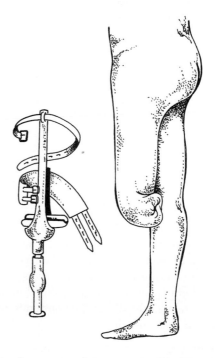

Figure 4.27 *A young man from a remote village presents 5 years after trauma requesting an amputation of a useless flail extremity. There is a flexion deformity of the knee, an ununited fracture of the tibia and a deformed foot in fixed equinus. He is already ambulant with a home-made prosthesis in which he kneels. The limb fitting services are rudimentary. A high below-knee amputation, although unconventional, may be the best solution. Individual patient requirements and local prosthetic facilities should influence the choice of amputation.*

The operation may be performed with equal medial and lateral skin flaps, or with unequal anterior and posterior flaps. The patient is placed prone, and the flaps raised. The access to the joint is from the popliteal fossa where the artery is ligated and nerves divided. The posterior muscles and joint capsule are divided, and the knee flexed before the division of the patellar tendon at its attachment to the tibia. After division of the cruciate, medial and lateral ligaments the amputation is complete. The patella is retained. The patellar tendon is sutured to the cruciate ligaments, and the remains of the extensor retinaculum to the hamstrings.

Variations

Variations of this operation include the classical *Gritti–Stokes* amputation (Fig. 4.28) and various subsequent modifications of it. The Gritti–Stokes operation is normally performed with the patient supine. Unequal anterior and posterior flaps are raised. The long anterior flap extends down to the patella tendon insertion, which is divided and the knee joint entered. All soft tissue posteriorly is divided, and the femur is then divided immediately above the femoral condyles. The patella, from which the articular surface has been removed, is swung over so that the patella lies over the divided femur. Stabilization can be achieved with wire sutures, passed through drill holes in the bone of the patella and femur, and the patella tendon is sutured to the hamstrings. This amputation lost popularity because of difficulties with prostheses but, with this overcome, there has been some renewed enthusiasm.[11] The removal of the femoral condyles makes it more suitable than a through-knee amputation if the tissue perfusion is marginal. An oblique division of the femur with a 30° angle has been a useful recent variant giving better early stability (Fig. 4.28b).

Above-knee amputations

These are common amputations for ischaemia, and for trauma, and the priorities for the surgeon in different circumstances vary. In general, the longer the stump the better the control of the prosthesis, and ideally 70 per cent of the femur (or around 25–30 cm as measured from the tip of the greater trochanter) should be retained. If the stump is longer than this, the same problems arise with the knee joint of a prosthesis as with the through-knee and Gritti–Stokes amputations. In a child every effort should be made to preserve the whole femur, as already discussed. The underlying pathology sometimes dictates an amputation in the upper third of the femur, but if less than 10 cm of femur can be preserved then disarticulation through the hip joint may be preferred in a younger patient in order to fit a more satisfactory prosthesis. In contrast, a short femoral stump, even one with a flexion deformity, is better for the wheelchair-bound amputee.

The operation can be performed with equal anterior and posterior myocutaneous flaps, or unequal flaps with a longer anterior flap (Fig. 4.29). The quadriceps muscle is sutured to

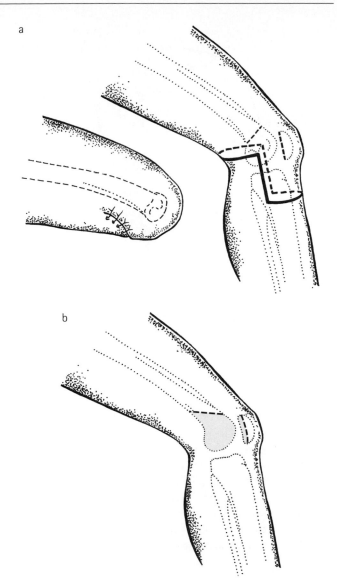

Figure 4.28 *(a) Gritti–Stokes amputation. A long anterior flap brings the scar posteriorly. The femur is transected immediately above the condyles. The patella is retained, but its articular surface is removed, before it is fixed to the divided femur. (b) A modification in which the femur is transected at an angle to give superior early stability.*

the hamstrings so that muscle action on the stump remains balanced. In a younger patient some form of more formal myodesis should be carried out.

Gas gangrene is a much feared postoperative complication, particularly after an above-knee amputation for ischaemia. Prophylactic antibiotics must be chosen which are effective against *Clostridium welchii*.

Disarticulation at the hip joint

This radical amputation may sometimes be indicated if insufficient femur can be preserved to make a satisfactory

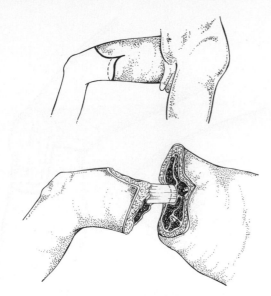

Figure 4.29 *An above-knee amputation. A two-flap technique is suitable for an amputation through the lower, middle or upper femur. A slightly longer anterior flap avoids a terminal scar.*

femoral stump. Two classical methods have been described: the method of the anterior racquet; and that of the single posterior flap. The second method may yield a better stump for limb fitting. The incisions for the two methods are shown in Figure 4.30. In the anterior racquet incision the 'handle' is placed in the line of the femoral vessels, and the medial flap is longer, so that the scar will fall away from the perineum. In the alternative single posterior flap method, the length of the flap should be 1.5 times the anteroposterior diameter of the limb at the level of the hip joint; the anterior part of the incision is 2.5 cm below and

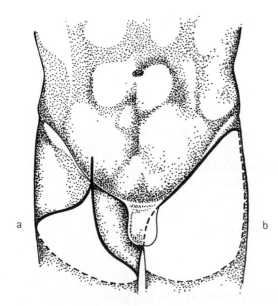

Figure 4.30 *Incisions that may be used for amputation at the hip. (a) A racquet incision with a longer medial flap. (b) A single posterior flap.*

parallel to the inguinal ligament. In each method the first part of the operation consists of exposure and ligation of the femoral vessels. The anterior muscles are divided in the line of the incision, and the joint is opened from the front. The adductors, the hamstrings and gluteus maximus are cut so that portions of them remain in the flaps. The sciatic nerve is found deep in gluteus maximus and is cut short. Disarticulation is completed by division of the capsule and of the remaining short muscles which are inserted into the trochanteric area. The flaps and muscles are trimmed to give reasonable bulk, without flabbiness, to the stump.

Hindquarter amputation

This mutilating radical amputation is fortunately seldom performed, but is occasionally indicated for locally advanced malignancy[12] or, in exceptional circumstances, when an above-knee amputation has failed in a patient with peripheral arterial occlusive disease. An elliptical incision affords access, first to the anterior abdominal muscles which are divided in line with the incision. The deep epigastric vessels are ligated and the symphysis pubis divided. The peritoneum and ureter are swept medially to expose the common iliac vessels which are ligated in continuity to reduce blood loss during dissection. Alternatively, this initial ligation can be solely of the internal iliac artery, distal to the origin of the superior gluteal artery, to safeguard the blood supply of the posterior buttock flap. The ilium is divided through the greater sciatic notch, and the major portion of gluteus maximus is retained. The remaining soft tissue is divided and all nerves are cut cleanly. The external iliac, obturator, gluteal and pudendal vessels must be ligated before division, even if the common iliac was ligated, as there is usually considerable cross circulation from the other side.

REFERENCES

1. *Campbell's Operative Orthopaedics*, 10th edn. ST Canale. St Louis: Elsevier Mosby, 2003.
2. *Standard Orthopaedic Operations*, 4th edn. JC Adams, CA Stossel. Edinburgh: Elsevier Churchill Livingstone, 1992.
3. *The Closed Treatment of Common Fractures*. J Charnley. London: Greenwich Medical Media, 2002.
4. *Manual of Internal Fixation – techniques recommended by the ASO-ASIF group*, 3rd edn. ME Muller, M Allgower, P Schneider, H Willennegger. Berlin: Springer-Verlag, 1990.
5. Bircher MD. Indications and techniques of external fixation of the injured pelvis. *Injury* 1996; **27** (Suppl. 2): S-B3-19.
6. Mucha P, Welch TJ. Haemorrhage in major pelvic fractures. *Surg Clin North Am* 1988; **68**: 757–73.
7. Ateşalp AS, Erler K, Gür E, *et al*. Below-knee amputations as a result of land-mine injuries: comparison of primary closure versus delayed primary closure. *J Trauma* 1999; **47**: 724–7.
8. Swanson AB. The Krukenberg procedure in the juvenile amputee. *J Bone Joint Surg* 1964; **46A**: 1540–8.

9. Chissell HR, Corner NB. Syme's amputation: a neglected procedure. *J R Coll Surg Edinb* 1993; **38**: 365–7.

10. Robinson KP, Hoile R, Coddington T. Skew flap myoplastic below-knee amputation: a preliminary report. *Br J Surg* 1982; **69**: 554–7.

11. Yusuf SW, Baker DM, Wenham PW, *et al*. Role of Gritti–Stokes amputation in peripheral vascular disease. *Ann R Coll Surg Engl* 1997; **79**: 102–4.

12. Clark MA, Thomas JM. Major amputation for soft-tissue sarcoma. *Br J Surg* 2003; **90**: 102–7.

5

VASCULAR SURGICAL TECHNIQUES: VASCULAR ACCESS AND TRAUMA

ANATOMY

An **artery** consists of three coats:

- The outer coat or *tunica adventitia* is composed of fibrous and elastic tissue, and contains the periarterial sympathetic nerves; it is attached only loosely to the middle coat, and can be stripped from it without difficulty.
- The middle coat or *tunica media* constitutes the main thickness of the arterial wall; it is composed of smooth muscle with a proportion of elastic tissue, this proportion being greater in the large vessels.
- The inner coat or *tunica intima* lines the lumen of the vessel. In a healthy artery, without atheromatous plaques, it is a thin layer consisting only of endothelial cells, supported on a basement membrane of elastic tissue which lies in contact with the tunica media.

A **vein** has a structure very similar to that of an artery, except that all coats – especially the tunica media – are much thinner.

DISSECTION OF VESSELS

When exposing an artery it is important to mobilize enough of the vessel and its branches to allow proximal and distal control. The best plane of dissection for this arterial mobilization is deep to the adventitia. Veins should be mobilized by dissection directly on the surface of the vein. This plane is usually outside the adventitia. All vessels should be handled gently, since trauma to the wall commonly leads to throm-bosis, and in particular they should never be grasped or clamped with an instrument likely to cause damage. Any clamp should be applied with the minimal compression required to control flow. Remember that the intima can be split without visible damage to the adventitia.

HAEMORRHAGE AND VASCULAR CONTROL

Vascular surgery may have to be undertaken in an emergency for situations such as vascular trauma or spontaneous rupture of an aneurysm. The initial overriding concern is to arrest exsanguinating haemorrhage. Major bleeding in limb trauma can normally be controlled by elevation combined with firm local pressure by pad and bandage to occlude the vessel at the point of injury. This temporary control allows the patient to be resuscitated and prepared for a definitive operation with adequate lighting and necessary facilities. No attempt should be made in an emergency to apply artery forceps blindly within a profusely bleeding wound as it is impossible to identify the damaged vessel with any accuracy, and there is a serious risk of injuring neighbouring structures.

When haemorrhage is from an intrathoracic or intra-abdominal vessel, local external pressure is impractical. Maintenance of circulating volume is essential, but surgery to gain proximal vascular control must proceed alongside resuscitation. This initial control may have to be more proximal than is ideal, but speed is important. It can be revised for more appropriate control closer to the site of damage as soon as possible.

The focus of management then shifts to the restoration of distal perfusion by repair or reconstruction of vessels. The surgical conditions for this should now approximate the elective situation. Vascular surgery requires precision and gentle handling of tissue which is not possible in the presence of haemorrhage from open vessels.

Limb tourniquet

A limb tourniquet will arrest haemorrhage and give excellent operative conditions but, as it prevents any distal limb perfusion from other undamaged vessels, tissue ischaemia is more profound than when the injured vessel alone is controlled. In an emergency, local pressure will usually suffice, and once the damaged artery has been isolated, proximal and distal control of the damaged section of vessel is then preferable to a tourniquet. A tourniquet is therefore normally reserved for situations where a bloodless operative field is necessary for the repair of tendons and nerves in addition to the repair of blood vessels.

Vascular clamps or tapes

Vascular clamps or tapes placed above and below the site of an arteriotomy or injury are the most versatile method of control (Fig. 5.1). Great care must be taken to avoid injury to a thin-walled vein lying in close proximity to an artery; for example, the inferior vena cava (IVC) is easily damaged during cross-clamping of the aorta. Vascular occlusion clamps are designed to hold a vessel occluded but with minimal crushing damage to the vessel wall. Unfortunately, if a vessel is diseased the distortion of its shape by the clamp can fracture an atheromatous plaque, and a flap of intima and atheroma may lift away from the vessel wall. It may then occlude the vessel, or detach as an embolus. Alternatively, the plaque fracture is a potential focus for thrombosis, or a possible initial entry point for a dissection. Damage often occurs when a clamp twists after application. Securing the handles of clamps to the drapes reduces the likelihood of this. Slings

of tape, fine silastic tubing or heavy silk ties are alternatives to a clamp, and are safer on the smaller distal arteries. A side clamp on a major vessel may be sufficient and has the advantage that distal flow is preserved (Fig. 5.2).

A temporary cross-clamp – placed at some considerable distance proximal to the site of injury – is occasionally indicated for major haemorrhage if immediate access to the damaged vessel is problematic. For example, the aorta can be cross-clamped above, or just below, the diaphragm for the initial control of life-threatening upper abdominal haemorrhage. Opening the chest to control intra-abdominal haemorrhage adds significant morbidity, and has little advantage over an aortic clamp applied just below the diaphragm.

Intra-luminal balloon

An intra-luminal balloon is a solution to vascular control if the vessel is inaccessible for the application of a clamp or sling above or below the site of surgery (Fig. 5.3). A Foley

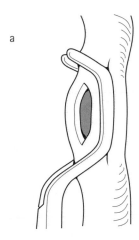

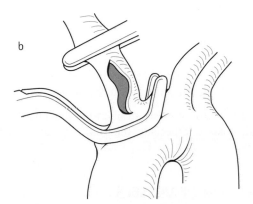

Figure 5.2 *An angled or curved side clamp can isolate part of the circumference of a large vessel while maintaining patency. (a) The control of an iatrogenic laceration in the inferior vena cava (IVC) with a Satinsky clamp. The laceration can now be repaired without continuing haemorrhage. (b) A curved side clamp is isolating the root of the brachiocephalic artery with its traumatic tear. Flow through the aortic arch is maintained.*

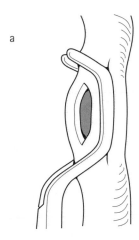

Figure 5.1 *Methods of controlling blood vessels. (A) Fogarty soft jaw clamp; (B) bulldog clamp; (C) atraumatic metal-jawed vascular clamp; (D) double ligature sling; (E) sling with snub.*

catheter is suitable for a large vessel, and a Fogarty catheter for a smaller vessel. The central lumen of the Foley catheter can be used as intravascular access for resuscitation.

Dangers of vascular occlusion

The surgeon must be aware of the deleterious effects of vascular occlusion. A proximal aortic clamp increases peripheral resistance and may precipitate severe cardiac failure. The release of such a clamp has even more profound cardiovascular effects. Skilled anaesthetic care is required, especially as many patients are arteriopaths with compromised coronary and cerebral vasculature.

The surgeon must remain aware of the deterioration which occurs distal to the operative field. An excellent technical reconstruction, capable of restoring long-term perfusion, is wasted if irreversible damage to distal tissue has been allowed to occur during the perioperative period. Speed is important to reduce ischaemic time. The circulation can sometimes be restored before completion of the procedure. For instance, after completion of the proximal anastomosis in a femoral-popliteal bypass, perfusion can be restored to the profunda system before the distal anastomosis is completed.

Stasis in the vascular tree distal to a clamp is inevitable, and thrombosis may follow. *Heparinized saline* (5000 units of heparin in 500 mL saline) should be instilled into the vessel distal to the clamp, often in addition to systemic heparinization.

TISSUE ISCHAEMIA

The sensitivity of different tissues to ischaemia varies. Irreversible ischaemic damage to cerebral cortex occurs within minutes, but a limb remains salvageable for several hours after total vascular occlusion. The kidneys, liver and gut form an intermediate group. It is often difficult to predict whether vascular occlusion is complete, or whether perfusion continues at a slightly, or significantly, reduced level. There are anatomical variations in arterial arcades. In addition, there may be changes in other arteries secondary to disease which may take the form of additional stenoses, or enlarged compensatory collateral channels. An alternative route for perfusion may be adequate when the patient is normotensive, but inadequate if the patient is shocked. If there is a danger that during temporary arterial occlusion distal perfusion may be inadequate to prevent damage to distal tissue a temporary shunt should be considered (see below).

Ischaemic damage to muscle results in swelling and a rise in pressure within a closed fascial space. Perfusion decreases as interstitial pressure approximates perfusion pressure and secondary ischaemic damage from *compartment syndrome* follows, as discussed in Chapter 3. It is of particular concern in the management of vascular lower-limb trauma, especially in a crushing injury where there may be additional muscle

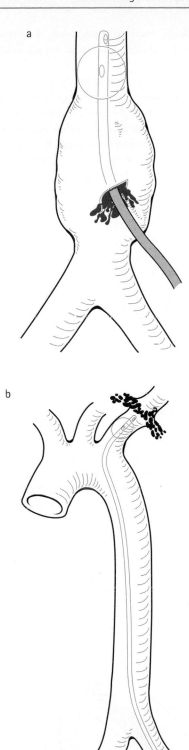

Figure 5.3   *An intra-luminal balloon catheter is valuable for proximal arterial control in situations where direct access to the artery is difficult. In (a) the catheter has been introduced through a ruptured aortic aneurysm to occlude the inflow, while in (b) it has been introduced through the femoral artery to occlude the root of the subclavian artery proximal to a traumatic rupture.*

swelling as a direct result of the trauma. A *fasciotomy* should always be considered after a vascular repair in these circumstances.[1]

Renal function is often compromised after major vascular surgery, and especially after emergency surgery for a ruptured aortic aneurysm.[2] It has sometimes been necessary to cross-clamp the aorta above the renal arteries, even if only for a few minutes, with some resultant renal ischaemic damage. More often, the renal insult has been partly that of hypovolaemic shock followed by an 'ischaemia–reperfusion' insult. Any ischaemic tissue below the aortic cross-clamp releases inflammatory cytokines, free radicals, activated white cells and other toxic metabolites into the circulation. These substances invoke a cascade of damaging reactions throughout the body, and in particular cause damage to the lungs and kidneys. Impairment of renal and pulmonary function greatly increases postoperative morbidity and mortality. Skilled anaesthetic care, fast but meticulous surgery with a short ischaemia time and good intensive care facilities all improve results.

Temporary shunts

Temporary shunts are indicated when there is concern that irreversible damage may occur to distal tissue during the period of ischaemia (Fig. 5.4). They are frequently employed during carotid surgery (see Chapter 6). Even though a normal Circle of Willis will maintain adequate perfusion to the whole cerebral cortex from a single carotid artery, this cannot be guaranteed in an individual patient. They also have a place in the severely damaged limb with unstable skeletal damage. The fractures should, if possible, be stabilized prior to vessel reconstruction, or damage to the

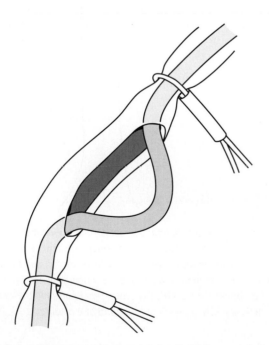

Figure 5.4 *A temporary shunt maintains distal tissue perfusion while still allowing the surgeon good access in a dry field.*

reconstructed vessel may occur during manipulation of the fracture. However, any further delay before revascularization of the distal limb is critical when there has already been several hours of ischaemia during transfer to hospital. A temporary shunt – both arterial and venous – followed by skeletal fixation and finally a meticulous vascular reconstruction undertaken in optimal circumstances may be the best solution.[3] Silastic tubing is satisfactory for a temporary shunt, but a specially designed shunt has either a balloon cuff which when inflated fits snugly against the intima (Pruitt–Inahara shunt), an expanded end with specially fitted clamps (Javid shunt) or, alternatively, a shunt with a groove at which point an external tape, when tightened, will form a good seal.

BASIC ARTERIAL SURGICAL TECHNIQUES

Surgery to repair or reconstruct arteries is delicate, and must be undertaken in optimum conditions. Sterility, adequate access, a good light and control of haemorrhage are all essential. Non-absorbable monofilament sutures are used which will slide atraumatically through the vessel wall and create the least tissue reaction. Soft, pliant, monofilament polypropylene is most favoured. A useful standard size of suture for femoral and popliteal arteries is 5/0. Finer sutures are used for smaller vessels, whilst as large as 2/0 may be used for the aorta. Round-bodied needles are the most suitable for normal vessels, but a tapercut needle may be better for suturing dense graft material or heavily diseased arterial wall. During closure, special care must be taken to include the intima in every stitch (unless of course an endarterectomy has been performed) as the dissection of an intimal flap is probably the commonest cause of early thrombosis after reconstruction. A needle passed from without-in is in more danger of lifting a flap of diseased intima than a needle passed from within-out. When a needle has to be passed from without-in, the intima should be supported against the vessel wall as the needle is inserted (Fig. 5.5). Sutures with a needle at both ends (*a double-armed suture*) are extensively used in vascular surgery. Fine monofilament sutures are easily damaged, and if one end is to be held temporarily a rubber-shod clamp should be employed. Monofilament sutures must not be handled with metal instruments as they tend to fracture and are then prone to breaking with minimal strain.

Arterial ligation

A ligature of appropriate diameter and strength for the size of the artery must be selected. A transfixion ligature gives extra security, especially if the stump of an artery beyond the ligature is short. An over-sew technique will give an even more secure closure than a transfixion ligature when a very major vessel must be closed. For example, there is the danger

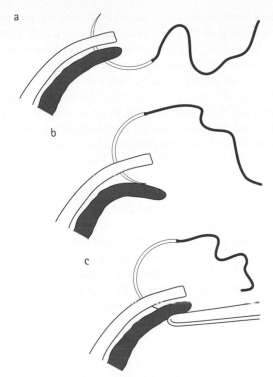

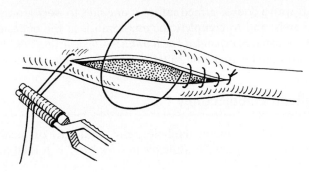

Figure 5.6 *Closure of an arteriotomy.*

Figure 5.5 *(a) A needle passed from within-out presses an intimal atheromatous plaque safely against the vessel wall. (b) When passed from without-in, it may separate off the plaque and initiate a dissection. (c) This separation is prevented by supporting the intima with an instrument.*

of a 'blow-out' of the aortic stump when the aorta has to be divided and the distal perfusion restored with a bypass graft with inflow from a more proximal site.

Arteriotomy

This should, as a general rule, be made longitudinally, allowing the surgeon to see a greater area of the inside of the vessel. It can be extended and it provides access to the orifices of branches – advantages which outweigh the only benefit of a transverse incision, which is that it can be closed with less tendency to narrow the lumen. However, in vessels of 4 mm diameter or less – especially if made simply for the purposes of embolectomy – a transverse incision may be preferable and, unlike an arteriotomy in a large vessel, it should be closed with interrupted sutures. Closure of an arteriotomy is most commonly performed with a continuous suture seeking to obtain slight eversion of the cut edges, and to encourage intimal apposition with exclusion of the non-intimal layers from the lumen. As the end of the closure is approached, it may become more difficult to ensure that all layers are included in the stitch. It is therefore advisable that a separate end stitch should be placed at the opposite end of the incision, as shown in Figure 5.6. When dealing with medium to small vessels (as distinct from microsurgery), the

use of magnification (×2–4) by means of loupes, or spectacles fitted with binocular lenses, is often advisable. Accurate suturing is more important in vascular surgery than in most other areas.

A clean sharp injury to an artery may occur iatrogenically during surgery on adjacent structures, or may be the result of penetrating trauma. Repair is as for the closure of an arteriotomy, but see the section on vascular trauma below.

Vein patch

Closure of an arteriotomy must not result in any significant narrowing. Simple sutured closure of a longitudinal incision in any artery smaller in diameter than the common femoral will commonly cause unacceptable narrowing. Unacceptable narrowing will also occur on the closure of an arteriotomy in a segment of diseased common femoral artery. A vein patch should be used in any such closure (Fig. 5.7). Autogenous saphenous vein is the most suitable material for a vein patch as the thinner-walled jugular or cephalic veins are less able to withstand arterial pressure. The proximal part of the long saphenous vein should not be sacrificed for this as it may be required for future reconstructive vascular surgery. A suitable patch can be harvested from the ankle, or often more conveniently from one of the groin tributaries to the sapheno-femoral junction. The ends of the patch are where technical difficulties arise. It is therefore recommended to

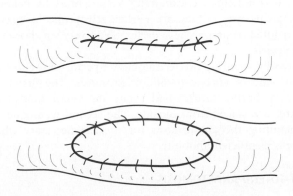

Figure 5.7 *Simple closure of an arteriotomy may result in a stenosed segment. This can be avoided by using a vein patch.*

start with a double-armed suture at one side, to work around the ends, and to complete the anastomosis at the opposite side. A patch of *expanded polytetrafluoroethylene* (*e-PTFE*) or Dacron can be used if no suitable vein is available.

Balloon embolectomy

The slender balloon embolectomy catheter, originally designed by Fogarty,[4] is available in sizes 3 to 7 F. It is 80 cm long and has a delicate inflatable balloon close to its tip. The catheter is threaded into the artery through an arteriotomy, to a level beyond which no clots are thought to be present. The balloon is then inflated with sterile saline until slight resistance is felt, and the catheter is withdrawn with the balloon inflated, bringing with it any clots present within the lumen. The inflation should be gradually increased to match the widening calibre of the artery if the catheter is being withdrawn from the distal arterial tree. If it is being withdrawn from larger proximal arteries, the balloon must be gradually reduced in size. Gentleness is essential to minimize intimal damage. Atheromatous plaques can be felt as areas of roughness as the balloon is drawn up or down the artery. The artery may narrow significantly at these points, and if the operator does not actively let fluid in or out at each point significant damage can result, including stripping of the endothelium. A similar technique can be employed for thrombotic occlusion of a bypass graft. In a synthetic graft, which lacks an intimal lining, successful clearance can be achieved even after several days have elapsed.

Vascular anastomoses

There are many different techniques for joining blood vessels to each other, or to synthetic grafts. In constructing an end-to-end anastomosis, care must be taken to avoid narrowing the lumen, and it is always preferable, except in the largest vessels, to bevel the ends (see Fig. 5.9). It is usually more convenient to use continuous sutures, but interrupted sutures should be used in children where subsequent growth is anticipated. Children's vessels must be handled with great care as they are particularly prone to spasm. Interrupted sutures are also preferable in very small or delicate vessels.

Broadly, there are two techniques for performing either an end-to-end or an end-to-side anastomosis. The first is to place anchoring sutures and rotate the vessel so that all sutures are placed from outside. The second technique, of parachuting the anastomosis together, is necessary when there is insufficient mobility.

END-TO-END ANASTOMOSIS

In an end-to-end anastomosis, three interrupted anchoring sutures are placed equidistantly around the circumference

and used to rotate the vessel for access during the remainder of the anastomosis (Fig. 5.8). This technique is only possible where the mobility of the vessel is not impaired by branches. More commonly, a posterior row of continuous sutures is initially placed intra-luminally, with the cut ends of the vessel still some distance apart (Fig. 5.9). The frictionless quality of polypropylene allows the ends to be *parachuted* together. The front of the anastomosis is then completed from without, using both ends of the double-armed suture. The clamp is released before the two ends of the suture are tied together. The returning blood distends the anastomosis and prevents too tight a tie causing a 'purse-string' stenosis. Minor leakage from an anastomosis will cease after local pressure. A significant leak will require a further suture, and clamps should be reapplied before doing this as the vessel may tear and the situation worsen. Areas of leak in an anastomosis can be sutured with a figure-of-eight or a mattress suture. The suture can be buttressed with a Dacron or e-PTFE pledget. This is a particularly helpful manoeuvre if the reason for leakage is that the vessel is tearing, and it is commonly used for leaks at the top end of an aortic graft.

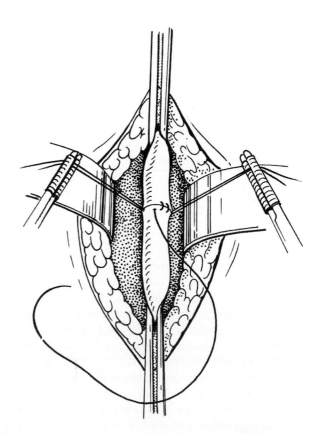

Figure 5.8 *Interrupted anchoring sutures are placed first to unite the vessel equidistantly around the circumference. The ends of these sutures are left long and held in forceps. The anastomosis is then performed with a continuous suture between these anchoring sutures which are used to rotate the vessel for access. The continuous suture should slightly evert the edges.*

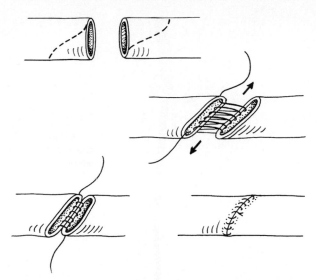

Figure 5.9 *When access or mobility is too poor for the technique illustrated in Figure 5.8, a running, posterior monofilament suture draws the ends together and is continued around the front of the vessel.*

END-TO-SIDE ANASTOMOSIS

An end-to-side anastomosis follows similar principles. It is commonly placed between a diseased vessel and a bypass graft of either vein or synthetic material. An arteriotomy in the vessel – the length of which is two or three times the diameter of the graft – forms the 'side' for the anastomosis. The 'end' of the artery, vein or synthetic graft is bevelled, as this allows it to lie naturally, reduces the angles of flow both into and out of it, and produces a wider end for the anastomosis. An incorrect angle will predispose to folding or kinking. If access is unrestricted a double-armed suture is placed first at the 'heel' and a second similar suture at the 'toe' (Fig. 5.10). All sutures can then be placed from without. If access is more restricted, a double-armed suture is placed at the heel and then the back row of continuous sutures placed from within before the ends are 'parachuted' into apposition. The anterior portion of the anastomosis is then completed from without (Fig. 5.11).

Endarterectomy

The atherosclerotic pathology which occludes arteries is mainly within the intima, with a variable extension into the media. It is possible to find a surgical plane of cleavage between the atheromatous plaques and the relatively healthy vessel wall. A variable thickness of media will thus be excised with the atheroma. Endarterectomy is undertaken through an arteriotomy with proximal and distal arterial control, as described above. It is important to leave a smooth interior to the cleared artery. This can be difficult when there is thickened, but less severely affected, intima beyond the limit of the excision. In particular, any intimal step at the distal extent of the excision must be avoided as the blood flow will

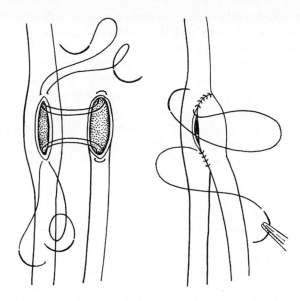

Figure 5.10 *The initial anchoring sutures have been placed at the heel and toe of the anastomosis between the native artery and the vein graft, and as access is unrestricted the remainder of the anastomosis will be completed from without.*

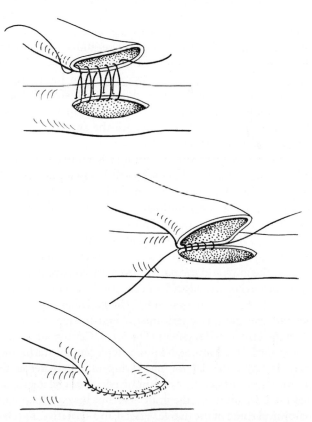

Figure 5.11 *When access is limited, the initial stitch with a double-armed suture should be at the heel, and the back of the anastomosis is completed from within in a similar fashion to that illustrated in Figure 5.9. The front of the anastomosis is performed from without and on completion the two ends of the suture are tied together.*

tend to lift residual plaque off the vessel wall, with the risk of dissection. If a gently shelving intimal plaque edge cannot be achieved then fine sutures may have to be used to hold this thickened intima against the vessel wall. The arteriotomy is then closed, most frequently with a vein patch. Endarterectomy has now been superseded in most situations by reconstructive arterial surgery with bypass grafts, or alternatively by angioplasty. It is, however, still the most appropriate operation for carotid stenosis, and carotid endarterectomy is described in more detail in Chapter 6.

VASCULAR RECONSTRUCTION

Vascular reconstruction with grafts may be required for a long congenital stenosis or for trauma where a segment of vessel wall has been lost or severely damaged. In these situations the surgeon is handling healthy artery above and below the area that has to be replaced. However, the commonest indication for reconstructive arterial surgery is, unfortunately, in patients with degenerative arterial disease causing stenosis, occlusion or aneurysmal dilatation. The patient has generalized disease throughout the arterial tree. The arteries to which the surgeon has to anastomose a graft are often affected at least to some degree by the same process. Vessels both proximal and distal to the operation site are also affected and outflow, or inflow, may be compromised. Most importantly, the patient is by definition carrying an increased risk of complications due to occlusive disease in vessels supplying vital organs – the brain, kidneys and heart. All of these factors should influence the surgical decisions and are discussed further in Chapter 6.

Vascular reconstruction in trauma is commonly with a replacement graft of vein, or prosthetic material, used to bridge the defect between undamaged proximal and distal portions of the artery. Autologous vein is preferable if there has been penetrative trauma. This is best harvested from the contralateral limb in order to avoid exacerbating any potential venous compromise. Two end-to-end anastomoses between the graft and the native vessel are constructed.

Vascular reconstruction for occlusive degenerative disease is more often with a bypass graft. The native artery is left *in situ* and the graft is anastomosed end-to-side above and below the obstructed segment (Fig. 5.12). Certain advantages are claimed over an end-to-end replacement technique. There is less potential for narrowing of the vessel at the anastomoses, dissection is minimized, and collaterals are preserved. In addition, the graft does not have to follow the anatomical route of the native vessel if an alternative is preferable. In-flow above the graft must be adequate, and a good run-off into distal vessels is essential for success. Vascular reconstruction for aortic aneurysmal disease is commonly with an *in-lay* technique. The aneurysm is opened and the graft placed within it. The anastomosis is end-to-end, but half of its circumference is sutured from within (Fig. 5.13).

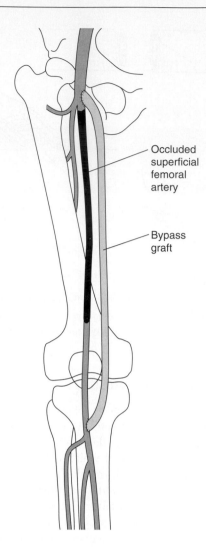

Occluded superficial femoral artery

Bypass graft

Figure 5.12 *A bypass graft with end-to-side anastomoses is frequently used for reconstruction in occlusive vascular disease. The diseased native vessel is left* in situ.

Autologous vein

Autologous vein is the material of choice for reconstruction of small and medium-sized arteries. A successful vein graft quickly becomes thickened to take on many of the characteristics of an artery. A normal long saphenous vein is the ideal substitute for an artery of comparable size. If the long saphenous vein is unavailable, or diseased, then alternative superficial arm veins can be used, and for coronary artery surgery the internal mammary vein is a suitable alternative. The vein may be used to bridge a gap resulting from the excision of an injured segment, or to bypass a diseased segment.

'Vein harvest' must be meticulous to avoid unnecessary trauma to the vein, and is described in more detail in Chapter 6. All tributaries must be identified and ligated

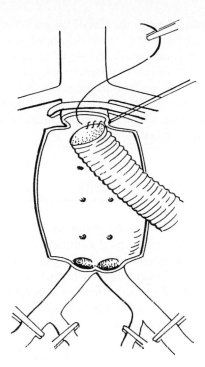

Figure 5.13 *An in-lay technique is suitable for the graft replacement of an aortic aneurysm. The aneurysm is opened and the graft laid within it. The back of both the proximal and the distal anastomosis is sutured from within.*

2–3 mm from the main vein in order to avoid crimping of the adventitia. When the vein is removed from its bed, it is then commonly *reversed* to avoid the effect of its valves. It is sutured end-to-end to bridge a traumatic defect, or end-to-side as a bypass for obliterative disease. The suturing methods are described above. The vein should be sutured under a moderate degree of tension, otherwise it stretches when arterial blood is admitted, becomes tortuous and prone to thrombotic occlusion. A vein graft, which is to be used for a bypass in the thigh, may be left 'in situ'. It is exposed, isolated and its tributaries ligated in a similar manner, but it is not lifted from its bed in the subcutaneous fat. The proximal end-to-side anastomosis is then performed and the vein graft is allowed to fill from above, which shows the locations of the venous valves. The valves are then cut with a valvulotome inserted into the vein from below. Valvotomy can also be performed under direct vision using angioscopy.

Prosthetic grafts

Prosthetic grafts are satisfactory for the reconstruction of large arteries in situations where a vein graft is seldom practical due to considerations of size. They are inferior to vein grafts for the reconstruction of small arteries, but are an alternative for smaller vessels when a vein graft is not possible. Indeed, with recent improvements in graft material and surgical techniques, the long-term patency of synthetic grafts, even when carried down to the ankle, continues to improve. They are more prone to clotting at low flow velocities and, in addition, platelet adhesion is a greater problem than in vein grafts. This will occur especially where blood flow is turbulent, and the distal end-to-side configuration on a small vessel is particularly vulnerable.[5] Cuffs and patches of vein have been incorporated into these distal anastomoses in an attempt to improve patency (Fig. 5.14), and when insufficient vein is available for a whole bypass a composite graft can be formed reserving the vein for the distal portion. Prosthetic grafts do not become lined by endothelium, but a smooth inner luminal surface develops which consists mainly of collagen.

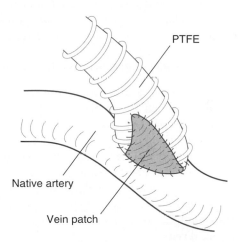

Figure 5.14 *Vein is the ideal graft material for distal reconstruction, but insufficient vein may be available. A cuff or a patch of vein incorporated into the anastomosis between the synthetic graft and the native vessel may improve long-term patency.*

DACRON

Dacron has proved a durable replacement for the aorta and iliac vessels. It is less suitable for distal vessels as it becomes less flexible with time, and damage to its structure occurs where it crosses joints. The inert polymer thread is woven or knitted to form a straight tube, or bifurcated graft, of varying sizes. Knitted grafts have the advantage of greater porosity which allows more in-growth of native tissue, but the initial porosity necessitates pre-clotting unless they have already been sealed during the manufacturing process with collagen, gelatin or albumin. These sealing agents prevent initial porosity and leakage, but as they are absorbed tissue in-growth can occur. These grafts are now in routine use, and most operating theatres in the UK do not stock grafts that require pre-clotting. *Pre-clotting* may still have to be performed by those surgeons working under financial restrictions. About 20 mL of the patient's own unheparinized blood is passed through the prepared unsealed knitted Dacron graft to coat the interior. The residual blood is left in a dish and, after about 4 minutes this residual blood will be seen to have clotted. This indicates that blood will also have clotted in the pores of the graft and partially sealed them. The procedure is then repeated twice more with further unheparinized blood. On each occasion clotting occurs faster as activated clotting factors accumulate in the graft wall. The pores of the graft are now sealed with fibrin and platelets, and any excess clot is squeezed out of the lumen. Heparin (20 000 units) is then mixed with 50 mL of blood and flushed through the graft. This both reverses the thrombogenic potential of the build-up of mural activated clotting factors and checks for residual leaks.

Dacron is also valuable as a patch when vein is unavailable. A small piece can be used as a buttress over which a suture is tied when suturing friable diseased arterial wall, and a collar of Dacron can be placed over an aortic anastomosis to support the vessel wall.

EXPANDED POLYTETRAFLUOROETHYLENE (E-PTFE)

e-PTFE retains flexibility and is usually preferred for infrainguinal bypass, although recent trials have shown little difference between the patency rates of e-PTFE and Dacron. The material is non-compliant and stitch holes will leak. Small-diameter needles should therefore be used. It also has no longitudinal elasticity, and tension must be avoided – in contrast to the technique with a vein graft where tortuosity is of greater concern. Research continues into other graft material and into modifications of biological material such as human umbilical vein.

Assessment of vascular reconstruction

Assessment of flow at the end of any reconstructive procedure is important, and on-table angiography is the 'gold standard'. Failure of a graft in the first few hours is usually due to a technical failure which could have been detected before the wound was closed. The graft may be twisted, kinked or tortuous. Alternatively, there may be residual undetected clot in the distal vasculature, or an anastomosis may be leaking and the resultant haematoma is compressing the graft. Re-exploration is mandatory.

Failure of a vein or prosthetic graft may occur early or late as a result of thrombosis. Long-term patency of vein grafts is superior to that of prosthetic grafts, and this difference increases in smaller vessel reconstructions. Late atheroma and stenosis can develop within a vein graft, but more commonly there is disease progression in the native vessels that impedes the inflow or the outflow. Aneurysmal change, in which the vein becomes tortuous and dilated, can also occur. Sluggish flow then predisposes to thrombosis. Tortuosity, dilatation and atheromatous stenosis do not occur within prosthetic grafts. However, the bond between the prosthesis and the native vessel remains vulnerable and late anastomotic disruption and false aneurysm formation may occur. Infection is a major concern with prosthetic grafts, but less so with vein grafts.[6] Once established, infection is very difficult to eradicate and usually heralds the loss of the graft. Grafts impregnated with antibiotics have been developed in an attempt to overcome this complication. Prophylactic antibiotic cover is routine for all reconstructive vascular surgery.

Grafting techniques in different anatomical locations and varying circumstances are discussed in Chapter 6, where the surgical challenges of the occluded, disrupted and infected graft are also addressed.

MICROVASCULAR SURGERY

Advances in operating microscopes, miniature instruments, suture materials and surgical techniques have led to the development of microsurgery, mainly as a subspecialty of plastic surgery. It has enabled reconstruction of arteries previously considered too small for any attempt to be worthwhile. Digital vessels can be repaired, and the small nutrient arteries of free flaps anastomosed to allow free tissue transfer. This is discussed in more detail in Chapter 1. Microvascular surgery is restricted to specialist units, where the volume of work is such that expertise can be developed, and patients should be transferred to these centres.

RADIOLOGICAL INTERVENTIONAL ALTERNATIVES

Minimally invasive endoluminal vascular interventions have found an increasing place in the management of vascular pathology.[7] *Angioscopy* is performed by some vascular surgeons, but for most intra-luminal procedures reliance is placed on radiological imaging. The minimally invasive intra-luminal techniques have in the main been developed by radiologists, as an extension to their diagnostic angiography skills. Interventional radiologists work in close cooperation with vascular surgeons and there is considerable cross-over between the disciplines. The most appropriate management for an individual patient will depend not only on the vascular lesion which is present but also on the patient's overall condition and on the skills and facilities that are available.

A femoral artery approach is the most versatile for interventional procedures, but the brachial artery is an alternative. Floppy-ended catheters can be passed up the femoral artery into the aorta, or any of its branches, under X-ray control. They can be advanced into the left heart. The catheter can be used for injection of contrast for angiography. In the *Seldinger* technique a floppy-ended guide wire is advanced to the appropriate position and a catheter is then introduced over the guide wire. This is a standard method of delivering a balloon catheter or stent through a stricture.

Angioplasties

Angioplasties are a satisfactory alternative to reconstructive surgery for many arterial stenoses. Inflation of the balloon splits the atheromatous plaque and enlarges the lumen. In general, this approach is more successful in short stenoses. The success of a false lumen created by the accidental sub-intimal passage of the balloon has led to deliberate sub-intimal angioplasties with superior results in some centres for long strictures. Angioplasty is also appropriate for fibromuscular stenoses. However, these frequently re-stenose quickly and consideration must be given to primary stenting or surgery.

Stents

Stents can be introduced using a similar technique and allowed to expand once in position. They may be employed to maintain a lumen after dilatation of a large artery. Intraluminal stenting of aortic aneurysms is now an established technique, though its value is still under review. Venous stents (introduced through the femoral vein) may maintain iliac venous patency when the vein is compressed by malignant pelvic lymph nodes.

Fibrinolysis

Fibrinolysis is now often a superior alternative to surgery in an acutely ischaemic limb, provided that the limb is not so acutely threatened that any further delay would be critical to tissue survival. *Streptokinase* and other newer agents are delivered into the clot via a catheter sited at angiography. Streptokinase is strongly antigenic, and repeat treatment risks anaphylactic reactions. The more expensive *tissue plasminogen activator* (*t-PA*) is safer, and is widely used by vascular surgeons because it is much more effective in clearing both occluded grafts and the large vessels of the lower limbs. A variety of regimes have been developed with slow infusion, pulsed-spray delivery and high-dose bolus infusion. In some methods there is a mechanical element to the clot disruption in addition to the pharmacological. During treatment there is often an initial deterioration in perfusion and a worsening of ischaemic pain as the clot fragments, and careful monitoring and pain relief are essential. Although the fibrinolytic agent is delivered locally, there is a systemic risk of haemorrhagic complications, exacerbated by the need to keep the patient fully anticoagulated with heparin. These have to be balanced against the alternative risk of operative intervention. Trial data suggest that female patients over 80 years of age are particularly prone to haemorrhagic complications.

Embolization

Embolization of arteriovenous malformations and inaccessible bleeding arterial vessels is another area where the interventional radiologist may be able to achieve better results than conventional surgery. In both situations vascular obliteration is desired at the site of the pathology, but at open operation the surgeon can often only ligate feeding vessels. This is less satisfactory as inflow is re-established from collateral vessels.

BASIC VENOUS SURGICAL TECHNIQUES

Many of the basic vascular techniques are similar for arteries and veins. Principles of proximal and distal vascular control are similar. Venous bleeding may be profuse but local pressure – and the utilization of gravity to reduce venous pressure – will normally control the immediate problem. A small vein can then nearly always be safely ligated. A large vein can be sutured in a similar fashion to an artery, but the wall is more delicate, and more elastic. Venous thrombectomy and embolectomy have been virtually replaced by intra-vascular thrombolytic techniques.

Vein has, however, proved to be the ideal material for arterial reconstruction. A small piece of long saphenous vein can be harvested and shaped into a patch or cuff, as discussed above. A short segment of vein can form a bridge between arterial ends severed by trauma, and a longer length of long saphenous vein is the ideal bypass graft for infra-inguinal occlusive arterial disease. These techniques are discussed in more detail above and in the relevant sections of the next chapter.

Venous reconstructive surgery has been disappointing in comparison with the results for arteries, as the low velocity flow in veins predisposes to thrombus formation. Sophisticated techniques, sometimes involving the creation of a controlled arteriovenous fistula to increase flow, have however been associated with success and are discussed in more detail in Chapter 6. Arteriovenous fistulae are also created for venous access for renal dialysis and are described in Chapter 6.

VARICOSE VEINS

Patient demand for the treatment of varicose veins is high. Many patients are only troubled by the unsightly dilated superficial veins, but others complain of aching legs on standing. A minority have complications of chronic venous insufficiency, including venous eczema, lipodermatosclerosis and chronic venous ulceration. Varicose vein surgery should be strongly advised for those who are developing signs of venous hypertension, when it can be shown that venous reflux into superficial veins is a major contributory factor. In 40 per cent of cases varicose veins will be the sole cause, and in a further 40 per cent there is a mixed superficial and deep component. However, venous hypertension in 20 per cent is due to deep venous incompetence and insufficiency alone. These patients may attribute their symptoms to their coexistent varicose veins, but simple varicose vein surgery will offer little benefit, and may even harm these patients.

Careful preoperative assessment of patients with varicose veins is essential.[8]

AETIOLOGY AND ASSESSMENT

The majority (80 per cent) of varicose veins originate from the long saphenous vein (LSV). Either the entire LSV or the segment below the mid-thigh perforator is incompetent. However, the remaining 20 per cent of varicose veins originate from the short saphenous vein (SSV) and therefore require a different approach. The proportion of limbs demonstrating calf perforator and SSV reflux grows as the burden of chronic venous insufficiency increases,[9] such that over one-third of patients with a leg ulcer will have SSV disease on duplex scanning. Careful preoperative assessment is therefore essential. Given the labour-intensive nature and often limited availability of colour-flow Doppler scanning, a pragmatic approach is to perform a clinical and hand-held Doppler assessment on all patients with varicose veins in the out-patient department, referring those with either ambiguous distribution of reflux, or audible venous reflux in the popliteal fossa to the vascular laboratory for further imaging. Reflux heard while insonating over the popliteal fossa or the posterior aspect of the calf is difficult to interpret, even by the most experienced clinicians. Furthermore, an unnecessary exploration and/or failure to find an unusually situated sapheno-popliteal junction are hazards that can be minimized by the judicious use of preoperative duplex.

Duplex scanning provides anatomical and physiological information that is invaluable, and is increasingly employed in the routine preoperative assessment. In patients with recurrent varicose veins and those with complications of chronic venous insufficiency this assessment has increasing importance. It is only after a full assessment that optimum treatment can be planned.

ANATOMY

The *great saphenous vein* is almost universally known to surgeons in the UK as the *long saphenous vein*, and this more familiar name is therefore used in the text. It commences on the medial aspect of the foot and lies along the medial aspect of the limb in the subcutaneous fat until its termination at the sapheno-femoral junction. It passes in front of the medial malleolus at the ankle, and behind the femoral condyle at the knee. Superficial tributaries, and connections with the short saphenous system are variable. There are, however, always several tributaries to the proximal few cm of the vein. There are also connections with the deep venous system via *perforators* (veins which perforate the deep fascia). In the thigh, perforators form a junction with the long saphenous vein itself; in the leg the junction is with a posterior tributary of the LSV, the posterior arch vein (Fig. 5.15).

The *small saphenous vein* is also more commonly known by its old name of the *short saphenous vein*. It is formed on the lateral side of the foot, ascends behind the lateral malleolus, and lies on the lateral and then posterior aspect of the leg until its termination at the sapheno-popliteal junction. To reach its termination, the vein must pierce the dense deep fascia of the popliteal fossa, and this occurs at a variable point

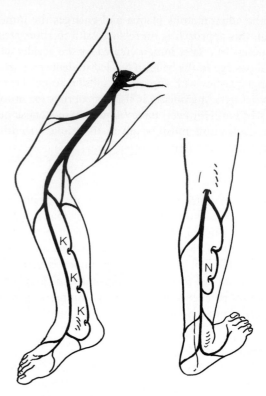

Figure 5.15 *The anatomy of superficial veins is very variable except for the main long and short saphenous trunks. The thigh perforators communicate directly with the long saphenous vein (LSV). Below the knee the perforators marked N and K communicate only with tributaries of the main trunks.*

from the upper mid calf to just above the skin crease behind the knee. The sapheno-popliteal junction is also variable in position, as is the length of vein lying beneath the fascia. This anatomical variation is itself a strong indication for routine duplex scanning prior to short saphenous surgery.

Sclerotherapy

Injection sclerotherapy was widely practised for many years, but its use declined when it became clear that lasting benefits were rare and that there were frequent skin complications. Good results can, however, be obtained by injection sclerotherapy alone in a selected group of patients who have minor cosmetic varices that are not associated with an incompetent sapheno-femoral or sapheno-popliteal junction. Incompetent junctions require surgical ligation, after which sclerotherapy can be successful in closing any residual varices. A delay of around 6 weeks will allow any natural improvement to occur and avoid unnecessary treatment. However, as most of the dilated superficial veins can be removed at the time of surgery by a combination of venous stripping and avulsions, many vascular surgeons have abandoned sclerotherapy entirely.

Sapheno-femoral ligation (Trendelenberg)

The incision is centred 1 cm below and 2 cm lateral to the pubic tubercle. If the groin crease is at this level it is often convenient to use this as it gives a superior cosmetic result. However, in obese patients the skin crease may not be at the desired level for exploration and it is often affected by intertrigo and more prone to infection. The vein is usually palpable with the patient standing and can be marked pre-operatively. Alternatively, pulsation of the femoral artery lying immediately lateral is a useful landmark. The incision is deepened through the subcutaneous fat, and then through a membranous layer of superficial fascia (Scarpa's fascia). The vein lies in the fat, deep to this layer. The vein is cleared proximally and distally, either by sharp dissection or by gentle blunt dissection, until its termination in the femoral vein and all its tributaries are exposed (Fig. 5.16a). The saphenous vein must not be divided until it has been unequivocally identified. The common femoral vein must be clearly seen to continue both proximally and distally to the sapheno-femoral junction. It is usually a different colour to the LSV and a small external pudendal artery usually – but by no means always – crosses transversely between the two veins. The medial and lateral sides of the common femoral vein should be exposed, both to confirm the anatomy and to ensure that the medial tributaries that can cause vulval varices are divided (or simply ligated if space is restricted). The multiple tributaries to the sapheno-femoral junction and the proximal LSV are then ligated and divided. The counsel of perfection suggests that these tributaries should be pursued to the first division and then each tributary ligated separately at this level. Dividing the tributaries out at their first division makes recurrence from the formation of collateral channels less likely than if the ligated tributaries are lying in close proximity to the saphenous stump. The LSV is then divided between artery forceps close to the sapheno-femoral junction, so that the stump can be suture ligated in such a way that that there is no deformity of the common femoral vein (Fig. 5.16b). Pinching this vessel with a stitch, or leaving an over-long stump of LSV, are both likely to increase the risk of deep venous thrombosis. The distal cut end of the LSV is then ligated if no strip is to be undertaken.

If at any stage major venous bleeding occurs, the greatest danger is that the surgeon – in his or her anxiety to arrest haemorrhage – may apply artery forceps blindly in the depths of the wound, and by so doing may cause damage to the femoral artery or vein. Firm pressure with a gauze swab and reduction of venous pressure by lowering the head of the table should be initiated instead, and maintained for *5 minutes,* before the damage is reassessed. By this time bleeding will have almost ceased and the application of artery forceps to a vessel from which a clip or ligature has slipped, or the repair of a femoral vein tear, will be relatively easy.

Most surgeons combine this operation with a strip of the LSV between the groin and the knee, as if it is left *in situ* the chance of recurrent varicose veins is higher.[10] If the strip is extended much below the knee, the risk of damage to the

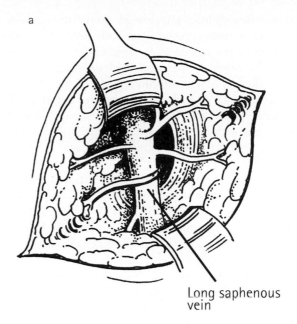

Long saphenous vein

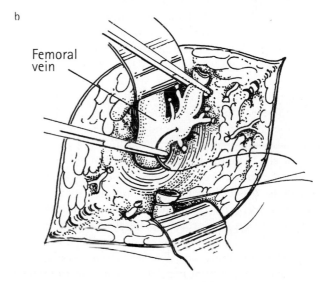

Femoral vein

Figure 5.16 *Sapheno-femoral ligation. (a) The terminal few centimetres of the LSV and its tributaries are exposed. (b) The tributaries are ligated and divided. The proximal end of the LSV is lifted forwards to display the sapheno-femoral junction and any remaining tributaries. Finally, the LSV is transfixed flush with the femoral vein.*

great saphenous nerve increases significantly. A few surgeons pursue a selective policy and preserve the vein if it is of small diameter and the thigh perforators are competent. This decision should be based on accurate preoperative assessment, including duplex scanning. The removal of a relatively normal LSV deprives the patient of a potential donor vein.

Groin surgery for recurrent varicose veins

Surgery for recurrent varicose veins is associated with significantly more morbidity and poorer patient satisfaction than varicose vein surgery in an unoperated groin. The commonest causes of recurrence associated with reflux from the groin include failure of complete sapheno-femoral disconnection at the original operation, and neovascularization that has resulted in new connections between the common femoral vein and a LSV which was not stripped but left *in situ* in the thigh.[11] Recurrence can also occur through a mid-thigh perforator with reflux carried up to the groin in a persistent LSV. Preoperative imaging by duplex – or less commonly now, by varicography – is essential. If a significant connection at the groin is demonstrated, then re-exploration of the groin should be considered. However, if the groin component is trivial and the LSV is being fed by a thigh perforator, stripping from the level of the knee to the perforator, leaving the groin untouched, should be considered.

Re-exploration of the groin is indicated when there are recurrent varicose veins associated with significant groin reflux. The saphenous vein may not have been tied flush at the original operation and juxta-femoral tributaries may have been left *in situ*. Reflux is continuing through these and still filling the distal superficial veins. Alternatively, there may have been failure in the identification of the LSV at the original procedure, and a large tributary – or one arm of a double saphenous system – may have been mistaken for the LSV itself. In these instances re-exploration can be fairly straightforward, but it must be remembered that the surrounding scar tissue has greater tensile strength than these veins, which are easily torn – particularly if blunt dissection is used. Veins formed by neovascularization are thin-walled vessels and are thus very difficult to dissect. They also lie anterior to the femoral vein. It is therefore recommended that in re-exploration the femoral vein is approached laterally through unscarred territory.

The skin incision is usually placed transversely, though some advocate a vertical incision, just medial to the pulsation of the artery, allowing a greater longitudinal exposure of the common femoral vein. During dissection it is important to remember that a lymph leak is a frequent complication. The lymphatic vessels run in the line of the blood vessels, and transverse division of tissue without ligation should be avoided. The anterior surface of the femoral artery is identified first and this leads the dissection to the correct level to identify the anterior surface of the femoral vein. All tissue passing anteriorly from the vein can then be isolated and divided. One way of doing this is to identify a clear portion of the common femoral vein above and below the level of the recurrence, and then pass a tie or suture around the mass of scar tissue lying anteriorly. This will contain any remaining sapheno-femoral junction, whether veins missed at the original operation or thin-walled veins from neovascularization. In recurrent groin surgery for varicose veins, the LSV should always be stripped if it was left *in situ* at the original operation.

Vein stripping

The stripper consists of a length of wire or plastic which can be passed along a vein from one opening into the vein to another. The portion of vein between is then stripped out under the intact skin (Fig. 5.17). A rigid metal 'pin-stripper' is favoured by some surgeons. The technique is used most frequently for the removal of the LSV in the thigh after the completion of a sapheno-femoral ligation, but the technique is also applicable to other lengths of superficial vein. Stripping down from the groin distally is considered by some surgeons to be preferable to stripping towards the groin, but the traditional strippers can be introduced from either end as the heads are detachable and interchangeable (Fig. 5.17). Stripping techniques that invaginate the vein are gaining popularity as they cause less trauma to adjacent tissue.

A long saphenous strip is performed after completion of the groin dissection. The LSV should be exposed in the groin for as much length distally as is possible as there is often a large medial upper thigh tributary, which can be ligated

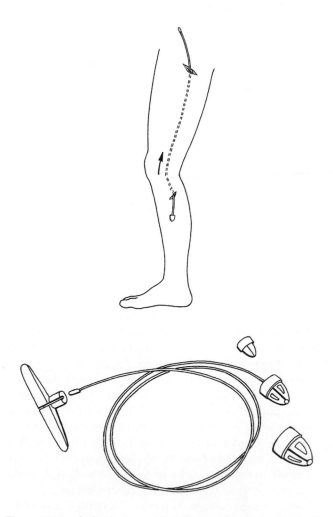

Figure 5.17   *A plastic disposable stripper with a range of sizes of 'olive' or 'acorn' heads. The subcutaneous route of the stripper, in a strip of the LSV from knee to groin, is shown with a dotted line.*

reducing the chance of a groin haematoma. Identification also lessens the likelihood of entering this tributary with the stripper if it is passed from above.

Traditionally, the LSV is exposed below the knee by a small incision over a skin mark placed preoperatively to mark a suitable site. The vein is isolated, an artery forceps insinuated beneath it, and a second artery forceps applied across the vein. A loose ligature is then placed around the vein above this point and held in artery forceps. A small incision is made into the vein between the artery forceps and the loose ligature. The stripper, with a small blunt head attached, is introduced and advanced beyond the loose ligature which is then ligated snugly to prevent bleeding (Fig. 5.18a). The vein has then to be fully divided and the distal end ligated (Fig. 5.18b). It may however be preferable to delay this until the stripper has been successfully threaded along the whole length of the vein, as it provides additional stability. The stripper should be palpable through the skin throughout its course. If it catches in a trib-

utary or varix, then guidance by pressure from without, combined with partial withdrawal and rotation of the stripper, will usually allow it to pass. If this manoeuvre is unsuccessful, an additional incision may be made over the vein at the point where the stripper has stuck, and the vein may have to be removed in segments. A stripper which becomes impalpable may have entered the deep veins and must be withdrawn with great care to avoid damage.

The stripper head finally presents in the groin wound within the distal stump of the LSV to which the artery forceps is still applied. A loose ligature is placed around the vein a few centimetres below the forceps, and a small incision made through which the head can be delivered (Fig. 5.18c). The ligature is then tied. A larger acorn- or olive-shaped head is then attached to one end of the stripper and traction on the other end will deliver the stripper, with the avulsed vein attached, out through the wound (Fig. 5.18d). Tributaries and perforators will be avulsed, and it is important to reduce

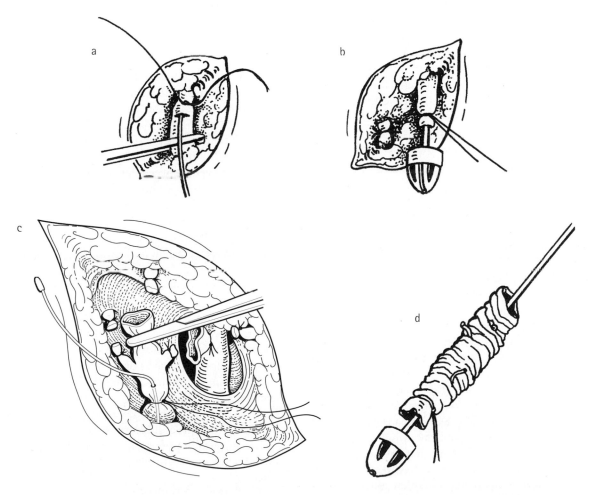

Figure 5.18 *(a) A ligature has been placed around the LSV, which has been isolated just below the knee. The stripper is passed through a small incision in the vein and guided through the loose ligature. (b) The ligature has been tightened to prevent back-bleeding, and the stripper has reached the groin. The vein is fully divided and the distal end ligated. (c) A loose ligature has been placed around the LSV in the groin, just below the forceps on the divided distal end. The stripper is guided through this ligature, which is then tightened, and then delivered out through a small incision in the vein. (d) The stripper has been pulled out and the whole length of the avulsed vein is telescoped against the stripper head.*

haemorrhage by tilting the table head down a few minutes prior to stripping if the entire operation has not been performed in this position. The limb is either bandaged, or has a compression stocking applied, as soon as the wounds are closed. Therefore, if any additional surgery is necessary, such as multiple phlebectomies, the final delivery of stripper and vein should be postponed until this has been completed.

Retrograde introduction of the stripper from the groin has the advantage that only a very small incision is needed at the distal end. After completion of the groin dissection, the stripper is introduced into the LSV, with a single throw tie around the vein to control bleeding. The stripper is advanced down the vein. Often, the first valve is partially intact and this must be broken. If this area of vein can be visualized this can reassure the surgeon that the sudden 'give' was not the stripper passing out of the vein. The stripper can be followed by palpation as it passes to just above, or below, the knee and here a small incision is made for retrieval of the stripper. At this point the tie on the proximal end should be completed. Artery forceps are passed through the small distal incision and the LSV, with the stripper within it, is grasped and firmly pulled. The vein may tear but the stripper will come through the skin. If the vein is intact, a small venotomy is made and the distal portion of the stripper delivered. The stripper is then pulled down and, without an acorn head the vein will invert and come through a very small cut in the skin. Some surgeons use a large acorn and strip down, but do not deliver the vein and acorn out through the lower incision. Instead, before the vein is stripped, a long heavy tie is attached to the acorn. This allows the vein to be pulled back up again, after stripping and distal division, for delivery in the groin.

Short saphenous ligation

The position of the sapheno-popliteal junction is very variable and, as the upper portion of the SSV is no longer easily palpable after it has pierced the fascia, it is important to mark the vein and its termination preoperatively by ultrasound. Patients must be anaesthetized in such a way that the airway is secure as they are turned into a prone position to afford surgical access to the popliteal fossa.

A transverse skin incision is made over the vein about 2 cm below its termination. The vein can be seen as a blue line through the deep fascia. The deep fascia is then divided in line with the skin incision, or vertically which gives better access. The vein is isolated by careful sharp dissection until an artery forceps can be passed deep to it, with care taken to avoid including the accompanying, and often adherent, sural nerve. The vein is divided between artery forceps and the distal end is then ligated. The proximal end is then followed deep into the popliteal fat to the sapheno-popliteal junction, and ligated flush with it. The finding of multiple tributaries from muscles heralds the approach of the junction. These are easy to tear, and tying them off is time-consuming and often difficult. There is frequently a superior tributary to the last

1 cm which is the termination of a superficial vein, and which may also communicate with the long saphenous system. It is important to ligate and divide this tributary as, if left, it is a source of recurrence. The sapheno-popliteal junction is not always a distinct T-junction as found in the groin, and the vein may terminate amongst a plexus of thin-walled deep veins. Over-zealous dissection may damage these and cause resultant haemorrhage which is difficult to control. There is also great anatomical variation. The SSV may enter the popliteal vein well above the popliteal skin crease, and on occasion an incompetent short saphenous vein may have no communication with the popliteal vein. The superior branch may be so large that it appears as a continuation of the main vein and there is only a short wide side communication between superficial and deep veins at the level of the popliteal skin crease. This variant must be considered as it can be damaged by rough passage of an instrument deep to the saphenous vein, especially if the preoperative marking has been misleading.

Perforating veins

A thigh strip will avulse all the significant thigh perforators. Alternatively, isolated incompetent perforating veins in the thigh can be ligated through a small incision after careful preoperative marking. The LSV is isolated above and below the junction with the perforating vein, which is also defined. Artery forceps are applied to the three limbs of the T-junction and the vein between divided. The ends are then ligated.

Perforating veins in the calf do not join the long saphenous vein directly, and stripping of the main vein to the ankle does not treat them (see Fig. 5.15). When surgery is indicated for incompetent calf perforators there are usually severe skin changes in the area, and incisions directly over the vessels are unlikely to heal satisfactorily. The skin is often also adherent to the underlying fascia. For these reasons a *sub-fascial* approach is preferable. The incision through skin and deep fascia is placed in healthier adjacent tissue, and the plane between the muscle and deep fascia developed. The perforating veins crossing this plane are ligated and divided. Preoperative marking of the perforators is unnecessary if the operation is to be performed using a minimal access technique. This subfascial endoscopic perforator surgery can be performed with fewer complications than the open operation, but the long-term benefit of either procedure has yet to be demonstrated.

The surgical options in chronic venous insufficiency including reconstructive venous techniques are discussed in Chapter 6.

VASCULAR TRAUMA

The proportion of a surgeon's vascular work which is related to trauma is extremely variable. Vascular injury is common in war situations, but is also frequent where there is a high level of urban violence. In many of these scenarios the conditions for complex vascular surgery may be sub-optimal, and the management of the vascular injuries will have to be tailored to the level of surgical and support facilities available and the vascular experience of the surgeon. In the UK, most vascular injuries are iatrogenic.

Iatrogenic vascular injuries

Vascular injuries that occur during open surgery are normally immediately obvious because of haemorrhage. Many are clean arterial incisions which can be closed as an arteriotomy, once vascular control has arrested the haemorrhage. Injuries to large veins can be repaired in a similar fashion, but it is often more appropriate simply to ligate a smaller vein. Iatrogenic injuries to the aorto-iliac vessels have been reported from the initial entry into the peritoneal cavity with a Veress needle at the start of laparoscopic surgery. These injuries may extend through the back wall of the vessel, and it is important to mobilize the vessel sufficiently so that the posterior wall can be checked and repaired if necessary.

The cannulation injury to an artery at angiography usually seals and heals uneventfully. However, a *false aneurysm* can form after femoral angiography, or more commonly after cardiac catheterization and angioplasty. If distal flow is satisfactory an operation can often be avoided. Ultrasonography is used to verify the connection with the artery. Local pressure with the ultrasound probe for 15–20 minutes over the leaking point can then induce thrombosis in the aneurysm. Many radiologists will inject thrombin, under ultrasound guidance, into a suitably sized aneurysm. However, larger lesions and those that are actively bleeding often require surgery. The associated co-morbidity – which is often the reason for the intervention in the first place – means that actively bleeding patients are often under-resuscitated, and this must be carefully corrected during the preoperative period. The co-morbidity also explains the high mortality in those patients who require surgical intervention. The smaller brachial artery is more likely to thrombose and occlude. The forearm is seldom threatened with critical ischaemia as there is a good collateral anastomosis around the elbow. However, long-term symptoms of forearm claudication may be troublesome, and if forearm muscle ischaemia is more severe a Volkman's contracture may ensue. Therefore, an occluded brachial artery after angiography should not be ignored. A balloon thrombectomy will usually restore flow, after which a formal repair can be undertaken. This will most often involve the repair of an intimal flap.

Trauma

Penetrative trauma may traverse a blood vessel wall. The damage can vary from a clean incision with a sharp knife to extensive destruction from a high-velocity bullet injury (see Chapter 3). Vascular injury can also occur in *blunt trauma*.

A spicule of fractured bone may lacerate a vessel, or a crushing, shearing or stretching force may contuse or tear the vessel wall. An adventitial haematoma from a crushing injury is relatively harmless, but an intimal split – which is common with a shearing injury – predisposes to the formation of secondary thrombus, or dissection of the arterial wall. Distal blood flow may be satisfactory on initial examination, but is then lost as thrombosis or dissection develops at the site of injury. If both the intima and media split, the vessel is held only by the adventitia and delayed rupture can occur, or occasionally a late aneurysmal dilatation develops.

Surgical intervention

The decision to explore an artery is straightforward if there is an overlying wound with profuse arterial bleeding and distal ischaemia. Often, the decision is more difficult and has to be based on the probabilities of an arterial injury. An arteriogram is invaluable in these circumstances and should be performed if at all possible.

EXPLORATION OF AN ARTERY

The exploration of an artery for traumatic damage is often a compromise between the exploration of the wound already present and the standard approach to the vessel described below. If there is profuse haemorrhage, this must be held in check until the vessel has been mobilized sufficiently to gain proximal and distal control. Surgical access may therefore be required first to a major vessel proximal to the site of injury for temporary inflow control. Brisk bleeding usually indicates a partially severed artery which is unable to contract. A completely severed artery will often close with intense spasm, and the contracted ends are found lying within a haematoma. Proximal and distal tapes should therefore be in position before an arterial haematoma is explored.

'Arterial spasm' associated with an injury is an unsafe diagnosis, and if good distal flow is not restored within 2–3 hours the artery must be explored, unless angiography has been performed which confirms continuity of the vessel and no evidence of arterial trauma. Discontinuity on an angiogram is not spasm. When an apparently intact, but contracted, artery is found at exploration it should be viewed with great suspicion. There is almost certainly damage to the intima in the form of a transverse split, and the spasm is secondary to this. Application of local vasodilator drugs may abolish the spasm and temporarily restore some distal flow, but this should not reassure the surgeon that there is no significant damage. Deterioration may occur later as the distal edge of an intimal tear rolls up to form a partially occluding flap on which thrombus develops. When an intact – but contracted and contused – artery is found it must be explored. The damage will be at the proximal end of the contracted segment. The damaged section of artery at the junction between the normal and contracted segments should be excised and continuity restored. In most situations a short venous bridging graft will be necessary.

Sometimes at exploration a large expansile haematoma or false aneurysm is encountered, associated with a small arterial wound. The haematoma should be evacuated and the artery repaired.

SIMPLE LIGATION

Simple ligation of a damaged artery is always an alternative to repair, and is occasionally the only solution even for proximal arterial injuries in combat conditions. The vessel is ideally ligated at the site of injury, but occasionally a more proximal ligation is the only possibility, due to problems of access. However, any arterial injury at or above the elbow or knee should be repaired or reconstructed, if at all possible, as simple ligation at this level risks significant ischaemia, even if the limb remains viable. (The subclavian and superficial femoral arteries constitute exceptions to this general rule, as good distal perfusion is maintained by collaterals.) Repair or reconstruction of arteries below the knee or elbow is desirable, but only necessary if more than one main artery is injured, or when there is compromised tissue perfusion as a result of anatomical or pathological variations in arterial arcades.

Intravenous drug abuse is associated with multiple punctures of both veins and arteries in the groin and antecubital fossa. Arteries are damaged both by the mechanical trauma to the vessel wall and repeated infections. Surgical intervention may be necessary for bleeding, or for an expanding pseudoaneurysm. Ligation is indicated as reconstruction in these circumstances is extremely difficult. Fortunately, the vessel has usually been damaged so many times that the collaterals are well developed.

ARTERIAL REPAIR OR RECONSTRUCTION

This first requires the clearance of thrombus from the proximal and distal arterial tree by the passage of a Fogarty catheter, followed by instillation of heparinized saline. A clean incision in a large artery may be sutured without narrowing the lumen, but it is often necessary to use a vein patch in a smaller artery, or when contused edges of the arterial wound have had to be trimmed. A completely severed artery can be repaired by direct end-to-end apposition if minimal trimming is required and there is no tension. More often, a short vein graft interposition is required after contused vessel wall adjacent to the injury has been excised. The proximal end-to-end anastomosis is completed and the graft allowed to fill. The vein graft is then cut to the appropriate length, and the distal anastomosis performed. If access to the injury is difficult, simple ligation followed by a bypass graft is an alternative. The foreign material of prosthetic patches and grafts should preferably be avoided in penetrative trauma as the operative field is contaminated.

The most frequent repair is a simple closure of a groin puncture site after an endovascular investigation or therapeutic intervention. The cannula has often been inserted into a diseased portion of the superficial femoral artery, or into its bifurcation. In these circumstances the puncture wound is held open and the bleeding is resistant to pressure. A vertical groin incision will usually be adequate, and the incision is extended proximally to expose the external oblique and the inguinal ligament. The common femoral artery is controlled with a vascular clamp immediately below the inguinal ligament. However, this may not be possible, or the bleeding may be coming from a puncture above the inguinal ligament. In these circumstances the external iliac artery must be clamped. The external oblique is split, then the internal oblique and transversalis layers, and usually the lateral portion of the rectus sheath. The peritoneum is not entered but is swept up to expose the retroperitoneal iliac vessels.

VENOUS REPAIR AND RECONSTRUCTION

This is often disappointing, as discussed above. However, a simple laceration in a large or medium-sized vein can usually be sutured successfully. More extensive repair or reconstruction is advisable when major axial veins (e.g. the femoral) are damaged. Distal veins are more appropriately treated by ligation except in the 'near-amputation' situation, when the restoration of venous drainage, in addition to arterial reconstruction, improves outcome.[3] Two veins should be rejoined for each artery. An oblique end-to-end technique with interrupted sutures is recommended.

EXPOSURE OF THE MAIN VESSELS OF THE TRUNK AND LIMBS

Exposure of the main vessels of the trunk and limbs is described below, and the emergency situations in which this might be required are discussed. Emergency exposure may have to be undertaken in acute occlusion, spontaneous aneurysmal rupture, or when arterial injury is suspected. However, the commonest indication for exposure of a main artery is for the reconstruction of stenosed or aneurysmal vessels damaged by chronic arterial disease. These elective operations are described, and their indications discussed, in more detail in Chapter 6.

The intrathoracic aorta and great vessels of the superior mediastinum

Any general surgeon working outwith a major centre will occasionally be required to gain emergency access to these vessels in a patient with major trauma for whom transfer to a thoracic unit is not an option (see Chapter 7). A median sternotomy exposes the aortic arch and the roots of the major arteries which arise from it.[12] The incision can be extended upwards along the anterior border of sternocleidomastoid to include more extensive access to the carotid vessels. Alternatively, a lateral extension above the clavicle provides further access to the subclavian vessels. The descending thoracic aorta is exposed through a left lateral thoracotomy.

Side occlusion of the arch of the aorta may allow repair to a localized area of damage (see Fig. 5.2b, page 72). This technique is often applicable in elective surgery for occlusive disease at the roots of the major arteries. Unfortunately, in trauma the anatomy is distorted by haematoma, and the damage may be extensive. Successful repair may require cross-clamping of the aorta and cardiopulmonary bypass techniques.

The carotid arteries

Endarterectomy for the prevention of stroke is the most frequent elective vascular operation in the neck, and is the commonest indication for surgical access to the carotid arteries. The operation is described in Chapter 6. A similar approach is required for excision of a carotid body tumour. Carotid artery exposure in an emergency is almost exclusively for penetrating trauma to the neck, the management of which is discussed in Chapter 9. The neck is arbitrarily divided into three zones (see Fig. 9.3, page 157) for the management of neck trauma. Zone 1 extends for 1 cm above the upper border of the manubrium, Zone 3 is above the angle of the mandible, and Zone 2 lies between. Lateral penetrating wounds in Zone 2 so commonly involve the carotids that some surgeons recommend exploration in all cases, although others are more selective.[13] Injuries in Zones 1 and 3 less frequently involve the carotid arteries, and both the exposure of the vessels and their repair are more difficult. Angiographic assessment of injuries in Zones 1 and 3 is therefore recommended before any surgical exploration. In Zone 1 the common carotid is deep to omohyoid, and any injury may also involve other major vessels in the superior mediastinum. A median sternotomy with extension of the incision up into the neck may be required (see Fig. 9.4, page 157). In Zone 3 the carotids are less accessible, lying deep to the posterior belly of digastric and the parotid gland; the external carotid may be within the gland. The involvement of a neurosurgeon may be essential as there may be no undamaged internal carotid artery outside the cranium.

Uncontrollable haemorrhage into a severely damaged face, maxillary antrum or larynx can be life-threatening. Ligation of the external carotid artery on the side of the injury can be life saving, and is approached by the exposure of the carotid bifurcation. The external carotid is the anteromedial branch (see Chapter 9).

ANATOMY

The *common carotid artery* begins its course in the neck behind the sternoclavicular joint. Thence, it passes upwards, deep to the sternocleidomastoid muscle, in a line towards the lobe of the ear but ends – usually opposite the upper border of the thyroid cartilage – by dividing into the external and internal carotid arteries. It is enclosed along with the internal jugular vein and the vagus nerve in the carotid sheath of deep cervical fascia; the vein is lateral to it, and the nerve lies posteriorly in the groove behind the two vessels. The *external carotid artery* runs upwards from the carotid bifurcation to end behind the mandible, by dividing into maxillary and superficial temporal arteries. It leaves the carotid triangle by passing under cover of the posterior belly of the digastric muscle, and its upper part occupies a groove on the deep surface of the parotid gland, or lies within the gland. The external carotid artery is the major vascular supply to the neck, face and scalp. There are three large anterior branches: the superior thyroid; the lingual; and the facial. The occipital and posterior auricular are posterior branches. The *internal carotid artery* ascends from the carotid bifurcation to enter the skull through the carotid canal, just posteromedial to the temporomandibular joint. It is at first posterolateral to the external carotid artery, and then deep to it. It is enclosed in the carotid sheath, with the internal jugular vein laterally, and with the vagus nerve deep to the interval between them; at the skull base the vein is posterior to the artery. There are no branches in the neck and it supplies purely intracranial structures. The superficial relations of the carotid vessels are in the description of the exposure.

EXPOSURE

Elective carotid surgery can be performed under local or general anaesthesia. In penetrating trauma, a general anaesthetic with control of the airway is important. The head is turned to the opposite side and slightly extended, and a sandbag is placed between the shoulder blades. The ideal cosmetic incision is placed in a skin crease, and in an elective situation this can usually be sited to give adequate exposure. If greater longitudinal exposure is required, the middle part of the incision should run parallel to the anterior border of sternocleidomastoid (Fig. 5.19). Maximum exposure of the carotid vessels in an emergency can be obtained by a long oblique incision along the anterior border of sternocleidomastoid (see Fig. 9.4b, page 157). In order to avoid damage to the cervical branch of the facial nerve the upper end of the incision should not approach nearer than 1.5 cm to the angle of the mandible. Platysma and deep fascia are divided in line with the skin incision, and the external jugular vein is ligated and divided. The flaps are dissected a little way to elevate them off the deeper tissues.

The anterior border of sternocleidomastoid is freed and the muscle retracted posteriorly. The common facial vein lies superficial to the common carotid artery and crosses it just below the bifurcation (Fig. 5.19). This is ligated and divided, after which the internal jugular vein can be displaced backwards to expose the carotid arteries more fully. The descending branch of the hypoglossal nerve is visible on the surface of the carotid artery. It can usually be preserved, but little harm ensues from sacrificing it if necessary. The main hypoglossal nerve crosses superficial to the carotid arteries, just above the bifurcation, and should be preserved. At the upper extremity of the dissection the posterior belly of digastric, the parotid gland and the great auricular nerve may be visible. If the thyroid gland and the strap muscles are retracted anteromedially,

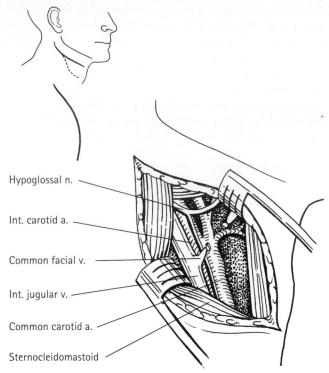

Hypoglossal n.

Int. carotid a.

Common facial v.

Int. jugular v.

Common carotid a.

Sternocleidomastoid

Figure 5.19   *A transverse skin crease gives limited access to the carotid bifurcation. Greater exposure is achieved by an S-shaped incision or even a long oblique incision along the anterior border of sternocleidomastoid. The sternocleidomastoid muscle is retracted posteriorly and the common facial vein divided to display the carotid bifurcation.*

the superior thyroid artery is exposed along with the superior laryngeal nerve which lies in a deeper plane.

The vulnerability of the cerebral cortex to ischaemia must be remembered, and consideration given to a temporary shunt during any period of proximal and distal arterial control. Repair of a carotid laceration will usually require a vein patch to avoid stenosis. A severely damaged external carotid can be simply ligated, but the common or internal carotid should be repaired or reconstructed.

Subclavian and axillary arteries

Exposure of these arteries may be required for reconstructive arterial surgery for obliterative and aneurysmal disease. In this elective surgery the precise area of the pathology is known preoperatively, and a limited exposure is often appropriate. However, in trauma, a more extensive exposure is usually necessary. Adjacent veins and nerves may also be damaged, and it is difficult to gain safe proximal and distal control amongst other vital structures when the anatomy is distorted by haematoma.[14]

ANATOMY

The *subclavian artery* crosses the front of the cervical pleura at the root of the neck. It arches from behind the sternoclavicu-

lar joint to the outer border of the first rib, where it becomes the axillary artery. It rises to a level of 1–2 cm above the clavicle, when the shoulder is depressed. Scalenus anterior crosses anterior to the artery. The first part of the artery is defined as the portion which lies medial to scalenus anterior; the second part lies behind this muscle, and the third part lateral to it. The subclavian vein lies in front of scalenus anterior, at a lower level than the artery, and behind the clavicle.

The *axillary artery* runs downwards and laterally behind the clavicle in the roof of the axilla, and continues as the brachial artery at the lateral border of the axilla. The axillary artery is divided into three parts by pectoralis minor which crosses anterior to the second part. The axillary vein lies just below and medial to the artery throughout its course, and the brachial plexus lies in close association with the artery.

The superficial relations of the arteries are in the descriptions of the exposures and are illustrated in Figure 5.20.

EXPOSURE

The *third part of the subclavian* artery is the most surgically accessible. In trauma, when extensive exposure of the artery

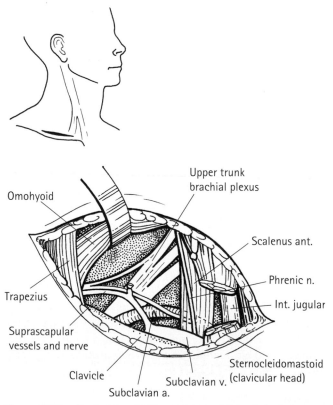

Omohyoid

Upper trunk brachial plexus

Scalenus ant.

Phrenic n.

Int. jugular

Trapezius

Suprascapular vessels and nerve

Clavicle

Subclavian a.

Subclavian v.

Sternocleidomastoid (clavicular head)

Figure 5.20   *The incision for the exposure of the subclavian artery is above and parallel to the clavicle. Omohyoid is retracted, and the subclavian artery is visible between the scalenus anterior and the brachial plexus. Division of scalenus anterior and medial retraction of the internal jugular vein exposes the proximal subclavian artery. When more extensive exposure of the vascular root is required the internal jugular can be retracted laterally, or the incision can even be extended to combine it with a median sternotomy.*

is required, the third part is often exposed initially and then the incision is extended medially. A limited exposure of the third part of the subclavian artery is occasionally indicated in trauma when there is uncontrollable haemorrhage from the axillary artery. A temporary clamp on the subclavian artery will then provide some proximal control during exploration of the axilla. Ideally, the damaged axillary artery is then repaired or reconstructed, but simple ligation of the third part of the subclavian artery is another possibility. The perfusion of the upper limb is safeguarded by an anastomosis around the shoulder, which is fed by branches arising from the proximal subclavian artery.

The arm is placed at the side and drawn downwards in order to depress the shoulder; the head is turned to the opposite side. An incision is made 1–2 cm above the clavicle from the sternal head of sternocleidomastoid to the anterior border of trapezius (Fig. 5.20). The superficial fascia and platysma are incised in the same line and the deep fascia divided. The external jugular vein may cross the operative field and have to be divided between ligatures. A supraclavicular nerve may also have to be sacrificed. Omohyoid is retracted upwards, and the third part of the subclavian artery is now exposed, with the upper and middle trunks of the brachial plexus lying supero-laterally. The suprascapular artery which arises from the thyrocervical branch of the first part of the subclavian artery crosses the operative field as it runs supero-laterally, anterior to the subclavian artery, with its accompanying vein and nerve.

Exposure of the first and second parts of the subclavian artery requires division of the clavicular head of sternocleidomastoid and division of scalenus anterior, followed by medial retraction of the internal jugular vein. The phrenic nerve lying on the surface of scalenus anterior should be preserved, and held in a sling to retract it out of the operative field. The common carotid artery is obscured by the internal jugular vein. Lateral retraction of the vein exposes the common carotid artery and, with both arteries in the operative field, a carotid–subclavian bypass graft is possible through this approach.

The supraclavicular incision can be combined with a median sternotomy in which case the sternal head of sternocleidomastoid is also divided (see Fig. 9.4a, page 157). This gives the extensive exposure necessary to gain control of the proximal subclavian or the brachiocephalic trunk in major trauma (see Chapters 7 and 9).

Axillary artery exposure is required both in trauma and for axillofemoral bypass grafts. The upper limb is partially abducted and supported on an arm board. The incision for an extensive exposure is along the deltopectoral groove from the lower border of the clavicle to the lower border of the anterior axillary fold (Fig. 5.21). Anterior branches of the axillary artery and the termination of the cephalic vein will be encountered. The cords of the brachial plexus lie around the artery, and the axillary vein lies infero-medially. The tendon of pectoralis minor is divided.

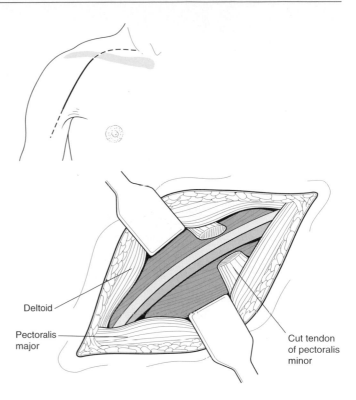

Figure 5.21   *The axillary artery is approached via an incision along the deltopectoral groove. It can be extended proximally if simultaneous access to the subclavian artery is required, or distally to expose the brachial artery. Division of pectoralis minor and retraction of pectoralis major and deltoid exposes the artery.*

This incision can be extended downwards to expose the brachial artery. The approach to the brachial artery is normally below the pectoral muscles (Fig. 5.22), but when extensive access is required pectoralis major may have to be divided. The incision can also be extended proximally to join with a supraclavicular incision and provide extensive simultaneous access to both the subclavian and the axillary artery. The clavicle crosses the operative field, but can often be left intact. However, the root of the neck is a hazardous area for an inexperienced surgeon. The subclavian artery is relatively thin-walled, and bleeding from it – or from one of the great veins – is very difficult to control. In emergency situations, when rapid control of both the third part of the subclavian and the first part of the axillary artery may be essential, there should be no hesitation in resecting the middle third of the clavicle.

A more limited exposure of the axillary artery, as may be required for an elective bypass graft, is described in the section on axillofemoral grafts in Chapter 6.

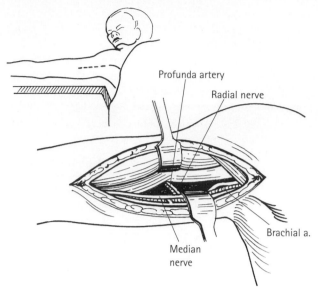

Figure 5.22 *Exposure of the brachial artery in the right upper arm.*

A transverse trans-axillary approach to the axillary artery as it crosses the first rib is used in the treatment of thoracic outlet syndrome (see Chapter 6). The rib can be resected through this incision and the artery released. Access to the artery is, however, very limited and it is an unsuitable approach for trauma or for any reconstructive procedure.

Brachial artery

The brachial artery may be approached with ease throughout its relatively superficial course. Exploration is most likely to be required for embolism, or for iatrogenic trauma inflicted in the course of cardiological investigations. Exposure may also be necessary to investigate possible damage associated with a fracture of the humerus or penetrating trauma.

ANATOMY

The brachial artery begins as a continuation of the axillary artery at the level of the lower border of teres major. It runs downwards and slightly laterally, at first medial to the humerus and then in front of it. It ends in the cubital fossa, at the level of the neck of the radius, by dividing into radial and ulnar arteries. The artery is accompanied by venae comitantes in its lower part, and by the basilic vein in the upper part.

In *the arm*, the median nerve – which at first is lateral – crosses in front of the middle third of the artery and then runs along its medial side. The ulnar nerve is on the medial side of the artery in its upper half, but diverges from its lower half. The median cutaneous nerve of the forearm also lies to its medial side in the upper half of the arm. At the *front of the elbow* the brachial artery enters the cubital fossa, with the tendon of biceps on its lateral side, and the median nerve on

its medial side. They are roofed over by the deep fascia containing the bicipital aponeurosis, which stretches from the tendon of biceps to blend with the deep fascia over the medial side of the forearm.

EXPOSURE

In *the arm*, exposure is by an incision along the medial edge of biceps. The arm is abducted and rotated laterally and supported on an arm board (Fig. 5.22). There may be a case for leaving the arm entirely free, supporting the limb only at the shoulder and at the elbow, as arm support displaces the muscles and renders the approach more difficult. The deep fascia is divided along the same line, and care is taken to avoid the basilic vein which pierces the deep fascia in this vicinity. The biceps is mobilized and drawn laterally to expose the artery and the median nerve. For *exposure at the elbow*, the arm is abducted and supported on an arm board in the position of lateral rotation. The deep fascia (including the bicipital aponeurosis) is incised vertically, and the bicipital tendon retracted laterally. This is illustrated in Figure 5.23 for the *left* arm. A vertical skin incision would not now be recommended across the flexor aspect of the joint. Similar access can be achieved by a transverse cubital fossa skin crease incision, enlarged by vertical extensions up from the medial end of the transverse incision, and down from the lateral end.

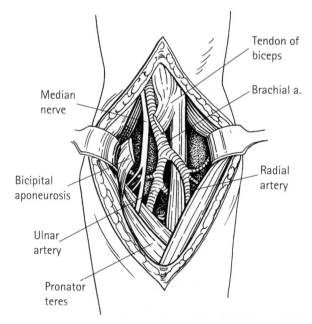

Figure 5.23 *Exposure of the brachial artery in the left cubital fossa. A vertical skin incision across the anterior aspect of the joint should be avoided, however.*

The abdominal aorta, renal vessels, and inferior vena cava

The abdominal aorta and iliac arteries are frequently involved in atherosclerotic degenerative pathology, which may take the form of either occlusive or aneurysmal disease. The approach to these arteries is required mainly for reconstructive arterial surgery, and this frequently occurs in an elective setting. However, the spontaneous rupture of an abdominal aortic or iliac aneurysm, or trauma which involves any of the major abdominal vessels, necessitates emergency surgery for the control of exsanguinating haemorrhage.

ANATOMY

The *abdominal aorta* enters the abdomen between the crura of the diaphragm, as a direct continuation of the descending thoracic aorta. It ends on the front of the body of the 4th lumbar vertebra, to the left of the midline, by dividing into right and left common iliac arteries (Fig. 5.24). The upper abdominal aorta is not easily accessible from the front. There are only a few centimetres of unexposed aorta above the pancreas, and the coeliac trunk arises from this short segment. The pancreas, the splenic vein, the left renal vein and the third part of the duodenum then all cross in front of the upper abdominal aorta and are closely applied to it. Three

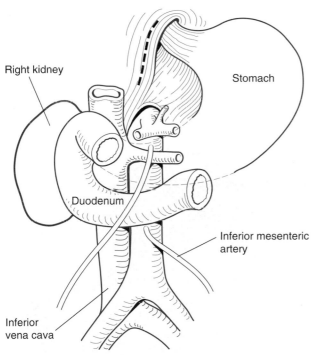

Figure 5.24 *In the upper abdomen the aorta is relatively inaccessible. Tributaries of the IVC cross it anteriorly, whereas more distally the iliac arteries lie anterior to the veins. The retroperitoneal duodenum and pancreas also impair access. A vertical incision in the posterior parietal peritoneum, lateral to the duodenum, enables the surgeon to mobilize the second or fourth part of the duodenum off the IVC or aorta respectively. A vertical incision in the right diaphragmatic crus exposes sufficient supra-coeliac aorta for the application of a temporary occlusion clamp. When more extensive exposure of the proximal abdominal aorta or IVC is required, a medial visceral rotation manoeuvre may be indicated.*

large arterial branches arise from the retro-pancreatic aorta; first the superior mesenteric artery from its anterior aspect, and then the renal arteries from the lateral aspects. The origins of these major arteries greatly hamper any upper abdominal aortic mobilization. The infra-renal aorta is more mobile and accessible. It has only the pre-aortic nerve plexus over its anterior surface, and in addition the only significant branches – the inferior mesenteric artery and the gonadal arteries – can be sacrificed as collateral anastomotic channels will normally prevent ischaemia of the tissue which they supply. The *inferior vena cava* (IVC) lies along the right side of the aorta until it diverges to the right and is separated from it by the right crus of the diaphragm.

EXPOSURE AND CONTROL

Fortunately, for most reconstructive aorto-iliac surgery – both in elective and emergency settings – infra-renal aortic access is sufficient as the upper abdominal aorta is relatively spared the degenerative pathology. A *trans-peritoneal aortic approach* is most commonly employed. Initially, on entering the peritoneal cavity, the retroperitoneum is obscured by bowel. The omentum and transverse colon are first swung upwards, after which the small bowel is displaced to the patient's right to expose the duodenojejunal flexure. An incision is made just lateral to the fourth part of the duodenum to gain retroperitoneal entry and expose the aorta. For infra-renal aortic occlusion, a vascular clamp is introduced with the blades on either side of the aorta, which is then compressed bilaterally. The IVC is to the right and the left renal vein is anterior, and care must be taken to avoid venous injury. The surgeon's fingers, when inserted either side of the aorta, are used to guide the clamp safely into position. When an aneurysm is present the clamp must be on the normal-calibre aorta above the aneurysm. A finger introduced into the retroperitoneum can feel the proximal extremity of the aneurysm.

Access to the upper abdominal aorta is restricted, and is more easily understood in relationship to the embryological folding of the bowel and the subsequent layers of retroperitoneal structures. This is described in more detail in Chapter 13. The standard access to the infra-renal aorta can be extended proximally by extending the incision to the left of the fourth part of the duodenum, and dividing the inferior mesenteric vein. The renal vein is then retracted in a sling to expose the renal artery lying behind it and the origin of the renal arteries from the aorta. Alternatively, mobilization of the splenic flexure of the colon will expose the left renal vein crossing the aorta just below the pancreas. When further upper abdominal aortic access is required – and in particular when there is a posterior penetrating injury – a left-sided medial visceral rotation may be necessary. The plane is entered lateral to the spleen and the dissection carried medially *behind* the spleen, kidney and pancreas to lift all the viscera off the retroperitoneal structures.

Proximal aortic control may be necessary in trauma, or for

an extensive aneurysm. The supra-coeliac aorta can be accessed by opening the lesser sac through the lesser omentum. A vertical incision is then made in the right crus of the diaphragm, as marked in Figure 5.24. The distal extremity of the descending thoracic aorta lies immediately deep to the crus. A finger is passed either side of it, and then a vascular clamp is applied. The thoracic aorta can also be cross-clamped at an initial 'emergency room' left thoracotomy (see Chapter 7). This manoeuvre is associated with significant morbidity, and is therefore reserved for occasions when the abdominal aorta is not accessible, or if there is doubt as to which side of the diaphragm the bleeding is coming from. A supra-coeliac clamp renders both kidneys and the whole bowel ischaemic, and is therefore only a temporary solution unless a shunt is employed to restore distal perfusion. Safe ischaemic time for the kidneys can be extended by renal cooling (see Chapter 25).

The alternative *retroperitoneal approach* to the abdominal aorta is an extension of the retroperitoneal approach to the iliac vessels.

Access to the *right renal artery*, as it crosses posterior to the inferior vena cava, and the infra-hepatic anterior aspect of the *inferior vena cava*, is achieved by first mobilizing the hepatic flexure of the colon, followed by 'Kocherization' of the duodenum so that the head of pancreas can be lifted forwards (see Chapter 13). If access is needed to the posterior aspect of the whole vena cava, a right-sided medial visceral rotation is required utilizing the plane behind the right kidney and the liver, which must also be mobilized forwards.

The iliac vessels

ANATOMY

The *common iliac arteries* are the two terminal branches of the aorta. They run downwards and laterally to the pelvic brim, where each divides into an internal and external iliac artery. The *internal iliac arteries* run backwards and downwards into the pelvis. They then divide into multiple named branches which supply the pelvic organs, in addition to the superior and inferior gluteal arteries which supply the gluteal muscles and form anastomotic collaterals within them with branches of the profunda femoris artery. The internal iliac artery can be ligated on one side, without any adverse consequences. The *external iliac arteries* continue downwards and laterally on the psoas muscle to end under the inguinal ligament by becoming the femoral arteries. The *external iliac veins* lie on the medial sides of the arteries. The distal inferior vena cava and the terminations of the common iliac veins lie deep to the right common iliac artery (see Fig. 5.24). This anatomical arrangement is ideal for reconstructive aorto-iliac surgery, but access to the common iliac veins in trauma can be very difficult. It is sometimes even necessary to divide the artery for access and re-anastomose it afterwards.

EXPOSURE

Exposure of the *iliac vessels* is seldom required in isolation, and additional exposure of either the aorta or the femoral artery often dictates the surgical approach. An *abdominal trans-peritoneal approach* is thus suitable for emergency surgery for iliac vessel trauma or aneurysmal rupture, or when aorto-iliac reconstructive surgery is planned. The distal aorta and right iliac vessels are exposed by division of the overlying peritoneum. The left iliac arteries are exposed by division of the peritoneum lateral to the pelvic mesocolon. The ureters must be identified and safeguarded. Some damage is almost inevitable to the autonomic plexi overlying the vessels, but with care this can be minimized. The *extra-peritoneal approach* to a unilateral iliac artery is often combined with the exposure of the femoral artery for an iliofemoral bypass graft reconstruction, an operation described in Chapter 6. In arterial trauma to the common femoral artery, a localized approach to the external iliac artery may be required for proximal vascular control. An oblique muscle-cutting iliac fossa incision is made parallel to the inguinal ligament, and a few centimetres above it, to avoid the inguinal canal and spermatic cord. The peritoneum is swept upwards and medially to expose the external iliac vessels lying on the pelvic brim on the medial edge of the psoas muscle (Fig. 5.25). Clamps on iliac arteries should be placed from the front with one blade either side. Attempts to encircle the artery increase the danger of iliac vein damage.

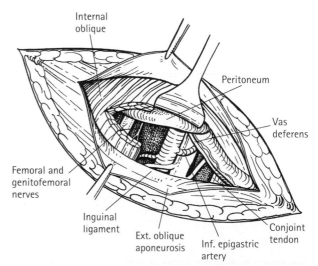

Figure 5.25 *Extraperitoneal exposure of the right external iliac vessels at the groin. Further retraction of the peritoneum would expose the termination of the common iliac artery and the ureter.*

The femoral arteries

The proximal portion of the femoral artery is superficial and easily accessible for percutaneous investigative and interventional techniques. It is also the favoured artery of access for lower limb, or iliac, embolectomy. Its superficial position renders it vulnerable to traumatic (and iatrogenic) damage. In addition, femoral artery access is required in iliofemoral or femorodistal reconstructive surgery for occlusive degenerative pathology.

ANATOMY

The femoral artery commences as a direct continuation of the external iliac artery under the inguinal ligament at the mid-inguinal point. It runs obliquely downwards through the femoral triangle and the sub-sartorial canal. Surgeons refer to the proximal portion, above the origin of the profunda, as the *common femoral artery*, and the distal portion as the *superficial femoral artery*. The femoral artery ends at the junction of the middle and lower thirds of the thigh, by passing through the opening in adductor magnus, to become the popliteal artery. At the inguinal ligament the femoral nerve lies lateral to the artery, and the femoral vein is medial. Distally the femoral vein lies posterior to the artery. The *profunda femoris artery* arises from the lateral side of the femoral artery 3–4 cm below the inguinal ligament; it runs medially behind the femoral artery to disappear between the adductor muscles.

EXPOSURE

The skin incision is made along the line of the artery. The LSV will be encountered in the subcutaneous fat, and should be preserved in case it might be required for reconstruction. The deep fascia is incised, and the sartorius muscle mobilized. Sartorius is then retracted laterally to expose the common femoral artery and the origin of the profunda femoris. To expose the distal superficial femoral vessels, sartorius is retracted medially and the underlying bridge of fibrous tissue which roofs over the sub-sartorial canal is divided.

The popliteal artery

Emergency access to the popliteal artery is occasionally necessary in trauma. More frequently, it is required in reconstructive surgery for degenerative vascular disease.

ANATOMY

The popliteal artery begins as a continuation of the femoral at the opening in the adductor magnus. It runs downwards in the popliteal fossa to end at the lower border of popliteus by dividing into the *anterior tibial* artery and the tibioperoneal trunk, which in turn divides into *posterior tibial* and *peroneal* branches. The popliteal vein is medial to the artery in its lower part but crosses it posteriorly to lie posterolateral to it in its upper part. The tibial nerve crosses the vessels posteriorly from the lateral side above to the medial side below.

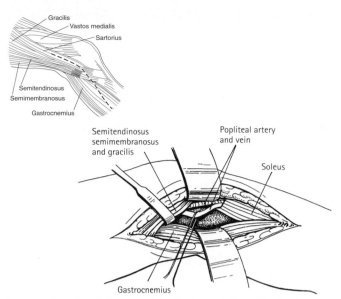

Figure 5.26 *Medial approach to the lower left popliteal artery. Only the lower half of the illustrated skin incision has been used, and the tendinous insertions into the proximal tibia are preserved and retracted anteriorly.*

EXPOSURE

A *posterior exposure*, which displays the anatomy as described above, only affords limited access to the vessels, but is suitable for the release of a popliteal entrapment or the excision of an adventitial popliteal artery cyst. The transverse popliteal skin crease incision can be extended by a vertical extension up from its medial end and down from its lateral end. This is followed by a vertical incision of the deep fascia into the fat of the popliteal fossa. The SSV may have to be ligated for access, or can be preserved and retracted with the popliteal vein to expose the artery.

A *medial approach* provides superior access for most situations. The patient is placed supine, with the hip externally rotated and the knee slightly flexed. The skin incision (Fig. 5.26) is commenced 1 cm posterior to the medial tibial condyle and is extended either upwards along the anterior border of sartorius, or distally 1 cm behind the posteromedial border of the tibia. The LSV lies close to the skin at this level, and inadvertent injury must be avoided if it is required for reconstruction. The tendinous insertions of sartorius, gracilis and semitendinosus all cross the operative field to their insertion into the tibia. If access is only necessary to either the proximal or the distal popliteal artery, these tendons can be left intact and retracted. For *exposure above the knee*, the deep fascia is incised along the anterior border of sartorius which is then retracted posteriorly. Alternatively, sartorius and gracilis are retracted anteriorly. The adductor magnus tendon can be divided to expose the femoropopliteal junction. For *exposure below the knee*, the deep fascia is incised to allow anterior retraction of the tendinous insertions into the tibia, and posterior retraction of the medial head of gastrocnemius (Fig. 5.26). When a more extensive exposure is required the full length of the skin incision is utilized and the tendinous insertions into the tibia divided. In addition, the medial head of gastrocnemius can be divided if access is still insufficient. The popliteal fat is gently separated and the fascia surrounding the neurovascular bundle incised longitudinally. The popliteal vein is retracted posteriorly and must be separated with great care as venous bleeding in the popliteal fossa can be difficult to control and even any minor damage to the vein is likely to lead to thrombosis; venous duplication in the form of venae comitantes is not uncommon. The artery is then separated from the tibial nerve and encircled with a sling. If more distal access is required to the trifurcation of the popliteal artery, the soleus muscle and the anterior tibial vein are divided.

The peroneal artery, anterior and posterior tibial arteries

The surgical approaches to these arteries are almost exclusively in the setting of distal reconstructive surgery for peripheral vascular obliterative disease. The approaches are therefore described in Chapter 6 in the section on infrapopliteal reconstructions.

REFERENCES

1. Abouezzi Z, Nassoura Z, Ivatury RR, et al. A critical reappraisal of indications for fasciotomy after extremity vascular trauma. Arch Surg 1998; 133: 547–51.
2. Brown MJ, Nicholson ML, Bell PR, et al. Cytokines and inflammatory pathways in the pathogenesis of multiple organ failure following abdominal aortic aneurysm repair. Eur J Vasc Endovasc Surg 2001; 22: 485–95.
3. Barrow AAB. Complex vascular and orthopaedic limb injuries. Editorial. J Bone Joint Surg (Br) 1992; 74-B: 176–8.
4. Fogarty TJ, Cranley JJ, Krause RJ, et al. A method for extraction of arterial emboli and thrombi. Surg Gynecol Obstet 1963; 116: 241–4.
5. Stonebridge PA, Prescott RJ, Ruckley CV. Randomised trial comparing infrainguinal polytetrafluoroethylene bypass grafting with and without vein interposition cuff at the distal anastomosis. The Joint Vascular Research Group. J Vasc Surg 1997; 26: 543–50.
6. O'Brien T, Collin J. Prosthetic vascular graft infection. Review. Br J Surg 1992; 79: 1262–7.
7. Minimal Access Therapy for Vascular Disease. AL Leahy, PRF Bell, BT Katzer (eds). London: Martin Dunitz, 2002.
8. Bailey and Love's Short Practice of Surgery, 24th edn. RCG Russell, NS Williams, CJK Bulstrode (eds). London: Hodder Arnold, 2004.
9. Stuart WP, Adam DJ, Allan PL, et al. The relationship between the number, competence, and diameter of medial calf perforating veins and the clinical status in healthy subjects and patients with lower-limb venous disease. J Vasc Surg 2000; 32: 138–43.
10. Sarin S, Scurr JH, Coleridge Smith PD. Stripping of the long saphenous vein in the treatment of primary varicose veins. Br J Surg 1994; 81: 1455–8.
11. Stonebridge PA, Chalmers N, Beggs I, et al. Recurrent varicose veins: a varicographic analysis leading to a new practical classification. Br J Surg 1995; 82: 60–2.
12. Prêtre R, Chilcott M, Mûrith N, et al. Blunt injury to the supra-aortic arteries. Review. Br J Surg 1997; 84: 603–9.
13. Demetriades D, Charalambides D, Lakhoo M. Physical examination and selective conservative management in patients with penetrating injuries of the neck. Br J Surg 1993; 80: 1534–6.
14. McKinley AG, Abdool Carrim ATO, Robbs JV. Management of proximal axillary and subclavian artery injuries. Br J Surg 2000; 87: 79–85.

OPERATIVE MANAGEMENT OF VASCULAR DISEASE

WESLEY STUART

VASCULAR PATHOLOGY

Arterial disease

While the spectrum of arterial disease includes tumour, infection and inflammation, the commonest pathological processes encountered by a vascular surgeon are aneurysmal disease, occlusive disease and embolic events.

Aneurysms

Aneurysms can be divided into true aneurysms, in which every layer is dilated but in continuity, and false aneurysms, in which there is a breach in the layers and rupture is prevented by thrombus, a single intact layer and the surrounding tissues. False aneurysms are either post-traumatic or post-infective, and in the UK are most commonly iatrogenic. The aorta, the iliac, common femoral, popliteal and common carotid arteries are the most common extra-cranial arteries to be affected by true aneurysms. Other vessels may become aneurysmal, but this is unusual. Frequently, discovery is an incidental finding when either clinical examination, or an investigation, is performed for another reason. Aneurysms may present as a mass, or a pulsation, of which the patient is aware, and pressure from the expanding aneurysm can cause a range of relatively minor symptoms. Unfortunately, a significant number of aneurysms come to light as a result of a complication: rupture, thrombosis, distal embolism, fistula formation or infection.

Occlusive disease

Occlusive disease may present with an insidious development of symptoms, or with sudden critical deterioration in the circulation. Typically, occlusive disease in the lower limbs has a relapsing, remitting course. The initial symptoms of claudication diminish as collaterals develop, and then return as further segments of artery narrow or occlude. Many patients do not report symptoms until more than one segment is affected, or long occlusions have developed, such is the compensatory capacity of a well-developed collateral bed. Only 5 per cent of the patients who present with claudication will ultimately lose the limb. By far the commonest occlusive disease in the developed world is atheroma which predominantly – but by no means exclusively – affects the arteries to the lower limb. However, the vascular surgeon may also have to consider arterial occlusive disease of the upper limb, the cerebral cortex, the kidneys and the gut.

Embolus

An embolus presents as a sudden arterial event. The effect will depend on the size of the embolus and whether the collateral circulation can maintain sufficient distal perfusion to maintain viability. These collaterals may be normal anatomical anastomotic arcades, or anastomotic channels which have enlarged secondary to coexistent occlusive pathology. Large emboli can arise from the left atrium in atrial fibrillation, or from the left ventricle in association with a ventricular aneurysm or a subendocardial myocardial infarction. Emboli can also arise from the thrombus within an aneurysm in a more proximal part of the arterial tree. Atheromatous emboli, which have detached from an unstable atheromatous plaque in a proximal artery, are usually smaller and often multiple.

Vascular trauma

Vascular trauma includes iatrogenic vascular injury, and also the injuries sustained in a range of situations including military conflict and civilian violence. The relative importance of the various aetiologies will depend on the environment within which a surgeon is practising. Vascular trauma is discussed in Chapter 5.

Venous disease

Venous disease accounts for a significant proportion of the healthcare budget. The standard operations for varicose veins are described in Chapter 5. Varicose vein surgery is widely performed for ill-defined and quite varied symptoms and signs. Surgery is associated with high recurrence rates, modest patient satisfaction and frequent litigation.[1] Varicose vein surgery should not be assigned to an unsupervised, inexperienced junior surgeon as such practice has commonly resulted in poor outcomes.[2] Although for the majority of patients varicose veins remain a cosmetic problem, associated with a variable degree of discomfort, approximately 5 per cent will develop skin complications of chronic venous insufficiency, namely ulceration and lipodermatosclerosis.

Deep venous thrombosis is common, and once more the consequences are wide and varied. Pulmonary emboli are life-threatening emergencies, venous claudication from a chronically obstructed system can be incapacitating, and venous ulcer disease is a highly morbid condition. Fortunately, the natural history of an adequately treated deep venous thrombosis is thrombus resolution with minimal symptoms. Venous gangrene, which results from massive occluding proximal thrombosis, is rare. Incipient venous gangrene can be managed by aggressive leg elevation with the salvage options of thrombolysis or surgical thrombectomy. The surgical interventions in chronic venous insufficiency are discussed later in this chapter.

INFRARENAL AORTIC ANEURYSMS

Infra-renal aortic aneurysms first became amenable to successful surgical repair during the 1950s, and aortic surgery is now dominated by this condition.[3] The aneurysmal dilatation may be confined to the aorta or it may extend into the iliac arteries. Aneurysmal dilatation which involves the supra-renal or thoracic aorta is fortunately less common as the surgery for thoraco-abdominal aneurysms is extremely challenging. Degenerative aortic disease can also be occlusive, and a mixed pattern of occlusive and aneurysmal disease may be encountered. Occlusive aortic disease can also occlude or stenose the origins of arteries arising from it.

SELECTION

In the elective setting the repair of an infra-renal abdominal aortic aneurysm carries a 5–10 per cent mortality, although some units report rates of less than 5 per cent. After rupture, the mortality rate of the minority who survive the initial rupture to reach hospital and are then selected for repair is in the region of 40–60 per cent.[4] It therefore seems appropriate to identify those at risk of rupture and to offer surgery before rupture occurs. Many areas of the world – including some parts of the UK – have commenced screening programmes based upon good quality evidence of benefit.[5] However, the true natural history of aneurysms remains the subject of debate, and evidence from the UK Small Aneurysm Trial suggests that the rupture rate of abdominal aortic aneurysms less than 6 cm in antero-posterior diameter on ultrasound scan has been overestimated in the past.[6] What is widely accepted is the need to consider intervention when the diameter exceeds 5.5 cm. Still open to debate is whether conventional surgery or endovascular aneurysm repair offers the best outcome.

Patient selection is a contentious area, and the preoperative investigations are determined by local protocols that are often dependent upon availability and cost. It would appear sensible to suggest that patients being considered for elective abdominal aortic aneurysm repair require a cardiac assessment over and above simple exercise tolerance estimation and electrocardiography; for example, echocardiography and an assessment of renal and pulmonary function (spirometry). More detailed anatomical information is required than that provided by simple ultrasound scans in order to exclude supra-renal extension of the aneurysm, to verify the position and number of renal arteries, and to identify iliac artery aneurysmal or occlusive disease. If available, a computed tomography (CT) angiogram is the current optimal investigation.

THE OPERATION

The patient is placed in a supine position, and should be prepared in such a way that there is access to the femoral vessels. Prophylactic antibiotics are administered according to local protocol. The abdomen is opened using a midline or transverse incision. The latter incision affords satisfactory access and may be associated with less postoperative pain. The transverse colon is lifted up and packed superiorly, while the small bowel is displaced to the right into a bowel bag outside the abdomen or tucked away within the abdomen. The third part of the duodenum is mobilized from the front of the aorta, leaving sufficient peritoneum as a cuff to allow restoration of peritoneal continuity afterwards. The peritoneum is divided in front of the aneurysm and the aneurysm neck is approached, dividing the pre-aortic tissue by diathermy, or between ties. The inferior mesenteric vein is routinely encountered to the left of the aneurysm, and this can either be divided between ties or displaced upwards. The dissection often needs to be taken up to the level of the left renal vein to create sufficient room to clamp above the aneurysmal tissue and exclude it completely when securing the graft (Fig. 6.1a). Occasionally it is necessary to divide the left renal vein. Some authorities advocate that it should always be reconstituted to avoid deterioration in renal function. Division of the left renal vein is certainly associated with a greater mortality. It must be remembered that aortic aneurysms rotate and lengthen as well as expand in girth, and the sides of the aorta need to be exposed carefully to avoid damage to the paired testicular and lumbar arteries, as well as a variable accessory renal artery; and also to avoid tearing the left ilio-lumbar and gonadal veins. Sometimes it is easier to divide these vessels between titanium clips, rather than attempt to preserve them.

Once the neck of the aneurysm has been adequately exposed, the iliac arteries must be exposed. It is not necessary to pass tapes or slings round these vessels. In fact, this can be hazardous due to the risk of damaging the iliac veins, and is best avoided as a routine. The right common iliac artery is covered only by a single layer of peritoneum and retro-peritoneal fat. Be aware of the course of the ureter, as outlined in Chapter 25. The first part of the left common iliac artery is immediately deep to the peritoneum, and this allows adequate access for clamping if the aneurysm is confined to the aorta or proximal common iliac artery. However in more complex situations, requiring more distal clamping of the iliac vessels, the sigmoid colon may require mobilization, or the clamp may need to be applied just proximal to the inguinal ligament. It is a fairly common scenario that the

aneurysmal process, on one or the other side, extends up to – or beyond – the iliac bifurcation. This presents two problems. First, the internal iliac artery must be exposed, again not necessarily slung, to allow occlusion during the reconstruction. Second, a decision may be required with respect to perfusion of the pelvic organs. Overt rectal or distal colonic ischaemia requiring surgical intervention occurs at a rate of 1–2 per cent after abdominal aortic aneurysm repair, and subclinical colonic ischaemia may be more common than was suspected several years ago. It is generally considered to be reasonable to aim to have one out of the three vessels (inferior mesenteric artery or either internal iliac artery) in circulation at the end of the procedure. Sometimes the distal limb of a bifurcated graft can be fashioned to include the origin of the internal iliac artery, but occasionally a vessel must be formally re-implanted or a jump graft performed.

After adequate exposure of the vessel above and below the aneurysm, 5000 IU of unfractionated heparin is administered intravenously, and after 2 minutes the vessels can be clamped. Some authorities advocate clamping the distal circulation first in order to minimize the risk of embolization – an essential sequence if the patient presented with distal embolic phenomena.

The aorta is opened longitudinally at a convenient site, and care is taken to incise to the right of the inferior mesenteric artery (Fig. 6.1b). The arteriotomy is extended up and down the vessel, to a distance 1–2 cm short of the supposed

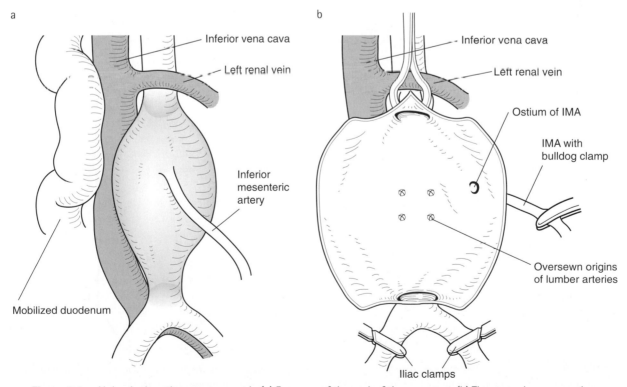

Figure 6.1 *Abdominal aortic aneurysm repair. (a) Exposure of the neck of the aneurysm. (b) The opened aneurysmal sac.*

neck proximally, and 1–2 cm short of the bifurcation distally. The final extent of the incision – top and bottom – is not made until the inside of the vessel has been inspected, and the correct levels of the neck and bifurcation confirmed. The thrombus, which is almost invariably present, must be scooped out and the aneurysm sac wiped clean with a swab. This will usually – though not always – reveal sites of back bleeding from the lumbar, inferior mesenteric or median sacral vessels. A self-retaining retractor can be placed within the sac itself. The inferior mesenteric artery should be gently occluded with a bulldog or other light clamp at the sac edge, but the other vessels can be oversewn from within, with a strong suture (2/0 or 3/0 silk or polypropylene) using a fig-ure-of-eight technique. Often the back wall of the aorta – particularly the distal end – is very calcified, and a controlled local endarterectomy may be needed to allow a stubborn ves-sel to be adequately sutured.

The longitudinal arteriotomy incision is then extended to just beyond the proximal limit of the aneurysm. Incisions are then made at 90 degrees to the longitudinal line of the aorta above the aneurysm (Fig. 6.2a). At this level, in the presence of a large aneurysm, even normal aortic tissue may arch ante-riorly and care must be taken not to cut directly backwards as this can make the proximal anastomosis unnecessarily diffi-cult. The distal end is completed following similar principles, and a decision reached as to whether a 'tube graft' or bifur-cated 'Y-graft' is more appropriate. If the aorta is of normal calibre for a portion below the aneurysm – or if the common iliac arteries are truly normal and not at all separated – then a tube graft may be used (Fig. 6.2b). Otherwise, a Y-graft is needed (Fig. 6.2c). The diameter of the graft to be used is now estimated, based upon the use of sterile 'sizers' or sim-ply by 'eyeballing' the neck and comparing this with the size drawn on the unopened graft box. Modern grafts, whether woven or knitted, are pre-sealed and no longer require 'pre-clotting' with the patient's own blood.

The graft is laid within the opened aneurysmal aorta as an inlay graft (see Fig. 5.13, page 79). The body of a bifurcated graft must be trimmed before the top end is sutured. It is cut to within 3 cm of the diverging limbs in order to avoid kink-ing. There are a variety of techniques used for the proximal anastomosis. Most frequently the anastomosis is performed with a continuous 2/0 or 3/0 monofilament, non-absorbable, double-ended suture which is commenced posteriorly. The suture is continued in both directions, around the posterior and lateral aspects of the anastomosis, before it is tightened and the graft parachuted into position. The anterior aspect of the anastomosis is then completed and the two ends of the suture tied together, to one or other side of the midline. An anterior knot over the convexity of the aorta should be avoided as it is more likely to come into direct contact with bowel, thereby increasing the likelihood of infective compli-cations. Interrupted evenly spaced mattress sutures may be a better alternative when the aortic wall is grossly thickened and friable, but unless the posterior aortic wall has been tran-sected the posterior sutures will have to be placed from within and the knots will lie in the lumen. Importantly, the posterior wall must be secured with deep bites – often into, and including – the anterior longitudinal ligament of the spine. When the proximal anastomosis has been completed the graft is clamped 2–3 cm distal to the anastomosis and the aortic clamp is released to test the anastomosis. Any bleeding points which are identified need to be dealt with as deemed appropriate, after reclamping the aorta. Figure-of-eight sutures, or sutures tied over a pledget of Dacron to prevent them cutting through a friable aortic wall, are standard tech-niques. A cuff of Dacron, cut from the graft, can be used over a vulnerable anastomosis to provide additional support.

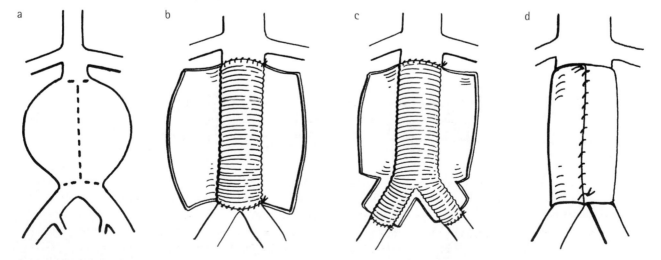

Figure 6.2 *Diagrammatic representation of an aortic graft. (a) The arteriotomy incisions. (b) An opened sac with an in-lay tube graft in position. (c) An opened sac with an in-lay Y-graft in position. (d) The sac has been closed over the graft.*

The graft is then cut to length. There should be a very modest degree of tension which prevents the prosthesis from bowing forwards or kinking. The distal anastomosis is performed in a similar fashion to the proximal, but before completion the graft is flushed to remove any thrombus that has formed within it. When the distal circulation is restored, a fall in systemic blood pressure and perfusion is likely. This is due to a sudden reduction in systemic vascular resistance and the return of cold, deoxygenated blood laden with free radicals, activated white cells, carbon dioxide and lactic acid, all of which are cardio-depressant and also cause pulmonary vascular vasoconstriction. Therefore, the anaesthetist must be warned before releasing the clamps, in order to ensure that the patient's intravascular compartment has been adequately filled, and that the necessary fluids and pressor agents are to hand to deal with a sudden fall in systemic blood pressure. Furthermore, the iliac arteries should be released sequentially, allowing flow to one limb at a time. The surgeon must pay attention to the effects on systemic blood pressure. If the pressure drops precipitously, it can be brought up again by partially or fully occluding the graft by finger pressure. A 10- to 20-mmHg drop in blood pressure and rise in end-tidal CO_2 is reassuring which, together with the return of a palpable femoral pulse, indicates the restoration of blood flow to the lower limb.

Before closing the aortic sac and reconstituting the peritoneum over the graft, the following should be checked. Is the colon still well perfused and is the inferior mesenteric artery back bleeding, and if so, does the origin of the inferior mesenteric artery require suture ligation? Have any lumbar arteries started bleeding now that the distal circulation has been restored? Are both femoral pulses present (if they were palpable preoperatively), and are the feet pink? If all is well, the small bowel and omentum can be eased toward their normal positions and the aortic sac closed (Fig. 6.2d). The opened aneurysm sac is sutured over the graft and the peritoneum is then also closed over it. Care must be taken to ensure that no part of the graft is left exposed. Adjacent gastrointestinal tract can adhere to exposed graft with an increased risk of infection or fistulation.

RETROPERITONEAL APPROACH

This is an alternative approach for an elective abdominal aortic aneurysm repair. The patient is positioned supine but tilted with the left side elevated. A left oblique muscle cutting incision is made through the abdominal wall muscles, and the peritoneum is retracted medially to give good access to the retroperitoneal abdominal aorta. This approach may be associated with less ileus, and reduced haemodynamic and respiratory stress with a resultant faster postoperative recovery. In addition, other intra-abdominal pathology – including adhesions from previous surgery – can be avoided. Access is superior if visceral reconstruction is also necessary. The main disadvantage of a retroperitoneal approach is the poor access it affords to the right iliac vessels. The principles

of the operation and the crucial operative steps are otherwise similar to those of the transperitoneal approach.

Inflammatory aneurysms

Around 5 per cent of abdominal aortic aneurysms are inflammatory. The main clinical feature is the pearly white appearance to the aortic wall that extends up to the duodenum. The inflammatory component involves the surrounding tissues and organs by adhesions, and this condition is related to the more diffuse inflammatory process of retroperitoneal fibrosis. In the majority of cases, the diagnosis is made at operation, although certain features support a preoperative diagnosis. For example, the patient may have presented with a systemic illness including fever and malaise, and a raised erythrocyte sedimentation rate (ESR). The appearance of a halo around the aneurysm, or an associated hydronephrosis, may have been detected on imaging. In addition, some patients with inflammatory aneurysms present with symptoms from ureteric obstruction, and the aneurysm is detected during urological investigations.

As the surrounding inflammation offers the aneurysm no protection from rupture, the indications for surgery are similar as for other abdominal aortic aneurysms. At operation the patient is more likely to require a supra-renal clamp and the surrounding structures – and in particular the duodenum – are at greater risk of damage. It may be necessary to clamp the aorta without separating the duodenum from the aneurysm. The patch of aortic wall adherent to the duodenum can then be circumcised after the aorta has been opened. The adherent patch of aneurysm wall is then left on the duodenum, thus avoiding the risk of duodenal damage if separation is attempted. Ureterolysis is advocated by some, but the risk of ureteric damage is high. It is usually unnecessary as, after the aneurysm has been repaired, the natural history is for the inflammation to settle and for any ureteric obstruction to resolve. Temporarily, ureteric obstruction can be managed by ureteric stents. Those patients who present with impairment of renal function may come to surgery with stents already *in situ*, and this will make identification of the ureters at operation much easier.

Ruptured abdominal aortic aneurysm

PREOPERATIVE MANAGEMENT

The diagnosis may be straightforward. A history of collapse and the clinical, or ultrasound, finding of an abdominal aortic aneurysm are sufficient grounds upon which to proceed to emergency repair. Occasionally, diagnostic difficulties occur either regarding the presence of an aneurysm or whether rupture has occurred. A CT scan may be helpful, but cannot be completely relied upon to differentiate the symptomatic from the ruptured aneurysm. A preoperative chest X-ray is desirable, as this may indicate a thoracic component to the aneurysm. An ECG is usually performed, and a difficult decision may ensue if it transpires that the patient is actually having a myocardial infarction at the time of presentation.

The surgical principles for repair of the ruptured abdominal aortic aneurysm differ little from that of the elective case. However, mortality is higher and it is unwise to subject every patient to surgery, especially if the prospects for survival are non-existent.[7] Scoring systems may aid these difficult decisions.[4,8]

After the decision has been made to proceed, the following steps are essential. Intravenous access through a large-bore cannula in the antecubital fossa is required. A urinary catheter should be inserted. The blood transfusion service must be alerted, blood cross-matched, and fresh-frozen plasma and platelets organized. If there is a delay in transfer to an appropriate centre, or to theatre, it is best not to resuscitate the patient too vigorously. Whilst the patient remains conscious, the blood pressure can be left with a systolic as low as 70 or 80 mmHg. Aggressive fluid infusion may raise the arterial blood pressure at the cost of displacing the thrombus at the rupture site and restarting the bleeding. Central venous cannulation can wait until after induction of anaesthesia. However, if there is time an arterial line is helpful. There is often a dramatic fall in blood pressure on induction, as the paralysing agent eliminates abdominal muscle tone and any element of tamponade. It is because of this particular possibility that it is common practice to prepare and drape the patient before the anaesthetic is administered, so that there is no unnecessary delay before the haemorrhage can be controlled surgically.

THE OPERATION

The operative procedure is essentially the same as described above for the elective situation. A transverse incision may still be chosen over a midline as access is usually adequate, but bleeding may occur from divided epigastric vessels when the blood pressure is restored.

It is rare for a patient to survive long enough to reach the operating theatre with a free intraperitoneal rupture. When a free rupture is encountered at laparotomy, pressure may be required directly onto the neck of the aneurysm to control the bleeding. Alternatively, a Foley catheter with a 30-mL balloon can be passed into the aorta, and up beyond the neck of the aneurysm (see Fig. 5.3a, page 73). The balloon is inflated to control the bleeding. The catheter lumen must be spigotted or clamped. If control at the neck is still difficult, then the aorta can be temporarily clamped through the lesser sac. A window is opened in the lesser omentum and the aorta can be exposed and clamped by separating the fibres of the diaphragmatic crura from the aorta (see Fig. 5.24, page 93). This manoeuvre will render more tissues ischaemic, and the effects of clamp release are more profound. Therefore, the clamp should be moved down to an infra-renal position, if and when this is possible.

Fortunately, the situation is usually a stable one, the haematoma is contained by the peritoneum, and a careful dissection can be performed. The duodenum is most frequently displaced to the right by the haematoma and is already partially mobilized. Dissection can proceed with division of the peritoneum over the aneurysm, followed by exposure of the aneurysmal aortic wall itself. The aorta should be followed superiorly, dividing the inferior mesenteric vein as it is encountered. Bleeding – either active or from the haematoma – will inevitably obscure the view, and the assistant needs to be active with the sucker in one hand and retractor in the other. Care must be taken to identify the neck of the aneurysm, and this often requires dissecting all the way up to the renal vein as in the elective case. The clamp must be carefully placed after clearing both sides of the aorta. It is easy to damage the inferior vena cava (IVC) or renal vein by hastily forcing a clamp into place. Routinely, the aorta is clamped before exposing the iliac vessels. If the iliac arteries are also aneurysmal then these must be treated and excluded by the repair. It is also possible that the rupture has occurred through the wall of an iliac artery.

If the situation is truly stable and the haematoma modest in size, some surgeons will administer heparin once the aorta is clamped, as the patient is more likely to suffer a thrombotic than a haemorrhagic complication once this stage has been reached. Other surgeons flush heparinized saline down each iliac system in order to reduce the possibility of iliac or femoral thrombosis while the repair is being performed.

Repair proceeds as for elective abdominal aortic aneurysm surgery. The graft is inserted as usual, and care must be taken to ensure that the iliac arteries are back-bleeding before completing the distal anastomosis. If there is no back-flow of blood from the legs it is prudent to sweep the distal vessels with a Fogarty catheter at this stage. As with the elective situation, perfusion of the feet must be checked before the abdomen is closed.

Inevitably there are occasions when the situation is not salvageable. Intraoperative complications may occur. The patient may arrest, or suffer a myocardial infarction with loss of cardiac output, despite the use of inotropes. An irreversible coagulopathy may develop or there may be purely surgical problems. The aneurysm may extend high above the renal arteries, there may be multiple dense adhesions that make it slow and difficult to gain access to perform a repair, or the aortic defect may be exposed by dissection and rapid and uncontrollable haemorrhage ensue. Whatever the circumstances, a decision to abandon the procedure may have to be made. This is best made in conjunction with other colleagues present.

AORTO-CAVAL FISTULA

Occasionally, when operating on a ruptured abdominal aortic aneurysm an aorto-caval fistula may be encountered. This may have been suspected preoperatively if the patient presented with 'high output cardiac failure', and was noted to have mottling of the lower torso and lower limbs despite apparently adequate upper body perfusion. An abdominal bruit or thrill may have been detected. The proximal aortic clamp is applied and the aorta opened. The fistula is then oversewn from inside the aorta with a heavy suture. Temporary control can be gained by local digital pressure on the IVC above and below the fistula.

Mixed aneurysmal and occlusive disease

It is normal to be able to perform elective aneurysm surgery from within the abdomen. However, the additional complication of coexistent occlusive disease frequently requires a unilateral or bilateral groin exploration to identify suitable outflow vessels for the graft. This is just one reason for an excess of morbidity and an increase in the reported mortality, to approximately 10 per cent, when compared with simple aneurysmal disease. However, the most important reason for the increase in observed mortality is that the presence of occlusive disease indicates a higher risk of latent, or overt, coronary and other atheromatous disease, and therefore an increased risk of perioperative myocardial and cerebral infarction, and of renal failure.

Planning the procedure requires adequate arterial imaging. A CT angiogram may suffice, but digital subtraction angiography (DSA) is still considered desirable by many surgeons. For the bypass to be symptomatically effective it is important to know that there are patent vessels at groin level. The bypass can be performed to the common, superficial or profunda femoral artery. However, as with aneurysmal disease, some thought must be given to the pelvic circulation at the end of the procedure. If there are no internal iliac vessels visible on imaging, and the inferior mesenteric artery is patent, then this vessel may need reimplanting. If an internal iliac artery is patent and the external iliac artery is patent from the groin up, then retrograde perfusion can be expected to be sufficient. However, difficulties arise if the external iliac artery is occluded, and both the internal iliac arteries (or the only remaining patent internal iliac artery) are perfused by patent common iliac arteries that will be excluded by the bypass. In this situation, if the inferior mesenteric artery is also chronically occluded, a jump graft may be needed to the internal iliac artery.

The above description of surgery for abdominal aortic aneurysm applies for cases of mixed arterial occlusive and aneurysmal disease. However, if a bypass to the femoral system is planned, it is usual to explore the groins first before opening the abdomen. A suitable site for the distal anastomosis is chosen, and the tunnels for the graft are prepared next. An index finger is gently inserted, nail down, in front of the common femoral artery and a space created into the pelvis. Beware of the deep circumflex iliac vein as it runs over the distal external iliac artery as it can easily be torn. Once this space has been fully opened to the limit of the finger, the tunnel is completed from above once the abdomen has been opened. The index finger is gently advanced in front of the common

iliac artery, pushing peritoneum and, more importantly, the ureter in front of the proposed tunnel. The two fingers will meet and a little, gentle, circular action of the fingertips may be required to break down the last intervening connective tissue. A long instrument – for example, a Roberts clamp – is then passed up from the groin, and from there a tape can be pulled down to the thigh and clipped to ensure that the track can be found again when the time comes to pass down the limbs of the graft. The tunnels are usually formed before the administration of heparin and, therefore, before the proximal anastomosis has been performed.

Each limb of the graft is then anastomosed end-to-side onto the segment of femoral artery which is most appropriate. One last consideration when performing these procedures is closure of the proximal ends of the iliac segments. The common iliac arteries are usually clamped at the start of the procedure, as for simple abdominal aortic aneurysm repair. After the top end of the graft is secured, the origins of the common iliac arteries, or other convenient site, must be sutured closed. This closure requires a double row of non-absorbable, heavy, monofilament suture, and this must be checked for haemostasis at the end of the procedure. Otherwise, even in the unusual case of chronic total occlusion of the iliac segment, there is a chance of back bleeding when the clamps are released at the completion of the distal anastomoses.

Endovascular aneurysm repair

Since the first published reports of endovascular aneurysm repair by Parodi in 1991, there has been a revolution in the management of abdominal aortic aneurysm.[9] The advantages offered by endovascular repair are lower morbidity and mortality, and a shorter postoperative stay in hospital. There is therefore the possibility of offering repair to less-fit patients. The major disadvantages are cost and problems with the reliability of new technologies, the need for long-term device surveillance, and the high incidence of often-minor problems that nonetheless require reintervention. The principle of this technique is aneurysm exclusion, rather than the conventional aortic replacement.

Preoperative assessment of the aneurysm morphology and measurements of the dimensions at the neck and distally are crucial. A variety of devices and systems are marketed. Most are delivered after a femoral cutdown, but there are now low-profile products that can be delivered percutaneously. The whole process is performed under radiological control. The femoral artery is cannulated and an initial angiogram performed, confirming the positions of renal arteries. The prosthesis is secured proximally first, usually below the renal arteries, although there are now fenestrated devices that allow supra-renal deployment. Following this the ipsilateral limb is secured distally. The contralateral common femoral artery is cannulated and the prosthesis for the contralateral limb delivered and positioned through the long component (Fig. 6.3).

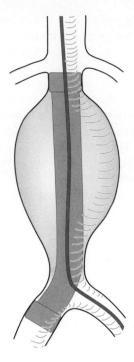

Figure 6.3   *Endovascular aneurysm repair. One component of the stent graft is already positioned. The guide wire is in place through the left iliac system and the second component will be delivered over this.*

Aortic graft complications

The true rate of graft complications is not known but it is estimated that approximately 1–2 per cent of aortic grafts will become infected. This may manifest as a systemic illness due to graft-sourced sepsis. Alternatively, it may present as a local graft problem in the form of a pseudo-aneurysm, or pus formation at an anastomotic site, most frequently in the groin. More serious local manifestations include fistula formation or haemorrhage due to anastomotic disruption. It seems reasonable to consider aorto-enteric fistulae in the same category as infective complications because the graft is inevitably infected at this stage, the aetiology is considered by many to be infection, and the treatment options are similar.

Diagnosing graft infection is often far from straightforward. If the patient presents with torrential gastrointestinal bleeding, sepsis or with an obvious septic focus and a CT scan demonstrates perigraft fluid, ectopic gas or intravenous contrast medium in the bowel lumen, the diagnosis is simple. However, much more difficult is exclusion – or confirmation – of graft infection in a patient with more insidious symptoms, for example weight loss, lethargy, pain or gastrointestinal blood loss. CT scans, or angiography, may show focal bowel thickening, inflammation of the perigraft tissues or minor anastomotic dilatation, but none of these alone will secure a diagnosis. Labelled white cell scans and magnetic resonance imaging (MRI) have a role, but reported sensitivities vary widely. Upper and lower gastrointestinal endoscopy

are often unhelpful unless there is active bleeding, but an ulcer in the third or fourth parts of the duodenum should be treated with suspicion. The patient may present many years after the original surgery, and the bacteria implicated range from a destructive *Staphylococcus aureus* to a low-virulence *Staphylococcus epidermidis*.

Operative strategy in all infected grafts is defined by two aims: (i) excision of infected material; and (ii) restoration of circulation to the tissue which was perfused by the graft. This is particularly challenging in aortic grafts where perfusion of the whole lower part of the body needs to be considered and, in addition, in some patients occlusive disease may have been all (or at least part) of the reason for the original surgery. The mortality of surgery for infected aortic prostheses is reported at up to 50 per cent, with major amputation rates in the survivors also approaching 50 per cent. A major concern is recurrent infection in a newly implanted prosthesis, either by direct or haematogenous seeding.

Occasionally a local procedure can be performed. The limb of an infected, aortic bifurcated graft can be excised, and this may be sufficient if the patient presented with a chronic problem and the upper part of the graft is incorporated into the surrounding tissues. Some surgeons advocate that if any part of a graft is infected then it must be assumed that the whole is affected. Pragmatically, an elderly or frail patient may survive a local graft excision if the infection is low grade, and there may not be a further problem within that patient's lifetime.

The options for definitive surgery, either urgent or planned, can be considered in three main ways:

1. The method of reconstitution of flow must be decided upon, anatomic or extra-anatomic (Fig. 6.4). The extra-anatomical route has the major advantage that there is a lower risk of infection in the new graft. Axillo-femoral bypass is described in the section on limb salvage surgery below.
2. The material for the replacement conduit must be chosen. The choice includes prosthetic material, prosthetic material with microbial retardant adjuvant (e.g. rifampicin or silver coating) or autologous vein. Long saphenous vein is unsuitable for this purpose, but a graft can be fashioned using both superficial femoral veins. The popliteal vein can form an extension to this free vein graft if further length is required. Problems with venous return are minimal if the profunda femoris vein is left intact. In addition, a small number of surgeons have reported work using arterial allografts.
3. It should be considered whether the procedure might be staged. This is occasionally an option even in aortic grafts if the original bypass was performed for claudication and the collaterals are sufficiently well developed to allow the limbs and pelvic organs to remain viable after graft excision. It has the advantage that the infected graft can be excised and all residual sepsis eradicated before a new graft is inserted.

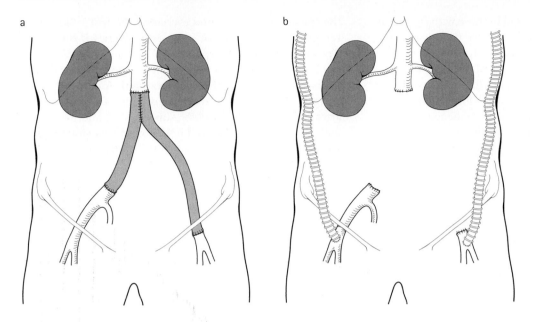

Figure 6.4 *Reconstruction for infected aortic grafts. (a) The infected graft has been excised and replaced with a deep vein graft to the common iliac artery on the right and to the common femoral artery on the left. (b) After excision of the infected aortic graft, the aortic stump and the right common iliac artery have been oversewn. Bilateral axillo-femoral grafts can restore distal perfusion.*

When an infected aortic graft is excised and an extra-anatomical replacement graft has been chosen, the stump of the proximal native aorta must be closed. This is a vulnerable end closure of a large artery which has a wall made friable by both the underlying degenerative disease and the infection. Monofilament mattress sutures are usually recommended before the aortic clamp is released, followed by a further continuous suture. Distally, the iliac stumps must also be oversewn (Fig. 6.4b). When, in order to safeguard distal perfusion, an extra-anatomical bypass has to be performed at the same time as the excision of the graft, the axillo-femoral bypass is created first. Great care is needed to isolate the clean from the infected operative field.

SURGERY OF THORACO–ABDOMINAL ANEURYSMS

These aneurysms are subdivided into types I to IV, and are illustrated diagrammatically in Figure 6.5. The nomenclature is superficially confusing, as type IV aneurysms – despite extending up to the diaphragm – are still confined to the abdominal aorta. However, the additional technical challenges they pose, compared with infra-renal abdominal aortic aneurysms, justifies their inclusion with the other thoraco-abdominal aneurysms.

The surgery for any of these aneurysms is a very major undertaking, with significant mortality and morbidity. In

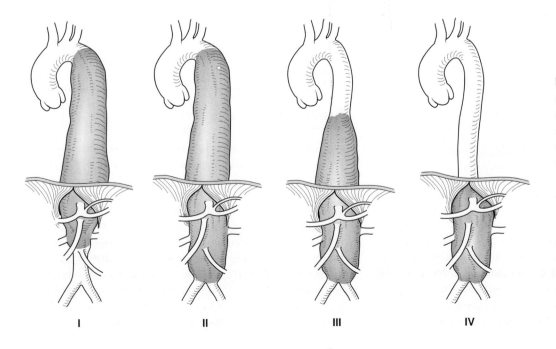

I   II   III   IV

Figure 6.5 *Thoraco-abdominal aneurysms are classified into four types. Type I is a thoracic aneurysm which extends down to involve the origins of the visceral vessels. Type II is a diffuse aneurysm involving the whole of the thoracic and abdominal aorta. Type III involves the whole abdominal aorta but only the lower thoracic aorta. Type IV in which the suprarenal portion of the abdominal aorta is involved, but the aorta is normal above the diaphragm.*

many elderly and frail patients – and in those with significant co-morbidity – surgical intervention will not be justified. Surgery has been centralized to tertiary referral units in order to improve outcome, and most general vascular surgeons will refer potentially suitable patients to these centres for assessment and surgery. It is however still important that the additional technical and physiological challenges of these operations are understood by those dealing with the commoner vascular problems. Further reading on the subject is recommended.[10]

ACCESS

The patient is usually positioned supine, but is rotated so that the left chest and shoulder are raised. The left arm is raised on a support. A long thoraco-abdominal incision is needed to expose the whole length of the thoracic and abdominal aorta. In type IV aneurysms the incision does not need to be extended so far proximally, but access into the chest will still be required. This incision alone is associated with significant postoperative respiratory morbidity. If the transperitoneal approach to the infradiaphragmatic aorta is chosen the aorta, spleen and left kidney are swung anteromedially. The alternative retroperitoneal approach is also satisfactory unless an endarterectomy will be needed on a visceral or right renal artery, when access may be inferior.

VASCULAR CONTROL

It is the high cross-clamping of the aorta which is mainly responsible for the mortality and morbidity of this surgery. Complications include ventricular strain with an intraoperative myocardial infarction, renal damage both from ischaemia and from reperfusion injury, and paraplegia from spinal cord ischaemia. Prior to closing the proximal clamp, the patient is systemically heparinized. The kidneys may be additionally protected by the administration of a diuretic, in addition to local cooling. Temporary shunts to maintain distal blood flow have been employed in attempts to reduce left ventricular strain, acute tubular necrosis and paraplegia, but these have not been universally successful. A left heart bypass is also used on occasion, and this can maintain distal perfusion if segmental clamping is employed. For example, the proximal anastomosis can be performed with clamps on the aorta at the diaphragm and at the junction of the aortic arch and descending aorta. Meanwhile, inflow from the left heart bypass to a femoral artery can maintain perfusion through all branches of the abdominal aorta by retrograde flow.

RECONSTRUCTION

The aneurysmal sac is opened and the top end of a long prosthetic graft is secured in place in a similar fashion to that employed in an infra-renal aneurysm repair. There is then the additional challenge of restoring inflow to the important branches of the thoracic and abdominal aorta. Except in the lower type IV aneurysms, the high cross-clamp endangers

the spinal cord. Sometimes therefore, the first vessels to be reimplanted are a pair of intercostal arteries if these were demonstrated on a preoperative CT angiogram. When this has been done, the cross-clamp can be moved more distally so that spinal cord perfusion is restored. A patch of native aorta is then cut to encircle the origins of the right renal artery, the coeliac axis and the superior and inferior mesenteric arteries. A similar-sized hole is cut in the graft and the patch of native aorta sewn into it. The left renal artery is reimplanted into the graft in a similar fashion with a second patch (Fig. 6.6). The occlusion clamp can then be moved again to a more distal site to allow renal and visceral reperfusion before the distal anastomosis is fashioned. Occasionally, the renal and visceral arteries cannot be simply reimplanted on a patch of native aorta. There may be an atheromatous stenosis of the origin of the artery. An endarterectomy may be successful in restoring patency, but a separate bypass graft may have to be fashioned.

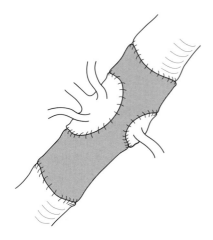

Figure 6.6 *Discs of native aorta are cut to include the origins of the renal and visceral arteries. These discs are anastomosed into holes cut in the graft.*

OCCLUSIVE DISEASE OF THE VISCERAL ARTERIES

Renal artery revascularization

Occlusive disease of the renal arteries, with resultant ischaemic renal tissue, can result in two main complications. The ischaemic tissue may cause renovascular hypertension by alterations in the renin/angiotensin homeostatic balance, and renal function can deteriorate. When these complications ensue, but the kidney has retained some useful function, revascularization is an option. If function is extremely poor, a nephrectomy may be the better alternative if the other kidney is normal. Renal revascularization should be considered in poorly controlled hypertension if one kidney has a renal artery stenosis of >70 per cent, and it may also be indicated for deteriorating renal function, especially when acute renal failure is precipitated by angiotensin-converting enzyme inhibitors.

Revascularization by angioplasty and endoluminal stents is increasingly a simpler option than surgery, especially in elderly patients with significant cardiovascular co-morbidity. In younger patients the stenosis is more commonly either post-traumatic or from fibromuscular dysplasia. Angioplasty with stenting may be better for fibromuscular dysplasia than surgical revascularization, due to fewer complications. Surgical options include endarterectomy and bypass grafts, either alone or in conjunction with aortic replacement.

ENDARTERECTOMY

A transaortic renal endarterectomy, as illustrated in Figure 6.7, is a satisfactory approach which is usually possible without a full aortic cross-clamp. The incision is transverse and extends into the renal artery. Closure is with a vein patch.

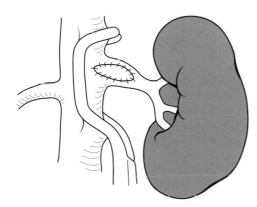

Figure 6.7   *A renal endarterectomy. A side clamp is maintaining distal flow. Closure is with a vein patch.*

RENAL ARTERY GRAFT

The choice between infra-renal and supra-renal aorta as the donor site depends mainly on the distribution of any concomitant aortic atheromatous changes. The anastomosis is end-to-side onto the aorta and, if there is no atheroma and the aorta is pliable, it may be possible to construct this anastomosis with a side clamp on the aorta whilst preserving distal flow. A cross-clamp will be necessary if the aorta is thickened and atheromatous. The distal anastomosis of graft to native renal artery beyond the stenosis is end-to-end (Fig. 6.8).

When the abdominal aorta is too heavily diseased for a graft to be taken from the region of the kidney, there are several alternative operative strategies. A graft can be taken from the hepatic artery or, after a splenectomy, the splenic artery can be anastomosed end-to-end to the renal artery (Fig. 6.9). Alternatively, the kidney can be mobilized and autotransplanted into the iliac fossa. This will require an arterial and a venous anastomosis, but the ureter – after mobilization – can be left undisturbed. Unfortunately, if the aorta is heavily diseased the iliac arteries are often similarly affected.

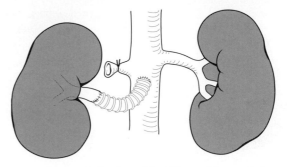

Figure 6.8   *Revascularization of the kidney with a graft from the infra-renal aorta. This is an end-to-side anastomosis onto the aorta, but an end-to-end anastomosis to the renal artery distal to the stenosis.*

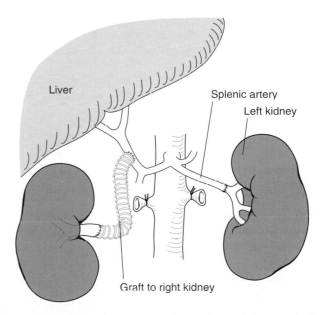

Figure 6.9   *Alternative donor arteries can be used to revascularize a kidney. Right: a graft has been taken from the hepatic artery. Left: the spleen has been removed and the splenic artery itself used for an end-to-end anastomosis.*

SIMULTANEOUS AORTIC AND RENAL ARTERY RECONSTRUCTION

This more major procedure, with a significantly higher mortality rate, should however be considered when there is significant aortic pathology in itself justifying surgery (Fig. 6.10).

Mesenteric ischaemia

Acute mesenteric ischaemia, presenting as an intra-abdominal emergency with ischaemic or infarcted bowel, is discussed in Chapter 22. Acute presentation is usually after infarction has occurred, and revascularization of the bowel is therefore seldom a practical option. However, those patients

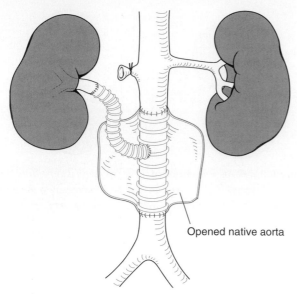

Figure 6.10 *Right renal revascularization has been combined with an infra-renal aortic tube graft.*

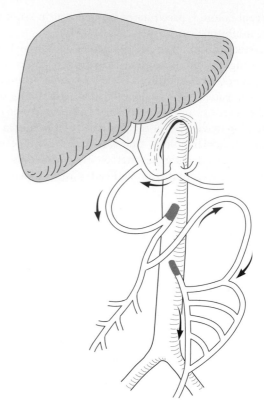

Figure 6.11 *Extensive collateral circulation allows the whole gut to be perfused through a single patent visceral artery.*

who present with chronic or critical mesenteric ischaemia can be viewed in a similar fashion to those requiring revascularization for limb salvage. The occlusions in the visceral arterial tree are almost always segmental and multiple. For a considerable period compensation is possible as there is already an anatomical communication between the three visceral arteries to the gut, and these channels open up as alternative routes for perfusion. It is not uncommon to maintain adequate perfusion of the bowel with only one of these visceral arteries still patent (Fig. 6.11).

Patients with chronic mesenteric ischaemia classically complain of non-specific post-prandial abdominal pain and weight loss. Diagnosis depends on an initial suspicion followed by vascular investigations. In critical ischaemia an urgent multidisciplinary approach is essential to save the ischaemic bowel.[11] Revascularization options include thromboembolectomy, endarterectomy and bypass grafts. Superior mesenteric artery embolism and embolectomy are described in the section on mesenteric vascular emergencies in Chapter 22.

ACCESS

The visceral arteries are usually isolated via a transperitoneal anterior abdominal approach. The *coeliac artery* is reached by an incision into the lesser sac through the lesser omentum. The aorta emerges into the abdomen just to the right of the oesophagus, which is easily identified if a nasogastric tube has been passed. The origin of the coeliac artery is very close to the diaphragm, and additional aorta above it can be exposed by an incision in the right crus of the diaphragm (see Fig. 5.24, page 93). The origin of the *superior mesenteric artery* can be reached by the same approach as that required for the coeliac artery, which is convenient when surgery is

planned on both vessels. It can also be reached a few centimetres from its origin, where it emerges from the pancreas, by displacing the transverse colon up, and the small bowel to the right. Access to the *inferior mesenteric artery* only requires incision of the posterior peritoneum over the anterior surface of the aorta.

The alternative posterior approach to all three arteries relies on a medial visceral rotation of the splenic flexure of the colon, spleen and tail and body of the pancreas.

ENDARTERECTOMY

Endarterectomy requires suprarenal aortic cross-clamping, with its associated risks. A trapdoor of aortic wall – including the origins of the coeliac and superior mesenteric arteries – is then raised to expose their origins. Good results have been reported with endarterectomy, but most surgeons favour bypass grafting or the reimplantation of a visceral artery.

BYPASS GRAFTS

Vein or prosthetic graft can be used as a bypass. Vein may be more liable to kink, but is preferred if any reconstruction is to be performed when there is also the need to resect a segment of infarcted gut. Inflow can be taken from the supra-coeliac aorta forming an antegrade graft, or from the infra-renal aorta forming a retrograde graft. The advantages of the latter are easier access, and the avoidance of a suprarenal aortic clamp which may be necessary in a supra-coeliac graft if the aortic wall is too stiff to allow a side clamp. Disadvantages include an increased danger of occlusion from kinking, but the risk of this can be reduced by using a stiffer prosthetic graft which is also long enough that it can enter the superior mesenteric artery in an antegrade direction (Fig. 6.12). As discussed above, it is usual for all three visceral arteries to be affected by occlusive pathology at the time of presentation, and for a large collateral network to have become established. Grafts are therefore seldom performed to all three arteries, and grafting to the superior mesenteric artery alone is often sufficient. There is however a good argument for performing a graft to two of the visceral vessels if only to ensure alternative inflow into the visceral arterial system if one graft should fail. A second limb of an infra-renal graft can be tunnelled up behind the neck of the pancreas for an anastomosis onto the coeliac artery.

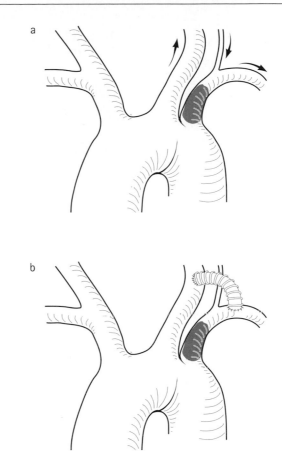

Figure 6.13 *(a) The proximal subclavian occlusion has resulted in 'subclavian steal', in which the upper limb perfusion is dependent on retrograde flow down the vertebral artery. (b) Revascularization with a bypass graft from the carotid artery.*

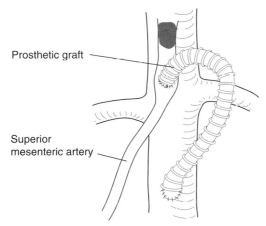

Figure 6.12 *A retrograde bypass graft from the aorta to the superior mesenteric artery. The wide curve reduces the risk of kinking, and aligns the flow with the recipient vessel.*

OCCLUSIVE DISEASE OF THE ARTERIES OF THE AORTIC ARCH

Although stenoses of the roots and proximal portions of the large branches of the aortic arch can occur in atheromatous disease, arteritis is an alternative underlying pathology which classically affects young women. Patients with carotid occlusion usually present with neurological symptoms. Those with subclavian occlusion may present with claudication, or critical ischaemia, of the upper limb. However, they may also present with neurological symptoms, when the only perfusion of the limb is from retrograde flow down the vertebral artery with subsequent deleterious effects on cerebral perfusion (Fig. 6.13a). This is known as *subclavian steal.*

Occlusion of the roots of these vessels is a comparatively rare disease, and an endovascular approach with angioplasties and stents is increasingly the first line of management. Surgery is therefore practised relatively infrequently, and

those patients who do require surgery are usually referred to surgeons with a special interest. Thus, these operations do not form part of the standard surgical practice of most vascular surgeons. However, the principles are similar to other vascular reconstructive challenges. Bypass grafts are fashioned to restore perfusion. When several vessels are involved, the proximal anastomosis may have to be taken from the aortic arch (Fig. 6.14). A median sternotomy or a 3rd space right anterolateral thoracotomy, will be necessary for access.

When the stenosis affects only one or two large arteries, extra-thoracic bypass techniques will be practical. Two such grafts are illustrated in Figures 6.13b and 6.15. In Figure 6.13b, a graft has been taken from the common carotid artery to the patent portion of the ipsilateral subclavian artery distal to the obstruction. The supraclavicular approach which allows simultaneous access to both these arteries is described in Chapter 5, and illustrated in Figure 5.20. Figure 6.15 illustrates a bypass from a patent axillary artery to a contralateral axillary artery which has an inflow obstruction. A bilateral infraclavicular approach, as described for an axillobifemoral bypass and illustrated in Figure 6.17, is used. The graft is tunnelled subcutaneously across the anterior chest wall.

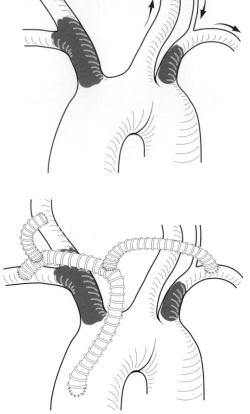

Figure 6.14 *A graft from the thoracic aorta to the arteries of the aortic arch which are occluded near their origins.*

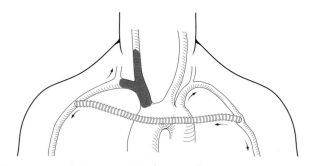

Figure 6.15 *A bypass graft from one axillary artery to the other to restore upper limb perfusion.*

OPTIONS IN LIMB SALVAGE SURGERY

The options for limb ischaemia include a conservative approach based upon best medical therapy, an endoluminal radiological approach, a reconstructive surgical approach, amputation if there is no possible reconstructive option (see Chapter 4), or a palliative approach, accepting that the ischaemic limb is a manifestation of end-stage cardiovascular or malignant disease.

- Best medical treatment comprises antiplatelet therapy, lipid management with diet, statins and the optimization of antihypertensive therapy. Advice and support should be given both regarding the cessation of smoking and the maintenance of regular exercise. In some centres exercise programmes are available.
- Radiological approach: endoluminal therapy has opened new avenues for limb salvage. Thrombolysis is an alternative to surgery in acute limb ischaemia from thrombus or embolus, either within a native vessel or within a graft. Balloon angioplasty – with or without stenting – offers many advantages over surgery, particularly in the aorto-iliac segment. In many situations endoluminal procedures alone are sufficient to salvage a limb. Percutaneous procedures can also be used in conjunction with reconstructive surgery to improve inflow, and allow a crossover graft or a femoral-popliteal graft to function. Angioplasty can also be used to help salvage a failing graft.

ACUTE LIMB ISCHAEMIA

In the absence of protective collaterals, a sudden occlusion of an artery can present as acute limb ischaemia. Limb salvage will usually require emergency intervention to restore distal perfusion, whether this is by thrombolysis, by surgical thromboembolectomy or by an emergency vascular reconstruction. No attempt should be made to restore the circulation to a limb that is non-viable as this will merely hasten the death of the patient from multiorgan failure. The only alternative is amputation, but in those patients who are already terminally ill, supportive palliative care is usually more appropriate.[7]

Diagnosis and assessment

Classical presentation of acute limb ischaemia is with the five 'Ps': a sudden onset of Pain, followed by Perishing cold, Pallor, Parasthesia, and ultimately Paralysis. The marble white leg is not seen universally as venous reflux disease, or a trickle of blood via collaterals, can colour the skin and confuse the situation. Hand-held Doppler assessment is very helpful, as is a clinical comparison with the pulse pattern of the contralateral limb.

Having made a diagnosis of acute limb ischaemia, the question is raised as to whether this is an embolic phenomenon, or an acute deterioration on the background of existing pathology, with thrombosis *in situ* due to atheroma, aneurysm or a thrombotic tendency. Ultimately, the biggest decisions in acute limb ischaemia are with respect to the time available for investigation, and then the most appropriate salvage procedure. A good history will reveal the rate of change. If the symptoms of pain have progressed to sensorimotor deficit within 2–3 hours, then the patient has little in the way of protective collaterals and the limb is imminently threatened. Consideration should therefore be given to urgent exploration with a view to thromboembolectomy and on-table imaging, all of which can be performed under local anaesthesia.

However, the patient in whom symptoms and signs have developed over a day or so, with a history of claudication and evidence of contralateral peripheral arterial occlusive disease, merits urgent imaging in order to plan the best treatment. In addition, in acute ischaemia of more insidious onset, interventional radiology may provide the best initial therapy in the form of thrombolysis (see Chapter 5), even if it has to be followed by later angioplasty or definitive surgery. The groups of patients for whom lysis is particularly suitable are those with graft occlusion, those with emboli arising from a popliteal aneurysm, and those in whom there is a specific underlying anatomical abnormality, such as a popliteal entrapment syndrome. In each of these scenarios, lysis can be used to retrieve a difficult ischaemic problem and allow definitive corrective surgery at a later date. Be wary of a patient presenting with a complication of a thrombosed or embolizing popliteal aneurysm (see below). Some 50 per cent of patients presenting in such a way will ultimately lose their leg, due – at least in part – to a failure of timely diagnosis.

The limitation of thrombolysis in acute limb ischaemia is the delay after the start of treatment before there is any improvement in perfusion. There is often even an initial worsening of both the symptoms and signs of ischaemia in the first few hours. This makes it an unsuitable treatment when the initial assessment indicates limb loss within 4–6 hours unless the circulation is restored.

Thromboembolectomy

The need for preoperative imaging is dictated by the nature and onset of the presenting signs and symptoms, and also the facilities available for on-table angiography. Anticoagulation is commenced with 5000 IU of unfractionated heparin.

The two commonest sites for this procedure are the common femoral artery in the groin, and the distal brachial artery at the elbow. In both cases this represents a site of arterial bifurcation where an embolus may lodge. Following the lodgement of an embolus, there is propagation of thrombus both proximal and distal to the occlusion. This must also be addressed before perfusion can be restored. The diagnosis of embolus is more secure in the upper limb, as in the lower limb there is a greater likelihood of an iliac or superficial femoral artery thrombosis occurring on a background of pre-existing disease. Thrombectomy may be successful in this situation but, if it is not successful in restoring distal perfusion, there may be a need for a salvage bypass.[12]

BRACHIAL EMBOLECTOMY

This can easily be performed under local anaesthesia in a cooperative patient. Most patients tolerate this procedure well, but it is advisable to have an anaesthetist present as an acute cardiorespiratory deterioration can occur during the procedure. Often a pulse can be felt all the way down the brachial artery to just above the bifurcation in the antecubital fossa. This is the site to infiltrate with 10–15 mL of 1 per cent lignocaine, in the anaesthetic room before scrubbing.

The skin should be prepared from the shoulder to the wrist, and the hand is placed in a see-through bowel bag, or draped in such a way as to allow ready assessment of the return of perfusion. A lazy-S incision is made from just medial to the distal portion of the biceps muscle, over the tendon and then down onto the forearm. After incising the skin, a few subcutaneous veins are usually encountered; these should be divided between ties or pushed to the side with a self-retainer. The brachial artery lies between the biceps tendon and the median nerve and deep to the bicipital aponeurosis. The latter structure can be incised to allow further exposure (see Fig. 5.23, page 92). The brachial artery is slung, and this can be used to retract it forwards to find the bifurcation. Both the radial and ulnar arteries must be slung to allow proper clearance of these vessels. Note that the interosseus artery often arises close to, or at the bifurcation. This vessel may produce troublesome back-bleeding.

The arteries are clamped and a transverse arteriotomy is performed about 1 cm proximal to the bifurcation. A Fogarty balloon is passed, proximally first and then distally, down both the radial and ulnar arteries separately. Good inflow must be established, as well as good back-bleeding from each of the distal vessels. The Fogarty catheter must be used with care. Do not over-inflate the balloon, and carefully adjust the pressure as resistance changes, feeling the pressure through your thumb holding the syringe.

Completion angiography is desirable. Ideally, this is achieved with a C-arm image intensifier system. Modern machines can produce subtraction images in theatre. Once satisfied, the arteriotomy is closed with interrupted 5/0 or 6/0 monofilament sutures, inserted so that the needle passes from deep to superficial on the distal part of the artery.

FEMORAL EMBOLECTOMY

Most femoral explorations can also be performed under local anaesthesia. However, because of the number of cases that require fasciotomies, and the occasional need for salvage crossover or bypass grafts, it is essential that the duty anaesthetist has seen the patient preoperatively. Once more, it is better to inject the operative field with 1 per cent lignocaine (20 mL) before scrubbing. The groin should be shaved, and consideration must be given to the possible need for a crossover graft. The skin of the limb is prepared down to the ankle, after which the foot is placed in a transparent bowel bag. Make sure that the landmarks are exposed. The inguinal ligament runs between the anterior superior iliac spine and the pubic tubercle, and these points of reference must be in view. The approach to the common femoral artery is described in Chapter 5, but to summarize, a vertical or oblique incision is made and the subcutaneous fat divided down to Scarpa's fascia. The fascia is incised and deep to this level, veins and lymphatics must be divided between ties as encountered. The lymphatic channels are commonly seen just anterior to the common and superficial femoral arteries. The common femoral artery is slung at the level of the inguinal ligament, and tapes are then also passed around the superficial and profunda femoral arteries. Be careful not to damage the profunda femoris vein when dissecting the profunda femoral artery. The posterior aspect of the bifurcation must be carefully inspected to avoid missing a 'first perforating branch' of the profunda. A lateral or medial circumflex artery may also come off the common femoral artery rather than the profunda as usual.

Pay careful attention to the quality of the vessels. The superficial femoral artery may be chronically occluded, the origin of the profunda may be narrowed, or there may be a posterior plaque running down into the common femoral artery from the external iliac artery. All of these features will influence the direction and nature of the arteriotomy. The common femoral artery is opened, longitudinally if the vessels are disease-free and large or if the common and superficial femoral arteries are heavily diseased and a vein patch is considered necessary. A transverse arteriotomy is preferable if the vessel is diseased posteriorly, but is widely patent and soft anteriorly. An oblique arteriotomy down into the profunda femoral artery is best if the superficial femoral artery is chronically occluded and the origin of the profunda is hard and therefore in need of patch angioplasty closure. If in doubt, a transverse arteriotomy is perhaps best as this can be converted into a diamond opening and either patched if necessary, or closed primarily if a simple embolectomy is performed.

Inflow must be established first. The iliac system is swept with a large (size 4) Fogarty catheter. Good inflow, once gained, must be protected by flushing dilute heparinized saline solution (2000 IU heparin in 500 mL saline) up the iliac system. Occasionally, inflow cannot be established. Are the iliac arteries hard and craggy when the catheter is passed? Perhaps the catheter cannot be passed up at all. Is this due to a blockage or non-negotiable kink? At this stage active consideration may be given to a salvage extra-anatomical bypass.

Once inflow is established, attention is turned to the distal arterial tree. A size 3 Fogarty catheter is passed down the superficial femoral artery. In the case of a classic embolus, the major fragment will be found on opening the common femoral artery, but there will be smaller fragments and a ribbon – often an arterial cast – of propagated thrombus down the superficial and profunda femoral arteries. Keep passing the catheter up and down until there is no further return of thrombus. There should be good back-bleeding, and the catheter should have been passed down to 40 cm at least. At this stage many advocate a completion angiogram. If this can be accomplished it certainly should be, but in some theatres there is no C-arm facility with image intensification. An alternative is to close the arteriotomy and watch for a healthy reperfusion of the foot. An awake patient will often report a return of feeling and warmth.

Completion angiography is always desirable in femoral embolectomies, and if the clinical result of reperfusion is poor – or if the catheter cannot be passed beyond the adductor hiatus – then an angiogram really is essential. It may be that there is chronic obliterative disease with a stenosis or occlusion at the femoropopliteal level, or the thrombus may be strongly adherent to the vessel wall. Alternatively, there may be a slightly unusual cause for acute ischaemia, for example a thrombosed popliteal aneurysm or an acute presentation of an entrapment syndrome.

If the problem is adherent clot, either in the distal circulation or on the wall of a major vessel, then thrombolysis can be considered. Tissue plasminogen activator (t-PA) can be administered directly into the artery. The usual dose is 10 mg made up to 20 mL and instilled for 20–30 minutes before repeating the angiogram. If there is a chronic superficial femoral artery block, collaterals will be well developed. In this situation, clearance of both the acutely blocked iliac system – and of the common and profunda femoral arteries – may be sufficient to restore perfusion to the limb. It is worth closing the arteriotomy and watching what happens to the foot. A patch angioplasty of a narrowed profunda origin may be sufficient to prevent rethrombosis.

Sometimes a salvage bypass is required, as is performed for chronic ischaemia and described below.

SADDLE EMBOLI

Even a large embolus which lodges in the aortic bifurcation can be cleared by femoral embolectomy. This must be carried out through both femoral arteries, as illustrated in Figure 6.16.

CHRONIC LIMB ISCHAEMIA AND ARTERIAL RECONSTRUCTION

The management of a chronically ischaemic limb requires a holistic approach from the outset, carefully balancing the patient's general condition and co-morbidity against the severity of the limb ischaemia and the level of symptoms. Available bypass material and the potential for success, based on imaging, must be considered.

Although a patient with a chronically ischaemic limb can often be managed conservatively, there are some who – although the limb is not threatened – will seek intervention for claudication that might inhibit their active lifestyle.

Despite the relatively benign course of chronic limb ischaemia, a proportion of patients will develop *critical limb ischaemia*. Pragmatically, this can be considered to be a limb which is actually threatened with loss of viability if left untreated. By definition, it is a chronic situation resulting in rest pain and/or tissue loss in the form of ulceration or gan-

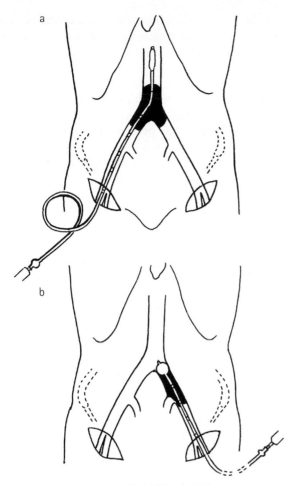

Figure 6.16 *Embolectomy of a saddle embolus at the aortic bifurcation. (a) The catheter tip is above the embolus after introduction through the right femoral artery. (b) Residual clot is then removed via the left femoral artery.*

grenous digits. Typically – but not exclusively – the ulcers affect the bony prominences of the foot. The development of sensorimotor signs (altered sensation and/or power), or calf tenderness which implies muscle necrosis, both indicate impending limb loss. Intervention – either radiological, in the form of angioplasties or stents, or surgical in the form of bypass grafts – becomes necessary if amputation is to be avoided. Endarterectomy, although a standard treatment for atheromatous stenosis of the carotid artery, has a diminishing role in the treatment of chronic ischaemia of the lower limb.

Before examining individual scenarios, it is helpful to consider the principles governing the choice of procedure, conduit and anatomical route taken to connect the recipient and donor vessels. Essentially, a graft will fail if the inflow is inadequate, the outflow vessels are too diseased or narrowed, or the conduit is inadequate in terms of quality, diameter or material. The most frequently used conduit for infra-inguinal bypass is the long saphenous vein (LSV). If the bypass is only going to the above-knee popliteal segment, a prosthetic material probably produces similar patency and limb salvage rates. However, for longer bypasses it is generally accepted that prosthetic material is inferior. The absence of a suitable LSV results in a choice between the hunt for a suitable vein, the use of a prosthetic material, or the use of a biological material such as human umbilical vein. Although the ipsilateral LSV is usually the preferred option, other suitable superficial veins include the contralateral LSV, a short saphenous vein or an arm vein. A deep system vein, such as the femoral vein, can also be considered. Dacron and expanded polytetrafluoroethylene (e-PTFE) are the standard prosthetic materials used for arterial conduits, and these can be used with or without a distal cuff of vein.

A graft may be routed in a way that mimics the vessel that it is replacing, *anatomical bypass*, or in a way that does not, *extra-anatomical* bypass. Examples of anatomical bypasses are the femoropopliteal bypass, the aorto-bifemoral bypass and the ilio-femoral bypass. Extra-anatomical bypasses include femoro-femoral crossover grafts and axillo-femoral grafts. The reasons for choosing a particular route include the choice of inflow and outflow vessels, the choice of anaesthetic technique, and the patient's general health. For example, an axillo-femoral graft obviates the need to open the abdomen, while a femoro-femoral crossover graft can be performed under regional or even local anaesthesia.

It is helpful to think of the lower limb blood supply divided into three segments, namely, the *aorto-iliac* segment, the *femoro-popliteal* segment and the *distal vessels*. Clinical examination will give a fairly good indication of the segments affected by occlusive disease. In general, it is unusual for a limb to become critically ischaemic if only one segment is involved. However, if the patient is diabetic the foot may develop ulceration and web space sepsis in the presence of an arterial tree that is, to all intents and purposes, normal to the level of the distal calf. Similarly, a patient may develop rest pain or tissue loss if relatively mild arterial disease is compounded by poor cardiac function.

Adequate imaging is essential before planning salvage procedures. Usually a limb can be dramatically improved by simply dealing with the most diseased, and usually blocked, segment, whether this is by radiological or surgical means. As indicated above, the requirements for a successful procedure are adequate inflow and an appropriate landing site for a bypass graft. The operations, segment by segment, are described below, but it must be borne in mind that radiologists can help – especially in aorto-iliac disease – with either a definitive treatment or by improving inflow to allow a more distal bypass. Furthermore, there is increasing evidence that femoro-popliteal disease can be managed effectively by a radiological endovascular procedure, even in critical ischaemia. A randomized controlled trial addressing this particular issue is currently in progress.

Aorto–iliac disease

Aorto-iliac segment disease can be dealt with very successfully by an interventional radiologist, and as a result the number of surgical procedures on this segment has fallen significantly over the past twenty years. Extra-anatomical and anatomical bypass are however still necessary. The most commonly performed procedures are aorto-bifemoral grafts, axillo-femoral grafts and crossover grafts.

The groin dissection is described above. Usually, this is performed first – before the inflow procedure – to establish that the graft is a viable proposition. The common inflow sources are the aorta, the axillary artery, the contralateral femoral system or, less commonly, the ipsilateral or contralateral iliac systems. Small modifications of the groin approach may be necessary according to the donor source, for example, the direction of the skin incision and the line of the arteriotomy.

AXILLO–BIFEMORAL GRAFTS

The advantages of the axillo-bifemoral graft are essentially related to the level of surgical insult to which the patient is subjected. No major muscle groups are incised, the abdomen is not opened, and the aorta is not clamped. Axillo-femoral grafts also have a role when there is a need to avoid a site of infection in the abdomen. Before surgery it is wise to check that the donor artery is disease-free. Measuring the blood pressure in both arms can be enough, but many prefer the reassurance of a duplex scan to confirm normal flow patterns. An axillary artery approach which gives extensive access is illustrated in Figure 5.21. However, as only limited access is required for this procedure, a small transverse incision, located 1–2 cm below the central portion of the clavicle, is suitable. Laterally the incision extends to a point just below the medial limit of the delto-pectoral groove (Fig. 6.17). Once through the skin, the pectoral fascia is encountered. This fascia and the underlying pectoralis major muscle are incised along the lines of the fibres and held open with a self-retaining retractor. Deep to this is the clavipectoral fascia,

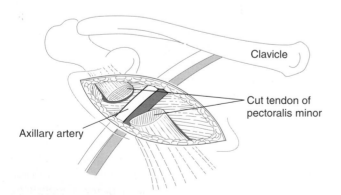

Figure 6.17 *A small transverse infra-clavicular incision will provide good access to the axillary artery for an axillo-femoral bypass.*

which is incised. In so doing, a free edge of the pectoralis minor is exposed. This muscle can be retracted, divided at this stage, or divided later. The pulsation of the axillary artery can usually now be felt clearly. The artery and vein are closely related, the artery running slightly superior and deep to the vein. The tributaries to the vein can be ligated and divided. The artery must be slung with great care as this is a very soft vessel and can be torn, and branches avulsed, easily. It may be advisable to ligate the minor branches, especially those arising posteriorly, to prevent back-bleeding when the vessel is opened. Passing a sling around the artery as soon as is safe will allow the application of some gentle traction which will be helpful during the more distal dissection.

Make the tunnel and pass the graft into place before heparin is administered. This is done by first running a finger deep to pectoralis major and onto the chest wall. If the graft is only to one groin, then it is often possible to push the tunnel device from here all the way to the groin. The graft should run in the mid-axillary line before being directed medially to pass in a gentle curve, medial to the anterior superior iliac spine (see Fig. 6.4b). If the groin is infected, the graft can be directed laterally for longer to allow passage through healthy subcutaneous tissue to the superficial femoral or mid-thigh profunda artery. If the graft is to go to both groins, an additional incision is often helpful. The surgeon has the choice of using a commercially prepared bifurcated graft, or suturing a crossover piece to pass from the groin, or higher, to the other side. The additional incision allows the crossover portion to be placed carefully without kinking. Tunnelling in the subcutaneous plane of the abdominal wall carries a real risk of entering a body cavity or coming through the skin. It is important that the drapes are carefully placed at the start to allow as much view of the planned track as possible. Despite this, the fact that many patients are obese or very frail means that mishaps are a well-recognized occurrence.

The anastomosis at each end can be performed in a standard fashion, but make sure that there is enough length in the graft so that it is not tight even at the extremes of movement of the very mobile shoulder joint.

AORTO–BIFEMORAL GRAFTS

In occlusive disease these grafts are performed in a fashion similar to that described above for aneurysms. Many surgeons prefer an end-to-side arrangement in the abdomen. This may be less haemodynamically favourable and more difficult to cover with peritoneum at the end, but it keeps more collaterals in circulation, especially to the pelvic organs, and so probably offers some protection to the limb in the event of graft occlusion. In many cases of aortic occlusion, the graft itself may be sited lower down the aorta than the angiogram first suggests. The top part of the occlusion is often fairly fresh thrombus that can be pulled out like a champagne cork using a Fogarty catheter. This is especially the case if the level of the occlusion extends up to the origins of the renal arteries and the aorta feels soft.

FEMORO–FEMORAL CROSSOVER GRAFTS

This extra-anatomical graft is a simple procedure that may be performed quickly, under regional anaesthesia. The groin dissections are performed as described above. The graft is tunnelled subcutaneously just above the pubis. Sometimes it is helpful to arrange that each arteriotomy is slightly oblique so that the graft lies in a gentle curve (Fig. 6.18a). Be careful when tunnelling; the abdominal wall and even the bladder can be penetrated, especially in patients with previous abdominal surgery.

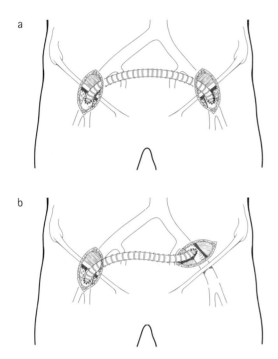

Figure 6.18   *Crossover grafts. (a) Femoro-femoral. (b) Ilio-femoral.*

ILEO–FEMORAL GRAFTS

This is very similar to the femoro-femoral graft, except that the common or external iliac artery is used as an alternative inflow (Fig. 6.18b). The approach to the iliac arteries is by retroperitoneal dissection through a muscle-splitting incision. The external oblique aponeurosis is split first, up to the edge of the rectus sheath. The internal oblique and transversus muscle fibres are then split to reveal the peritoneum, which is swept up by blunt dissection. The retroperitoneal vessels are exposed and the arteries are easily dissected if this is an untouched field. The graft can be run out through the corner of the wound to the contralateral groin, or under the inguinal ligament for an ipsilateral graft.

Femoro–popliteal segment: femoro-popliteal bypass

Despite recent advances in endovascular techniques, the femoro-popliteal bypass – as shown diagrammatically in Figure 5.12, page 78 – remains a procedure that is performed regularly by vascular surgeons. A randomized controlled trial comparing this procedure to angioplasty in critical ischaemia (BASIL Trial) has now finished recruiting, and the results are awaited.

The patient with chronic, severe lower-limb ischaemia affecting the femoro-popliteal segment will usually have a superficial femoral artery occlusion stretching from its origin to the above-knee or, more commonly, the below-knee popliteal segment. During the preceding months, or years, the patient will have developed collateral circulation through the profunda system, but at some point disease will have developed at another site with resultant incapacitating claudication, or critical limb ischaemia. The site of this disease progression is important because there may be implications for inflow and outflow of any bypass which is planned. Occasionally, it is the origin of the profunda that has become stenosed, allowing the possibility of a profundoplasty for limb salvage.

Before embarking on a femoro-popliteal bypass, it is important to establish that there is adequate flow through the iliac segments. If it is inadequate it should be improved with an endovascular procedure either before, or ideally at the same time as, surgery. The distal circulation may be compromised, but providing that there is at least one calf vessel in continuity to the ankle joint a femoro-popliteal bypass has a reasonable chance of success. Even in the absence of a complete calf vessel some surgeons will still perform a bypass into a 'blind' popliteal segment, relying on a bed of small collaterals to provide run-off.

If the graft is to be taken to the above-knee segment of the popliteal artery, there is probably little difference in the success rates of prosthetic grafts and autologous vein. However, vein is almost certainly superior in terms of both patency and limb salvage rates if the graft is to be taken more distally.

OPERATIVE PROCEDURE

The patient is positioned supine with the limb prepared from the level of the umbilicus down to the ankle. Some surgeons place the foot in a clear bowel bag to aid the final check of perfusion following revascularization. The leg must be free enough to allow repositioning during the procedure. Usually, the recipient artery is dissected first, as this vessel is more likely to define whether bypass is possible. The common femoral artery is then isolated by a standard groin dissection, modified by an angled incision to allow access to the LSV. After both the inflow and outflow vessels are exposed, the tunnel for the graft should be made prior to the administration of heparin. The order of the anastomoses then depends on the techniques employed. For example, the distal anastomosis is completed first in a reversed vein graft, but the proximal anastomosis is first in an *in-situ* vein graft.

Exposure of the above-knee segment popliteal artery is achieved through a medial incision starting level with the upper part of the femoral condyle and extending proximally for 10 cm or so, a hand's breadth behind the patella (see Fig. 5.26, page 95). This is the surface marking of the LSV. The exploration proceeds through the groove between the vastus medialis muscle mass and the medial hamstrings (semitendinosus and semimembranosus). Sartorius and gracilis are retracted forwards with vastus medialis. The muscles are held apart by a self-retaining retractor, and the artery is found on the underside of the femur having just passed through the adductor hiatus. The popliteal fossa at this level is often quite fatty. The artery and vein are easily separated and, when mobilized, the popliteal artery can be brought to the surface. There are usually large genicular branches and these should be protected and preserved.

Exposure of the distal segment of the popliteal artery is also most commonly approached from the medial side. The skin incision is placed parallel and 1 cm posterior to the medial subcutaneous border of the tibia. The exposure is easier to perform if the knee is bent to 90 degrees and the hip is flexed and abducted as much as the joint will allow. The LSV often lies directly under these markings, and there is frequently little subcutaneous fat to protect against damage at the time of skin incision. It must be freely mobilized and protected, and then the medial head of the gastrocnemius is retracted posteriorly, dividing the dense fascia connecting it to the tibia. The plane between the bone and muscle is opened and access to the distal popliteal fossa is quickly gained. Occasionally, the insertions of the tendon of semitendinosus, semimembranosus and gracilis restrict access (see Fig. 5.26). Some authorities advocate division of these structures, but space can usually be gained by full mobilization and retraction of the tendons. The artery is lateral to the vein, and the two vessels must be separated with some care, as venous bleeding at this stage can be difficult to control. If the popliteal artery is soft it may be enough to pass slings around this artery alone. However, the proximal part of this artery is often diseased and therefore it is frequently necessary to place the arteriotomy slightly more distally than this. For this reason, it is common to tie, or suture ligate, and divide the anterior tibial vein to allow the anterior tibial artery and tibio-peroneal trunk to be slung (Fig. 6.19). Clamping these vessels can be difficult. Ideally, a light bulldog clamp will suffice but sometimes it is necessary to double-loop and tighten the slings, with or without the use of a vessel occluder.

Vein graft

The LSV can be used either *in situ* or as a free reversed graft. In either case, the broad proximal segment of the LSV makes an ideal hood in terms of both size and shape for either the proximal or the distal anastomosis. For this reason the LSV must be divided as close to the common femoral vein as is safe, using a Satinsky clamp to maximize the length of the vein graft (Fig. 6.20).

All tributaries of the LSV must be accurately ligated with a 1-mm stump length. Care must be taken not to impinge upon the vein by catching the adventitia in a knot and kinking the graft.

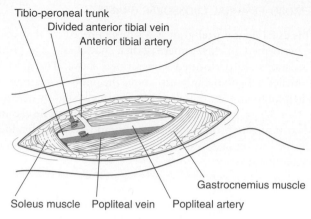

Figure 6.19 *Medial approach to the below-knee segment of the popliteal artery. Note the divided anterior tibial vein which has increased distal access and enabled the tibio-peroneal trunk to be isolated.*

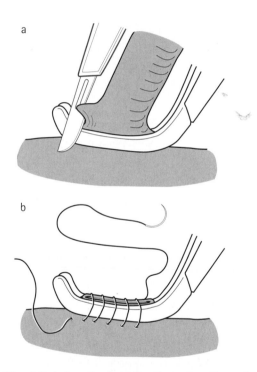

Figure 6.20 *A technique for dissecting the saphenofemoral junction and maximizing the length of the graft without compromising the lumen of the common femoral vein. (a) A clamp is applied at the junction and the vein cut flush against it. (b) The common femoral vein is closed by suturing over the clamp. This suture is left loose and then the clamp is wriggled free, before returning with a second row of stitches to tie the suture to itself.*

In-situ grafts These have the advantage of their size matching the vessels to be anastomosed, and the graft is also left undisturbed for a good portion of its length. However, occasionally the saphenofemoral junction is much lower than the first usable portion of common femoral artery and therefore the LSV must be mobilized for some length down the thigh to allow a tension-free proximal anastomosis. Sometimes it is not possible at all. Disadvantages of *in-situ* grafts include the valves which must be destroyed, and the action of passing a valvulotome to destroy them can seriously damage the graft intima. In addition, each tributary is a potential fistula. After the proximal anastomosis is completed the femoral artery clamp can be released. This allows some flow down the vein graft as far as the first competent valve, and also allows the profunda system to perfuse the limb. The valvulotome is then passed up from the distal end of the vein through a small venotomy, as it is convenient to do this before dividing the distal end of the vein. The valvulotomy device must be passed several times, rotating it through 90 degrees each time. Care must be taken when passing the device to minimize trauma to the intima. The proximal anastomosis must also be protected, usually by the assistant's fingers pinching the graft. If the valvotome passes unintentionally through the anastomosis the sutures may well snag and be cut. There are then three ways of dealing with the tributaries. The first is to expose the entire length of the vein and inspect it for tributaries, particularly on its deep aspect. The second is to perform an angiogram and, using commercially available tape with distance markers, identify the sites of tributaries seen on the pictures and cut directly onto them. In the third option the vein is exposed through a series of short skip incisions, and a pocket Doppler probe applied. If the graft is pinched distal to the probe and flow can be heard, then there must be a patent tributary more proximally. This can be hunted for and tied off. This process is repeated until the distal end of the graft is pinched and no flow is detected.

Free reversed grafts If the LSV is to be a free reversed graft, then it must be harvested, reversed and tested. There is some benefit to be gained from preoperative duplex marking of the vein. This will indicate with some reliability the course of the vein and its distal diameter and sites of confluence. The vein can be harvested, and its tributaries ligated, through a long single incision or through a series of interrupted, or skip, incisions. The latter approach takes longer, but it may reduce the wound complications. It is important not to cut obliquely onto the vein as this undermining increases the risk of skin necrosis and wound problems. The proximal end of the vein is divided at the saphenofemoral junction, as described above, but the distal end of a free graft is best not divided until the arteriotomy site at both ends is decided, even if this means waiting until arteries are opened. Further vein length may be needed. The harvested vein is tested by gentle distension with heparinized saline. Do not over-distend the graft as this will damage the adventitia. Small holes, caused by the avulsion of tiny tributaries, may require repair with a figure-of-eight stitch. Be careful not to narrow the vein.

Tunnelling

The graft can be tunnelled deeply following an anatomical pathway, or superficially, essentially occupying the site of the LSV. A synthetic graft – and even an externally supported graft – may be best placed deeply in order to avoid graft-occluding bends and kinks. A free vein graft can go deep, but this does mean that access to any stenosis detected by surveillance is difficult to reach. For the above-knee popliteal graft, the vein can simply be placed in the track from which it was harvested and then directed through the distal wound to the popliteal artery. However, the below-knee popliteal graft can be kinked by the hamstring tendons and has to turn through a more acute angle when passing from superficial to deep. One option here is to run the graft superficially along the thigh and then pass it deep into the above-knee popliteal fossa, guiding it down into the distal space from below. This technique requires a further – albeit limited – dissection of the superior portion of the popliteal fossa.

The possibility of creating a twist in a vein is very real. If the proximal anastomosis is performed first, the clamp can be released and the pulsatile pressure down the vein will often show any twists missed by simple inspection. Care must then be taken not to introduce any twist as the graft is manipulated into position. A completion angiogram will not only indicate anastomotic problems, but is likely to show a twist.

The anastomoses

The anastomoses are usually end-to-side, both proximally and distally. These can be performed by fixing the heel with a mattress suture first, but many find that a parachute technique works best and allows the precise placement of each suture without the need to lever up on the graft, risking a tear.

The recipient portion of the popliteal artery has already been isolated at the start of the operation. The slings or bull-dog clamps are applied for arterial control as described above. The arteriotomy is placed according to the atheroma in the popliteal vessel, but this can be a very difficult anastomosis. One way of carrying out the distal anastomosis is to parachute down the heel of the graft before completing the distal fashioning of the vein. The extra portion can be trimmed as the toe is approached, but before this it can be clipped and used to hold the graft in a suitable position to allow the back wall of the anastomosis to be sutured more easily (Fig. 6.21).

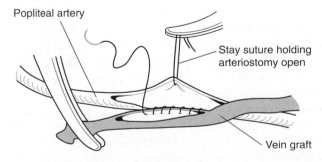

Figure 6.21 *Popliteal anastomosis. A stay suture holds the artery open, making the suturing of the far side of the anastomosis easier. The vein graft is held by mosquito forceps, but this damaged portion of vein will be excised to shape the toe of the graft.*

Distal bypasses

When arterial occlusive disease in the lower limb involves the distal segment, arterial reconstruction may no longer be possible. Reconstruction is however still an option if there is a patent artery to offer adequate outflow from a graft. The sites for distal anastomoses are the anterior tibial artery, the posterior tibial artery and the peroneal artery. A graft is also occasionally taken to the dorsalis pedis artery.

Anterior tibial artery

The anterior tibial artery is most commonly exposed in the middle or distal third of the calf. The incision is made halfway between the lateral subcutaneous border of the tibia and the anterior border of the fibula. The tibialis anterior muscle is separated from the extensor hallucis longus and extensor digitorum longus muscles. The anterior tibial artery runs between these muscle groups on the interosseus membrane, and then on the tibia for a short distance before it crosses the ankle into the foot underneath the superior extensor retinaculum. A graft to this vessel can be run subcutaneously, medial to lateral across the thigh, to pass behind the lateral aspect of the knee, and then down the lateral aspect of the calf. Alternatively, it can be channelled more like an *in-situ* graft down the medial aspect of the thigh. It then has to cross the tibia before meeting the recipient artery, or it can be passed through the leg, after incising the interosseus membrane and creating a tunnel medial to lateral from the popliteal fossa to the lateral compartment.

Posterior tibial artery

The posterior tibial artery is easily exposed along its distal third by a vertical incision starting 1 cm or less posterior to the medial subcutaneous border of the tibia, extended in a 'hockey stick' fashion under the medial malleolus if necessary. The posterior tibial artery is found quite superficially situated in a groove between flexor hallucis longus and flexor digitorum longus. Bypasses to this artery are ideally suited to the use of *in-situ* LSV graft.

Peroneal artery

The peroneal artery may be approached from either the medial or lateral side. With the lateral approach it is possible to run a graft around the back of the fibula and lift the flexor hallucis longus muscle back off the bone to create a space, but mostly, the lateral approach involves removing a segment of the fibula to expose the artery. Some authors describe a sub-periosteal excision of the bone to allow it to be reimplanted at the end.

It is also possible to approach the peroneal artery from the medial side. This helps the harvesting and placement of the graft quite considerably. Taking an approach similar to that for the posterior tibial artery, the flexor hallucis longus is mobilized and the peroneal artery runs lateral to the tibial nerve in the groove between the fibular origin of flexor hallucis longus and tibialis posterior.

Dorsalis pedis artery

It is possible to bypass onto the dorsalis pedis artery, although the opportunities for this are few in number. Frequently, the patients with severe calf vessel disease also have foot vessel occlusions, or have diabetes and the micro-circulation is therefore dubious. However, the vessel is easily exposed and the distal end of the LSV runs anterior to the medial malleolus and is therefore very nicely placed to provide a conduit.

Popliteal artery aneurysms

Popliteal artery aneurysms are a particular problem. If identified asymptomatically, elective surgery is indicated. It was traditionally taught that the threshold for intervention was 2 cm, but more recent investigations have suggested that up to 3 cm is relatively safe. Limb threat due to popliteal aneurysm is usually due to either an acute thrombosis within the aneurysm or embolization of thrombus fragments. Up to 50 per cent of patients presenting with acute complications of popliteal aneurysms ultimately lose the limb, and this is often due to a failure in diagnosing the problem.

Full diagnostic imaging is very important to establish the extent of the aneurysm and to confirm that there are distal vessels to receive a bypass. The aim of surgery is to exclude the aneurysm from circulation, but before this can be achieved a period of treatment with a thrombolytic agent may be necessary to open the calf vessels. Occasionally, the process of lysing an occlusion may result in distal embolization as blood starts to flow past partially lysed thrombus. For this reason, regular and frequent review is essential up to the time of surgery.

There are two commonly used approaches to a popliteal aneurysm. In the truly elective situation, some surgeons advocate operating on the patient in the prone position through a lazy-S incision. This has the advantage of allowing excellent exposure of the popliteal system in order to get above and below the aneurysm. However, harvesting a piece of vein for use as a graft is difficult, and it may be necessary to turn the patient during the procedure. A medial approach to the popliteal fossa means that a conventional LSV harvest is possible, but the lower end of the aneurysm may be relatively inaccessible as the aneurysmal expansion pushes the trifurcation of the artery distally. The medial approach to the above- and below-knee segments of the popliteal artery is described above. As access is required to both segments, the two incisions can be combined as a single long incision. A vein graft bypass is anastomosed end-to-side onto the popliteal artery, both above and below the aneurysm. Ties are then placed around the popliteal artery above and below the aneurysm to exclude it from the circulation (Fig. 6.22).

THORACIC OUTLET SYNDROME

The vessels and nerves to the upper limb must traverse the narrow cervico-axillary canal to enter the axilla, and the

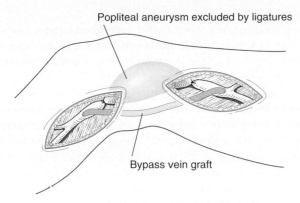

Figure 6.22 *Popliteal aneurysm. The popliteal artery has been approached from the medial aspect and ligated above and below the aneurysm. Distal perfusion is restored with a bypass graft.*

vessels in addition have to turn over the first rib from their intrathoracic origin. The wide range of movement of the shoulder joint changes the shape and size of this channel. Not surprisingly, a range of arterial, venous and neurological symptoms are reported from impingement on these structures.[13] Few patients, however, develop severe symptoms or complications, and the great majority can be managed conservatively. Many surgeons believe that thoracic outlet syndrome is both over-diagnosed and over-treated. Surgical opinion though is divided, and others believe that many patients with milder symptoms can be helped by surgery.

- **Neurological symptoms**, of pain, parasthesia and paresis, are caused by pressure on the cords of the brachial plexus. The pressure is more often from the scalene muscles which are attached to the first rib rather than from the rib itself. Aberrant scalene bands to a rudimentary cervical rib are also implicated.
- **Vascular symptoms** are much less common than neurological symptoms and account for only 5 per cent of the cases. The fulcrum for the compression is the first rib. Vascular compression may give rather non-specific symptoms, but complications such as a venous thrombosis or an arterial stenosis or aneurysm can occur.

Surgical approach

Surgery for thoracic outlet syndrome is an uncommon operation in vascular surgical practice, and many patients will be referred to those surgeons with a special interest, both for their assessment and for their surgery. Surgery consists of enlarging the space for the neurovascular bundle. This includes the removal of a cervical rib (and any attachments to it) if one is present. More often the skeletal anatomy is normal, and the surgery is focused on the removal of the middle portion of the first rib, the release of the scalene muscle attachments, or a combination of the two procedures. Operations for thoracic outlet syndrome can either be

transaxillary or supraclavicular. The choice of approach is dependent on what structure is predominantly implicated in the compression. For example, accessory rib excision, and the more extensive scalenectomy advised for upper brachial plexus compression, require a supraclavicular incision. Lower brachial plexus compression and vascular compression are satisfactorily released by an excision of the middle portion of the first rib and the release of the scalene attachments to it. This is most commonly undertaken from an axillary approach. However, if arterial reconstruction – necessitated by a stenosis or aneurysm – is anticipated a supraclavicular approach will provide superior vascular access. Details of the surgery of thoracic outlet syndrome are available in specialist vascular textbooks,[10] but the two standard operations are summarized below.

THE AXILLARY APPROACH

The patient is anaesthetized and stabilized in a lateral position with the arm abducted and supported. A transverse incision is made in the axilla, overlying the third rib. An axillary tunnel is developed up to the first rib on the surface of serratus anterior. Intercostal brachial nerves will usually have to be sacrificed. The dissection is then over the first rib, taking great care not to damage the subclavian artery, the subclavian vein and the brachial plexus (Fig. 6.23). The vessels are gently separated from the rib, and from scalenus anterior, which is then divided. The distal portion of the muscle should be excised, because if it is simply released adhesions from the cut end can cause recurrent symptoms. Scalenus medius and the tendon of subclavius can also be divided for additional release. The rib is then divided posteriorly, behind the T1 and C8 nerves which must be identified and protected, and finally anteriorly near the costochondral junction, while the subclavian vein is gently held out of the way.

THE SUPRACLAVICULAR APPROACH

An incision above the medial half of the clavicle is deepened through platysma, and the subclavian artery exposed as

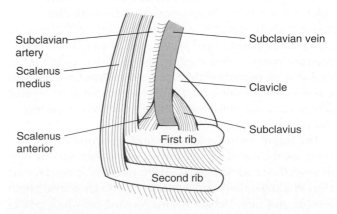

Figure 6.23 *The view of the first rib, and the subclavian artery and vein from the axillary approach.*

described in Chapter 5 and illustrated in Figure 5.20, page 90. The phrenic nerve on the surface of scalenus anterior is identified and held in a sling while the underlying muscle is separated from its attachment onto the first rib and excised. Scalenus medius is also excised. The central portion of the first rib can also be excised from a supraclavicular approach, but access is more limited and this can be technically more challenging than via the trans-axillary approach. When an accessory rib is present it is usually surrounded by scalenus medius with tendinous attachments both to it and to the first rib. The rib is cleared of muscular attachments, disarticulated anteriorly and divided posteriorly level with the transverse process. Great care is necessary to avoid damage to the T1 nerve root during this manoeuvre.

CAROTID ARTERY SURGERY

Carotid artery stenosis

One area of vascular surgery which has been examined extensively by randomized controlled trials is the management of carotid artery stenosis. Since the late 1980s a series of reports have provided vascular surgeons with help and guidance about patient selection for carotid endarterectomy.[14,15] In summary, carotid endarterectomy is indicated for symptomatic carotid territory embolic disease if the degree of stenosis is >70 per cent and the vessel remains patent. Evidence also suggests that patients with asymptomatic lesions, but with a similar degree of stenosis, may benefit from carotid endarterectomy.[16,17] Furthermore, there is now CT evidence of carotid territory infarcts which indicate that patients may be experiencing subclinical embolic episodes. However, the number of patients to be treated to prevent one stroke is much greater, and the place of asymptomatic carotid surgery continues to be debated. Carotid endarterectomy is one operation in which quality control is paramount. Some centres have published impressively low perioperative stroke rates, but each practising surgeon must be able to quote to patients a personal stroke rate. Furthermore, a vascular surgeon must always remember that both arms of the major trials included best medical therapy in the form of anti-platelet therapy, lipid profile therapy and optimal blood pressure control. Best medical therapy itself continues to evolve; most recently with evidence of benefit from the routine use of ACE inhibition,[18] and it may be that data collected fifteen years ago will need reappraisal or even repeating in due course.

The major controversies surrounding carotid endarterectomy are the use of shunts, the use of patches, and the type of anaesthesia administered. More recently, it has become clear that angioplasty and stenting of carotid lesions are both feasible and safe. Debate is now focused on which procedure – endovascular or operative – is safer and more durable.

Shunts

The placement of a shunt during carotid endarterectomy is routine in some centres, but is used on a selective basis in others (Fig. 6.24). Several methods exist of estimating cerebral perfusion during the period that the internal carotid has to be occluded. These include transcranial Doppler and internal carotid artery stump pressures. However, none has given a completely reliable measure of adequate oxygenation. Although a shunt should improve cerebral perfusion during this period, shunt insertion itself carries some risk of vessel dissection, and even with a shunt in place there is an argument that estimations of cerebral perfusion are still necessary to ensure that the shunt is working.

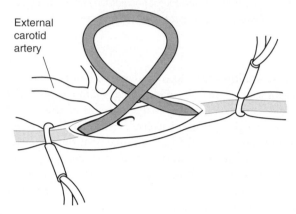

External carotid artery

Figure 6.24 *A shunt as used in a carotid endarterectomy.*

Anaesthesia

Many surgeons perform carotid endarterectomy under regional anaesthesia, using both superficial infiltration and a deep cervical plexus block. This has the advantage of allowing selective shunting of patients based upon deteriorating neurological status following the application of a clamp. The patient's motor and sensory functions can be assessed objectively, and the higher functions can be gauged by simple conversation. It may be that these patients benefit from the avoidance of general anaesthesia in other ways, in the form of quicker postoperative recovery, reduced rates of cardiovascular complications and a less labile blood pressure profile in the recovery period. These outcome measures are currently under investigation by randomized controlled trials of general versus local anaesthesia (GALA trial).

Patches

The use of patches by surgeons also varies. Some never patch, others patch selectively, and some always patch. There is a view that every artery will be narrowed by primary closure and that a patch is required no matter how skilful the surgeons may consider themselves to be. Others take the view that if the disease is adequately cleared and the internal carotid artery is >6 mm in diameter, then a primary closure is acceptable. The restenosis rate is higher in female patients, and therefore the threshold for the use of a patch is lower. Many surgeons who are selective with male patients will routinely use a patch on female patients. The material used for patching is also subject to discussion. A prosthetic patch (either Dacron or e-PTFE) has the advantage of being available 'off the shelf' and does not require harvesting but it occasionally becomes infected. Vein needs to be harvested – either the LSV from the groin or the external jugular vein from the neck – and this is a possible problem if the procedure is being carried out under local anaesthesia. Although the potential complication of a prosthetic graft infection has been avoided, the vein patch is occasionally subject to rupture or aneurysmal change.

Operative procedure

A description of the exposure of the carotid arteries is given in Chapter 5 and illustrated in Figure 5.19. In summary, the sternocleidomastoid muscle is retracted laterally to reveal the internal jugular vein. This is then mobilized and the common facial vein and other tributaries to it are divided. The carotid arteries lie beneath the vein. The common carotid artery is exposed first. Note the vulnerable position of the vagus nerve shown on the illustration for carotid body tumours (Fig. 6.25). The recurrent laryngeal nerve is in double jeopardy from clamping on both its downward and return journeys. This is the cranial nerve most frequently damaged during carotid endarterectomy. The external carotid is the next vessel to be exposed and slung, followed by the superior thyroid artery. The internal carotid artery can then be exposed and slung. Note the position of the hypoglossal nerve. This cranial nerve can be mobilized if necessary by dividing the occipital branch of the external carotid that prevents the hypoglossal from being pushed up out of the way. The common and internal carotid arteries require adequate exposure to allow a shunt to be placed easily and quickly if necessary. It is also important to expose the internal carotid to a sufficiently distal level to enable a clamp to be placed above the disease. The upper limit of the disease is often visible from the outside of the artery. The patient should now receive 5000 IU of unfractionated heparin and the clamps can then be applied – internal carotid artery first, then common and external.

The common carotid artery is opened with a longitudinal arteriotomy. The incision is extended up into the internal carotid artery, and should extend both proximal and distal to the atheromatous plaque. If a shunt is to be used it is inserted at this stage. The endarterectomy plane is then entered. This is easiest to identify at the proximal end of the arteriotomy, and gentle outward traction on the artery wall using forceps can be helpful in providing the initial separation in the correct plane. The dissection in this plane is continued up into the internal carotid artery. The plaque normally thins distally and can be followed to its end, avoiding an intimal step in the internal carotid artery at the limit of the dissection. If however an intimal step is unavoidable it should be secured with fine Prolene sutures to prevent dissection. Closure is either with or without a patch, as discussed above.

Carotid body tumour (chemodectoma)

The carotid body usually lies on the posterior aspect of the bifurcation of the common carotid artery. The chemodectoma, which arises within it, is therefore closely applied to the carotid bifurcation. Although frank malignancy and metastases are uncommon, the histological appearance does

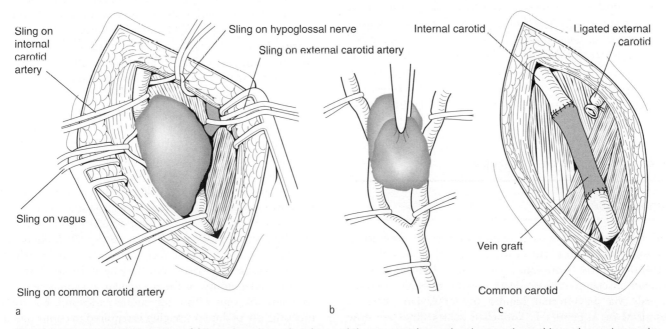

a

b

c

Figure 6.25 *Carotid body tumour. (a) Tapes have been placed around the common, internal and external carotid arteries, and around the vagus and hypoglossal nerves. (b) The tumour is dissected off the vessels in the sub-adventitial plane. (c) When the arteries have to be excised with the tumour, the external carotid is ligated but a graft is interposed between the common and internal carotid arteries.*

not predict either local invasion or metastatic potential. As the tumour can become progressively more difficult to separate from the carotid arteries as it enlarges, early excision is usually recommended. Clinical diagnosis depends first on clinical suspicion, and many are thought initially to represent a malignant lymph node as they are very firm on palpation. Further investigations include CT, MRI and angiography.

OPERATIVE PROCEDURE

The approach to the carotid bifurcation is similar to that for a carotid endarterectomy, and is described in more detail above and in Chapter 5. For large tumours an oblique vertical incision at the anterior border of sternocleidomastoid will provide more extensive access than a skin crease incision. The hypoglossal nerve is separated from the tumour and held in a sling. A sling is passed around the common carotid artery, and if it is possible further slings are placed around the distal internal carotid and external carotid arteries, before dissection is commenced. Dissection at the outer boundaries of the tumour allows the isolation, ligation and division of large thin-walled tumour vessels, and increased mobility of the tumour is achieved. Rotation forwards of the tumour enables the vagus to be identified and separated from the tumour. It is then also held in a sling (Fig. 6.25a).

The tumour is then dissected off the carotid arteries. In most cases there is a subadventitial plane of cleavage which can be followed (Fig. 6.25b). The arterial wall is left otherwise intact, and aneurysmal dilation is not a complication. When the tumour is circumferential it may have to be transected until the correct plane is reached. However, in some tumours this subadventitial plane cannot be followed, and a segment of the carotid arteries must be resected with the tumour. A carotid reconstruction is then performed with a vein graft anastomosed to the common carotid below the tumour and to the internal carotid above it. The external carotid is simply ligated and divided (Fig. 6.25c). During the resection and reconstruction a temporary shunt is usually established to maintain inflow into the internal carotid artery and safeguard cerebral perfusion.

VASCULAR ACCESS SURGERY

Venous access

Peripheral venous access is almost universally established percutaneously, but a 'cut-down' procedure, as described in Appendix I, is sometimes necessary. Central venous catheter insertion is now nearly always possible percutaneously via an internal jugular or subclavian route as described in Appendix I. Tunnelled central lines are now routinely established by similar manoeuvres for a range of clinical indications (see Fig. 11.5, page 195). Central venous lines can also be inserted through the cephalic or external

jugular vein, by a cut-down technique, and then threaded proximally. This is a method that is now seldom employed. The cephalic vein is exposed in the deltopectoral groove. It joins the axillary vein after piercing the clavipectoral fascia. The external jugular vein can be exposed by an oblique incision lateral to the lateral edge of the sternocleidomastoid, 2 cm above the clavicle. A cannula can be directed through it into the internal jugular vein.

The internal jugular can also be cannulated directly using an open surgical approach. It lies immediately deep to the lower third of the sternocleidomastoid muscle, and can be approached via a small transverse incision at the lateral border of the muscle, which is then retracted medially. The danger of air embolism must be remembered when the vein is entered.

Arteriovenous fistulae

There is little doubt that an adequately functioning arteriovenous fistula remains the preferred access for haemodialysis. The majority of patients in the UK requiring long-term haemodialysis do so on a background of chronic renal failure associated with the complications of metabolic, cardiovascular or autoimmune disease processes. The need for access can therefore often be predicted for many months before dialysis is indicated. A permanent indwelling central catheter or an external shunt are alternative methods of access, but these have significant disadvantages – most notably sepsis and central vein thrombosis. The widespread use of central catheters often reflects the difficulties encountered by nephrologists when seeking to arrange a functioning arteriovenous fistula before a patient actually needs renal replacement therapy.

The rules for arteriovenous fistula formation are simple. Prosthetic material should be avoided as much as is possible. A patient's first fistula should be as distal as possible; some surgeons will perform an anatomical snuffbox fistula, but others start at the radial artery. The non-dominant arm is preferable as this makes home dialysis easier, and also allows the patient more freedom during dialysis. A distal fistula that fails to mature is not necessarily a disaster as the more proximal veins have often enlarged and thickened, and this increases the chances of success at a higher level.

As always, careful patient assessment and choice of procedure are the keys to success. Palpate a donor artery carefully, not only for a good volume pulse but also for evidence of calcification. Many patients will have occlusive arterial disease, and this may affect the upper limb – especially if the patient has diabetes. The potential recipient veins – particularly the cephalic vein at the wrist – may have been damaged over the years by phlebotomy, or the placement of venous cannulae. Assessing the vein with a tourniquet is helpful, but sometimes the use of duplex imaging is required to confirm that a vein is patent and in continuity. Similarly, a patient in whom a central catheter has been used for a prolonged period may have a central venous stenosis or occlusion. Suspicion of this needs investigation as it will ultimately lead to failure of the arteriovenous fistula.

The procedure can be performed under local anaesthesia or, preferably, a regional block. At the wrist level, a longitudinal incision – placed halfway between the radial artery and distal cephalic vein – will allow both vessels to be mobilized. The choice is then made, according to surgical preference, between a side-to-side and an end-to-side anastomosis. To fashion a side-to-side Cimino fistula, a parallel longitudinal arteriotomy and venotomy are made, and the vessels sutured side-by-side with a continuous 6/0 monofilament, non-absorbable suture. A similar procedure can be performed at the elbow level.

Alternative techniques, in the face of unsuitable, absent or damaged superficial veins, involve the harvesting of a segment of LSV and placing this subcutaneously in the upper arm, connecting the distal brachial artery to a proximal segment of the brachial vein (Fig. 6.26). A variation of this procedure that spares the LSV is mobilization of the brachial vein, disconnecting it proximally, rerouting it through a subcutaneous tunnel, and then anastamosing it to the distal brachial artery. Finally, a loop of e-PTFE can be used between two vessels.

Once all sites of upper limb bypass have been used, explored or discounted, the lower limb can be considered. The options here include forming a loop on the anterior thigh from mobilized LSV or e-PTFE. If more urgent access is required – for example in a patient with central venous occlusion requiring dialysis – consider the Scribner shunt, which does not have to await maturity before it can be used. The Scribner shunt is the original arteriovenous 'fistula', and has several disadvantages compared with the techniques described above. Infection can track in at the exit site of the shunt, and skin erosion over the subcutaneous tubing can occur. It does, however, occasionally still play a role. Teflon pipes are inserted into an adjacent artery and vein, at one of a variety of sites including the ankle or the wrist. The pipes are then connected externally, and this connection is broken to attach to dialysis.

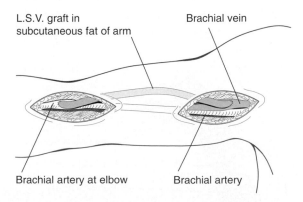

Figure 6.26 *Subcutaneous long saphenous vein (LSV) can be used for an arteriovenous fistula in the arm. Alternatively, the brachial vein can be mobilized, tunnelled subcutaneously, and then sutured to the brachial artery.*

L.S.V. graft in subcutaneous fat of arm

Brachial vein

Brachial artery at elbow

Brachial artery

SURGERY OF CHRONIC VENOUS INSUFFICIENCY

The management of patients with chronic venous insufficiency starts with a full venous assessment. This assessment is a large and important subject, and cannot be covered completely in an operative text. As discussed in Chapter 5, the majority of patients with signs and symptoms of chronic venous insufficiency have reflux from their deep into their superficial veins. In some patients this is the sole cause of their venous hypertension, and in others it is a significant factor. Many of these patients will therefore benefit from varicose vein surgery, and the standard operations are described in Chapter 5.

However, in 20 per cent of patients with chronic venous insufficiency the pathology is confined to the deep veins, while in a further 40 per cent deep venous pathology is a contributory factor. These patients may be very symptomatic with a swollen heavy leg and incipient, or established, venous ulceration. Investigations will usually confirm either deep venous incompetence or obliteration of the deep veins. Previous deep venous thrombosis is the commonest underlying pathology. Management is in general non-operative, and concentrates on measures to improve venous return such as elevation of the limb when at rest, and support stockings.

VARICOSE ULCERS

Those patients who develop varicose ulceration may require surgery to the ulcer itself, but the mainstay of management starts with a vascular assessment, in which it is particularly important to exclude any arterial component to the ulceration. If reflux into superficial veins is a contributing factor to the venous hypertension, then varicose vein surgery should be considered. Occasionally, reconstructive surgery to deep veins – as discussed below – may be appropriate. However, successful treatment is most frequently that of non-operative measures to improve venous return. When this has restored healthy granulation tissue to the base of a large ulcer but re-epithelialization from the edges is slow, a split skin graft (as described in Chapter 1) can speed the final healing. In patients with severe liposclerosis surrounding an ulcer, conservative measures may fail even to produce a healthy granulating base. In these patients it may be better to excise the whole area and place a skin graft directly onto the deep fascia. This approach is also indicated for those patients who develop a squamous carcinoma within a long-standing varicose ulcer.

Venous reconstruction

Operations to restore competence to the valves of deep veins have been attempted but have not been widely adopted as the results are often disappointing. Similarly, venous bypasses have not been particularly successful. The comparatively sluggish flow in veins and the propensity for thrombosis at least partly explains the disappointing results of reconstructive venous surgery when compared with arterial reconstruction. In addition, many patients with chronic venous insufficiency are thrombophilic.

VALVE REPAIR

This can be attempted in primary valvular incompetence, but not when incompetence is secondary to valves damaged by a previous deep venous thrombosis. It is most commonly attempted on a valve in the common femoral or popliteal vein. The vein is exposed and the valve identified. The anatomy of the insertion of the cusps is important, as the vein must be opened longitudinally exactly at the cusp insertion to prevent any iatrogenic damage to the cusps. The internal anatomy can usually be visualized by emptying the vein of blood, clamping it, and then filling it with heparinized saline. Fine Prolene sutures with the knots tied on the outside are then used to take the tucks (Fig. 6.27).

VENOCUFF

This technique has the advantage of simplicity but, again, it is only suitable for primary incompetence. A Dacron cuff is sewn around the vein to support it and reduce its diameter at the level of the incompetent valve. The decrease in vein diameter restores competence to the valve.

VEIN TRANSPOSITION

An isolated segment of brachial vein, with its intact valves, has been used as a replacement bypass graft for a segment of lower limb vein in which the valves have been destroyed by thrombosis.

SAPHENOUS CROSSOVER GRAFT (PALMA PROCEDURE)

This operation can restore venous drainage when there is a unilateral iliac vein occlusion. Although only a minority of patients with chronic venous insufficiency have isolated occlusion at this level, they usually have particularly severe symptoms and wish to consider surgery. The LSV on the

affected side is used as the bypass, and is isolated from groin to knee. It is divided distally, but the sapheno-femoral junction is left intact. In addition the tributaries around the junction are preserved to maintain the normal alignment of the vein and prevent kinking. The valves must be destroyed within the vein as blood flow will be in the reverse direction. The femoral vein on the opposite limb is exposed in readiness to receive the vein graft. A suprapubic subcutaneous tunnel is created and a small sterile sigmoidoscope is inserted along it, through which the vein graft can be passed. An end-to-side anastomosis is then performed (Fig. 6.28).

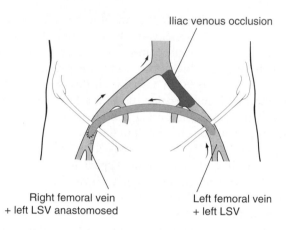

Iliac venous occlusion

Right femoral vein + left LSV anastomosed

Left femoral vein + left LSV

Figure 6.28 *A Palma crossover vein graft for an occluded left common iliac vein. The left long saphenous vein (LSV) has been brought across for an end-to-side anastomosis onto the right femoral vein.*

Temporary arteriovenous fistula

This addition to the procedure described above is favoured by some surgeons. The rationale for the approach is to increase flow through the graft in the early postoperative period when the danger of thrombosis and graft occlusion is highest. Once this period is over, the arteriovenous fistula is closed by interventional radiology. A separate vein or prosthetic graft can be used to create the arteriovenous fistula or the end of the LSV used, as illustrated in Figure 6.29.

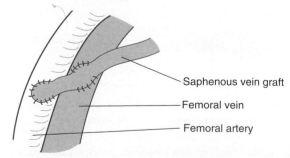

Saphenous vein graft

Femoral vein

Femoral artery

Figure 6.29 *An arteriovenous fistula has been created by anastomosing the vein graft onto both the common femoral vein and artery.*

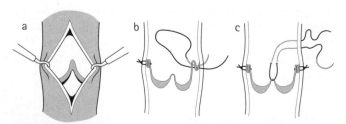

a b c

Figure 6.27 *Repair of a venous valve. (a) The vein is opened longitudinally exactly at the attachments of the valve cusps. (b) The first suture to plicate the valve is already tied, and the second is being inserted. (c) The final suture is inserted.*

LYMPHOEDEMA SURGERY

Lymphoedema may be either primary or secondary. Secondary causes include local obliteration of lymphatic channels by tumour, surgical excision and radiotherapy. These are the main forms encountered in the Western world, and most patients will present early so that preventative measures can be instituted before the swelling is far advanced. Over 90 per cent of patients with lymphoedema can be managed by conservative means. Compression garments and intermittent pneumatic compression devices can limit the swelling of the limb and will also contribute to preventing any deterioration in the skin. These patients are prone to streptococcal cellulitis, which causes further deterioration. Any infection must be promptly and aggressively treated.

A great many surgical options have been developed in attempts to restore lymphatic drainage. They may be applicable in lymphoedema secondary to a local obstruction, and they have also been used for the forms of primary lymphoedema where an obstructive rather than an obliterative pattern prevails. A large number of procedures have been devised, but most have been disappointing. All are based on the principle of providing an alternative route for the drainage of lymph:

- *Thompson procedure (buried dermal flap)*. A full-length calf incision is made and the subcutaneous tissue is debulked. A long skin flap from one side of the incision is de-epithelialized and buried into the deep muscle compartment.
- *Omental transposition*. Omentum is mobilized and brought into the subcutaneous tissue of the affected limb. This procedure was generally abandoned as it was of doubtful benefit and postoperative complications were frequent.
- *Enteromesenteric bridge*. An isolated loop of ileum, which has been denuded of mucosa, is brought into the affected limb instead of omentum.
- *Lymphatico-venous anastomoses*. Early attempts at this consisted of anastomosing a transected lymph node to a vein. More recently, success has been claimed with direct lymphovenous anastomoses between dilated lymphatic channels and small veins using microsurgical techniques.[19]

Surgeons practising in the developing world are more likely to encounter patients who present late with advanced swelling of a limb and skin changes. In addition, in areas where filariasis is common this will be the prevalent underlying pathology. Filariasis causes mainly obstruction at the level of the lymph nodes, but damage is more diffuse than in other forms of secondary lymphoedema and there is also lymphatic reflux.

Excisional surgery to reduce the size of the limb may be the most appropriate initial treatment.

- *Charles procedure*. Skin and subcutaneous tissue are excised circumferentially from knee to ankle. Excision is either down to, or includes, the deep fascia. The underlying surface is then skin grafted. Good results can be obtained, but the grafted skin may be unstable and is liable to ulceration.
- *Homan's procedure*. The original operation has been serially modified and is now usually performed as a staged procedure. A longitudinal strip of skin, and a larger volume of lymph-laden subcutaneous tissue, is excised and the wound closed. Significant reduction in limb girth can be achieved by repeated surgery, without the skin complications associated with the Charles procedure. In some very advanced cases however a Homan's procedure may no longer be technically feasible.

REFERENCES

1. Campbell WB, France F, Goodwin HM. Research and Audit Committee of the Vascular Surgical Society of Great Britain and Ireland. Medicolegal claims in vascular surgery. *Ann R Coll Surg Engl* 2002; **84**: 181–4.
2. Lees T, Singh S, Beard J, *et al*. Prospective audit of surgery for varicose veins. *Br J Surg* 1997; **84**: 44–6.
3. DeBakey ME, Cooley DA, Crawford ES, *et al*. Clinical application of a new flexible knitted Dacron arterial substitute. *Am Surg* 1958; **24**: 682–9.
4. Hardman DT, Fisher CM, Patel MI, *et al*. Ruptured abdominal aortic aneurysms: who should be offered surgery? *J Vasc Surg* 1996; **23**; 123–9.
5. Ashton HA, Buxton MJ, Day NE, *et al*. The multicentre aneurysm screening study (MASS) into the effect of abdominal aortic aneurysm screening on mortality in men: a randomised controlled trial. *Lancet* 2002; **360**: 1531–9.
6. The UK Small Aneurysm Trial Participants. Mortality results for randomised controlled trial of early elective surgery or ultrasonographic surveillance for small abdominal aortic aneurysms. *Lancet* 1998; **352**: 1649–55.
7. Campbell WB. Non-intervention and palliative care in vascular patients. Leader. *Br J Surg* 2000; **87**: 1601–2.
8. Prance SE, Wilson YG, Cosgrove CM, *et al*. Ruptured abdominal aortic aneurysms: selecting patients for surgery. *Eur J Vasc Endovasc Surg* 1999; **17**: 129–32.
9. Parodi JC, Palmaz JC, Barone HD. Transfemoral intraluminal graft implantation for abdominal aortic aneurysms. *Ann Vasc Surg* 1991; **5**: 491–9.
10. *Vascular Surgery*, 5th edn. Rutherford RB (ed.). Philadelphia: Saunders, 2000.
11. Bradbury AW, Brittenden J, McBride K, *et al*. Mesenteric ischaemia: a multidisciplinary approach. Review. *Br J Surg* 1995; **82**: 1446–59.
12. Myre HO. The 'failed' embolectomy. Clinical dilemma. *Br J Surg* 2000; **87**: 136–7.
13. Thompson JF, Jannsen F. Thoracic outlet syndromes. Review. *Br J Surg* 1996; **83**: 435–6.

14. Randomised trial of endarterectomy for recently symptomatic carotid stenosis: final results of the MRC European Carotid Surgery Trial (ECST). *Lancet* 1998; **351**: 1379–87.

15. North American Symptomatic Carotid Endarterectomy Trial Collaborators. Benefit of carotid endarterectomy in patients with symptomatic moderate or severe stenosis. *N Engl J Med* 1998; **339**: 1415–25.

16. The CASANOVA Study Group. Carotid surgery versus medical therapy in asymptomatic carotid stenosis. *Stroke* 1991; **22**: 1229–35.

17. The Veterans Affairs Cooperative Study Group. Efficacy of carotid endarterectomy for asymptomatic carotid stenosis. *N Engl J Med* 1993; **328**: 221–7.

18. Bosch J, Yusuf S, Pogue J, *et al.* and the HOPE investigators. Use of ramipril in preventing stroke: double blind randomised trial. *Br Med J* 2002; **324**: 699–702.

19. Campisi C, Boccardo F, Zilli A, *et al.* Peripheral lymphedema: new advances in microscopic treatment and long-term outcome. *Microsurgery* 2003; **23**: 522–5.

7

CARDIOTHORACIC SURGERY FOR THE GENERAL SURGEON

INTRODUCTION

Every general surgeon should have the ability to open the chest of a patient in an emergency. Surgeons working in hospitals without cardiothoracic units, may have to perform an emergency thoracotomy for trauma in a patient who is too severely injured to allow stabilization for transfer to a specialist unit. In addition, the upper gastrointestinal surgeon may require more extensive access to the intrathoracic oesophagus than can be achieved trans-hiatally, while the vascular surgeon may require access to the intrathoracic aorta and its branches. However, in the elective situation, subspecialization has resulted in much of the intrathoracic oesophageal and vascular surgery being transferred to tertiary referral centres.

Truly isolated general surgeons who are unable to transfer either elective or emergency cardiothoracic cases are unfortunately unlikely to have the necessary anaesthetic, or intensive care, facilities available to justify embarking on major intrathoracic surgical procedures. However, they may have to deal with other problems that are now rarely encountered in the developed world, and for which simpler surgical solutions are still appropriate.

The importance of a team approach to cardiothoracic intervention cannot be over-emphasized. This is routine in specialized units, but the diagnostic and interventional skills within the armamentarium of the cardiologist, chest physician, radiologist, anaesthetist and intensivist must also be remembered by the general surgeon when faced unexpectedly with a cardiothoracic challenge.

The success of all but the most minor cardiothoracic surgery is linked to the perioperative anaesthetic support available. The physiological changes associated with opening the chest require skilled anaesthesia. Once a hemithorax is open in a patient who is breathing spontaneously, the lung on that side collapses, while adequate spontaneous ventilation of the remaining lung is also severely compromised. Any inspiratory effort that can be achieved is wasted on moving the mediastinum further towards the uninjured side, and drawing air backwards and forwards from the other lung. A cuffed endotracheal tube and positive-pressure ventilation under the control of the anaesthetist overcomes these mechanical problems, but the lung in the opened hemithorax will inflate and obscure the operative field. A lung retractor can be used to hold the lung partially deflated and out of the way. The lower-lying 'good' lung, however, remains vulnerable with this technique during a thoracotomy. Without the protection of double cuffs, blood or other material from the operation field may trickle across the carina down into the uninjured lung. A double-lumen tube (Fig. 7.1) which allows separate ventilation of either lung will solve both problems, but its accurate insertion requires anaesthetic skill that may not be available. Whichever method is employed, there will be some blood

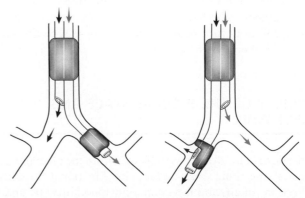

Figure 7.1 *Double-lumen endotracheal tubes serve a dual role. In addition to allowing separate ventilation of either lung, the double cuffs protect the good lung from overspill across the carina from the other lung.*

which passes through the non-aerated lung and will not be oxygenated. This creates a temporary functional right to left shunt and a depressed arterial oxygen saturation. The shunt, however, is short-lived and seldom a major obstacle because, as the lung collapses or is retracted, the blood flow through it diminishes by hypoxic autoregulation.

If the chambers of the heart, ascending aorta or pulmonary trunk are injured, or have to be opened, circulatory arrest will greatly diminish the blood loss. Snares are placed around the superior vena cava (SVC) and inferior vena cava (IVC) to occlude inflow and produce circulatory arrest. Unfortunately, unless a surgeon is familiar with operating in the chest, placing a snare around the SVC in the face of a crisis may be an insurmountable obstacle. A further challenge in an emergency is that, whereas a circulatory arrest can be safe for a minute or so in the well-perfused patient with a high oxygen saturation, it can be the last straw for a hypovolaemic and desaturated patient.

As even in optimal circumstances, circulatory arrest can be undertaken for such a short time, only very limited intracardiac surgery is possible with this manoeuvre alone. In addition, surgery on the heart and great vessels may require the heart to be kept still for fine work to be undertaken safely. Specialized techniques which include hypothermia to extend the time of safe circulatory arrest, arrest of the heart, in addition to extracorporeal circuits which maintain perfusion during the operation, have greatly expanded the scope of cardiac surgery. However, as they are not options for the general surgeon, they are not described further.

In elective and emergency surgery on the intrathoracic aorta, even if the proximal clamp can be placed so that cerebral perfusion is maintained, the spinal cord and kidneys will be ischaemic. The haemodynamic effects of occluding the major part of the cardiac outflow in a beating heart is another relevant consideration. Limited shunts to maintain perfusion to vital organs may occasionally have a place, but are seldom a practical solution in an emergency outside a cardiothoracic unit.

General surgeons are therefore restricted in what they can realistically offer within the thorax with limited facilities. Those surgeons who have least access to specialist cardiothoracic help are unfortunately often also those with the least facilities in their own hospital.

SURGERY OF THE PLEURAL SPACE AND CHEST WALL

Collections of fluid, air, pus or blood within the pleural space displace the lung and reduce its functional capacity. Collections of air, and less commonly blood, may be under tension, and the mediastinum will be displaced towards the opposite side. This has two further adverse, mechanical cardiorespiratory effects. The displacement and kinking of the IVC and SVC obstruct the venous return, with reduced car-

diac filling and a resultant drop in cardiac output. In addition, the displaced mediastinum reduces the functional capacity of the contralateral lung.

Thus, the collection must be drained, the urgency depending on whether the collection is under pressure.

ASPIRATION

This is a simple technique that is suitable for the drainage of a serous pleural effusion. With the patient sitting, an appropriate posterolateral site is chosen. It should be remembered that the hemidiaphragm on the side of an effusion may be elevated and that, in the presence of inflammation, the two layers of pleura in the costo-diaphragmatic recess are often adherent. If too low a site for aspiration is chosen it is easy to enter the abdomen and damage the liver or spleen (Fig. 7.2). Local anaesthesia is infiltrated down to the level of the parietal pleura. An aspiration needle, connected to a syringe by a two-way tap, is introduced close to the superior border of a rib to avoid damage to the neurovascular bundle (Fig. 7.3). The two-way tap permits aspiration into, and emptying of, the syringe without disconnection of the needle. Simple aspiration is insufficient for the drainage of blood or thick pus.

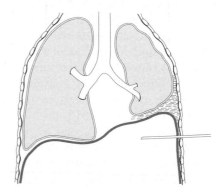

Figure 7.2 *A basal pleural effusion is often associated with an elevated hemi-diaphragm and fused peritoneum in the costo-diaphragmatic recess. If too low a site is chosen for aspiration the abdomen is entered inadvertently.*

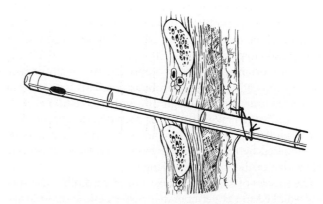

Figure 7.3 *The intercostal neurovascular bundle is partially overhung by the rib above. Damage should not occur during the insertion of an intercostal drain placed immediately above a rib.*

Air is easily aspirated through a needle, but this may not be appropriate. In a small simple pneumothorax, observation alone may be sufficient, while in a more major pneumothorax a chest drain is more effective, and safer.[1] Release of a tension pneumothorax with a large-bore needle can, however, be a temporary life-saving manoeuvre. In an emergency, although it is recommended that the needle is introduced through the second intercostal space in the midclavicular line, the proximity of the superior mediastinal vessels must be remembered, and the alternative site in the 'safe triangle' (see below) has advantages. Air escapes when under pressure until there is no longer any tension, the mediastinum returns to the midline, and the other lung can inflate. A tension pneumothorax has been converted to a simple pneumothorax and a chest drain is then inserted with the patient no longer in severe respiratory distress.

CHEST DRAIN INSERTION

This is the standard treatment for a pneumothorax or a haemothorax, and an intercostal drain may be required with some urgency following thoracic trauma. Positive-pressure ventilation can convert a small undetected simple pneumothorax into a tension pneumothorax. This should be remembered in any patient with multiple injuries who requires a general anaesthetic, or ventilation, as part of the management of their other injuries. Prophylactic chest drain insertion before induction of anaesthesia should therefore always be considered, even after apparently insignificant chest trauma. A chest drain is also usually indicated at the end of an operation in which the pleural space has been entered, to drain any postoperative collection of blood, or leak of air. In these circumstances a chest drain is inserted in a supine patient. The 'safe triangle', recommended for insertion of a drain, is bounded by the mid-axillary line posteriorly, the lateral border of pectoralis superiorly, and inferiorly by a line projected from the 5th intercostal space anteriorly. In an elective setting a chest drain can be inserted with the patient sitting, with the arm held across to the opposite shoulder. The drain can then be sited lower, and more posteriorly, if this is felt to be beneficial in, for example, the drainage of basal pus. A posterior drain, however, may cause problems if the patient then lies on the skin exit wound. It is often possible to position the internal portion of the drain posteriorly but still bring the skin exit round towards the mid axillary line.

Local infiltrative anaesthesia is satisfactory. Trochar techniques for the insertion of a drain are inherently dangerous. The sudden loss of resistance as the parietal pleura is entered allows the momentum to carry the trochar point into the substance of the underlying lung, and potentially even into hilar structures. In the safer open technique, a small incision is made through the skin and intercostal muscles immediately above a rib and the incision is carried through the parietal pleura. The intercostal vessels lie immediately under each rib and, by inserting a drain immediately above a rib,

damage to the vessels can usually be avoided (Fig. 7.3). When the parietal pleura is breached the lung collapses away from the chest wall and a finger is inserted into the pleural space to check for, and release, any adherent lung. The chest drain can then be introduced safely into the pleural space. It can be angled up towards the apex for a pneumothorax, or down to the lung base for a haemothorax.

The chest drain must be securely held in place with a suture, which will also prevent any air leakage around the tube. A further untied suture can be inserted at this stage and will be tied as the drain is removed to prevent air entry through the track (Fig. 7.4). Underwater drainage is established immediately after the drain is in the pleural cavity (Fig. 7.5). Air is expelled with each breath, and bubbles through the water. No air can

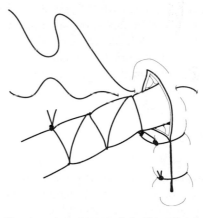

Figure 7.4 *The chest drain is securely held in place by a skin suture which is also snugging the skin around the drain. It can be cut so as to release the drain but so that it still holds the skin in apposition. An additional untied mattress suture is in position. This will be tied as the drain is withdrawn to prevent air entry into the pleura along the drain track. Purse-string sutures are no longer recommended.*

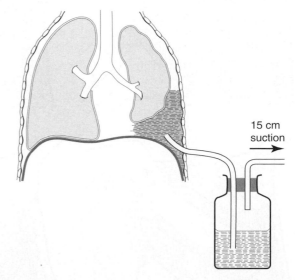

15 cm suction

Figure 7.5 *Under-water seal drainage, with or without suction, is a simple well-tried system of chest drainage.*

be drawn back into the pleural space, and there is no danger of the fluid in the bottle being drawn back if the bottle remains below chest level. Low-pressure suction can be added for more efficient drainage. The indications for chest drainage, and the management of chest drains, is covered in more detail in the British Thoracic Society Guidelines.[2]

Surgery for empyema

An empyema is treated with the appropriate antibiotics plus adequate drainage. Drainage can be more effective if the skill of a radiologist is harnessed, and drains are placed accurately into localized collections using image-guided techniques. Often, neither repeated aspiration nor continuous drainage with a chest drain are sufficient if the pus is thick, and a chronic empyema forms. Early referral of a patient with this type of empyema to a thoracic surgeon is important to secure optimum treatment, with good re-expansion of the underlying lung and a satisfactory functional recovery. This may require decortication of the abscess cavity after any active sepsis has been controlled. Alternatively, some form of open drainage may be necessary.

DECORTICATION

Decortication involves the excision, at thoracotomy, of the thickened visceral and parietal pleura which form the walls of the abscess. Chronic empyemas, whether secondary to an untreated pneumonia or a tuberculous infection, will be encountered relatively frequently in areas where health resources are limited. Surgeons practising in these areas, however, are unlikely to have the anaesthetic facilities for a safe major thoracotomy. Decortication is never an urgent operation and ideally it should not be performed outside a thoracic unit; thus, patient transfer is indicated. For the isolated surgeon without the possibility of specialist referral, an open drainage procedure will be a safer alternative.

OPEN DRAINAGE

These are safe procedures for *chronic* empyemas with a thick cortex. The lung is adherent to the parietal pleura, and will not collapse when a limited thoracotomy into the abscess alone is performed. In the absence of skilled anaesthesia and the facilities for a major thoracotomy, they are a safer option than a decortication. Intra-pulmonary pus can also be drained in the same manner if the inflammation has extended out to the pleura with resultant pleural adhesions preventing lung collapse.

Drainage with rib resection is performed when more conservative management has failed, and can be undertaken under general or local anaesthesia (Fig. 7.6). The classical descriptions describe a subperiosteal resection of approximately 5–8 cm of rib, but a smaller incision is now considered adequate. The deep periosteum and parietal pleura are then incised to enter the empyema and a drain is inserted.

Thoracostomy is a more permanent skin lined drainage into the chest. An H-shaped incision, with each limb approximately 8 cm in length, produces two horizontal skin flaps. Two adjacent ribs, their periosteum and the intervening

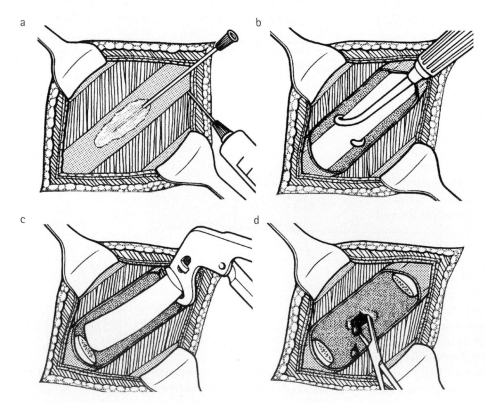

Figure 7.6 *Drainage with rib resection. (a) When performed under local anaesthesia, lignocaine must be injected under the sensitive periosteum. (b) The periosteum is incised longitudinally and elevated from the rib. The deep surface can be stripped of periosteum with a curved periosteal elevator. (c) A section of rib is resected. (d) The posterior periosteum and pleura are incised.*

intercostal muscles, neurovascular bundle and parietal pleura, are excised to produce a chest wall defect 8 cm square. The skin flaps are then sutured to the parietal pleura.

MINIMAL ACCESS TECHNIQUES IN THE CHEST

These techniques are valuable for both diagnostic and interventional purposes, and may avoid the necessity for a thoracotomy.

Bronchoscopy

This is currently mainly performed with flexible fibre-optic instruments which are easier to pass without traumatizing the airway. A laceration of a main bronchus can be confirmed, or a tumour visualized and a biopsy taken for histological examination. The simplest intervention is the aspiration of a mucus plug from a main bronchus, though intensive physiotherapy combined with suction will usually result in re-expansion of the lung without recourse to this procedure. Foreign bodies within the bronchial tree can be removed using a bronchoscope, and palliative tumour reduction with diathermy or laser destruction can also be carried out endoscopically. Much of this work is undertaken by chest physicians and intensivists, whose help should be recruited by the surgeon when faced with a challenge. For example, in an emergency the anaesthetist can pass a double-lumen tube and, while maintaining ventilation of one lung, the chest physician can pass the flexible bronchoscope through the endotracheal tube to assess bronchial damage in the other.

A general surgeon who has to perform a bronchoscopy, whether to retrieve a foreign body or mucus plug, will almost certainly have to do this with a rigid bronchoscope. The lubricated rigid scope should be passed in a patient anaesthetized with a general anaesthetic except in critical circumstances. The patient is first positioned with the neck only slightly extended, and the scope is advanced to the cords. The tip of the scope is passed behind the epiglottis, and used to lift it forwards to expose the vocal cords. The bronchoscope is then rotated so that its tip can be passed through the vocal cords into the trachea. Ventilation through the bronchoscope should maintain adequate gas exchange. The patient's neck must then be fully extended as the scope is advanced down the trachea (Fig. 7.7).

Mediastinoscopy

This is the visualization of the mediastinum. A telescope is introduced into the anterior superior mediastinum through a small transverse incision above the suprasternal notch. Tissue biopsy samples may also be taken for histological assessment. Mediastinoscopy is of particular value in the

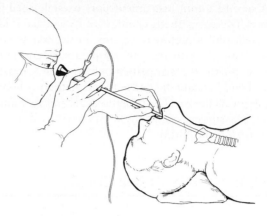

Figure 7.7 *Rigid bronchoscopy.*

assessment of a superior mediastinal mass, and in the pre-treatment lymph node staging of a bronchial malignancy. It is a procedure which should probably only be performed by thoracic surgeons. If a general surgeon requires histology of upper mediastinal nodes a small second interspace incision (a mediastinotomy) is a safer alternative.

Video-assisted thoracoscopic surgery (VATS)

This procedure is based on the same principles as laparoscopy, and has followed a similar evolutionary development, so that it can now be used for an increasing range of intrathoracic operations. In its earliest forms, diagnostic visualization and biopsy of pleural lesions was possible through a rigid endoscope with a telescope and biopsy channel. Diathermy was possible if an insulated scope was used, and the first thoracoscopic cervical sympathectomies were performed in this way. Much more complex cardiothoracic surgery can now be undertaken with multiple instrument ports, and a separate high-quality light source with video camera. VATS is also increasingly an option for surgery on the intrathoracic oesophagus.

General anaesthesia and a double-lumen endotracheal tube are essential. The initial pneumothorax is established either with a Veres needle, or by an open technique similar to that for the insertion of a chest drain, and the first port for the camera is inserted. At the end of an operation, the last port is kept open until the anaesthetist has reinflated the lung. A chest drain is not always necessary unless further bleeding is anticipated, or there is a danger of an air leak from the lung. Port site closure only requires secure skin closure.

THORACOSCOPIC SYMPATHECTOMY

The indications and extent of sympathetic ablation are discussed in more detail in Chapter 3. This operation is now most frequently performed as a VATS procedure using a two-port technique. The first port is usually placed in the axilla in the 3rd intercostal space, and is a 10-mm camera port. A second 5-mm instrument port is established in the 5th space. The sympathetic chain, with its ganglia, is identified as a pale pink structure traversing the necks of the ribs. It is found lying deep to the parietal pleura, which must be incised to isolate the sympathetic chain. The sympathetic chain is then lifted and divided with the diathermy hook. On the right, great care must be taken to avoid injury to the azygos vein. The surgery can be undertaken with a short hospital stay and low morbidity.[3]

SURGICAL ACCESS TO THE CHEST

Access for open surgery within the thorax may be anteriorly through the sternum, laterally between the ribs, or from below through the diaphragm. There is also limited access from the neck. In an emergency, most general surgeons will feel more comfortable with a lateral thoracotomy than a median sternotomy, unless they have had some exposure to cardiac surgery during their training.

Median sternotomy

This is the incision which is performed most frequently for elective cardiac surgery and provides excellent access to the heart. It may also be the most appropriate incision in an emergency when damage to the heart or to the great vessels of the superior mediastinum is suspected. The incision can be extended up into the neck along the anterior border of sternocleidomastoid for injuries of the carotid root, or laterally above the clavicle for access to an injury to the subclavian root (see Chapters 5 and 9).

A vertical midline skin incision is made from the suprasternal notch to the xiphisternum, and deepened down to bone. The manubrium and sternum are then divided in line with the skin incision, using an electric oscillating saw designed specifically for this purpose. If this is not available, a longitudinal substernal tunnel is made close to bone with long forceps and a Gigli saw is passed underneath the sternum with the aid of a long artery forceps (see Chapter 4). There is danger of injury to the underlying heart, and it is also easy to breach the right pleura. Opening the sternum in repeat surgery is hazardous as the heart may be adherent to the sternum. It should only be attempted with an oscillating saw, which cuts through the outer table first, then the inner table without jeopardising adherent structures beneath the sternum. Bleeding from the sternal marrow is reduced by the application of bone wax, and bleeding from the periosteal edges is controlled with diathermy coagulation.

The sternum should be separated from underlying structures before attempts are made to separate the edges widely with a self-retaining retractor. The pleural sacs are swept off the pericardium, and no entry into either pleural space is required. The thymus, lying on the pericardium in the superior mediastinum, is divided in the plane between the lobes,

avoiding the innominate vein superiorly. The pericardium is then incised vertically.

After surgery within the pericardium, drains should be left both inside the pericardium and in the anterior mediastinum. The two halves of the sternum are then drawn together. Stainless steel wire sutures can either be introduced through the sternal bone with a heavy needle, or the sutures can be placed further laterally through the intercostal fascia at the lateral sternal edge. The latter are easier to insert, but there is a danger of injury to the internal mammary artery.

Postero-lateral thoracotomy

This is the standard approach for elective surgery of the lung. A right thoracotomy also affords excellent access to the thoracic oesophagus, and a left lateral thoracotomy to the descending thoracic aorta. Access to the hilum of a lung and the mediastinal structures is good, but only on the respective side. In an emergency it is the incision of choice for a rapidly collecting unilateral haemothorax. In elective surgery, the level of the incision may be dependent on the underlying pathology, but in an emergency the 5th intercostal space is the most satisfactory. The patient is positioned on his or her side with pelvic and upper arm support to secure stability, and a posterolateral thoracotomy incision is made (Fig. 7.8). The alternative semi-prone position affords excellent stability for a posterolateral thoracotomy in an extreme emergency, but adequate ventilation may be more difficult.

The incision is made through the skin and latissimus dorsi in the same line (Fig. 7.9), and should be two finger breadths below the tip of the scapula. Posteriorly, the skin incision may turn up to divide the angle between the spine and the medial edge of the scapula. Anteriorly, it extends into the submammary fold. It is then deepened through the latissimus dorsi, the fibres of which are at about 90 degrees to the incision. The plane deep to latissimus dorsi is then developed upwards, under the scapula. The ribs and intercostal muscles are now exposed, so that it is possible to count the ribs, and plan the appropriate level for the thoracotomy. The edge of the second rib is the highest rib which can be felt under the scapula, and the flat surface of the third is then palpable

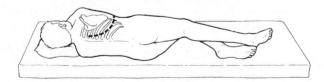

Figure 7.8 *A patient lying on his side and slightly prone is stable for an emergency postero-lateral thoracotomy. In the full lateral position the patient is unstable and must be securely supported and strapped. In addition, the uppermost arm requires support on an arm board.*

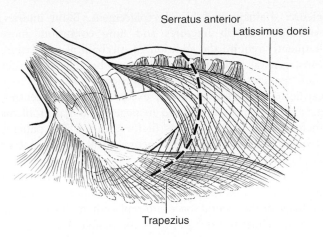

Figure 7.9 *Landmarks for a lateral thoracotomy.*

below it. Having identified the chosen space for the thoracotomy, the lower border of serratus anterior is freed by coagulation diathermy from the fascial and fatty plane and divided as low as is practical to preserve innervation. If more space is needed the trapezius can be divided.

Entry into the chest may then be through the intercostal muscles, directly along the upper border of the rib to avoid damage to the neurovascular bundle, or it can be through the bed of a rib. The former route is quicker in an emergency. If the incision is to be through the bed of a rib, the periosteum is incised along the length of the rib with diathermy, and stripped off its upper border (Fig. 7.10a). A periosteal elevator as shown in Figure 7.6(b) can be used for this. Stripping should be from back to front as the fibres of the intercostal muscles then keep the dissection on the upper border of the rib. The pleural cavity is then entered through the posterior periosteum. Care must be taken to avoid injury to the underlying lung, and a moment's apnoea from the anaesthetist can be helpful. Rib resection is unnecessary but division of the costo-transverse ligament posteriorly allows greater mobility of the superior rib, reducing the risk of fracture when the self-retaining retractor is introduced.

The pleura is incised, and with a double-lumen tube in place, the anaesthetist can allow the lung to collapse out of the operating field. The chest wall edges are protected by large swabs and a Finochetti, or other self-retaining chest retractor, is inserted. Rib retraction puts the intercostal neurovascular bundle on stretch. Prophylactic surgical division of the neurovascular bundle should be performed if tearing appears likely.

One or two chest drains are commonly placed in the pleural cavity at the end of surgery before closure, and are brought out through separate stab incisions. Rib apposition can be held by four pericostal sutures spaced along the incision (Fig. 7.10b), followed by a continuous suture approximating the upper leaf of the divided periosteum to the fascia over the intercostal muscle in the space below (Fig. 7.10c). The chest wall muscles are then repaired with absorbable sutures.

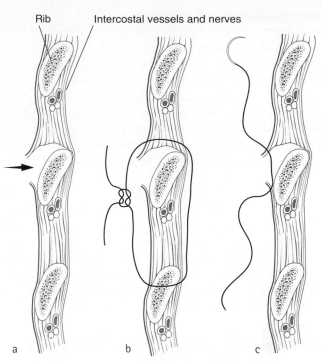

Figure 7.10 *Lateral thoracotomy. (a) The periosteum has been incised along a rib. The upper leaf of periosteum is elevated from the lateral surface and upper border of the rib to expose the posterior periosteum. The posterior periosteum and parietal pleura are then incised to enter the chest. (b) A pericostal suture passed over a rib will not damage the intercostal neurovascular bundle. Below a rib it can cause damage and it is preferable to pass it through the rib instead. (c) A continuous suture approximating the divided periosteum to the fascia overlying the intercostal muscles of the space below completes the closure of the chest wall.*

Transaxillary lateral thoracotomy

This is a limited lateral thoracotomy, performed through the medial wall of the axilla, which affords restricted access to the apex of the lung. It was a standard approach for a thoracic sympathectomy but it has now generally been superseded by VATS.

Antero–lateral thoracotomy

A left anterolateral thoracotomy is often the incision of choice for emergency access to the heart. Access to the posterolateral aspect of the left ventricle is superior to that obtained with a median sternotomy but, more importantly, it is a faster and safer approach, especially in the absence of the necessary saws. The patient is laid obliquely supine with the ipsilateral hip and shoulder raised. A left 5th space antero-lateral thoracotomy can be extended by a transverse or oblique division of the sternal body to a 5th or 4th interspace right antero-lateral thoracotomy if greater access is required. In this *clam-shell thoracotomy* both internal mammary arteries must be ligated and divided.

Thoraco–abdominal incisions

These incisions, which allow simultaneous access to the upper abdomen and chest, have lost popularity as both postoperative pain and respiratory complications are common. In general they can be avoided. A left thoraco-abdominal incision was routinely used for cancers of the gastric cardia and lower oesophagus. With the advent of minimal access techniques and circular stapling devices for anastomoses, it is now possible to perform both the dissection of the thoracic oesophagus and the anastomosis by using a trans-hiatal approach from below. When more extensive access to the intrathoracic oesophagus is necessary, a separate right thoracotomy incision is employed (see Chapters 16 and 17). A right thoraco-abdominal incision was used for liver surgery, but the alternative subcostal incision provides good access to the mobilized liver, with less morbidity. The thoraco-abdominal incision is described in Chapter 12.

Trans-diaphragmatic and trans-hiatal access

Access to the posterior mediastinum from below has the advantage that it does not necessitate entry into either pleural space. In addition, postoperatively there is no respiratory compromise from a painful thoracotomy wound. Trans-hiatal access to the oesophagus is now the routine approach for much of the laparoscopic surgery of oesophageal reflux and hiatus hernia. In surgery for cancer of the cardia and distal oesophagus, a similar approach for the dissection around the distal oesophagus can be combined with an open laparotomy (see Chapters 16 and 17). In the presence of a hiatus hernia access through the stretched hiatus may be ample. A normal hiatus can be enlarged, if necessary, by a diaphragmatic incision which is later closed.

Cervical access

Access into the superior mediastinum from incisions in the neck is limited. It is, however, usually sufficient to free a retrosternal goitre and lift it gently up but, occasionally a median sternotomy is necessary before it can be delivered safely. The cervical approaches to the roots of the vessels arising from the aortic arch are described in Chapters 5 and 9.

SURGERY FOR CHEST TRAUMA

The first priority in thoracic trauma is to re-establish the mechanical requirements for adequate circulation and blood–gas exchange, but only in a minority of cases is a thoracotomy necessary. Penetrating injuries, which are usually stab wounds, can almost always be managed by pleural drainage and blood replacement. Blunt injuries, with multiple rib fractures and lung contusion, more frequently require the addition of mechanical ventilation. Most general surgeons would hope to be able to transfer those patients requiring an emergency thoracotomy to a cardiothoracic unit. However, except in regional centres, general surgeons will have to manage the initial problems themselves to make patients fit for transfer. The patients frequently have other major neurological, abdominal or limb injuries.

Occasionally, the general surgeon will be faced with a patient who cannot be stabilized by mechanical ventilation, drainage of the pleural space and replacement of circulating volume. Thus, transfer becomes impossible and the only chance of survival is with an emergency thoracotomy. Surgeons in such a situation may have skilled anaesthetic and intensive care facilities, but no access to cardiopulmonary bypass, and will be operating in difficult conditions in an area in which they are probably unfamiliar. The confidence of general surgeons to open a patient's chest in an emergency will also depend on their experience during training, but in a stab injury, a thoracotomy on the side of the injury to control what is usually a chest wall bleed, and less commonly a simple laceration of the lung, is not an unduly difficult or hazardous procedure. The spectrum of injury after penetrating trauma differs from that encountered after blunt trauma.[4] In the depth of a stab wound the surgeon will usually encounter an injury similar to a surgical incision, and this can be sutured. In blunt trauma, general surgeons are less likely to find injuries which they can easily control or repair. The contused injury will not resemble a surgical incision, and it is seldom amenable to a simple sutured repair.

Infrequently this emergency surgery must be performed on an unconscious, un-anaesthetized dying patient in the accident department in a desperate attempt to control torrential haemorrhage. An immediate 'emergency room' thoracotomy forms part of the resuscitation of a patient in extremis following thoracic trauma. A cardiac laceration is the commonest remedial injury. In major trauma centres serving areas with a high level of civilian violence, these immediate thoracotomies have resulted in success in around 10 per cent of those with penetrating thoracic injuries.[5] Outside these centres the results from emergency room thoracotomies will be more disappointing, but nothing is lost in the attempt and an occasional life will be saved. If death is imminent, a low likelihood of benefit is tolerable.

The value of telephone advice from a cardiothoracic surgeon must be remembered in those situations where a general surgeon is unsure whether to transfer a patient or to proceed with a thoracotomy. An expert can sometimes talk another surgeon through an operation, or may offer to come and help; alternatively, transfer may be recommended with the specialist team already alerted, and the emergency operating theatre prepared.

Mechanical considerations

Inadequate gas exchange in the immediate aftermath of chest trauma is more often due to mechanical factors than to extensive pulmonary damage.

PLEURAL SPACE EXPANSION

Air or blood within the pleural space which is reducing respiratory capacity must be drained by the insertion of a chest drain (see above). In a severe case, the physical signs of major respiratory embarrassment, tracheal deviation, absent breath sounds and a dull or hyper-resonant hemithorax may necessitate action before even a confirmatory chest X-ray has been taken.

CHEST WALL STABILIZATION

The mechanical integrity of the chest wall is threatened by multiple fractured ribs as, on inspiration, an area between fractures may be drawn in as a flail segment of chest wall. Chest wall stabilization for such blunt injuries is by endotracheal ventilation with a cuffed tube and intermittent positive-pressure ventilation. This may have to be undertaken for some days before the patient can be weaned from the ventilator. Surgery to wire fractured rib ends together, or the insertion into a rib of a hook to which light traction can be applied to stabilize a flail segment, are now mainly of historical interest. However, such techniques may still be of value to a surgeon who is unable to transfer patients with chest trauma, and who has no facilities for ventilatory support. Simple strapping will partially support a rib fracture. Any improvement in ventilation is, however, mainly due to the pain relief which allows fuller diaphragmatic movement. This improvement far outweighs any reduction in rib movement from the splinting effect of the strapping. Local anaesthetic bupivicaine intercostal blocks and thoracic epidurals can be of great value in reducing pain, increasing voluntary respiratory effort, and thereby reducing secondary infection in poorly aerated lung bases.

Unfortunately, much of the problem of poor gas exchange after chest trauma is not explained on the basis of mechanical compromise, or secondary infection. The lungs themselves are injured, and deteriorating function in the few days after injury is more often related to lung contusion.

OPEN CHEST WOUND

Even an open chest wound, in which a pleural cavity is open to the environment, is manageable by using positive-pressure ventilation. If not immediately available, an airproof dressing restores the mechanical integrity of the chest wall and, with an underwater chest drain to release any tension from accumulating blood or air, allows re-expansion of the underlying lung.

DIAPHRAGMATIC LACERATION AND RUPTURE

The possibility of a diaphragmatic laceration should be considered in all penetrating injuries to the chest or abdomen. The incidence of diaphragmatic injury in association with stab injuries to the lower chest may be over 10 per cent. Small lacerations may be symptomless initially and the diagnosis is easily missed, only to present with late complications of herniation of an abdominal viscus through the defect. Positive-pressure ventilation may keep the abdominal contents down, but they then herniate through the defect when the patient breathes spontaneously with negative pressure. Repeat X-radiography during the initial hospital admission may therefore demonstrate a tear which was not apparent on an earlier radiograph. In addition, some patients present years after an injury, when a gradual increase in the size of the defect leads to late herniation of abdominal organs.

Blunt trauma which compresses the chest or abdomen can also rupture the diaphragm, which most commonly tears posteriorly on the left. A major rupture of the left hemidiaphragm can seriously impair respiratory function as the abdominal contents herniate into the chest. The situation is worsened by gaseous distension of the stomach, and nasogastric aspiration is worth instituting before transfer to theatre, though it will not always deflate the herniated stomach. A right-sided diaphragmatic rupture is less common, more difficult to diagnose, and seldom presents with early acute mechanical difficulties with ventilation. Diaphragmatic injury may be isolated, but is often associated with damage to the liver, spleen or left colonic flexure. A ruptured spleen lying within the chest and causing a haemothorax can cause diagnostic confusion.

In an acute presentation the diaphragm is most often repaired from below at laparotomy. Herniated organs must be gently extracted from the chest, and it may be necessary to enlarge the diaphragmatic defect to do this. This should be done with consideration of the orientation of the branches of the phrenic nerve to minimize denervation of the diaphragm. The edges of the laceration are then securely approximated with strong interrupted sutures. After each suture is tied it can be used to lift the edges of the diaphragm and thus make the placement of the next suture easier. This manoeuvre will also reduce the potential for damage to the underlying heart or lung.

If diaphragmatic injury is suspected, and there is no other indication for a laparotomy, a laparoscopy can confirm or exclude it. However, at diagnostic laparoscopy both the surgeon and anaesthetist must be aware of the potential risk of a tension pneumothorax due to the communication between the thoracic and abdominal cavities. If this occurs, the gas of the pneumoperitoneum is released. If this does not produce an instant improvement, then needle chest decompression followed by chest drain insertion is required. A video-assisted thoracoscopy, as described above, is a useful diagnostic alternative, especially as in experienced hands a repair can also be carried out using this minimally invasive approach.

Injuries which present some months, or years, later will require a careful dissection to free the abdominal viscera from within the chest, in order to return them to the abdominal cavity, before the diaphragmatic defect is sutured. For late injuries a thoracic approach is thus often preferred and, as it may no longer be possible to bring the edges together, a mesh must then be used to bridge the defect.

Surgery for intrathoracic bleeding

The indication for surgery may be the magnitude of the bleeding, usually through a pleural drain, but occasionally directly to the exterior. Other indications include cardiac tamponade, and evidence of mediastinal bleeding suggesting a significant major vessel injury.

BLEEDING INTO THE PLEURAL SPACE

An initial drainage from the pleural space of a haemothorax of more than 1500 mL, or once the chest drain is in place a continuing blood loss of >200 mL per hour, suggests a source of bleeding which is unlikely to stop spontaneously and will require a thoracotomy. The risks and benefits of transfer to a cardiothoracic centre have to be individually weighed. The rate of haemorrhage, the distance for transfer, the local expertise and the likely source of haemorrhage may all be factors in the decision. For example, a patient with a stab injury to the lateral chest is probably bleeding from a severed intercostal artery or a simple lung laceration. In contrast, a patient who has a haemothorax following a blunt deceleration force, or a bullet wound in the superior mediastinum, is more likely to have complex injuries to vital structures which will require bypass facilities and surgeons with experience in the field. More may be lost in a stable patient by a thoracotomy without these essentials than by the delay incurred in transfer. The benefit of a telephone discussion with a cardiothoracic surgeon must not be forgotten in these situations.

A postero-lateral thoracotomy on the side of the haemothorax is most often the incision of choice. However, it must be remembered that, particularly in penetrating trauma, an injury to the heart or mediastinal vessels may present with early major bleeding into the pleural space. If a cardiac injury is suspected, an antero-lateral thoracotomy is more appropriate than a postero-lateral thoracotomy.

A severed intercostal vessel is simply ligated. A bleeding lung laceration will usually have within it a vessel which can be secured. The remaining laceration is then oversewn or stapled to reduce haemorrhage and air leak, and the chest closed with chest drains. A severe injury to a lung hilum may be from penetrating trauma, or a deceleration shearing force. The vessels and bronchus may be partially avulsed, and the only way of controlling haemorrhage may be to complete the pneumonectomy. A Satinsky clamp applied around the vessels and bronchi in the hilum may give temporary control, but pulmonary veins avulsed from the left atrium are particularly difficult to control, repair or close. A general surgeon faced with this situation can do little more than follow general surgical principles in attempting to secure control. The anatomy of the hila is shown in Figure 7.11.

CARDIAC TAMPONADE AND CARDIAC INJURY

A small laceration to the heart from either penetrating or blunt trauma can bleed into the pericardial sac, but this may remain contained by the pericardium. Blood collects under pressure, compresses the heart, and prevents cardiac filling.

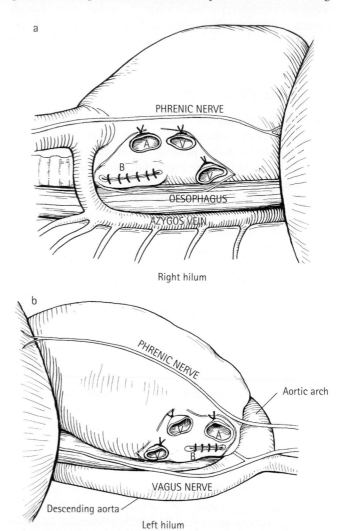

Figure 7.11 *Hilar anatomy. The bronchi (B) lie posteriorly and are shown closed in a linear fashion. The pulmonary arteries (A) lie immediately anterior to the bronchi, and the upper and lower pulmonary veins (V) lie more inferior. All vessels are shown ligated. The phrenic nerves lie anterior to the hila, on the pericardium. The vagus nerves lie posterior to the hila, in association with the oesophagus. (a) Right hilum; the azygos vein curves over the hilum to the superior vena cava. It lies lateral to the right vagus nerve and obscures it from view. (b) Left hilum; the aortic arch curves over the hilum to continue as the descending aorta. It partially obscures the oesophagus but the left vagus and recurrent laryngeal nerve (RLN) are vulnerable as they cross the lateral aspect of the aortic arch.*

In a classic case of cardiac tamponade, there is severe shock, dilated neck veins and muffled heart sounds. An X-ray shows clear lung fields and a bulbous outline to the cardiac shadow. More often, the situation is confused by multiple intra-thoracic injuries, and may be missed until it presents acutely with electromechanical dissociation in a 'cardiac arrest'. The pulseless patient with a beating heart has either exsan-guinated, or has a failure of cardiac filling due to cardiac tam-ponade. Without release of the tamponade the patient will die of what might be only a minor cardiac injury. Pericardial aspiration is inappropriate in trauma, as the underlying car-diac laceration will almost certainly re-bleed. The correct management is exposure of the heart, either through a left (or right) antero-lateral thoracotomy, depending on the side of the injury, or better still, through a vertical sternotomy if the surgeon is confident with the technique. A vertical median sternotomy will give superior access to the vessels of the superior mediastinum and can, if necessary, be extended into the neck (see Fig. 9.4, page 157).

The pericardium is opened anteriorly and parallel to the phrenic nerve, and blood under pressure is released. Once the pericardium is opened, the tamponade is relieved, and cardiac output increases with a resultant fall in venous pres-sure. Bleeding from the laceration is therefore often very minimal, and suturing of the laceration may be relatively simple. Cardiac wounds can be controlled initially by digital pressure. The commonest site for bleeding is the right atrium, which is thin-walled and easily sutured. Occasionally, it may be possible to isolate an atrial laceration with a side occlusion clamp while it is repaired. A 4/0 Prolene vascular suture is suitable for the atrial wall. A buttressed, pledgetted suture of heavier 3/0 Prolene is recommended for the closure of a laceration of ventricular muscle.

MEDIASTINAL BLEEDING AND MAJOR VESSEL TRAUMA

Particularly in non-penetrating trauma, bleeding from the disruption of a major vessel may be contained initially by intact adventitia and surrounding tissue. At this stage there is no gross loss of circulatory volume. An X-ray finding of a widened superior mediastinum from haematoma may be the only indication of a ruptured aorta, or of a major artery avulsed from the aortic arch. The challenges in interpreting emergency supine X-rays make the diagnosis more difficult, as a supine antero-posterior (AP) film, rather than the stan-dard postero-anterior (PA) view, makes the mediastinum look enlarged. Early diagnosis is essential if this window of opportunity for the transfer of such patients to a cardio-thoracic unit is not to be lost.

Occasionally, a general surgeon is forced by circumstance to operate. Unfortunately, the injuries encountered are com-monly beyond both the skills of a general surgeon and the limitations posed by the absence of cardiopulmonary bypass facilities.

The choice of incision will depend on the likely site of injury. For example, if the patient has an anterior bullet wound, a median sternotomy or an anterolateral thoraco-tomy which can be extended to a clam shell thoracotomy if necessary may be the most appropriate incision. Conversely, if an injury to the descending aorta is suspected, a left pos-terolateral thoracotomy will give superior access.

Major vessel trauma in the superior mediastinum is extremely challenging, and a surgeon inexperienced in tho-racic surgery will be most unlikely to succeed. The anatomy will be distorted by haematoma, and the trauma is seldom confined to the vessels. In penetrating trauma, the knife or bullet may also have transgressed the respiratory tree, the oesophagus or the spinal cord. In closed trauma, the shearing and traction forces may also have damaged adjacent struc-tures. For example, the avulsion injury of the subclavian artery from the aortic arch is frequently associated with a traction injury to the brachial plexus.

A deceleration injury is common in the relatively inacces-sible junction between the arch and descending aorta. Transfer is usually possible if this injury is diagnosed whilst the bleeding is still contained. If this opportunity is lost how-ever, a general surgeon may have to attempt a repair, though success is rare outside a cardiothoracic unit. Isolation of the injury for haemorrhage control, and repair, is hampered by the origins of major arteries, the need to maintain carotid perfusion and the problems associated with high aortic cross-clamping (see Chapters 5 and 6). A proximal clamp is placed across the base of the left subclavian artery and the aorta. A large soft clamp as used in bowel surgery is suitable for this. A second clamp is placed on the descending aorta, and a vasodilator such as nitroprusside is used to lower the blood pressure while the lesion is repaired. Unfortunately, in most instances the tension on the suture line makes it essen-tial to use a prosthetic graft which is unlikely to be available in a non-thoracic centre. A temporary Gott shunt from the arch to the descending aorta should be considered, as cross-clamping the aorta at this level risks paraplegia.

Major vessel injury in the posterior mediastinum is more accessible. It may be possible to suture a simple laceration of the descending aorta or the inferior vena cava. When a more extensive reconstruction or repair is required, the aorta may require to be cross-clamped and again, a temporary Gott shunt should be considered.

Major air leak

Most air leaks from damaged lung seal spontaneously, and can be successfully managed in the interim by intercostal underwater seal drainage. A very major leak, however, makes maintenance of ventilation, even by positive-pressure endo-tracheal mechanical ventilation, impossible as the resistance preventing air from escaping into the pleural cavity is less than that required to inflate the contralateral lung. Such a leak is usually from a ruptured bronchus. Haemoptysis and mediastinal emphysema are variable additional signs. A bronchoscopy can confirm the diagnosis.[6]

Temporary control of the situation, to allow transfer of the patient, may be possible with a double-lumen endotracheal tube, or even a single-lumen tube into the intact side. A balloon can be passed down a double-lumen endotracheal tube and inflated to occlude a bronchial laceration. A balloon can also be used to tamponade haemorrhage into the respiratory tree from a penetrating major vessel injury. These skills may be available from radiologists, anaesthetists or chest physicians, and their involvement in a cardiothoracic surgical emergency outside a regional cardiothoracic centre is invaluable. Rarely, the situation cannot be controlled for transfer, and the general surgeon will have to operate him/herself. A postero-lateral thoracotomy and repair of the bronchus with interrupted non-absorbable sutures is required. Wire was favoured, but an inert non-absorbable suture such as Prolene is now recommended. When there is also major hilar haemorrhage from a partially avulsed lung a pneumonectomy may be the only solution.

A mucosal tear in a bronchus allows the escape of air into the bronchial wall. There may be no pneumothorax or mediastinal emphysema, but the intra-mural air, haematoma and oedema may obstruct the bronchus. Presentation is with collapse of the lung distal to the bronchial obstruction. The diagnosis is confirmed bronchoscopically and the patient is transferred to a thoracic surgeon for repair of the bronchus.

A major broncho-pleural fistula can also occur as a post-operative complication of a pneumonectomy or lobectomy when the bronchial stump 'blows'. As an early complication, this will probably indicate a technical failure in the closure of the main bronchus, and repeat closure with non-absorbable sutures is practical. A late 'blow' is usually associated with infection, and the friable tissue will be technically difficult to repair. Small air leaks after lung resections can be managed conservatively and settle spontaneously.

Oesophageal injuries

The surgical management of intrathoracic oesophageal injuries, including iatrogenic and spontaneous perforation, is discussed in Chapter 17.

NON–TRAUMATIC EMERGENCY AND ELECTIVE CARDIOTHORACIC SURGERY

Cardiac surgery

No general surgeon practising in the developed world would even consider this surgery still to be within his or her remit. However, some generalists practising in remote areas of countries where resources prevent referral to cardiothoracic centres, may wish to consider appropriate cardiac procedures. Any cardiac surgery which requires cardiopulmonary bypass will obviously be impossible, and even simpler procedures will usually be impractical due to a

lack of intensive care and anaesthetic facilities. In addition, it must be remembered that many of the simpler cardiac, and extra-cardiac, procedures which can be performed without bypass have been superseded by superior, but more sophisticated, operations. Transfer of suitable patients to a specialist centre must therefore always be the main objective.

Two non-traumatic emergencies are, however, relatively common in the developing world. Both present with severe cardiac failure from a remedial mechanical cause, and often occur in young people. As neither require open-heart surgery, intervention can be considered if transfer is impossible.

CONSTRICTIVE TUBERCULOUS PERICARDITIS

This condition presents with worsening heart failure as the heart is prevented from filling by the fibrous constriction of the pericardium. Surgery consists of stripping off the adherent pericardium overlying the left heart through a left thoracotomy incision. Care must be taken to avoid injury to the coronary arteries. Unfortunately, a left thoracotomy without skilled anaesthetic and intensive care facilities may be an unsurvivable insult to these very sick patients. A more complete operation can be achieved through a median sternotomy, but the dense adhesions over the heart may make this approach more hazardous, especially if an oscillating saw is unavailable.

MITRAL STENOSIS

This presents with symptoms of left heart failure. The onset may be very sudden, and can be precipitated by the increased cardiac output in the mid trimester of pregnancy. Pulmonary oedema may be uncontrollable and, without intervention, death inevitable. A balloon valvotomy is now an option if the radiological skills and endovascular equipment are available. When they are not, and referral for specialist assessment and intervention is not possible either, the old technique of closed mitral valvotomy may still be appropriate. The stenosis in these young patients is a sequel of rheumatic fever, and the valve cusps, although fused, are pliable and otherwise free of degenerative disease. The cusps can be split along the line of fusion, either by a dilator introduced through the apex of the left ventricle or by a finger inserted through a left atrial purse-string, or a combination of the two techniques (Fig. 7.12).

Surgery of the intrathoracic aorta and great vessels of the superior mediastinum

This specialized field of surgery is divided between the cardiac surgeon, and the vascular surgeon with a special interest in intrathoracic work (see also Chapters 5 and 6). There are few situations in which a surgeon outwith these fields would be able to offer any useful surgical contribution.

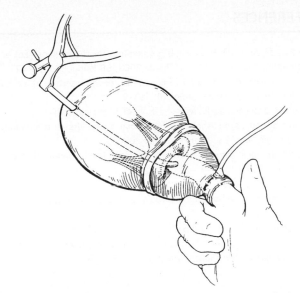

Figure 7.12   *A closed mitral valvotomy with a transventricular dilator guided by a finger in the left atrium.*

PULMONARY EMBOLECTOMY

This is an operation which many surgeons can describe but few have performed, or even seen undertaken, despite the fact that many patients die suddenly in hospital from a pulmonary embolism. The indications for surgery are, however, difficult to establish, and the window for useful intervention is very narrow. Surgery can only realistically be undertaken once the patient is sufficiently stable to be transferred to the operating theatre, and most patients who have survived the initial embolic event survive without surgery. Thrombolytic therapy is thus normally the management of choice. A median sternotomy is followed by isolation of the pulmonary trunk, around which tapes are passed for vascular control. An arteriotomy is performed and the clot aspirated, thereby relieving the acute right heart outflow obstruction. The arteriotomy is then sutured.

Thoracic surgery

Most of the thoracic surgery which a generalist can usefully undertake has already been described. There are, however, some surgeons who are able to offer a thoracic surgical service in addition to general surgery. These surgeons may wish to undertake elective lung resections for benign and malignant disease. However, descriptions of elective lobectomy and pneumonectomy, and discussion of the surgical management of bronchiectasis and lung cancer are outwith the remit of a textbook in general surgery. Further training and reading is essential for those generalists who wish to offer a more comprehensive thoracic surgical service.

Oesophageal surgery

Oesophageal surgery is shared between general surgeons with an upper gastrointestinal interest and thoracic surgeons. The issues involved and the operative solutions available are discussed in Chapters 16 and 17.

PAEDIATRIC CARDIOTHORACIC SURGERY

This surgery is, in the main, highly specialized and not within the field of the general surgeon. However, the surgical principles in the management of infection, including tuberculosis, are similar in the child and in the adult, and the surgical issues in thoracic trauma are also similar, although the spectrum of injury may differ. For example, in a thoracic crushing injury the greater pliability of the child's thoracic cage may allow serious damage to the intrathoracic viscera in the absence of fractured ribs.

General paediatric surgical practice includes the surgery of congenital diaphragmatic herniae and oesophageal atresia, and the surgical management of these conditions is described in Chapters 12 and 17, respectively. The paediatric surgeon with a large neonatal referral base will thus be familiar with intrathoracic surgical technique, but these neonatal intrathoracic operations are unlikely to be successful in conditions where general surgeons are forced to attempt them.

Congenital cardiac abnormalities

Congenital cardiac abnormalities are common, and most are managed optimally by early major surgery in which a definitive procedure is carried out before there is secondary tissue damage. The repair of a patent ductus arteriosus or a

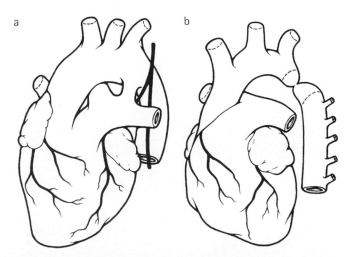

Figure 7.13   *(a) A patent ductus requires only a simple division for complete correction. The vagus nerve is vulnerable to injury. (b) Correction of a coarctation of the aorta requires excision of the short stenosed section and an end-to-end anastomosis.*

coarctation of the aorta might be achievable by a generalist when no referral is possible (Fig. 7.13). Surgical correction of other anomalies would not be a viable option in such surroundings.

The simple palliative procedures of the past included banding of the pulmonary artery, to limit excessive pulmonary blood flow, and the Blalock–Taussig shunt performed to increase it. The former was undertaken to limit the irreversible changes of pulmonary hypertension in those abnormalities with a large left to right shunt. The latter, in which the divided subclavian artery was anastomosed to the side of the ipsilateral pulmonary artery, was performed to improve oxygenation in cyanotic congenital heart disease. Although these may both be possible operations for a generalist, the indications for these procedures are dwindling, as better results are obtained with early definitive surgery.

REFERENCES

1. Henry M, Arnold T, Harvey J. BTS guidelines for the management of spontaneous pneumothorax. *Thorax* 2003; **58** (suppl. II): ii39–52.
2. Laws D, Neville E, Duffy J. BTS guidelines for the insertion of a chest drain. *Thorax* 2003; **58** (suppl. II): ii53–9.
3. Alric P, Branchereau P, Berthet J-P, *et al.* Video-assisted thoracoscopic sympathectomy for palmar hyperhidrosis: results in 102 cases. *Ann Vasc Surg* 2002; **16**: 708–13.
4. *Cardiothoracic Trauma.* S Westaby, JA Odell (eds). London: Hodder Arnold, 1999.
5. Ivatury RR, Kazigo J, Rohman M, *et al.* 'Directed' emergency room thoracotomy: a prognostic prerequisite for survival. *J Trauma* 1991; **31**: 1076–81.
6. Baumgartner F, Sheppard B, de Virgilio C, *et al.* Tracheal and main bronchial disruptions after blunt chest trauma: presentation and management. *Ann Thorac Surg* 1990; **50**: 569–74.

NEUROSURGERY FOR THE GENERAL SURGEON

The care of patients with head injuries is frequently undertaken by general surgeons who, with their anaesthetic colleagues, undertake both the monitoring and non-operative management of the patient with intracranial trauma. Only a small minority of patients will require transfer to a neurosurgical centre for surgical intervention. It is therefore important that those caring for such patients understand the pathology of injury to the brain, and the indications, benefits and limitations of intracranial surgical intervention. The operative management of scalp wounds associated with minor head injuries will remain the responsibility of the general surgeon, and it is again these surgeons who most frequently undertake minor elective surgery on the scalp.

Few general surgeons practising in the developed world anticipate a circumstance in which they will have to open the cranium. If such an emergency should arise, where transfer to a neurosurgical unit is not possible, almost certainly they would be able to benefit from telephone guidance from a neurosurgeon. However, the truly isolated generalist without the benefit of specialist support occasionally can offer a simple effective neurosurgical operation. It is for such surgeons that this chapter is predominantly written.

ANATOMY

SCALP

The various layers of the scalp are shown diagrammatically in Figure 8.1. The *galea aponeurotica* is a thin but dense aponeurosis, into which are inserted the frontal and occipital muscles. Its lateral margins blend with the strong temporal fascia. The skin of the scalp is bound to the underlying aponeurosis by a layer of dense fibrous connective tissue, in which lie the vessels and nerves. These three outer layers of the scalp move as one, and are separated from the pericranium by a layer of loose areolar tissue.

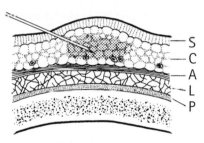

Figure 8.1 *The layers of the scalp.* Skin; Connective tissue; Galea Aponeurotica; Loose areolar tissue; Pericranium. *Local anaesthetic injections should be superficial to the aponeurosis.*

CRANIUM AND DURA MATER

In the adult the individual skull bones are fused and form the boundaries of the rigid intracranial compartment. The pericranium is the periosteum on the external surface of the skull. It is continuous with the outer layer of the dura at the foramen magnum, and is attached to the cranium at the sutures between skull bones. Unlike periosteum elsewhere, it is easily stripped off the underlying calvarial bone, and has little share in providing its blood supply, which is mainly from meningeal arteries. The dura forms a dense fibrous covering to the brain and spinal cord. Within the cranium the dura consists of two layers closely bound together, the outer of which represents the periosteum on the internal surface of the bone. The meningeal arteries lie extra-durally on the outer surface of the dura between the dura and the bone. Folds of the inner layer of the dura partially divide the intracranial space into supra- and infra-tentorial compartments, and the supra-tentorial compartment into two right and left spaces. The two layers of intracranial dura separate to enclose the cranial venous sinuses (Fig. 8.2). The subdural space is a potential space between the dura and the arachnoid mater.

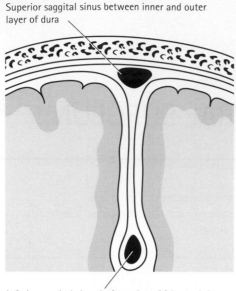
Superior saggital sinus between inner and outer layer of dura

Inferior saggital sinus in free edge of falx cerebri

Figure 8.2 *The two dural layers split to enclose the venous sinuses. The folding of the inner layer forms the falx cerebri and the tentorium cerebelli.*

ARACHNOID MATER

This is a very thin membrane covering the brain and spinal cord. It is separated from the pia mater, which is on the surface of the brain and spinal cord, by the subarachnoid space in which cerebrospinal fluid (CSF) circulates. This space is in direct communication with the ventricular system of the brain.

SCALP SURGERY

Local anaesthesia

Minor surgery on the scalp includes the removal of skin lesions, and the debridement and closure of lacerations. Surgery is usually performed under local anaesthesia, which should be infiltrated into the connective tissue layer, within which lie the superficial nerves. If there is little resistance to the injection, it implies that the solution is diffusing into the loose areolar tissue beneath the aponeurosis and that skin anaesthesia will be poor.

Control of haemorrhage

The scalp has a rich blood supply, and brisk bleeding occurs from any incision. Individual bleeding points are often difficult to identify and control in the dense fibrous layer of the scalp. Fortunately, although initial bleeding from a scalp laceration may be profuse, it has often stopped spontaneously by the time a patient reaches medical attention. Whenever

possible, operative incisions should be made vertically, in line with the main vessels. Bleeding is reduced if the incision is made with the cutting diathermy, but larger vessels will still bleed and are difficult to pick up in forceps. In minor excisional surgery digital pressure on the scalp lateral to the wound while surgery is completed, followed by deep sutures and pressure to the sutured wound is often sufficient to control bleeding. In the more major scalp incisions for neurosurgical access (Fig. 8.3), bleeding from the scalp edges must be controlled during surgery. Initial control by finger pressure on the adjacent scalp can be followed by pressure with Raney clips (Fig. 8.4). Alternatively, a series of artery forceps are applied to the galea aponeurotica at 1-cm intervals and then pulled back so that the galea is drawn over the cut surface, stretching and occluding the bleeding vessels.

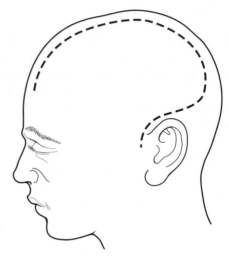

Figure 8.3 *A scalp flap which will allow extensive access to the lateral skull.*

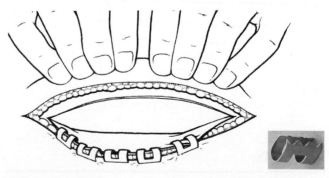

Figure 8.4 *Finger pressure will reduce bleeding from a scalp incision until Raney clips (shown in the inset) can be applied to the cut edge. Clips used to draw the aponeurosis over the skin edge are an alternative.*

Closure of scalp wounds

Similar principles apply to surgical incisions and traumatic wounds in the scalp. The scalp is thick, and the cut edges are often still bleeding when the surgeon is ready to close an incision. Therefore, deep full-thickness simple or mattress sutures, which compress the skin and subcutaneous fibrous connective tissue layer, are ideal. If the scar will later be covered by hair, any additional scarring attributable to the sutures will not be visible. Separate absorbable deep sutures in the galea are recommended in long wounds (Fig. 8.5). Scalp apposition, after either traumatic tissue loss, or after the excision of a skin lesion, can be surprisingly difficult, considering the apparent mobility of the scalp. Some tension on the suture line is permissible as the scalp has an excellent blood supply. However, if tension is unacceptable, a rotational flap may be used. A skin graft will give a bald patch which is often cosmetically unacceptable, but occasionally this may be the only immediate solution. A bald scar from the healing of a scalp defect or burn can be excised later: the defect may then be covered by adjacent hair bearing skin if the available tissue has been increased by an implantable tissue expander (see Chapter 1).

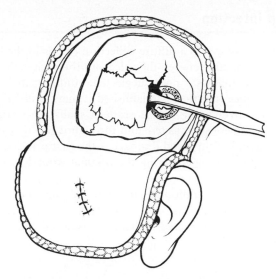

Figure 8.6 *A burr hole has been made adjacent to a compound depressed skull fracture. The displaced fragments can be levered back into position. This simple method of elevating a depressed skull fracture has great potential for increasing any initial brain injury. It is often safer to use rongeur bone forceps to nibble across the base of a depressed fragment before the fragment is lifted out.*

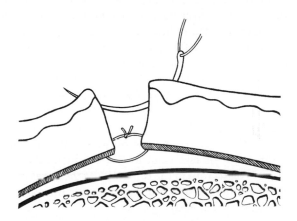

Figure 8.5 *Scalp wounds more than a few centimetres in length require separate closure of the aponeurotic layer.*

Scalp flaps for neurosurgical access

These U-shaped flaps are most commonly reflected on an inferior pedicle which is based on the vascular anatomy of the scalp. The incision through the aponeurosis is in line with the skin incision, and the flap is reflected in the subaponeurotic plane to expose a large area of cranium (Fig. 8.6). When frontal bone exposure is required, the incision for the flap should be sited within the frontal and temporal hairline, so that the scar is inconspicuous.

Scalp trauma

The significance of a small scalp wound is difficult to assess without knowing the nature of the injury. For example, a laceration with a broken glass bottle can confidently be assumed to involve only damage to the scalp, whereas a scalp split at the point of contact from a golf club, or similar small blunt object, may be associated with an underlying skull fracture.

This fracture will be compound and it may be depressed. In a major acceleration–deceleration injury, a scalp laceration at the point of contact with the ground, or a windscreen, may have no underlying fracture, or there may be an extensive 'eggshell fracture' involving a large area of cranium.

The possibility of a penetrating brain injury must not be overlooked. It may be obvious in a machete attack producing a large wound with extruding brain tissue, or external signs may be more subtle, and a reliable history not obtainable. The entry wound of a bullet may be small, and not easy to differentiate from an insignificant scalp laceration until the wound is cleaned and the hair shaved. An entry wound through the orbit, nose, ear or nasopharynx may not be immediately apparent.

Skull X-rays should be taken if there is any likelihood of a fracture underlying a scalp wound. A significantly depressed fracture, particularly one under a scalp wound, suggests a penetrating injury needing referral for specialist assessment. A scalp wound without an underlying fracture, or with a simple undisplaced fracture, usually requires only wound toilet and closure.

When dealing with an apparently simple laceration, an unsuspected fracture is occasionally found. If the fracture feels undisplaced, the scalp should be closed after wound toilet and debridement. If, however, the fracture appears displaced, or a penetrating injury is now suspected, no further wound toilet, exploration or probing is appropriate until a skull X-ray or CT scan is performed, and a review of the mechanism of injury is obtained, because neurosurgical referral may be more appropriate. Antibiotic prophylaxis should be started.

Scalp infection

A *subgaleal abscess* is a diffuse collection of pus in the loose connective tissue between the galea and the pericranium. It most often follows a deep, neglected, contaminated scalp wound. Once infection is established it may spread in this plane to involve the entire scalp. Usually, the original wound is obviously infected, and through it pus may drain spontaneously. Improved drainage is the first priority. This may be possible by enlarging the original wound and irrigating the whole space. Alternatively, and especially if there are loculations, additional incisions should be made. Antibiotic therapy is less important than adequate drainage, but is indicated if there is associated cellulitis of the scalp.

SURGERY OF THE CRANIUM

This surgery divides into the management of fractures, and the surgery of intracranial access.

Skull fractures

Skull fractures may involve the calvarium and/or skull base. A skull fracture is an indicator of a significant force imparted to the head. The only importance of the fracture itself is in its potential to damage the underlying brain, either directly or indirectly.

SIMPLE UNDISPLACED SKULL FRACTURES

No specific treatment is indicated. However, a fracture which traverses a vascular skull mark, such as that of the middle meningeal artery, increases the risk of an extradural haemorrhage.

COMPOUND UNDISPLACED SKULL FRACTURES

An overlying scalp wound is cleaned and closed, and the patient is started on broad-spectrum antibiotics as there is a danger of intracranial infection. It must be remembered that, even without an external wound, skull base fractures into the sinuses, middle ear and nasopharynx are compound with a risk of intracranial infection. Accordingly, antibiotic prophylaxis is usually given to any patient with a basal fracture of the skull or a fracture through the frontal sinus, and to any patient with a head injury who has bleeding from the ear or has CSF rhinorrhoea or otorrhoea. However, there is still some controversy over this antibiotic policy.[1] CSF rhinorrhoea or otorrhoea usually will cease spontaneously, but occasionally, if CSF leakage is persistent and profuse or when a pneumatocoele develops, it may be necessary to close the CSF fistula either intracranially (with a dural graft) or extracranially (as an ENT procedure).

SUBPERIOSTEAL HAEMATOMAS

A swelling, if accurately confined to the area of one skull bone, is usually associated with an underlying skull fracture. The haematoma is contained by the fusion of the pericranium to the underlying bone at the fissures. As the haematoma is organized and absorbed, palpable ridges develop at its edges which can mimic the edge of a depressed skull fracture. No action is required. A *subperiosteal abscess*, associated with osteomyelitis of a cranial bone, produces a similar localized swelling ('Pott's puffy tumour').Treatment is by drainage of pus, possibly removal of infected bone, and appropriate antibiotics.

DEPRESSED SKULL FRACTURES

In most instances these occur without a significant overlying wound, are not grossly displaced and, more importantly, the minor displacement has seldom resulted in spicules of inner skull table being driven through the dura into the brain. Elevation of these minor depressed fractures is recommended mainly for cosmetic considerations when they are in the frontal region. The indication for intervention by an isolated generalist is therefore somewhat tenuous. For the forehead, the most cosmetically acceptable scalp flap will be with the incision within the hairline. This can give extensive exposure of the frontal bone. Figure 8.6 illustrates the classical method of elevating a small depressed fracture through an adjacent burr hole. The burr hole is made on stable bone adjacent to the fracture, and not on the fracture line itself. Great care must be taken not to tear the intact dura. The technique is dangerous in the proximity of the dural sinuses. Many closed injuries which are suitable for this operation could be safely left alone.

Severe comminuted depressed skull fractures are an integral part of a penetrating head injury. The dura is torn, and spicules of bone will have been driven into the underlying brain substance. Exploration is indicated to remove spicules of bone, hair, missiles, metal and contaminated vegetable matter, and this is discussed further below. Very occasionally a skull X-ray indicates a similar fracture with spicules of in-driven bone but without an open wound. Exploration is again necessary for their removal. Severely displaced fractures with dural tears can not be simply levered back into position, and a craniotomy is usually necessary for adequate access.

Intracranial access

The simplest intracranial access is via a *burr hole*, but access is limited. This can be extended by enlargement of the burr hole with rongeur forceps to create a larger *craniectomy* (Fig. 8.7b). Access is still somewhat limited, and the larger defect in the cranium is unsatisfactory in the long term and may have to be addressed later. The alternative *craniotomy* involves removal of a plate of bone which is replaced at the end of the operation.

BURR HOLE

The temple is a common site for a burr hole. However, the principles are the same when burr holes are made in other parts of the cranium.

In the temple, *the scalp incision* is from the lower border of the zygoma, halfway between the eyebrow and the meatus, and runs upwards and slightly backward for about 5 cm (Fig. 8.7a). If a surgeon anticipates that he or she may be proceeding to a craniotomy, this incision, and those of any subsequent burr holes, should be modified so that they can be incorporated into a scalp flap incision. The superficial temporal artery may be either ligated or coagulated. In the lower part of the wound the temporalis muscle, covered by fascia, is incised and the muscle and periosteum split down to the bone. A strong self-retaining retractor is then placed to hold the muscle fibres apart (Fig. 8.7b).

The *burr hole* is made immediately above the midpoint of the zygomatic arch, using a perforator on a Hudson's brace (Fig. 8.8), or a more modern equivalent if available.

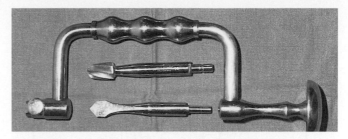

Figure 8.8   *A Hudson brace with skull perforator (below) and burr. These are the basic instruments which will probably be available to the general surgeon who has to open the cranium.*

The perforator should be turned rapidly with *gentle* inward pressure (at right-angles to the bone surface) to prevent sudden perforation of the bone. When the inner table is penetrated a characteristic rocking or juddering sensation is produced. The perforator should then be replaced with a burr, and the hole enlarged. Because the burr tapers and cuts a funnel-shaped hole it is safe to use, but the surgeon should still be careful not to plunge the instrument intracranially, especially through the thin bone of the temporal fossa.

At the end of the procedure, the bony defect of a burr hole can be ignored and the scalp closed in two layers over it. When a burr hole has been extensively enlarged as a craniectomy the defect may require a later cranioplasty.

CRANIOTOMY

A formal craniotomy is required when intracranial surgery requires access greater than that possible through a burr hole and limited craniectomy. Originally, a single osteoplastic flap, with the scalp left attached to the bone, was used, but it is now usual to raise scalp and bone flaps separately. The bases of the two flaps do not need to coincide. A scalp flap suitable for a large craniotomy is shown in Figure 8.3. It is reflected by separation through the loose areolar layer beneath the galea aponeurotica. To create a bone flap the calvarium is cut to connect a series of burr holes. The two holes at the base of the flap are placed closer than the others so that the narrow base can be nibbled across more easily with a bone rongeur. By means of a special guide, a Gigli saw can be passed between burr holes, with care being taken to avoid dural injury, and the intervening bone divided – with an outward bevel so that the freed portion of skull, when replaced, will not sink below its normal level. The bone at the base of the flap can be cut across, or fractured, but left attached by pericranium or temporalis muscle as a *pedicled bone flap* which is then lifted off the dura (Fig. 8.9). Alternatively, the skull bone and periostium are completely divided and the *free bone flap* lifted out of the wound and temporarily wrapped in moist gauze. At the completion of the operation, the skull flap is replaced and held in position with sutures joining the pericranium on the bone flap to pericranium on the adjacent skull.

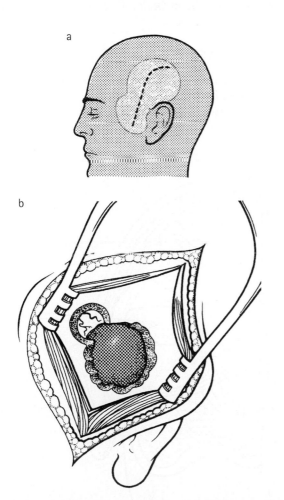

Figure 8.7   *(a) The surface marking of the incision for exploration of a suspected extradural haematoma in the temporal region. (b) The temporalis muscle is split and held apart by a self-retaining retractor to expose the temporal bone. The initial burr hole has been enlarged with a bone rongeur.*

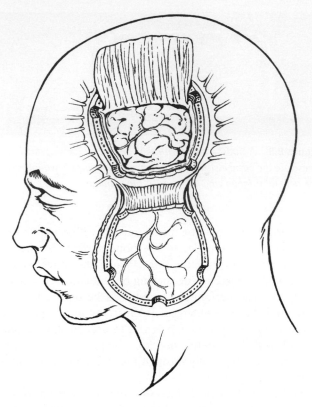

Figure 8.9 *A parietal bone flap has been raised by division of the skull between burr holes. It has been elevated as an osteoplastic flap still attached by the temporalis muscle. The dural flap has then been raised with its base towards the sagittal sinus.*

Cranial defects

These may be due to removal of bone fragments in comminuted or depressed fractures, or they may be the result of extensive enlargement of an exploratory burr hole. Repair by bone graft, or by the implantation of a titanium or acrylic plate, may be desirable to protect the brain from subsequent injury but this surgery should be postponed, commonly for at least 6 months, to minimize any risk of infection.

INTRACRANIAL SURGERY

The intracranial surgery of malignant, vascular and degenerative pathology is not included in this chapter, as it is a field in which the intervention of a general surgeon would be inappropriate. However, when confronted with cases of sepsis or trauma, a general surgeon who is unable to transfer a patient to a neurosurgeon may be able to offer an effective intracranial operation. This surgery includes the drainage of intracerebral pus, the exploration of a penetrating cerebral wound and the evacuation of a space-occupying, post-traumatic intracranial haematoma.

Drainage of intracranial pus

INTRACEREBRAL ABSCESS

These abscesses may develop by haematogenous spread from a distant source of infection such as an infective vegetation on a damaged aortic or mitral valve. They may also occur secondary to penetrative trauma, or to untreated infection in a fronto-ethmoid or mastoid sinus. Treatment consists of drainage of the abscess with a wide-bore needle introduced through a burr hole (Fig. 8.10). The wall of the abscess, which is often encapsulated, is felt as a characteristic resistance, and when this is penetrated the pus oozes out under pressure through the needle. An appropriate antibiotic regime is instituted and repeat aspiration may be necessary.

The major difficulty for a surgeon without sophisticated imaging is to confirm the diagnosis and localize the abscess. There may be localizing neurological signs, but there may only be evidence of infection and raised intracranial pressure. An abscess secondary to a sinus infection is commonly in the adjacent lobe of brain. This determines the site of exploratory burr holes.[2]

SUBDURAL EMPYEMA

Infected collections in the subdural space are mostly secondary to penetrative trauma, or occur as a result of the extension of an untreated infection in the air sinuses or middle ear. The patient classically shows evidence of an infective

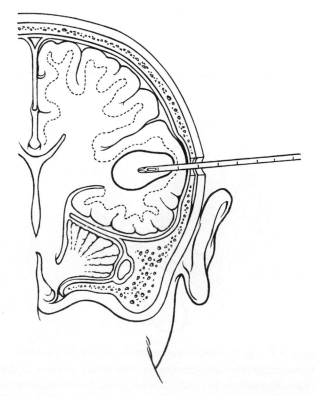

Figure 8.10 *An intracerebral abscess can be drained with a wide-bore needle introduced through a burr hole.*

pathology, and also has focal neurological signs such as a hemiplegia or epileptic convulsions; these are due to inflammation in the underlying cortex or thrombosis within underlying cortical veins. Treatment is by drainage of the pus, combined with antibiotic and anticonvulsant therapy. Commonly, a neurosurgeon will evacuate subdural pus through a craniotomy. For the general surgeon multiple burr holes[2] may provide adequate access for good drainage. The dura at the bottom of each burr hole is opened with a cruciate incision, the brain gently depressed (for example, with a smooth periosteal elevator or broad, curved dissector), and the subdural pus released.

Exploration of a penetrating cerebral wound

The neurological state and the external evidence of injury are highly variable in patients with penetrating brain injury. For example, a patient with a large open wound, and brain tissue visible within it, may be fully conscious with no apparent neurological deficit. Conversely, a deeply unconscious patient who has sustained a cerebral gunshot wound may have an insignificant entry wound which is missed at initial assessment. All penetrating wounds of the brain require urgent, skilled surgical attention. Exploration of an overlying wound should be avoided before the definitive surgery. The wound is covered with a sterile dressing, and the patient transferred to a neurosurgical unit if one is available. The initial resuscitation and assessment of the injured patient must not be overlooked, as inadequate resuscitation may compound the cerebral insult. In addition, other injuries may need more urgent attention than the cerebral wound. Exsanguination from a ruptured spleen, or ventilatory failure from a traumatic pneumothorax, can occur during transfer to a neurosurgical centre.

Surgeons who have no access to neurosurgical help will have to debride the penetrating wound themselves.[3] The surgery should be undertaken as soon as is practical, as any delay increases the risk of infection. Prophylactic antibiotic and anticonvulsant therapy should be started. The surgical aim is to remove all devitalized cerebral tissue, extravasated blood, bone fragments and any accessible foreign bodies, and to stop all haemorrhage. Complete debridement of this nature is dependent upon adequate exposure and good visibility.

OPERATIVE PROCEDURE

General anaesthesia with airway protection is recommended. The scalp should be shaved. A scalp flap will often afford better access to the area of injury than a simple extension of the external wound. A depressed fracture can be elevated through an adjacent burr hole (see Fig. 8.6), but this can be hazardous if there is a dural tear. Often it is safer to work from the burr hole using a bone rongeur to nibble along the base of a depressed fracture – that is, along its remaining attachment to the surrounding bone – thus converting the depressed fracture into a free fragment which can be lifted

more safely. When there is an extensive comminuted fracture with loose fragments, good intracranial access may be obtained by lifting these out. Larger fragments should be cleaned and replaced at the end of surgery. A small entry wound through the cranium can be enlarged with rongeur forceps, but access to the underlying brain will still be limited, and here a craniotomy is usually preferable.

The dura can be intact even with a severely depressed fracture. However, it may have been pushed in by bony spicules and stripped from the underside of the adjacent bone with associated extra-dural venous bleeding. This bleeding is best controlled by one or more hitch stitches, usually of absorbable material, between the dura and periosteum to pull the dura up against the bone, thus compressing the injured vessel (Fig. 8.11). Small dural lacerations, and contusion or lacerations of the underlying cortex, can be ignored if there is no significant bleeding or evidence of in-driven bone, hair or other contamination. When access beneath the dura is required, and the dura is not already extensively disrupted by the injury, the dura is opened with a U-shaped or cruciate incision and the dural flap(s) turned back to expose the cerebral cortex. The base of a dural flap should be towards the nearest venous sinus to reduce the risk of major venous bleeding (see Fig. 8.9).

Bleeding from a tear into a venous sinus can be extremely difficult to control. The operating table should be tilted to raise the patient's head and to reduce the venous bleeding – but not so much that bleeding stops and air enters the venous sinus, with resultant risk of major air embolus. An old technique which may still be of value in difficult circumstances is the use of a temporalis muscle graft which is hammered out into a thin sheet. This can be laid against a bleeding surface to which it adheres, and it is held in position with digital pressure for several minutes. Gelatin sponge or a similar preparation is also effective. Alternatively, pieces of muscle or gelatin sponge, that partly plug and buttress a sinus tear, may be held against the sinus by overlying stitches (e.g. of Vicryl 3/0) passed through the dura adjacent to one side of the sinus and through dura adjacent to the other side of the sinus. A sinus tear may be stitched directly, but sutures can tear easily through the thin sinus wall.

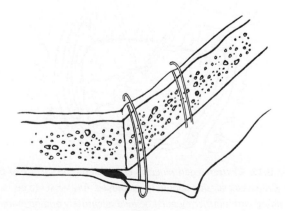

Figure 8.11 *Hitch stitches between the dura and the periosteum.*

Damaged cerebral tissue can be removed by irrigation and suction. A gentle jet of warm saline from a syringe and weak suction (25–35 cm Hg) through a fine-bore nozzle (3-mm lumen) will remove all devitalized brain matter and blood clot, but leave healthy brain tissue undisturbed. Any fragments of in-driven bone which become visible are gently extracted with forceps. The utmost gentleness must be observed as brain tissue is very delicate and, with rough handling, the surgeon is in danger of increasing the original injury. Meticulous attention must be paid to haemostasis. Bleeding vessels are coagulated with diathermy. They should be accurately held in fine forceps and the smallest effective current used to minimize damage to the underlying brain (Fig. 8.12). Bipolar diathermy is much safer than monopolar in this situation.

The exploration of *gunshot injuries* is particularly difficult. The entry wound is often small and may be mistaken for a simple scalp wound. The inner skull table is invariably fractured more extensively than the outer. Therefore, a craniotomy usually gives better access than simple enlargement of the cranial defect, especially as indrawn bone fragments are usually present. Access to the whole track is not possible without causing further damage, and a bullet in the depths of the brain should be left *in situ*. In through-and-through missile injuries the exit wound, which is usually larger and more impressive than the entry wound, should also be explored. The cavitation effect within the brain from any high-velocity bullet makes survival unlikely (see Chapter 3).

After completion of the debridement, and replacement of the dural flap(s), the dura is closed with fine absorbable

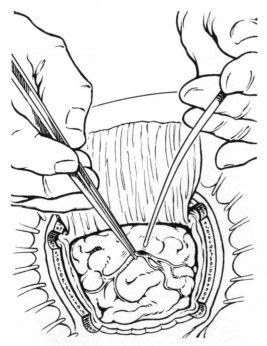

Figure 8.12 *Extreme gentleness is essential on the surface of the brain. Only weak suction should be employed. Any vessel to be coagulated with diathermy must be held accurately and no more current used than is necessary.*

sutures. When brain tissue is swollen, or there is a dural defect, it will not be possible to close the dura. Small tears can simply be covered with Gelfoam, but larger defects should have a transplant graft of pericranium or fascia lata stitched into place. If the patient's condition does not permit this, a large sheet of Gelfoam or Surgicel is applied over the surface of the brain and dural repair deferred for a later operation.

PATHOLOGY AND MANAGEMENT OF BRAIN INJURY

A post-traumatic haematoma, if unrecognized and untreated, can be fatal. For this reason many patients, even with apparently minor head injuries, are detained in hospital for observation. The main purpose of the observation is the early detection of this potentially remedial complication. A thorough initial clinical assessment, and the monitoring of any changes in neurological status, are pivotal in detecting a deteriorating situation.[4] Causes of any clinical deterioration must be sought, and the reasons, other than intracranial bleeds, must not be overlooked. In the UK, in most hospitals where general surgeons have patients under their care with head injuries, a potentially remedial intracranial cause of neurological deterioration can be confirmed or excluded by a CT scan before transfer to a neurosurgical centre.

The general surgeon may also have under his or her care patients who do not require transfer for neurosurgical intervention, but who have a significant brain injury. Many patients die, or suffer long-term sequelae, following head injuries in which there is no significant intracranial bleeding. Although no surgical intervention can alter the prognosis, the general medical care of these patients can be crucial to their outcome. This huge subject is outwith the scope of an operative surgical textbook, and further reading is essential.[5–8] However, a brief synopsis of the pathology of brain injury may be helpful.

Pathology of primary injury

The initial injury causes brain tissue to suffer direct contusional damage, or momentary stretching or distortion. In an acceleration deceleration injury, there may be no external evidence of trauma, but the brain, which is mobile within the cranium, impacts on the bone. The same mechanism, of mobile brain impacting on the skull, explains the contrecoup injury diametrically opposite the area of an impact. In addition, shearing forces tear the brain substance. No healing of disrupted neural cells within the CNS is possible, and the surgeon can do nothing to repair tears within the brain. An initial stage of neural shock, which lasts from a few minutes to a few days, resolves. Further neurological recovery involves the recruitment of other neural pathways and is not due to the 'healing' of brain cells which have been damaged irreversibly.

Pathology of secondary injury

Several factors are responsible for delayed ('secondary') brain injury, but the final pathway is mainly that of hypoxia,[7] to which brain cells are the most vulnerable tissue in the body. *Oxygen delivery is dependent on good perfusion by well-oxygenated blood.* Poorly oxygenated blood is often circulating after major trauma. The unconscious patient may have a partially obstructed airway and an inadequate respiratory effort, which can be further compromised by a concomitant chest injury. Brain perfusion, which is dependent on the *cerebral perfusion pressure*, may be poor in the patient with a head injury.

Cerebral perfusion pressure = Mean arterial pressure – Intracranial pressure

This relationship explains why it is extremely important to avoid hypotension in any patient with a head injury, especially as many will already have some increase in intracranial pressure. The commonest cause of hypotension in a patient with a head injury is hypovolaemic shock, usually attributable to coexistent multiple injuries.

CEREBRAL OEDEMA

Cerebral oedema after trauma is from the swelling of injured brain. Initially, a reduction in the volume of the CSF allows an increase in cerebral volume, without a significant rise in intracranial pressure, but the margin for compensation is small. Thereafter, intracranial pressure rises, with a resultant fall in cerebral perfusion. When this causes brain ischaemia there is an additional hypoxic insult to the brain, causing more cerebral oedema, and a deteriorating vicious circle is established. Hypercapnia dilates the cerebral blood vessels, causing a rise in intracerebral pressure, and must be avoided. Intracranial pressure can also be increased by obstruction of venous drainage, whether by the struggling of a confused patient, by the adoption of a head-down position, or by marked turning or twisting of the head to the side.

INTRACRANIAL HAEMORRHAGE

This occupies space within the closed intracranial compartment, causing intracranial pressure to rise with subsequent reduction in cerebral perfusion. Haematomas also displace the brain and put localized pressure on it.

Extra-dural haematoma

This often results from bleeding from a meningeal artery which runs in close apposition to the under-surface of the skull, and is torn when the skull is fractured. It may occur from a direct blow to the head, even if any primary brain injury is minor. The middle meningeal artery, under the relatively thin temporal bone, is the most vulnerable. Classically, after injury there has been only a transient loss of consciousness, a fracture which crosses the skull marking of the middle meningeal artery, and the patient has been kept in hospital for observation. A few hours later as the severed artery continues to bleed, and the haematoma increases in size, the intracranial pressure starts to rise steeply. Cerebral perfusion worsens and conscious level deteriorates. Displacement of the brain by the haematoma causes impaction on the tentorial opening. This first produces localizing signs which include a third nerve palsy, usually with a dilated pupil, on the side of the haemorrhage. Terminally, both pupils become fixed and decerebrate rigidity develops. Unfortunately, the classical early signs are the exception rather than the rule, and localizing signs can be misleading. However, the haematoma is usually on the side of the first pupil to dilate and/or to become fixed.

Acute subdural haematoma

Cerebral veins can be torn as they cross the subdural space to the venous sinuses by any shearing or deceleration force which temporarily distorts the intracranial anatomy. Such bleeding may be immediate and massive, especially if the tear extends into a venous sinus, and only specialist surgery can offer any realistic hope of success. A more minor injury may result in a haematoma which collects in the few hours after an injury, and may present clinically like an extra-dural haematoma. Unlike extra-dural haematomas, acute subdural haematomas more often occur in association with primary brain damage that is more major than the haematoma, and intracranially may be remote from the point of impact. Most areas of severe brain contusion will be overlain by small subdural haematomas of limited significance.

Chronic subdural haematoma

This occurs classically in an elderly patient who presents, some weeks after an apparently minor head injury, with altered consciousness, headaches and/or new neurological signs. There is some cortical shrinkage in old age, and the brain can move more freely within the cranium. A shearing force is thus more likely to tear a vein and cause a subdural bleed. In the elderly a fairly large haematoma can collect without any increase in pressure, as it is compensated for by a reduction in the larger volume of CSF that is associated with the ageing brain. When the haematoma liquefies it may expand significantly, so that compensation is no longer possible and neurological deterioration occurs.

Intra-cerebral haematoma

Tears of the brain substance may result in haemorrhage deep within the cerebral cortex – a situation which is unlikely to be amenable to a generalist's intervention. A surface laceration may produce haemorrhage into the ventricular system, or into the subarachnoid space.

General care of the patient with a head injury

A secure airway, adequate gas exchange and full resuscitation are vital in maintaining oxygen delivery to the cerebral cortex and preventing secondary brain injury. Sedation and mechanical ventilation are often necessary in order to obtain a CT scan in a patient with impaired consciousness. Mechanical ventilation is then often continued as, in addition to securing the airway and optimum ventilation, it also provides additional opportunities for maximizing cerebral perfusion.[8] Various agents to reduce brain swelling – including mannitol, diuretics and steroids – have been tried over the years. On the whole they have been disappointing, except as a temporary holding measure during transfer to a neurosurgical department or to an operating theatre for definitive treatment of a remedial cause of increased intracranial pressure. Antibiotic prophylaxis is usually given to patients with compound skull fractures. Any patient with a penetrating brain injury, an intracerebral haematoma or a compound depressed skull fracture is at risk of post-traumatic epilepsy. To prevent epileptic attacks these patients are usually given anticonvulsant treatment,[1] for example phenytoin, given at a loading dose of 15–20 mg/kg, followed by maintenance at 5 mg/kg per day.

DETERIORATION

When monitoring detects neurological deterioration, all remedial causes must be explored. Hypoxia, hypovolaemic shock, over-sedation and a post-traumatic convulsion should all be considered, in addition to an intracranial space-occupying haematoma. It must be remembered that generalized or localized brain oedema can also cause increased intracranial pressure, deterioration in conscious level, and even new focal neurological signs.

In patients in whom deterioration has been shown by CT scan to be due to an intracranial haematoma, urgent transfer to a neurosurgical unit is arranged. The general surgeon working in a remote area of the developed world may have to operate occasionally for a suspected extradural haematoma in a patient who cannot be evacuated to a neurosurgical unit. Almost certainly he or she will have the telephone support of a neurosurgeon, and may even have access to a CT scan. A CT scan will show accurately whether or not there is a haematoma. It will also indicate in which tissue plane a haematoma has formed and under which area of cranium, and whether it is small and incidental or the main cause of the increased intracranial pressure. However, diagnosis can be difficult especially in the absence of sophisticated imaging. Ultrasound can show deviation of the midline and, in the absence of CT scans, may help determine the side of a space-occupying haematoma.

A surgeon with no access to imaging has to rely on a clinical diagnosis,[9] and exploration may have to be through multiple burr holes.[3] Surgery may prove to have been fruitless, but as surgical evacuation of the haematoma is the only effective treatment for the life-threatening rise in intracranial pressure associated with an intracranial space-occupying haematoma, the attempt is justified.

EXPLORATION AND EVACUATION OF INTRACRANIAL HAEMATOMAS

Once a decision has been taken to operate, the patient should be given mannitol. A 20 per cent solution of mannitol is given intravenously over 5 minutes at a dose of 0.5 mg/kg. Intracranial pressure will fall temporarily, and although repeat doses can be given they become progressively less effective. Anti-seizure prophylaxis with phenytoin should be commenced, and the patient is ventilated to maintain a low P_aCO (ideally 4–4.5 kPa.). On transfer to the operating theatre, the patient is placed at a 20-degree head-up tilt to improve venous drainage, and the whole head shaved and prepared for surgery.

Emergency burr holes in trauma

A surgeon, who has the benefit of prior imaging, will plan to make a single exploration through the skull overlying the haematoma, and will know whether the blood will be encountered in the extradural or subdural space.

Urgent exploration, without the benefit of a scan, is best performed at the site of the fracture, or where there is external evidence of trauma.[2] If there is no sign of external trauma, the thin temporal region, with the underlying middle meningeal artery, is the most likely site of an extradural haemorrhage. Although the operation can be performed under local anaesthesia – or with no anaesthesia in an unconscious patient – a general anaesthetic with endotracheal intubation to control the airway and ensure adequate ventilation, is recommended. If there is a significant extradural haematoma, it will present at the burr hole under pressure.

TREATMENT OF THE EXTRADURAL HAEMATOMA

The haematoma needs to be fully evacuated and the bleeding vessel secured. Access must be increased by enlarging the burr hole in the direction indicated by the situation of the clot, usually towards the skull base. Alternatively, a formal craniotomy may be preferable. An actively bleeding vessel cannot be identified if there is overlying clot, or fresh bleeding, obscuring the view. A technique of irrigation and suction   similar to that employed for penetrating cerebral wounds and described above – is helpful. Ideally the artery is identified, and coagulated or ligated. If the middle meningeal artery is ruptured at the base of the skull, access may not be possible and a plug of bone wax pushed into the foramen spinosum will provide the necessary pressure to arrest the haemorrhage. Frequently, the site of the haemorrhage is obscure and active bleeding has ceased. After evacuation of the clot, and the arrest of any active bleeding, simple closure with an extradural vacuum drain is sufficient. Persistent venous extradural haemorrhage may occur from areas where the dura has been stripped from the bone by the expanding arterial haematoma. The bleeding is controlled by application of Gelfoam, and dural hitch stitches to compress the damaged veins (see Fig. 8.11).

TREATMENT OF AN ACUTE SUBDURAL HAEMATOMA

Unfortunately, the surgeon who has had to rely solely on clinical judgement may be faced with no extradural haematoma under the first burr hole. A subdural collection should then be suspected, especially if the dura is bulging and plum-coloured. The bulging dura is opened through a cruciate incision which allows evacuation of the clot. Gentle lavage and suction allows inspection of vessels on the brain surface, and any bleeding vessel is coagulated with diathermy. The burr hole can be enlarged if bleeding is continuing but the vessel has not been exposed. An acute subdural is often associated with a large area of underlying trauma to the brain, which can only be exposed by a craniotomy. The control of haemorrhage from dural veins and venous sinuses is described above (Exploration of penetrating cerebral wound, page 147).

MULTIPLE BURR HOLE EXPLORATION

Even if an extradural clot is discovered, there may be a contralateral subdural haematoma on the opposite side. When subdural clot is obtained, further collections may be present at other sites. When no significant extra or subdural clot is found at the initial burr hole, the underlying pathology is most frequently oedema from brain contusion, but there is also the possibility of extradural or subdural haematomas at other locations. A difficult decision must thus be made, in the absence of imaging, as to whether to explore through additional contralateral or ipsilateral burr holes.[3] Additional frontal and parietal burr holes should be positioned so that they can be joined to form a satisfactory bone flap for a subsequent craniotomy if this proves necessary (Fig. 8.13).

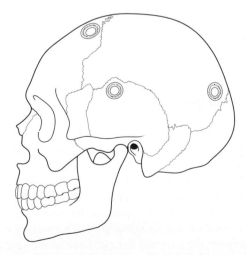

Figure 8.13   *When an initial temporal burr hole has not released clot, additional frontal and parietal burr holes may be successful.*

Burr holes for chronic subdural haematoma

The haematoma can be drained through a burr hole and, as all haemorrhage will have long since ceased, extended access to the underlying cortex is not required. The standard four burr hole exploratory approach, if imaging is unavailable, is shown in Figure 8.14. It must be remembered that these collections may be multifocal, and the discovery of a haematoma in one area does not exclude a second collection elsewhere.

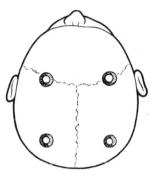

Figure 8.14   *Exploratory bilateral burr holes for a suspected chronic subdural haematoma.*

SPINAL CORD SURGERY

Spinal cord decompression

Elective surgery on the spinal cord and the vertebral column is the province of the neurosurgeon and the orthopaedic surgeon. Emergency surgery is indicated for clinically severe cord compression whether this is due to a haematoma, pus, a secondary deposit or a central disc prolapse. For most general surgeons, their responsibility for patients with these conditions is limited to the recognition of the pathology, and its confirmation, followed by urgent referral to the relevant specialist. Isolated generalists may on occasion have to operate themselves, and often without confirmatory imaging.

Tuberculosis of the spine may cause local compression from a mixture of pus, necrotic debris and bony sequestrae. Paraplegia is usually of insidious onset and fluctuant severity, and minor neurological symptoms may settle on antituberculous chemotherapy alone. Despite this, in some areas of the world, surgical decompression of a cord threatened by tuberculosis is still a common operation. However, it should be performed, if at all possible, by those surgeons who have had adequate training and experience in orthopaedic surgery or neurosurgery. Unlike surgery for an acute central disc prolapse threatening the spinal cord, surgery for tuberculosis is rarely a matter of great urgency. The disease process is located anteriorly, affecting an intervertebral disc and the adjacent two vertebral bodies, and therefore cannot be decompressed satisfactorily from the posterior approach.

POSTERIOR APPROACH

Emergency surgery by a posterior approach[10] may be performed to drain pus caused by pyogenic organisms or a haematoma compressing the cord. It is also a suitable approach for certain intervertebral disc lesions such as a large central disc prolapse compressing the cauda equina.

Surgery begins with a vertical incision over the spinous processes. The muscles are then stripped off the spines and laminae, and retracted laterally. *Fenestration*, in which a window is created into the spinal canal through the ligamentum flavum between two adjacent vertebral arches, should be sufficient to drain pus or blood in the epidural space and decompress the spinal cord. It is also possible very gently to retract the nerve root medially to approach a lateral disc prolapse (Fig. 8.15). However, the inexperienced spinal surgeon forced to operate on a prolapsed disc will almost certainly benefit from the safer, more extensive, access afforded by a *laminectomy*. Laminae are excised with bone nibblers, and care must be taken to avoid damage to spinal cord or nerve roots. Unfortunately, the more extensive the laminectomy the greater the risk of late instability of the spine. This is especially so if the anterior part of the spinal column – that is, the vertebral bodies and discs at the level of a laminectomy – is affected by disease impairing its stability.

ANTERIOR APPROACH

An anterior approach provides access to pathology of the vertebral bodies and discs compressing the cord from the front. It is a good approach for the anterior cord decompression required in tuberculosis. The excision of the necrotic vertebral body and disc is then followed by a cortical bone graft from the iliac crest to restore spinal stability, and correct the angulation deformity of vertebral body collapse. In the neck, the approach is between the thyroid gland and the carotid sheath (see Chapter 9). In the abdomen, the bodies of the lumbar vertebrae can be approached via a muscle-cutting loin incision and an extra-peritoneal dissection. In the thoracic spine, however, this approach necessitates a thoracotomy,[10] which will not be a viable option in a remote rural hospital with limited anaesthetic facilities. It is in such hospitals that general surgeons may find themselves forced to operate on patients with a worsening tuberculous paraplegia, and a costo-transversectomy is a safer compromise.[11]

COSTO-TRANSVERSECTOMY

This procedure allows the surgeon to decompress anterior pathology in the thoracic spine from a posterior approach. It avoids the necessity of opening the chest, and is performed through a vertical or curved incision a few centimetres from the midline. The incision is deepened to expose the transverse process of the vertebra and the posterior end of the rib which are then resected (Fig. 8.16). This will often result in entry into a paraspinal abscess. This abscess is in free communication, through a necrotic area of the vertebral body or the intervertebral disc, with the abscess which is compressing the cord. If, however, pus is not initially encountered, the anterior spinal canal abscess must then be entered through the infected and softened disc or vertebral body.

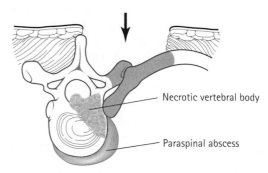

Necrotic vertebral body

Paraspinal abscess

Figure 8.16   *Spinal tuberculosis is primarily an anterior disease. In a costo-transversectomy via a postero-lateral approach, the initial bony excision of the costo-transverse joint affords entry into the paraspinal abscess compressing the cord through the necrotic area of a vertebral body or disc. The shaded area represents the bone that will have to be removed.*

Myelomeningocoele

This congenital abnormality is associated with severe neurological deficit below the lesion, often with musculoskeletal abnormalities. Urological complications are almost inevitable. In addition, many infants will develop progressive hydrocephalus requiring ventricular shunting, and associated mental handicap is common. Survivors will require long-term medical and social support. If no surgery is undertaken to cover the exposed neural tissue of the spinal cord, most infants develop infection and succumb within a few weeks. Therefore, the advisability of any surgical interven-

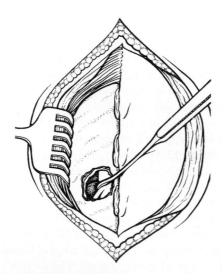

Figure 8.15   *The ligamentum flavum between two adjacent laminae has been* fenestrated. *The dural tube (theca) and the nerve root stretched over a disc protrusion may be retracted to expose it.*

tion should be carefully considered, especially where the availability of long-term medical care is minimal.

If surgery[10] is planned, it can be carried out within a few days of birth, and on occasion can even be performed under local anaesthesia. A skin incision is made round the exposed meninges, or round the neural plaque if the meningeal sac has already ruptured, and the plane developed between the skin and the dura until the neck of the sac is reached. The dura is then incised close to the neck but leaving sufficient dura to close it over the neural plaque. Any neural tissue entering the sac is dissected free and preserved, and the dura is closed. Primary skin closure may be possible or flaps may have to be mobilized.

REFERENCES

1. Dunn LT, Foy PM. Anticonvulsant and antibiotic prophylaxis in head injury. Review. *Ann R Coll Surg Engl* 1994; **76**: 147–9.
2. Meyer CHA. Intracranial Compression and Sepsis. In: B Ellis, S Patterson-Brown (eds). *Hamilton Bailey's Emergency Surgery*, 13th edn. London: Arnold, 2000, pp. 188–93.
3. Meyer CHA. Head Injuries. In: B Ellis, S Patterson-Brown (eds). *Hamilton Bailey's Emergency Surgery*, 13th edn. London: Arnold, 2000, pp. 175–87.
4. Advanced Trauma Life Support (ATLS) Course handbook.
5. *The Management of Head Injuries*, 2nd edn. DG Currie. Oxford: Oxford University Press, 2000.
6. Bartlett J, Kett-White R, Mendelow AD, *et al*. Guidelines for the initial management of head injuries; recommendations of the working party from the society of British neurological surgeons. *Br J Neurosurg* 1998; **12**: 349–52.
7. Chestnut RM, Marshall LF, Klauber MR, *et al*. The role of secondary brain injury in determining outcome from severe head injury. *J Trauma* 1993; **34**: 216–22.
8. Grant IS, Andrews PJD. ABC of intensive care; neurological support. *Br Med J* 1999; **319**: 110–13.
9. Morgan MR, Sparrow O. Surgical management of head injury with minimal investigation. *Trop Doct* 2001; **31**: 240–5.
10. Eisenstein S. The Spine. In: B Ellis, S Patterson-Brown (eds). *Hamilton Bailey's Emergency Surgery*, 13th edn. London: Arnold, 2000, pp. 194–206.
11. Bewes P. Spinal tuberculosis. *Trop Doct* 2001; **31**: 237–40.

SURGERY OF THE NECK

GENERAL TECHNIQUE

Anaesthesia and preparation

Local infiltrative anaesthesia is, in general, only suitable for very superficial surgery in the neck. Cervical plexus blocks have, however, proved to be both a safe and effective alternative to general anaesthesia for carotid endarterectomy. General anaesthesia given by facemask will often provide the surgeon with inadequate access; indeed, the mask itself and the anaesthetist will obstruct the surgeon, and turning the patient's head into a good position for surgical access can compromise the airway. The airway must remain secure in the position which is optimum for the surgery, and airway control from a distance, either by endotracheal intubation or by laryngeal mask, is more satisfactory.

The positioning of sterile towels so that they do not slip during surgery is important. A well-established method is illustrated in Figure 9.1. The head may then be turned to either side, or held straight with the occiput resting within a ring, or horseshoe, support. Extension of the neck is achieved with a sandbag beneath the shoulders, and supraclavicular access is improved by traction on the arm.

Even relatively superficial neck surgery can result in troublesome haemorrhage from anterior jugular veins and their tributaries. A steep head-up tilt will reduce venous bleeding, but at the risk of air embolus from negative intravenous pressure. Any hole in a large vein must be immediately occluded by digital pressure and the anaesthetist warned of the possibility of entry of air into the circulation.

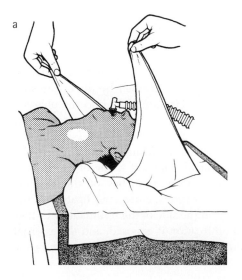
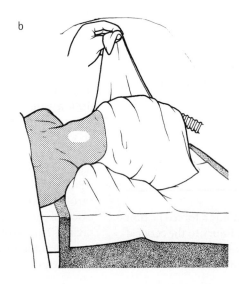

Figure 9.1 *(a) The patient's head is lifted. A sterile waterproof paper sheet and two sterile towels are laid beneath the head and neck. (b) The uppermost towel is folded across, over the chin, to cover the face and the anaesthetic tube.*

Neck incisions

Wounds in the neck can heal with disfiguring scars. Incisions must be planned, wherever possible, to follow the natural skin creases. These run approximately transversely, and most incisions can be placed along them (Fig. 9.2). When extensive longitudinal access is required a vertical incision can often be avoided by making two separate transverse incisions (see Fig. 9.8b), and this is particularly important anteriorly, where vertical scars will hypertrophy and contract. Even a horizontal incision anteriorly will hypertrophy in the suprasternal notch, and incisions for thyroid surgery should not be positioned too low for this reason.

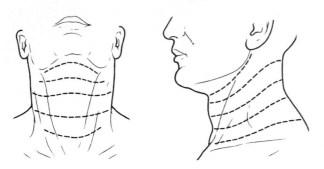

Figure 9.2 *Natural skin crease lines in the neck are approximately horizontal.*

If a vertical component to an incision is inevitable, it will cause less scarring if placed laterally either along the anterior border of sternocleidomastoid (see Fig. 9.4b), or along the anterior border of trapezius (see Fig. 9.8c, page 161).

Haemostasis is important before closure. A deep haematoma can threaten the airway from compression in the immediate postoperative period, and vacuum drainage for 24–48 hours is therefore routine. A superficial haematoma must also be avoided as it can increase subcutaneous fibrosis and scarring. Accurate apposition of skin and platysma is important for a good cosmetic result. Platysma is sutured with absorbable sutures, and provides considerable support to the skin closure. Clips or interrupted skin sutures can therefore usually be removed from the transverse anterior wounds used for thyroid surgery within 48 hours, without fear of wound dehiscence. The sutures in other neck wounds should normally be left *in situ* for around 7 days. If the surgeon prefers a subcuticular suture there is no urgency to remove it early, and removal will cause less discomfort if this is delayed for 10–14 days.

TRAUMA

Closed trauma to the neck is most commonly a forced flexion or extension injury, and is dominated by injury to the cervical spine and the cervical cord (see Chapter 4). Mechanical protection of the cervical spine is essential until an unstable cer-

vical fracture has been excluded. An intimal tear of a carotid artery can occasionally be caused by the same force. An anterior impact or crushing injury to the neck may inflict severe bruising and swelling, with progressive obstruction of the airway. Less commonly a fracture is sustained to the skeleton of the larynx, or the trachea is transected.

Penetrating and open trauma includes a wide range of injuries. There may be extensive soft tissue damage from a high-velocity bullet, or by fragments from a landmine explosion or shrapnel. In traffic accidents and falls from a great height, the patient's neck may have impacted on a protuberant object. In this scenario there may also have been a closed flexion–extension injury to the cervical spine.

Knife injuries include self-inflicted suicidal attempts. These are almost invariably long, anterior, profusely bleeding skin wounds. Occasionally, the wounds have opened into the larynx, through the thyrohyoid membrane or the thyroid cartilage. Since the head is thrown back at the time of wounding, the great vessels usually escape injury. Homicidal stab injuries are, however, more common and are encountered particularly in areas with a high incidence of urban violence. Guns are increasingly replacing knives as the weapons of choice, and in some areas are the most common cause of penetrating neck trauma.

Surgical management of neck trauma

Knowledge of the mechanism of injury is important in the assessment of any neck trauma. Even in an open injury, the possibility of an unstable cervical fracture may have to be considered. Mechanical protection of the spine until exclusion of a fracture will, however, make the assessment of the injury, the control of haemorrhage, and maintenance of the airway more difficult.

The *establishment of a secure airway* is the first priority. Endotracheal intubation is essential in any patient with neck trauma who is unconscious, or who has respiratory difficulty. The cuffed tube also protects the lower respiratory tract from further inhalation of blood. If endotracheal intubation is not possible an emergency tracheotomy may be required. A cricothyroidotomy may be a faster alternative in an emergency.

The *arrest of haemorrhage* is the next priority. External haemorrhage can usually be controlled by direct pressure until a wound is explored. Haemorrhage into the pharynx may be profuse, but once the airway is secure, either with an endotracheal tube or with a tracheotomy, pressure on the bleeding areas with pharyngeal packing will often bring the haemorrhage under control. The soft tissue of the neck is supplied almost entirely from branches of the external carotid artery. On rare occasions, emergency ligation of the external carotid artery on the side of the trauma may be lifesaving. The carotid bifurcation is exposed, and the external carotid is the *anterior division and has branches* (see below and Chapter 5).

The assessment of penetrating neck trauma can be difficult when there is only a small skin wound and the extent of any damage beneath is uncertain. If the patient is well, both the surgeon and the patient may be understandably reluctant to consider an unnecessary exploration. There is still debate as to whether all penetrating wounds should be explored or whether a more conservative policy of initial observation is more appropriate. Many of the principles of management have been evaluated in South Africa, where a selective policy on exploration is generally followed. Exploration is reserved for those who are judged to be at significant risk of having damaged important structures which require surgical repair. These can be divided into vascular, oesophageal and tracheal injuries. The history of injury, the direction of the track, the patient's symptoms and the physical examination are all important, in addition to more sophisticated investigations.

Vascular injuries

The neck is divided arbitrarily into three zones for the management of neck trauma in relationship to possible vascular injury (Fig. 9.3). Wounds in Zone I may have involved the major vessels in the superior mediastinum, and any exploration of such a wound will almost certainly require simultaneous access to the neck and mediastinum, with a supraclavicular incision extended down as a median sternotomy (Fig. 9.4a). A widened mediastinum on chest X-ray will alert the surgeon to a severe injury, and an angiogram should be performed before exploration unless haemorrhage forces immediate surgery. Angiography is desirable for all Zone 1 penetrating injuries, and surgery should be performed, if at all possible, by an experienced vascular surgeon (see also Chapter 5).

Penetrating wounds in Zone 3 are directly over the internal carotid artery. Access is difficult, and simultaneous access

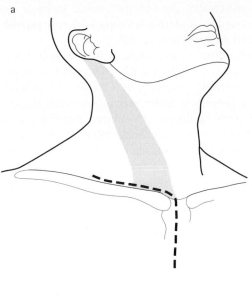

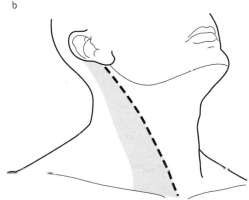

Figure 9.4 *(a) Zone 1 injuries to the carotid artery may require simultaneous access to the superior mediastinum. A median sternotomy incision can be extended as a supraclavicular incision or as an incision along the anterior border of sternocleidomastoid. (b) The incision along the anterior border of sternocleidomastoid may give superior access to the carotid artery in an emergency to that afforded by an oblique transverse skin crease incision.*

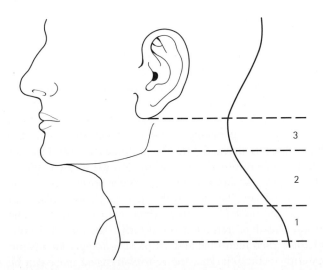

Figure 9.3 *Zone 1 extends for 1 cm above the upper border of the manubrium; Zone 3 is above the angle of the mandible; Zone 2 lies in between.*

intracranially may be necessary. A preoperative angiogram, together with the involvement of a vascular specialist, and occasionally also a neurosurgical specialist, is important.

Stab and bullet wounds are most commonly situated in Zone 2, and the risk of major vascular damage is obviously higher for lateral wounds. Some surgeons recommend exploration for all laterally placed Zone 2 injuries in order to exclude vascular damage, but a selective policy on exploration is favoured by others. Preoperative angiography is not routinely recommended. If a selective policy is followed, exploration should be undertaken of any lateral wound with evidence of significant haemorrhage, whether external or as an expanding haematoma. A bruit can also be further evidence of an arterial injury. Good access is essential, and the skin crease approach illustrated in Figure 5.19, page 90 may be insufficient. An oblique vertical incision along the anterior border of sternocleidomastoid will provide optimum arterial exposure (Fig. 9.4b).

At exploration a clean incision into a carotid artery can be sutured, but more frequently a vein patch is more appropriate to prevent stenosis (see Chapter 5). Consideration should be given to a temporary intraluminal shunt to preserve cerebral perfusion. An injured internal jugular vein can be ligated without adverse effect if the contralateral internal jugular is patent. On occasion it is necessary to tie off the external carotid artery. The surgeon must be sure that this is not the internal carotid artery. The carotid bifurcation may be quite rotated, so it is important to confirm that the artery believed to be the external carotid has branches before it is ligated. The internal carotid has no branches in this area.

If conservative management of a penetrating neck wound is undertaken, it is important that the vessels are imaged. A colour-flow Doppler ultrasound scan, performed the following day, is sufficient to exclude an intimal flap, a pseudoaneurysm or distal occlusion due to haematoma or contusion.

Tracheal and oesophageal injuries

Blunt trauma, with resultant haematoma and oedema, may obstruct the airway, and in a severe crushing injury there may be fractures of the skeleton of the larynx, which are best assessed on CT scanning when available. A fractured hyoid is usually managed conservatively, but if there is displacement of a thyroid cartilage fracture, this often requires repair with wires or mini-plates. Blunt trauma can usually be treated conservatively, and any threat to the airway managed by endotracheal intubation. Occasionally a tracheotomy is necessary. A history of anterior impact, associated with emphysema, requires a bronchoscopy to exclude a transected trachea as sudden asphyxia can occur if the divided ends become displaced. Formal repair is indicated for this injury.

Penetrating injuries will often heal spontaneously. A selective policy of only exploring those wounds through which air is bubbling, or those which are associated with major haemoptysis or haematemesis, appears safe.[1] All other patients with emphysema, or in whom there is any other reason to suspect injury to the pharynx or oesophagus, are given prophylactic antibiotics and given nil by mouth until a contrast swallow has excluded a leak. If a leak is demonstrated, oral intake must await a repeat contrast study showing the leak to have sealed. Further assessment of a tracheal injury includes laryngoscopy and bronchoscopy.

When repair is indicated, access to the superficial larynx and trachea is relatively straightforward. Simple closure, after wound toilet, with interrupted absorbable sutures is generally satisfactory. Access to the deeply placed pharynx and cervical oesophagus is difficult, especially when the anatomy is distorted with haematoma formation. The approaches described below for the drainage of retropharyn-

geal and parapharyngeal abscesses can be used, but a surgeon with limited experience in the neck will be reluctant to attempt any formal repair. Fortunately, arrest of haemorrhage, drainage of the parapharyngeal space and a strict nil-by-mouth policy until the breach has healed will often suffice.

Nerve injuries

Any penetrating injury to the neck may sever a nerve. Optimum operative conditions and surgical skill are more important than timing in repair, and referral to the relevant specialist is important (see Chapter 3).

INFECTIONS

Cellulitis in the neck requires prompt treatment with antibiotics. Careful monitoring of the airway is important as a tracheotomy may become necessary. Any associated infected collection or abscess should be drained. The underlying pathology must be sought as this may require surgical attention. Contamination from a breach in the wall of the hypopharynx, or cervical oesophagus, should be suspected in any patient who has had recent cervical trauma or surgery.

Abscesses can occur in any of the fascial spaces in the neck. The infection may be a direct extension of a primary infective process, or secondary to a suppurative lymphadenitis in the drainage nodes. Abscesses which present intra-orally are considered in Chapter 10, where the surgical managements of a *paratonsillar abscess* (quinsy), a combined *submental and submandibular abscess* (Ludwig's angina) and a childhood pyogenic *retropharyngeal abscess* are discussed.

Retropharyngeal abscess

The retropharyngeal space lies between the pharynx and the posterior layer of the deep fascia, and extends from the base of the skull to the level of the tracheal bifurcation in the posterior mediastinum. In the adult the abscess is usually tuberculous, secondary to cervical spine involvement. In contrast to the pyogenic retropharyngeal abscess in the child which is drained into the oropharynx (see Chapter 10), the tuberculous pus should be drained to the exterior. A horizontal incision is made, one finger breadth below the angle of the jaw. The tail of the parotid gland is dissected from the sternocleidomastoid, which is then retracted. The carotid sheath is retracted posteriorly. The superior constrictor is then identified and, by passing a finger lateral and posterior to the pharynx, the retropharyngeal space can be entered. Locules are broken down, the pus evacuated and a deep drain left into the cavity. Anti-tuberculous therapy is instituted.

Parapharyngeal abscess

The parapharyngeal space lies lateral to the pharynx. It is bounded laterally by the lateral pterygoid muscle and the parotid gland. It extends from the base of the skull to the level of the hyoid bone, where it is limited by the fascia over the submandibular gland. The carotid sheath lies posteriorly. An abscess in this space may be associated with a tonsillar infection and a quinsy, or with an infected lower third molar tooth. The primary pathology should be addressed first. However, drainage of pus will probably still be inadequate, and direct drainage of the parapharyngeal space may still be required. A horizontal incision is made over the anterior border of sternocleidomastoid, two finger breadths below the jaw. The sternocleidomastoid muscle is retracted posteriorly and the deep cervical fascia incised to enter the abscess cavity (Fig. 9.5). This abscess is deep, and often multiloculated, and is best explored with blunt finger dissection. It will also require a drain left *in situ* after initial drainage.

Acute mastoiditis

The surgical drainage of pus in the mastoid air cells is discussed in Chapter 10.

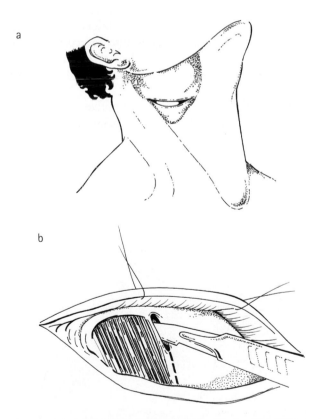

Acute parotitis

This, once common, complication in the postoperative surgical patient is now a rarity. It is associated with poor hydration, nutrition and mouth hygiene. In the early stages it may resolve on antibiotic therapy, but once pus has formed it must be drained. A small transverse incision, to minimize any risk to the branches of the facial nerve, is made overlying the area of greatest swelling. It is deepened until pus is encountered. Fortunately, the abscess usually occurs in the superficial portion of the gland and the facial nerve is safe, lying deep to the abscess cavity.

SURGERY OF LYMPH NODES

Surgical anatomy

The lymph nodes of the neck are somewhat arbitrarily divided into groups which are then described according to the position in which they lie (Fig. 9.6):

- *Submental* and *submandibular nodes* lie in these triangles and drain the floor of the mouth and the tongue. These nodes are described as level I cervical nodes.
- *Deep cervical nodes* lie deep to the sternocleidomastoid muscle and the deep cervical fascia. They lie both outside and within the carotid sheath, in contact with the internal jugular vein. They drain the tonsil, the pharynx, the larynx, the trachea and the thyroid gland. Inflammation within them is therefore common with upper respiratory infections, and carcinoma of the pharynx, larynx or thyroid may present with an enlarged metastatic node in this group. They are subdivided into level II, III and IV cervical nodes as representing the upper, middle and lower nodes of this group.
- *Pre-auricular, mastoid* and *occipital nodes* are superficial

Figure 9.5 *(a) The skin incision for drainage of a parapharyngeal abscess. (b) The deep cervical fascia is incised at the anterior border of sternocleidomastoid and the abscess entered. This approach is also used for access to the deep lymphatic tissue of the neck and for access to the upper oesophagus and hypopharynx.*

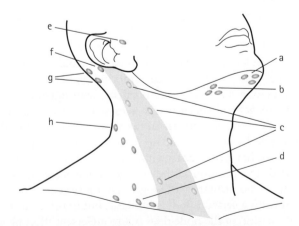

Figure 9.6 *The cervical lymph nodes.* (a) *Submental;* (b) *submandibular;* (c) *deep cervical;* (d) *supraclavicular;* (e) *pre-auricular;* (f) *mastoid;* (g) *occipital; and* (h) *posterior triangle.*

nodes which drain the skin and superficial tissue of the face and scalp.

- The *posterior triangle nodes* are deep to the investing fascia. They are classified as level V nodes.
- *Supraclavicular nodes* are continuous with the superior mediastinal nodes and with the axillary nodes. Metastatic involvement is seen in breast, bronchial and upper gastrointestinal cancer. Supraclavicular nodes are also classified as level V cervical nodes.
- *Anterior compartment nodes* surround the midline visceral structures, and include the retropharyngeal, paratracheal, prelaryngeal and pretracheal nodes. They are classified as the level VI group.

Drainage of purulent lymphadenitis

Purulent lymphadenitis can occur secondary to a tonsillitis, or other upper respiratory tract infection, and is encountered most frequently in infants. The upper deep cervical chain is the most commonly involved, but by the time it is apparent that there is pus and that the infection will not resolve with antibiotics, there is simply a collection of pus laterally in the neck which must be drained. A formal dissection with identification of the sternocleidomastoid and incision of the deep fascia to enter the deeper planes is seldom necessary. A small transverse incision over the most prominent part of the swelling, which is then deepened until pus drains, is normally sufficient. This incision will leave a satisfactory scar but will provide inadequate continuing drainage unless a drain is placed into the depth of the abscess and sutured to the skin, as illustrated in Figure 2.7, page 30.

Diagnostic lymph node biopsy

The differential diagnosis of an enlarged cervical lymph node includes inflammation, lymphoma and metastatic malignancy. Up to one in five patients with a carcinoma of the nasopharynx, oral cavity, oropharynx, larynx or hypopharynx present with a nodal metastasis. Such nodes should be excised en bloc with the other drainage nodes and the primary malignancy, to maximize the chance of cure. Nodal biopsy in isolation for diagnosis should be avoided as there is evidence that this increases morbidity, and possibly decreases long-term survival, in patients with squamous carcinoma. A general surgeon who sees a patient with an isolated neck node, particularly in the submandibular or in the deep cervical chains, should seek an ENT opinion prior to biopsy, so that malignancy within the drainage area can be excluded. The position of the enlarged node is a guide as to the site of the primary pathology.[2] Thyroid cancer can also present with a cervical node metastasis, but in this cancer an initial excision of the node does not so adversely affect prognosis. Malignant supraclavicular nodes are usually associated with advanced malignancies, often from a primary in the breast, chest or abdomen, which is no longer surgically

curable. Isolated excision biopsy is therefore oncologically harmless.

A fine-needle aspiration may be sufficient to confirm metastatic cancer cells, but cannot differentiate between inflammatory and lymphomatous changes, for which a node biopsy is necessary. The histologist must be able to study the architecture of the gland, and ideally a whole node is excised, with the dissection on the capsule of the node. If this is not possible due to the proximity of vital structures, or when nodes are matted together, a generous wedge excision is a safe compromise.

Occipital and **posterior triangle nodes** are relatively superficial and no large vessels are in the vicinity. Local anaesthesia is therefore suitable. The operation, however, should not be under-estimated, or undertaken for insignificant nodes. The surgeon must be aware of the surface markings of the accessory nerve when removing level V nodes, as the nerve crosses the posterior triangle at the level of the deep fascia (Fig. 9.7). The nodes lie in close proximity to the nerve, which is thus extremely vulnerable to injury, either from surgical division or diathermy damage. Accessory nerve injury results in significant shoulder dysfunction.

Deep cervical nodes are deep to sternocleidomastoid, and general anaesthesia and a protected airway are recommended. A transverse incision through skin and platysma, followed by posterior retraction of the sternocleidomastoid muscle after incision of the deep cervical fascia along its anterior border, will bring the surgeon into the correct plane. Care must be taken not to damage the internal jugular vein; its anterior tributaries, such as facial and thyroid veins, may have to be ligated and divided.

Supraclavicular nodes are often deceptive, and found at operation to be deeper than initially suspected. They may

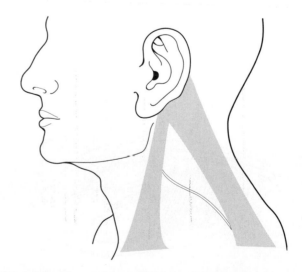

Figure 9.7   *The accessory nerve crosses the posterior triangle at the level of the deep fascia. The surface markings are from the junction of the upper and middle third of sternocleidomastoid to the junction of the middle and lower third of trapezius. Lymph nodes lie in close proximity to the nerve.*

merely be the only accessible part of a huge mass of matted mediastinal nodes, which are compressing the trachea and distorting the anatomy of the great vessels at the root of the neck. The surgeon should dissect with caution in optimum surgical and anaesthetic conditions. Tracheal compression in the superior mediastinum can make a general anaesthetic hazardous, but this is also a hazardous area for a surgeon to operate under local anaesthesia.

Radical neck dissection

The classical, *radical neck dissection* described by Crile in 1906 includes the en bloc excision of all cervical lymph nodes along with the sternocleidomastoid muscle, the internal jugular vein and the accessory nerve.[3] Many surgeons now prefer to preserve some of these non-lymphatic structures, even in the radical node excisions for ENT malignancies. Such dissections are described as *modified radical neck dissection*, and these are classified as:

- Type I, with preservation of the accessory nerve.
- Type II, with preservation of the accessory nerve and the internal jugular vein.
- Type III, with preservation of the accessory nerve, internal jugular vein and sternocleidomastoid.

Most surgeons perform a Type I modified neck dissection in preference to a classic radical neck dissection in an attempt to preserve function of the accessory nerve.

A *selective neck node dissection* preserves one or more lymph node groups in addition to the three non-lymphatic structures. For example, a level VI selective dissection is employed commonly in thyroid cancer.

The incisions for any form of radical neck dissection must be planned to afford good access and to leave inconspicuous scars. In addition, skin viability must be preserved, as a carotid artery exposed by skin breakdown has a risk of rup-

ture. The blood supply of the skin of the lateral neck comes from all directions, with a resultant relatively poorly vascularized central area directly over the common carotid artery (Fig. 9.8a). Vertical incisions and three point junctions in this central area should therefore be avoided, especially when radiotherapy has already been used, and salvage surgery is being undertaken. Two suitable incisions for radical neck dissections are shown in Figure 9.8, and the incision in Figure 9.8b is the method of choice after radiotherapy.

The skin flaps are elevated to include the platysma. In the submandibular area, in order to preserve the marginal mandibular branch of the facial nerve, the nerve is formally identified. If this is difficult, the flaps should be elevated by dissection in a deeper plane. This plane is on the body of the submandibular gland and the fascia over the gland is included in the flap.

Inferiorly the sternal and clavicular heads of sternocleidomastoid are divided to expose the carotid sheath. The internal jugular vein is isolated by dissection around it, and the vagus nerve, lying in a deep plane between the vein and the common carotid artery, is identified and preserved. The vein is then divided between ligatures. On the left, the thoracic duct is commonly divided at this point and will require oversewing to prevent leakage. The dissection is continued laterally, above the prevertebral fascia, to the anterior border of trapezius, elevating the fat pad overlying the scalene muscles and dividing the inferior belly of the omohyoid muscle which is included in the specimen. The external jugular vein and supraclavicular cutaneous nerves must also be divided. The transverse cervical vessels lie between the fat pad and the prevertebral fascia and should, if possible, be preserved. Underneath the prevertebral fascia the phrenic nerve runs medially and downwards on scalenus anterior. It is identified and preserved. The trunks of the brachial plexus are also beneath this fascia. Bipolar diathermy is therefore preferable to monopolar for this dissection so close to the nerves.

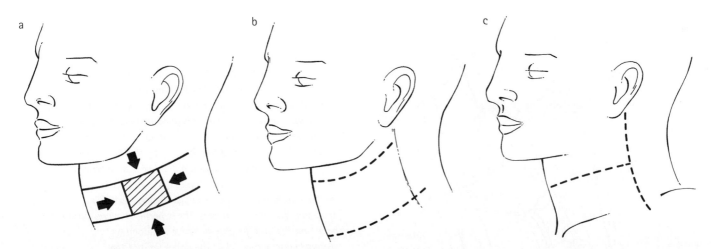

Figure 9.8   *(a) The shaded area has the poorest blood supply in the neck. It also overlies a relatively superficial segment of the carotid arteries. (b, c) Incisions which afford excellent exposure but avoid vertical incisions or three-point junctions in this area of skin.*

Posteriorly the limit of dissection is trapezius, and the dissection is continued up along its anterior border (Fig. 9.9a). The transverse cervical artery gives a vertical branch which runs up the anterior border of trapezius and requires formal ligation and division. The accessory nerve is divided in the classical radical dissection as it enters the muscle, but is preserved in all modified neck dissections. The upper third of the trapezius approaches the posterior border of the sternocleidomastoid muscle, the fibres of which are divided close to their mastoid insertion.

Anteriorly the superior belly of the omohyoid muscle forms the boundary of the dissection and is followed to its insertion into the hyoid bone and divided (Fig. 9.9b). The submental fat pad is dissected off until the anterior bellies of both digastric muscles are identified.

The *deep dissection* is commenced by reflecting forwards the posterior margin of the dissection and releasing the fat pad, with the nodes, off the prevertebral fascia and the underlying muscles, the levator scapulae and the scalenes. It is tethered down by the three cutaneous branches of the cervical plexus, namely the anterior cutaneous nerve of the neck, the great auricular nerve and the lesser occipital nerve. These nerves are identified and divided well away from the phrenic nerve. The internal jugular vein is dissected out of the carotid sheath up to the jugular foramen. The transverse process of the atlas is palpated and, just above this, the posterior belly of digastric will be found. This is retracted upwards, and the upper end of the jugular vein exposed where it is again divided between ligatures, with care being taken to preserve the vagus nerve. The hypoglossal nerve can be seen crossing lateral to the external carotid artery, and is in turn crossed by three small veins draining from the tissue to be excised. These vessels must be ligated and divided or they will tear, and attempts to stop the bleeding will endanger the hypoglossal nerve (Fig. 9.9c). The remaining sternocleidomastoid fibres are divided at the level of a line extending from the tip of the mastoid process to the angle of the jaw. A higher division

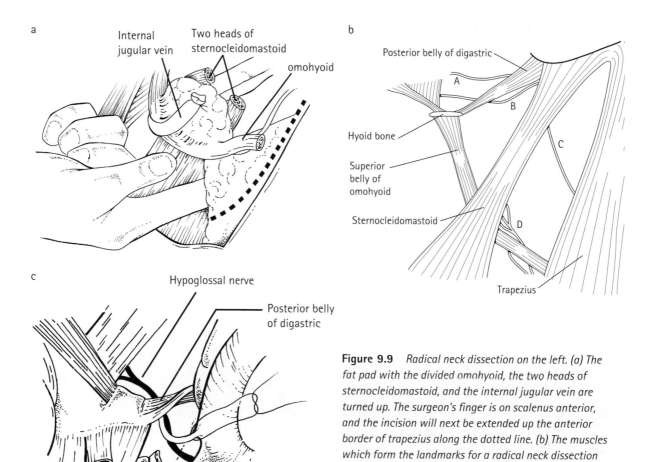

Figure 9.9 *Radical neck dissection on the left. (a) The fat pad with the divided omohyoid, the two heads of sternocleidomastoid, and the internal jugular vein are turned up. The surgeon's finger is on scalenus anterior, and the incision will next be extended up the anterior border of trapezius along the dotted line. (b) The muscles which form the landmarks for a radical neck dissection are shown with some of the nerves. (A) marginal mandibular branch of the facial; (B) hypoglossal; (C) accessory; (D) brachial plexus. The superficial nerves have been omitted and the phrenic nerve is hidden by sternocleidomastoid. (c) At the upper limit of the dissection the hypoglossal nerve is vulnerable. The small veins which cross it require individual ligation and*

places the facial nerve at risk, as it lies deep to the anterior border of the muscle.

Superiorly the submental fat pad, and the anterior edge of the submandibular gland, are dissected off the lateral surface of the mylohyoid muscle. The submental artery will require ligation and division. The posterior edge of mylohyoid is then retracted forwards, and the gland retracted inferiorly, to expose the lingual nerve which is freed and preserved. The submandibular duct is ligated. The facial vessels are ligated at the upper border of the gland, and the facial artery again at the inferior border.

COMPLICATIONS

Immediate complications include haemorrhage and pneumothorax, and raised intracranial pressure from compromised venous drainage. Necrosis of skin flaps, with exposure of the carotid artery, is a serious intermediate-term complication which requires further surgery at the earliest opportunity to cover the vulnerable vessel. A chylous fistula from injury to the thoracic duct is initially treated conservatively, but occasionally may require surgical intervention (see Chapter 17). Late complications include a frozen shoulder, in addition to the inevitable loss of function if the accessory nerve has been sacrificed.

Tuberculous cervical lymphadenitis

This condition is still encountered in areas of the world where bovine tuberculosis is common. Untreated enlarged nodes caseate and discharge. Cold abscesses with adherent overlying skin proceed to chronic discharging sinuses, and severe scarring. Surgery is seldom indicated if anti-tuberculous treatment is effective, although limited surgery in conjunction with effective chemotherapy is sometimes appropriate. The emergence of multi-resistant strains of tuberculosis, however, means that once again the surgeon may have to operate for this condition when no other treatment is effective. Tuberculous cervical lymphadenitis is almost invariably unilateral, and 90 per cent involve only one group of glands, the most common being the deep nodes beneath the sternocleidomastoid muscle, followed by the submandibular group.

When surgery is undertaken for resistant disease, it must include the excision of all diseased nodes if it is to offer a reasonable chance of eradication of the infection, and healing. This can, however, be a challenging operation when the deep cervical nodes are matted and adherent to the internal jugular vein, the wall of which may form the medial wall of the tuberculous abscess. A dissection similar to the radical neck dissection described above may be necessary to secure the internal jugular vein above and below the segment of involved vein, which has to be removed en bloc with the specimen. The accessory nerve and the sternocleidomastoid muscle can usually be preserved.

Cystic hygroma

These are congenital cystic abnormalities of the cervical lymph vessels. They present at birth and may be so large as to obstruct labour, or to compress and obstruct the newborn airway. The urgency of surgery will depend on size, but specialist referral to paediatric or ENT surgeons with experience of this condition is appropriate. Large lesions may extend down into the superior mediastinum. The deeper aspects of the lesion will have to be dissected off the internal jugular vein, and superiorly the multiloculated cyst may extend into the parapharyngeal space and the floor of the mouth. Dissection of the superior extensions places the facial nerve at risk, and a formal superficial parotidectomy may be necessary to safeguard its branches. Redundant skin is excised at the completion of surgery. Staged surgery or repeat resections are often necessary.

THE THYROID AND PARATHYROID GLANDS

Surgical anatomy

THYROID GLAND

This gland lies in the lower part of the front of the neck as a bilobed gland joined by an isthmus which overlies the second to fourth rings of the trachea. The lobes lie lateral to the larynx and trachea, and are in close apposition to them. A gland of normal size extends from the middle of the thyroid cartilage to just above the clavicle. The gland is enclosed in a sheath of pre-tracheal fascia, so that it moves on swallowing. Superficially it is covered by the sternothyroid and sternohyoid strap muscles.

Blood supply
The thyroid gland's blood supply is from the superior and inferior thyroid arteries. The superior thyroid artery is the first branch of the external carotid artery. It passes down to the upper pole of the thyroid lobe. The *inferior thyroid artery* arises from the thyrocervical trunk, a branch of the subclavian artery. It runs upwards and medially behind the carotid sheath to enter the middle of the back of the lobe. The *superior thyroid vein* leaves the gland with the superior thyroid artery and drains into the internal jugular or facial vein. The *middle thyroid veins* emerge from the lateral aspect of the lobe and cross in front of the common carotid artery to join the jugular vein. The *inferior thyroid veins* emerge from the isthmus and lower medial part of the lobe, and descend in front of the trachea to end in the left brachiocephalic vein.

Associated nerves
The associated nerves are in danger in any operation on the thyroid or parathyroid glands. The *external laryngeal nerve*, which is a terminal branch of the superior laryngeal branch of the vagus, runs downwards on the inferior pharyngeal constrictor, deep and medial to the upper pole of the thyroid

gland, to end by supplying the cricothyroid muscle. Near its termination it is in close proximity to the superior thyroid artery and is in danger of injury when this vessel is ligated. The *recurrent laryngeal nerve* supplies all the intrinsic muscles of the larynx. It arises from the vagus – on the right side as it crosses the subclavian artery, and on the left as it crosses the aorta. It hooks around the artery, and ascends in the groove between the trachea and the oesophagus. It enters the larynx below the lower border of the inferior constrictor, and is here closely related to the termination of the inferior thyroid artery where it is in danger of injury when this vessel is ligated. Anatomical anomalies, more common on the right, include a nerve following a more lateral course which then runs obliquely, or even horizontally, towards the larynx alongside, or anterior to, the inferior thyroid artery and is therefore more vulnerable to injury.

PARATHYROID GLANDS

The parathyroid glands consist of bilateral superior and inferior glands which lie behind the thyroid. Each is ellipsoid and pea-sized, and of a reddish-brown colour. The glands lie within 1–2 cm of the intersection of the recurrent laryngeal nerve and the inferior thyroid artery. The *superior glands* lie above and behind the nerve. The *inferior glands* lie below and ventral to the nerve. Considerable variation in position is common, however, and discussed further under parathyroidectomy.

Thyroid and parathyroid surgery

A secure airway and good access for the surgeon are essential. This is usually achieved by a general anaesthetic with endotracheal intubation and the head towelling technique shown in Figure 9.1a and b, page 155. The patient is positioned supine with a sandbag under the shoulders, the neck is extended, and the occiput supported on a head ring.

EXCISION OF A THYROGLOSSAL CYST

The thyroid gland develops from the thyroglossal duct, which grows down from the foramen caecum of the tongue. Incomplete regression of the duct results in a thyroglossal cyst or fistula. The cyst is in the midline – either above or below the hyoid – and moves with swallowing and tongue protrusion, unlike a thyroid swelling which moves only with swallowing. A fistula is usually secondary to spontaneous discharge or drainage of an infected thyroglossal cyst. The treatment of both a cyst and a fistula is excision. In order to prevent recurrence, the remnant of the thyroglossal duct must be traced towards the foramen caecum at the junction of the middle and posterior third of the tongue.

A horizontal incision is made over the cyst, or an ellipse is cut to include a fistula. The platysma is divided in line with the skin incision, the deep cervical fascia is divided vertically in the midline, and the strap muscles are separated. The cyst

is mobilized and the upward extension of the track is identified. This is followed upwards with ease until it disappears deep to the body of the hyoid bone to which it is densely adherent (Fig. 9.10). The hyoid must then be separated from the underlying thyrohyoid membrane. There is a space between these structures, and the surgeon's fears of encountering the endotracheal tube in the operating field are normally groundless. The central 1 cm of the hyoid bone is cleared of muscle attachments, and is then resected with bone nibblers so that it can be removed with the specimen. The dissection can then proceed into the tongue towards the foramen caecum. The track often disappears at this level and entry into the oral cavity is unnecessary. The wound is closed with vacuum drainage. When the cyst or fistula is low, and

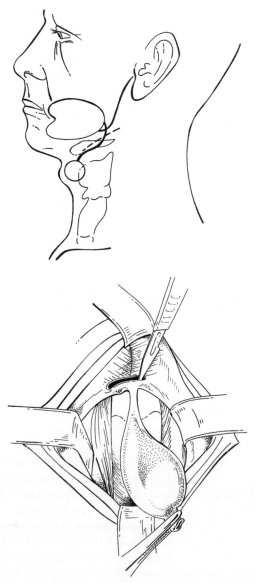

Figure 9.10 *The track from a thyroglossal cyst or sinus disappears behind the hyoid bone. If the central portion of the hyoid is not excised with the adherent track on its deep surface recurrence is likely.*

lying in the suprasternal notch, a second transverse incision higher in the neck may be required for access.

HEMITHYROIDECTOMY

This is undertaken usually for diagnostic purposes, when preoperative investigations of an apparently solitary thyroid nodule have neither excluded nor confirmed malignancy. Imaging with ultrasound scanning identifies whether the nodule is solitary or, as is quite common, a dominant nodule in a multinodular goitre. It also differentiates solid from cystic nodules. Technetium uptake scanning demonstrates whether the nodule is functioning and is described as 'hot', or non-functioning and described as 'cold'. Fine-needle aspiration cytology undertaken clinically, or with ultrasound guidance, can differentiate papillary from follicular tumours. Problems in differentiating benign from malignant follicular tumours limits the value of cytology in these lesions in all but a few specialist centres.

The most usual indications for hemithyroidectomy are a solitary cold nodule with follicular cytology, or a dominant cold nodule in a multinodular goitre with follicular cytology and where the multinodular changes are confined to one lobe. A hemithyroidectomy is required for definitive histological diagnosis. A peroperative frozen section is advocated by some, but most pathologists find that differentiating benign from malignant follicular tumours is again a particular problem, although the technique is useful in confirming a papillary carcinoma (which may be suspected but has not been proven on the basis of the preoperative cytology). Alternatively, a definitive pathology report within 48 hours allows a completion thyroidectomy to be undertaken in the same hospital stay if the tumour is malignant. If the tumour is benign the patient can be discharged home.

In young women, who form a lower risk group if they have papillary or follicular thyroid cancers under 1 cm in diameter, a hemithyroidectomy may be adequate definitive surgical treatment.[4,5]

The operation

A slightly curved transverse skin crease incision is made 2–3 cm above the sternum (it should not be positioned lower than this or the central portion of the scar will hypertrophy). The skin can be marked preoperatively using natural skin crease lines as a guide (see Fig. 9.2). Platysma is incised in line with the skin, and the skin and platysma flaps are elevated down to the sternum, and up to the thyroid cartilage. Traditionally, 40–60 mL of 1 in 400 000 adrenaline was infiltrated into the superficial tissue of the flaps prior to the incision to reduce bleeding, but this is of lesser value when diathermy coagulation is employed. A self-retaining Joll's retractor is then positioned to retract the flaps. The deep cervical fascia is incised vertically in the midline, and the strap muscles retracted laterally (Fig. 9.11a). Horizontal division of the strap muscles for access is seldom necessary, even in large goitres, as the muscles in this situation have already been stretched by the enlarged gland. If division is necessary

they should be divided high up as their innervation is from below. They are repaired at the end of the procedure.

The assistant retracts the strap muscles laterally, and away from the surface of the gland. Areolar tissue around the gland is divided and the middle and inferior thyroid veins are displayed. These require ligation and division. Skilled assistance is essential for this operation as these veins are unsupported by surrounding tissue and are very delicate. The artery forceps must be released with minimal movement of the tip as the surgeon tightens the ligature, or alternatively an aneurysm needle can be used. The deepest of the inferior thyroid veins may be in close proximity to the recurrent laryngeal nerve, and the final ligations in this area may have to wait until the nerve has been identified. Attention is next turned to the superior pole. With gentle traction on the now partially mobilized lobe it should be possible to pass a right-angled forceps behind the superior pole vessels and pass a mounted tie around them (Fig. 9.11b). An aneurysm needle is also very useful for this step. The external laryngeal nerve is endangered during this manoeuvre, and it is important to try and find the window medial to the superior pole vessels and stay a few millimetres lateral to the surface of the larynx. The ligature is then tied as low as possible. A second ligature is tied above it, and an artery forceps is placed immediately above this second ligature. The vessels are then divided between the ligatures and a further ligature tied on the superior thyroid pedicle before the forceps is released. Too high a tie of these vessels also endangers the external laryngeal nerve.

The lobe is then rotated medially out of its bed. The assistant is now retracting in a deeper plane, and the retractor is drawing the carotid sheath laterally. The inferior thyroid artery and the recurrent laryngeal nerve must now be displayed, and both lie beneath a fascial layer which must be incised. The inferior thyroid artery is ligated in continuity, but only after the nerve is identified and safeguarded. An aneurysm needle is the easiest method of passing the tie beneath the artery, which is then ligated as lateral as possible to minimize any danger to the nerve (Fig. 9.11c).

The final dissection of the deep portion of the gland off the recurrent nerve and the parathyroids is the most difficult, and must be performed with great precision. The medial surface of the lobe then separates easily from the trachea, and is finally only attached by the isthmus which is divided close to the contralateral lobe. A haemostatic continuous absorbable suture in the isthmus will control haemorrhage.

A deep vacuum drain is placed beneath the strap muscles before they are approximated. The platysma is sutured, and finally the skin is closed using sutures or staples.

TOTAL THYROIDECTOMY

This is performed for thyroid cancer and, increasingly for multinodular goitre and for the surgical management of thyrotoxicosis, as an alternative to subtotal thyroidectomy. It is also undertaken prophylactically in those patients who are

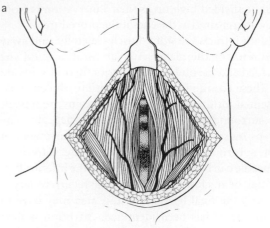

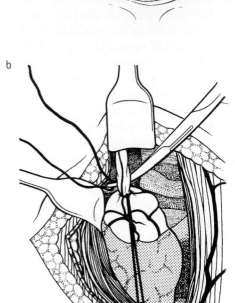

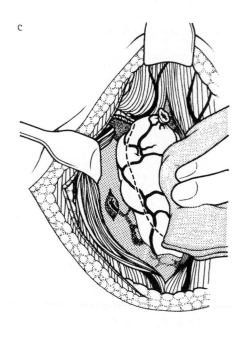

Figure 9.11 *A right hemithyroidectomy. (a) A horizontal skin and platysma incision is followed by elevation of the flaps. Vertical midline division of the cervical fascia and separation of the strap muscles exposes the gland. (b) The right strap muscles are retracted. Multiple small veins have been divided, and retraction has exposed the upper thyroid pole. The first ligature has been tied around the superior thyroid vessels close to the gland. (c) The retractor is now in a deeper plane and is retracting laterally the carotid sheath in addition to the strap muscles. Digital retraction over a swab draws the lobe medially. An incision through the posterior fascia allows identification of the recurrent nerve, running in a vertical or oblique orientation. The inferior thyroid artery crosses the nerve. The artery runs transversely and can be seen to pulsate. It is ligated in continuity.*

genetically at high risk of familial medullary thyroid cancer. The indication for excision of the whole thyroid in papillary and medullary cancer is the commonly multifocal pattern of the disease. In follicular cancer the rationale is complete eradication of thyroid tissue, so that any metastases can be identified and treated by uptake of radioactive iodine. If a definitive preoperative diagnosis is possible, as discussed in the section on hemithyroidectomy, a total thyroidectomy can be planned from the outset.

Operative procedure

Surgery is essentially a bilateral hemithyroidectomy, but the risks involved are higher. Unilateral recurrent nerve damage leaves a patient with a deeper voice of reduced strength. Bilateral damage results in the paralysed cords migrating medially to obstruct the airway, and a tracheostomy may be necessary. In addition, bilateral loss of parathyroid function, whether from excision or from ischaemic damage, may pro-

duce symptomatic hypoparathyroidism. Thyroid replacement therapy will of course be necessary.

LYMPH NODE DISSECTIONS WITH THYROIDECTOMY

Surgical opinion is divided on the prognostic value of the diagnosis of nodal metastases in differentiated thyroid cancer. It is also divided over the therapeutic value of prophylactic dissection of the clinically negative neck, whether such an operation should be a modified radical, or a selective, neck node dissection, and whether it should be preceded by frozen section histology of the nodes. There is also doubt over the relative merits of a modified radical neck dissection as compared with the selective removal of enlarged nodes in the clinically positive neck.

In *papillary thyroid cancer*, one view is that in addition to a total thyroidectomy the pre-tracheal and tracheo-oesophageal lymph nodes (level VI) are cleared, as this cervicocentral group is the most commonly involved. Frozen section histology is then obtained of a node in the middle portion of the ipsilateral deep cervical chain, as in the cervico-lateral region it is these level III nodes which most frequently will contain metastases.[6] If this node is positive, a modified radical neck dissection with preservation of the internal jugular vein, accessory nerve and the sternocleidomastoid muscle is performed. Many surgeons, however, would elect for a total thyroidectomy without any lymph node dissection in the clinically negative neck.

In *follicular thyroid cancer*, lymph node metastases are less common than in papillary cancer, and distant metastases are more common. Although this changes the balance of risk, the issues which dictate the surgical strategy in the clinically negative neck are similar.

In *anaplastic thyroid cancer* little is gained by radical surgery. Radiotherapy and chemotherapy may procure a short remission, and surgery is restricted to excision of the isthmus to prevent airway obstruction.

In *medullary thyroid cancer* the central and paratracheal lymph nodes (level VI) should be excised, and this dissection can be continued caudally to include upper mediastinal (level VII) nodes and the thymus gland. The deep cervical nodes may also contain metastases.[7] The advisability of a modified neck dissection can again be determined on frozen section histology of a deep cervical node.

SUBTOTAL THYROIDECTOMY

This has been the standard operation both for a large goitre, and for a toxic thyroid. More recently, total thyroidectomy has been advocated primarily to reduce the risk of recurrence of the goitre, or of thyrotoxicosis. This must be balanced against the greater risks to the recurrent laryngeal nerves and parathyroids. In a *large multinodular goitre* the aim may be purely cosmetic, but more commonly there are pressure effects on the trachea, and ultimately on the oesophagus. In subtotal thyroidectomy, the remnant is left mainly to safeguard the parathyroid glands and their blood supply, and to reduce the risk of injury to the recurrent laryngeal nerve.

Hyperthyroidism is primarily a medical condition. Surgery is indicated for those patients who relapse after medical treatment, and for those in whom the gland is nodular and enlarged in addition to being hyperactive. These patients should be managed in cooperation with a physician. Thyrotoxicosis must be controlled by medical means prior to surgery. Antithyroid drugs are now commonly combined with beta-receptor blockade to prevent the cardiovascular manifestations of an increase in circulating thyroxin. Following surgery, many of these patients will eventually become hypothyroid. Hypothyroidism is related more to the nature of the disease, and the immunological changes triggered by the surgery, than to whether the correct volume of thyroid remnant was retained. Traditionally, the surgical belief was that approximately one-eighth of the original gland should be retained.

Operative procedure

This proceeds in the same fashion as for a total thyroidectomy until after the inferior thyroid artery is ligated. The lobes are then transected, leaving a cuff of posterior thyroid tissue which lies on either side of the trachea from which the overlying isthmus has been removed (Fig. 9.12). A continuous haemostatic suture may be inserted in each transected remnant, but with great care as the residual thyroid tissue overlies the recurrent laryngeal nerve and the parathyroid glands.

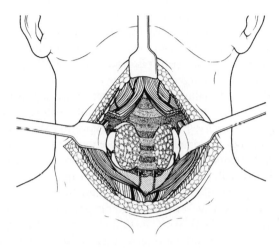

Figure 9.12   *Subtotal thyroidectomy. A small remnant of each lobe has been left bilaterally. The illustration shows a case in which partial division of the strap muscles proved necessary.*

RETROSTERNAL GOITRES

The whole thyroid gland may be lying retrosternally, or more commonly there is a retrosternal portion of a large goitre. The goitre is frequently symptomatic, and surgery is indicated for tracheal compression. The retrosternal goitre lies in the superior mediastinum above and anterior to the great vessels. It can usually be delivered up into the neck without difficulty. In situations where it cannot be delivered easily the proximity to these vessels must be remembered and force avoided. Occasionally, a median sternotomy is necessary for its safe mobilization (see Chapter 7).

PARATHYROIDECTOMY

This is undertaken for hyperparathyroidism. *Primary hyperparathyroidism* is usually the result of a secreting adenoma in one gland. The remaining glands are small and hormonally suppressed. However, a spectrum of adenoma and hyperplasia can occur, particularly in some forms of the multiple endocrine neoplasia (MEN) syndrome. In patients with renal pathology the initial hormonal abnormality is a compensatory *secondary hyperparathyroidism*, with hyperplasia affecting all four glands. Finally, the overactive glands may become autonomous and a *tertiary hyperparathyroidism* develops, which commonly involves more than one gland in hyperplastic or adenomatous change. When there is a solitary adenoma, only that gland should be excised, particularly when preoperative ultrasound and sestamibi scans correlate (see below). When a hyperplastic process involves all glands, it has been commonly advocated that three glands, and half of the fourth gland, should be excised. More recently, removal of all glands and maintenance replacement therapy with 1,25-dihydroxycholecalciferol has gained popularity, primarily to reduce the risk of recurrent hypercalcaemia. The operative strategy of surgeons operating on this condition will thus vary, depending on whether their referral practice is mainly of patients from a regional renal centre.

It is important to identify the side to be explored first in order to avoid unnecessary bilateral exploration in the majority of patients. An ultrasound, CT or MRI scan may demonstrate an enlarged gland. The subtraction scans with technetium and thallium, or the newer, more sophisticated sestamibi scans, have proved invaluable before routine parathyroid surgery. Prior to a re-exploration these can be repeated and additionally, selective venous sampling can be helpful. Patients with hyperparathyroidism secondary to renal disease will require a bilateral neck exploration, as will those with a familial predisposition and those whose preoperative scans suggest multi-gland disease. However, the 80 per cent of patients with suspected primary hyperparathyroidism only require a unilateral exploration on the side of the adenoma, as the removal of one enlarged gland and the identification of one normal gland is sufficient.

Operative procedure

Exposure of the parathyroid glands is achieved by mobilization of the lobe of the thyroid. Methylene blue is taken up selectively by the parathyroids, and the blue staining of the tissue is helpful in differentiating parathyroid tissue from lymph nodes or nodules of fat. It is administered in solution, as an infusion of 5 mg/kg over a 1-hour period. The colour differential diminishes after a further hour, and timing of the infusion can be difficult. Frozen section histology should be used for confirmation. The operation may be extremely straightforward, but sometimes parathyroid glands cannot be identified and may be lying in ectopic positions. A *superior* gland, which is not in its normal position, is often lying more *dorsally* and adjacent to the oesophagus, and may have migrated caudally as far as the posterior mediastinum. An *inferior* gland lies more *ventrally* but may have migrated caudally to lie in the anterior mediastinum, or cranially to lie close to the submandibular gland.[8] Parathyroid glands may also lie within the thyroid tissue.

RECURRENT SURGERY ON THE THYROID AND PARATHYROIDS

Reoperation, whether for excision of the remnant of a thyroid lobe, excision of a recurrent goitre or for a repeat exploration for recurrent hyperparathyroidism, carries a greatly increased risk of damage to the recurrent laryngeal nerve. The anatomy may be both obscured and distorted by scar tissue, and the planes for safe dissection are obliterated. The avoidance of these problems at subsequent surgery is one of the reasons why total thyroidectomy is gaining in popularity in expert hands. Surgery for a recurrent goitre may be requested on purely cosmetic grounds and should not be undertaken lightly. When reoperation is necessary the surgeon must take extra care during dissection, and the patient must be warned preoperatively of the increased risk of nerve damage. Referral to a surgeon with special expertise in the neck should always be considered in this situation.

POSTOPERATIVE COMPLICATIONS OF THYROID AND PARATHYROID SURGERY

Airway complications

Postoperative stridor can occur for several reasons:

- *Recurrent nerve damage*: an immediate problem with maintenance of the airway on extubation will occur if there has been bilateral recurrent nerve damage, as both paralysed cords drift medially. Laryngoscopy confirms paralysed adducted cords obstructing the airway. Re-intubation will have to be followed by a tracheostomy, which will usually be permanent unless the damage is no more than a temporary neuropraxia.

- *Tracheomalacia* is a complication of very large goitres and is therefore seldom encountered in surgical practice in the developed world. It presents with tracheal collapse after thyroidectomy. When it is recognized intraoperatively an elective temporary tracheostomy may prevent the need for an emergency tracheostomy for airway obstruction during the postoperative period.

- Haemorrhage deep to the strap muscles compresses, and finally occludes, the airway. Treatment consists of opening the wound to drain the haematoma and relieve the pressure. There is frequently some warning of this impending disaster, and the patient can be returned to the operating theatre for urgent intervention. When warning signs have been ignored, an acute emergency may present for which restoration of the airway in an unconscious anoxic patient must be achieved immediately. Sutures in the skin, platysma and strap muscle are cut at the bedside, the clot is evacuated, and the patient then returned to theatre for re-suturing of the wound. Clip removers should always be readily available at the patient's bedside for this emergency, if clips have been used for skin closure.

Biochemical complications

Early and late disturbances in thyroid and parathyroid endocrine balance are common:

- A *thyroid crisis* can occur postoperatively in a patient whose thyrotoxicosis was inadequately controlled preoperatively. Management is medical, with sedation and beta blockade. Preoperative control of thyrotoxicosis is therefore very important before surgery.

- *Hypothyroidism* is inevitable after a total thyroidectomy, and replacement thyroxin should be commenced. Hypothyroidism does not, however, pose problems in the immediate postoperative period, and replacement therapy should be delayed initially if thyroidectomy is undertaken for differentiated thyroid cancer, as postoperative radioactive iodine scanning is facilitated by thyroid stimulating hormone (TSH) stimulation. Many patients who have undergone subtotal thyroidectomy will eventually develop hypothyroidism.

- *Hypocalcaemia* is the manifestation of insufficient parathormone secretion. Parathyroid glands may have been excised, or rendered ischaemic by surgery. Presentation with tetany should be avoidable, as postoperative assessment of serum calcium is mandatory after thyroid and parathyroid surgery. This allows calcium, and if necessary 1,25-dihydroxycholecalciferol, support to be given should hypocalcaemia develop. Spontaneous recovery of parathyroid function is common.

THE SALIVARY GLANDS

Surgery of the parotid and submandibular glands requires a detailed understanding of the anatomy.

The parotid gland

Any surgery on the parotid gland risks injury to the facial nerve. The surgeon who operates infrequently in this area is more likely to injure the nerve, and for this reason a parotidectomy is now seldom undertaken by a generalist, who instead will refer a patient to a surgical colleague with a special interest in parotid surgery.

SURGICAL ANATOMY

The parotid gland lies in the space behind the mandible, below the external ear, in front of the mastoid process, and extends forwards on the lateral surface of the masseter. It overlies the posterior belly of digastric below, and deeply it is applied to the styloid process and its muscles. It is enclosed in a sheath which is derived from the deep cervical fascia, and which sends processes into the gland to divide it into lobules. The *upper pole* of the gland lies just below the zygomatic arch, and is wedged between the meatus and the mandibular joint. The superficial temporal vessels, temporal branches of the facial nerve, and the auriculo-temporal nerve are found entering or leaving the gland near the upper pole. The marginal mandibular and cervical branches of the facial nerve, and the two divisions of the retromandibular vein emerge from the *lower pole*. From the *anterior border* emerge the zygomatic and buccal branches of the facial nerve and, on a deeper plane, the parotid duct.

The *external carotid artery* ascends through the deep part of the gland. It terminates behind the neck of the mandible, by dividing into maxillary and superficial temporal arteries.

The *facial nerve*, after emerging from the stylomastoid foramen, almost immediately enters the posteromedial surface of the gland and after about 2 cm splits into two main subdivisions from which the terminal branches arise. The *retromandibular vein* forms within the substance of the gland by the union of the superficial temporal and maxillary veins, and it emerges from the lower pole usually as two trunks. The anatomy is remarkably consistent, with the nerve and its branches lying just superficial to the veins (Fig. 9.13). The *faciovenous plane,* in which the veins and the branches of the facial nerve lie, arbitrarily divides the gland into a superficial and a deep part. It was the appreciation of this anatomy that allowed surgery on the parotid with preservation of the facial nerve.[9]

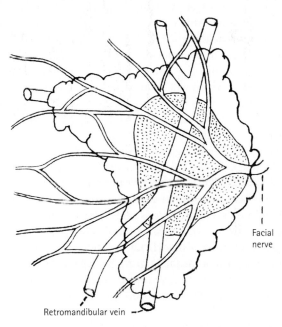

Figure 9.13   *The faciovenous plane as described by Patey. The retromandibular vein traverses the gland in a vertical direction, while the facial nerve trunk enters posteriorly and its branches fan out to leave the gland superiorly, anteriorly and inferiorly.*

DRAINAGE OF A SUPPURATIVE PAROTITIS

This was discussed earlier in this chapter.

REMOVAL OF A PAROTID DUCT CALCULUS

A calculus impacted in the duct, and obstructing the gland, is easily palpable from within the mouth. A temporary suture is placed around the duct, proximal and distal to the stone to prevent displacement, and a small incision is made directly over the stone to deliver the calculus as shown in Figure 9.16, for a submandibular calculus. After removal of the stone, no suture is required to close the opening in the duct. The buccal branch of the facial nerve accompanies the proximal segment of the parotid duct, and can be damaged during the removal of a calculus.

SUPERFICIAL PAROTIDECTOMY

This is most commonly undertaken for a lump within the gland. Fine-needle aspiration often indicates what the tumour is, but prior to the excision the malignant potential of the lump is not always known. Adenolymphomata are benign. Pleomorphic adenomas are locally recurrent if excision has been incomplete. One of the rarer salivary gland carcinomas may be suspected preoperatively if growth is rapid, or if there is any loss of facial nerve function. However, the majority of malignant parotid tumours do not present with abnormalities of facial nerve function. Pain is also an ominous feature, but can occur in benign disease from haemorrhage into a cystic space.

A nerve monitor, if available, is placed before the initial incision is made as this will warn the surgeon when the dissection is approaching the facial nerve. The anaesthetist must keep the patient non-paralysed for the device to be effective. The incision should give good access, with well-vascularized flaps and a scar which will lie inconspicuously in skin creases. A suitable incision is shown in Figure 9.14. It is deepened through the platysma until the surface of the parotid fascia is reached, and the anterior skin and platysma flap is elevated to expose the parotid gland with its covering fascia. Care must be taken to avoid injury to the branches of the facial nerve emerging from the anterior border of the gland. Some surgeons dissect above the platysma to avoid injury to the terminal branches, but there is said to be a higher incidence of Frey's syndrome with a flap superficial to platysma.

The dissection in a superficial parotidectomy is based on the identification of the facial nerve before it enters the gland and, by following the nerve and its branches, removing all tissue superficial to this faciovenous plane. The inferior pole

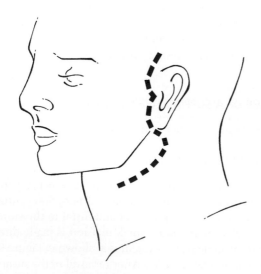

Figure 9.14 *A suitable incision for parotid surgery.*

of the parotid is lifted off the surface of the sternocleidomastoid muscle. The greater auricular nerve is found crossing the lateral surface of sternocleidomastoid, and is divided close to the gland. Sternocleidomastoid is then retracted posteriorly and the posterior belly of digastric identified. This is followed up to the mastoid process. The dissection is then carried deeply along the perichondrium of the tragal cartilage, and parotid tissue is separated from it. The cartilage ends in a 'pointer' which points to the facial nerve, 1 cm medially and inferiorly (Fig. 9.15a). A bridge of parotid tissue, overlying the facial nerve, lies between this pointer and the digastric muscle. This can now be elevated to expose the nerve which is very deep at this point.

Once the nerve has been identified it is followed forwards into the gland. It runs rapidly towards the surface, and account has to be taken of this obliquity during dissection. After about 2 cm it divides into upper and lower divisions. The upper division, and its branches, are dissected first. Fine artery forceps are inserted along the superficial surface of the nerve and the glandular tissue lifted forwards to display fine strands of tissue, between the nerve and gland, which are cut with scissors. The branches of the upper division are followed until they emerge from the gland. Between each branch of the nerve there will be a bridge of parotid tissue, passing between the superficial and deep portions of the gland, which must be divided (Fig. 9.15b). No major vessels should be encountered, but ligations of small vessels will be required – especially as diathermy dissection is dangerous in the proximity of the nerve. However, bipolar diathermy to individual small vessels is probably safe. A similar dissection is then performed along the lower division of the facial nerve and its subdivisions. The superficial part of the gland can now be removed leaving the deep portion of the gland, and the parotid duct, *in situ*.

As tumours are commonly in the superficial part of the gland, they can be removed by a superficial parotidectomy. However, the deep aspect of a tumour may be exposed by this dissection and great care must be taken to avoid breaching it. Occasionally a tumour extends deep to the faciovenous plane in the tissue bridge between the branches of the nerve. It is usually possible to retract the nerves with slings and excise the tumour intact without sacrificing nerves. A malignant tumour may invade nerve, and one or more of the branches may have to be sacrificed.

At the end of the dissection, the facial nerve and its branches lie exposed on the surface of the residual gland (Fig. 9.15c). From the upper division, there should be a temporal branch to the forehead and zygomatic branches, frequently two which cross the zygoma to the corner of the eye, and a large buccal branch which runs parallel to the duct and supplies the lower eyelid, nose and upper lip; an additional smaller buccal branch is often seen below the duct. From the lower division, there should be branches to the corner of the mouth and lower lip, and to the platysma. If all these branches have been identified and are anatomically intact the surgeon can be relatively reassured that any immediate post-

a

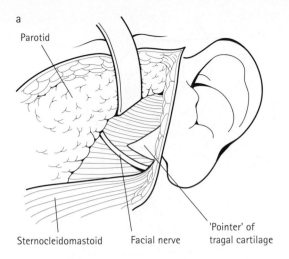

Parotid

Sternocleidomastoid   Facial nerve   'Pointer' of tragal cartilage

b

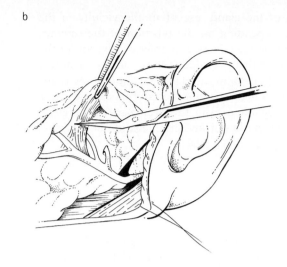

c

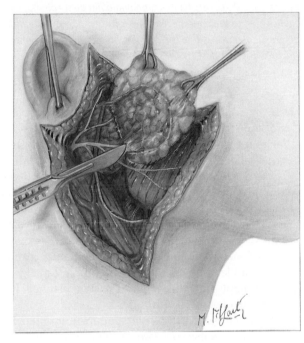

Figure 9.15 *Superficial* left *parotidectomy. (a) The facial nerve is identified by deep dissection on the surface of the tragal cartilage. (b) The superficial parotid tissue is lifted forwards and the tissue bridges, passing between branches of the facial nerve to the deep portion of the gland, are divided. (c) The facial nerve and its branches exposed at the end of a right superficial parotidectomy. (From an original drawing in the 1954 edition by Margaret McLarty, a founder member of the Medical Artists Association of Great Britain.)*

operative paralysis is no more than a neuropraxia and will recover, often within 48 hours but may persist longer. A severed nerve can be sutured, or if a portion has been excised, a nerve graft is a possibility, using the greater auricular or sural nerve. These techniques are discussed further in Chapter 3. A nerve stimulator, used at the end of the dissection, can demonstrate that the nerve is functionally, as well as anatomically, intact. The wound is closed over a suction drain with separate closure of the platysma and the skin.

TOTAL PAROTIDECTOMY

A total parotidectomy with sacrifice of the facial nerve may be unavoidable in the excision of a malignant parotid tumour which has extensively invaded the nerve. A facial nerve paralysis is inevitable, but a facial nerve graft – with the greater auricular nerve used to bridge the defect and sutured

using the operating microscope – offers the potential for some functional recovery, once regrowth of axons has occurred. In most instances it is possible to save some of the facial nerve branches, and only sacrifice those that are directly invaded, especially as no survival benefit has been shown for a pre-emptive radical parotidectomy with the sacrifice of uninvolved branches of the facial nerve. Sometimes, a total parotidectomy is combined with excision of the temporomandibular joint, the mastoid process, the external meatus and overlying soft tissue for a locally aggressive malignant tumour. Unfortunately, such radical surgery is disfiguring and seldom curative.

A total parotidectomy, with preservation of the facial nerve, is occasionally an appropriate operation for a tumour lying wholly, or partially, in the deep portion of the gland. The initial dissection is similar to that for a partial parotidectomy. The plane is developed between the superficial and deep portions of the gland, except in the vicinity of the tumour. Then, depending on the position of the tumour, retraction of either the superior or inferior division of the nerve off the underlying tumour allows access to dissect around the deep portion of the gland. Ligation of the retro-mandibular vein is necessary but the external carotid artery can usually be separated from the deep part of the gland unless there is direct tumour invasion. Ligation of the external carotid artery has no sequelae.

The submandibular gland

SURGICAL ANATOMY

The submandibular gland is situated partly below the mandible and partly deep to it. The body of the gland overlaps both bellies of digastric inferiorly. It is enclosed in a loose sheath of deep cervical fascia. The *inferolateral surface* is covered only by platysma and cervical fascia. The *medial surface* lies on, from before backwards, mylohyoid, hyoglossus and the pharyngeal wall. Between the gland and the hyoglossus are the lingual nerve, the submandibular ganglion and the hypoglossal nerve. The *deep part of the gland* is a prolongation extending from its medial surface, and lying under cover of mylohyoid. It lies alongside the *submandibular duct,* which also arises from the medial surface of the gland. The duct opens into the mouth on the sublingual papilla at the side of the frenulum of the tongue. The *facial artery* ascends in a deep groove medial to the posterior end of the gland, and then turns downwards and laterally between the gland and the mandible to enter the face at the anterior border of masseter. The facial vein descends on the infero-lateral surface of the gland.

REMOVAL OF A SUBMANDIBULAR DUCT CALCULUS

A calculus in the duct is palpable intra-orally and can be removed very simply under local anaesthesia. Two temporary stay sutures should, however, be placed around the duct on either side of the calculus and retracted upwards. This prevents displacement of the calculus back into the gland (Fig. 9.16). The thickened duct is then incised longitudinally over the calculus, which extrudes into the mouth. No attempt to suture the duct is necessary. If the stone is very far back in the duct, then it is usually safer to remove the gland, as attempts at per-oral removal of a posterior calculus risk damage to the lingual nerve.

SUBMANDIBULAR GLAND EXCISION

This is advised when the gland is chronically inflamed, or is the site of repeated stone formation. It is also a suitable operation for a pleomorphic adenoma. Tumours arising within the submandibular gland are less common than in the parotid, but are more likely to be frankly malignant. Excision for a malignant submandibular salivary tumour may require to be combined with a selective neck dissection, in which

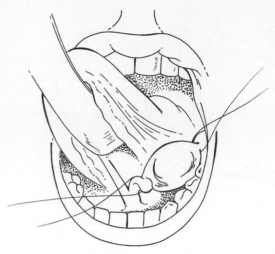

Figure 9.16 *Removal of a left submandibular duct calculus. The tongue is held to the opposite side and a suture placed around the duct, proximal and distal to the calculus, to prevent displacement. An incision is made directly over the calculus.*

there is the additional removal of the digastric muscle and the associated fat and lymph nodes up to the mastoid process and including the tail of the parotid (see also Radical neck dissections above).

Secondary carcinoma of the submandibular lymph nodes is commonly encountered, and may initially be mistaken for a primary salivary gland tumour. Many of these nodes are inseparable from the gland and, if excision is planned, the gland must be removed en bloc. However, the correct management of metastatic malignant submandibular glands is that of the underlying pathology. The primary malignancy must be sought and an en bloc excision planned if the tumour is still operable.

A submandibular gland excision commences with a horizontal skin crease incision, two finger breadths below the ramus of the mandible, and the incision is deepened down to the body of the gland. A superior flap, consisting of skin, platysma and the investing fascia of the gland, is then raised up to the ramus of the mandible, and retracted to expose the whole superficial surface of the gland. The aim is to avoid damaging the marginal mandibular branch of the facial nerve which lies between the platysma and the fascia, 2 cm below the ramus of the mandible. It is easily injured if a more superficial upper flap is raised. In a submandibular gland excision for a pleomorphic adenoma, an extracapsular, rather than the subcapsular dissection described above, is recommended.

The facial vein crosses superficial to the gland and is ligated and divided. Although the facial artery can be dissected out of its groove on the deep surface of the gland, it is simpler to divide and ligate it above and below. It is divided first at the upper border of the gland as it emerges from behind the posterior pole. The gland can now be dissected off the ramus of the mandible and the submental vessels are secured. The anterior part of the gland is then dissected backwards off the surfaces of the anterior belly of digastric and the mylohyoid muscles. The posterior border of mylohyoid is identified and retracted anteriorly to display the deep part of the gland and its duct. Infero-posterior retraction of the partially mobilized gland will pull the lingual nerve down in a U-shape where it is attached to the gland by the submandibular ganglion (Fig. 9.17a). This attachment, and the accompanying small vessels, require ligation and division. The hypoglossal nerve may be visible inferiorly (Fig. 9.17b), but it is often lying in a slightly deeper plane, protected from the operating field. An absorbable suture is used for ligation of the duct which is divided as far anteriorly as possible to ensure removal of any small calculi dislodged into the duct. A small bridge of salivary gland tissue may have to be transected at this point if the

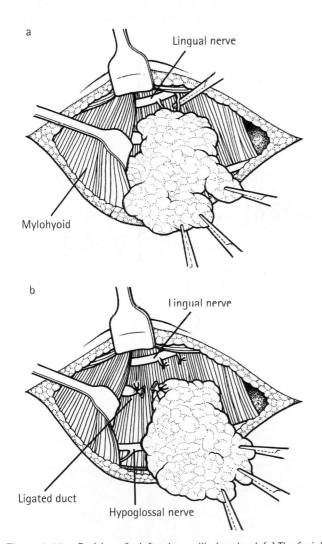

Figure 9.17 *Excision of a left submandibular gland. (a) The facial artery has been divided above the gland and the superficial portion of the gland has been dissected off mylohyoid which is now retracted forwards. The tented lingual nerve is visible. (b) The attachments to the lingual nerve have been divided, and the submandibular duct is ligated. The hypoglossal nerve is visible inferiorly.*

sublingual gland is continuous with the submandibular gland. The only attachment now is the facial artery which is ligated and divided for the second time at the lower border of the posterior pole. A short segment of artery is thus removed with the gland, and although this is not always necessary, it makes the dissection easier. A small suction drain to the bed of the gland is brought out posteriorly, and the wound closed with sutures to the platysma followed by skin closure.

SURGERY OF THE LARYNX, PHARYNX AND TRACHEA

Only the general surgeon who is unable to refer patients will expect to operate on these structures, all of which lie within the province of the ENT specialist.

Tracheostomy

This was once a common operation for life-threatening obstruction of the upper airway. The situation is now usually more satisfactorily managed by emergency endotracheal intubation, and it is only in exceptional circumstances that endotracheal intubation is impossible. Endotracheal intubation is the standard method for control of a patient's airway, and is used both for the patient who is deeply unconscious with no gag reflex to protect the lower airway, and for the patient requiring ventilatory support. Long-term intubation of the larynx is damaging however, and a decision regarding the need to convert to a tracheostomy should usually be made if the patient cannot be extubated within 2 weeks. This conversion to a tracheostomy is now commonly performed percutaneously in the intensive care unit by anaesthetists using specially designed kits. Most other tracheostomies are fashioned by ENT or faciomaxillary surgeons at the completion of a major resection. It is therefore now rare for a general surgeon working in a hospital with ENT surgeons, and a well-developed anaesthetic service, to undertake a tracheostomy either electively or in an emergency.

ANAESTHESIA

Ideal operative conditions include a general anaesthetic with the airway secured with an endotracheal tube. However, when a general surgeon has to perform a tracheostomy it will almost always be in an emergency in suboptimal conditions, on an unanaesthetized patient with no airway protection. In the unconscious, deeply cyanosed patient no anaesthesia is needed, and no further delay is justified. In the conscious distressed patient with partial airway obstruction, lignocaine with adrenaline is infiltrated deep to the proposed skin incision. In the developing world, the commonest scenario is a distressed baby or toddler with increasing airway obstruction from diphtheria, and no skilled anaesthetic personnel or facilities available. Secure restraint of the child is mandatory.

The child is wrapped in a sheet so that the arms are held firmly, and one assistant holds the child's body. A second assistant holds the child's head, comforts the child, maintains oxygen delivery and aspirates secretions from the upper airway.

OPERATIVE PROCEDURE

A transverse incision midway between the cricoid cartilage and the suprasternal notch is deepened through platysma (Fig. 9.18a). In an emergency a vertical incision is acceptable. The strap muscles are separated in the midline and the trachea palpated, with the overlying thyroid isthmus, under the cervical fascia. The thyroid isthmus is freed from the trachea, divided between clamps, and the ends oversewn with an absorbable suture (Fig. 9.18b). Inferior thyroid veins may cross the operative field, and require ligation and division. The cricoid and upper tracheal rings are now easily identified.

The inexperienced operator will tend to drift cranially as, in the adult, the trachea becomes progressively deeper as it is traced distally and, in the child, the innominate vein and the thymus may lie anterior to the trachea above the suprasternal notch. In addition, the apical pleura and the obstructed lungs will bulge up into the wound. It is important, however, that the tracheostomy is made at the level of the second to fourth tracheal ring as a more proximal tracheostomy damages the cricoid cartilage, and a sub-glottic stenosis may follow. The damage may be direct mechanical damage from a tracheostomy performed through the cricoid cartilage itself, but the cricoid can also be damaged by a perichondritis from an adjacent tracheostomy through the first tracheal ring.

A vertical midline incision in the trachea will allow insertion of the tube in a child or young adult. This is the technique least likely to cause a tracheal stenosis, or a failure of closure of a temporary tracheostomy. However, in an older

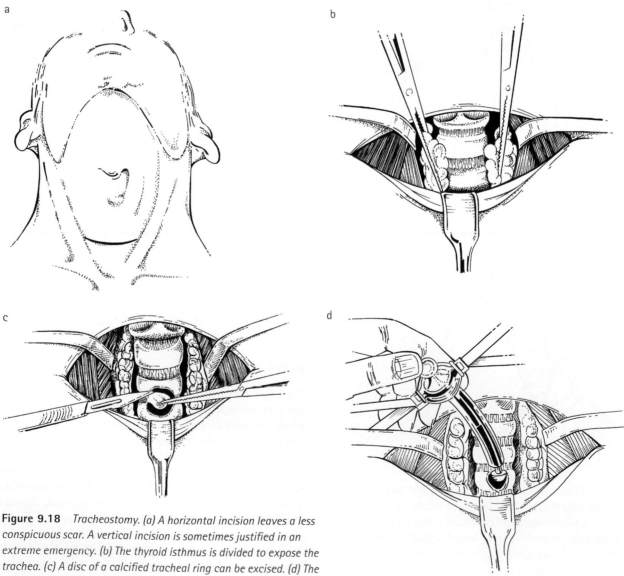

Figure 9.18 *Tracheostomy. (a) A horizontal incision leaves a less conspicuous scar. A vertical incision is sometimes justified in an extreme emergency. (b) The thyroid isthmus is divided to expose the trachea. (c) A disc of a calcified tracheal ring can be excised. (d) The tracheotomy tube is inserted.*

patient with calcification of the trachea, it is usually more satisfactory to remove a small disc of the second, or preferably the third ring (Fig. 9.18c). At this point the anaesthetist is advised to withdraw the endotracheal tube (if the procedure is being performed under general anaesthesia). Blood is aspirated from the trachea, the tracheostomy tube is inserted, and the wound closed (Fig. 9.18d). This should only be a loose closure or surgical emphysema may be troublesome. This initial tube should be sewn and taped in place as, if it becomes displaced, replacement in the first 72 hours before a track has been established is difficult.

Percutaneous tracheostomy

This is performed through an initial small skin incision. A needle with cannula is introduced into the trachea, the needle removed and a guide wire inserted through the cannula which is in turn withdrawn. After the track has been dilated by forceps, or by serial plastic dilators passed over the guide wire, the tracheostomy tube is inserted.

Branchial cysts and fistulae

These are congenital abnormalities associated with the failure of obliteration of branchial clefts. A branchial cyst presents most often in late childhood, or early adult life, as a deep cystic swelling at the anterior border of the sternocleidomastoid, between its upper one-third and lower two-thirds. A branchial fistula is apparent at birth, as an external opening near the anterior border of sternocleidomastoid, close to its distal insertion. The internal opening is in the tonsillar fossa.

A skin crease incision over a branchial cyst affords adequate access for its excision (Fig. 9.19a). The incision through skin and platysma should be at least 2 cm below the angle of the jaw in order to avoid the marginal mandibular branch of the facial nerve. The deep cervical fascia is incised along the anterior border of sternocleidomastoid. The cyst can then be carefully enucleated, but a search should be made for a deep extension. If present, this track will pass between the internal and external carotid arteries to the pharynx in the region of the tonsillar fossa, and must be excised (Fig. 9.19c).

A branchial fistula will frequently require two incisions as the first elliptical incision to excise the external opening will be too low for higher access (Fig. 9.19b). The track is often incomplete and ends blindly, but again the surgeon must be prepared to follow the track between the carotids if necessary. Branchial cyst and fistula surgery should not, therefore, be approached lightly by a surgeon operating infrequently in the neck.

Pharyngeal pouch

The common variety is an acquired posterior diverticulum between thyro- and crico-pharyngeus, in which food

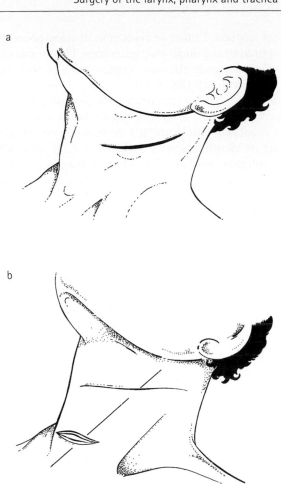

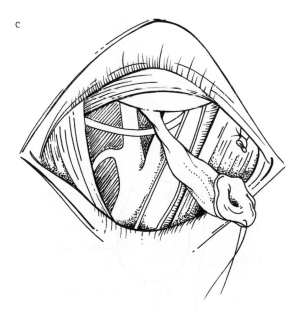

Figure 9.19 *Branchial cyst and fistula. (a) A single incision over a cyst is usually adequate. (b) The opening of a branchial fistula has been circumscribed by an elliptical incision, and the dissection of the fistula is commenced through this incision. Access for the proximal dissection will be inadequate, and a second higher incision as marked will be necessary. (c) The fistula track passes between the carotid arteries to the tonsillar fossa.*

becomes trapped. Failure of relaxation of crico-pharyngeus is thought to be the underlying pathology. The fundus of the pouch lies alongside the oesophagus which is then compressed by the pouch (Fig. 9.20).

Endoscopic stapling procedures are increasingly popular in expert hands but, if an open technique is required, the pouch is packed with gauze at a preliminary endoscopy to facilitate its identification. A standard cervical approach to the oesophagus (see below) brings the dissection onto the gauze-filled pouch lying behind the oesophagus, from which it must be separated. The plane around the fundus of the pouch is then followed up to its neck and the neck opened. A finger is inserted through the neck of the sac down into the oesophagus, putting the cricopharyngeus on stretch. A posterior vertical 4-cm myotomy of this muscle is then performed. The recurrent laryngeal nerves lie laterally and should not be endangered if the myotomy is performed in the midline posteriorly. The pharyngeal wall at the neck of the sac is closed, and a drain is placed adjacent to the closure.

Surgery for malignancy of the larynx, pharynx and trachea

Much of the radical surgery for cancers of the larynx and hypopharynx has now been centralized in specialist units. Close cooperation is essential between surgeon, radio-

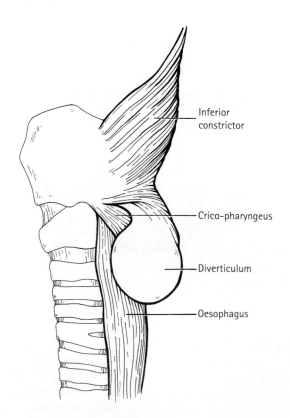

Figure 9.20   *The neck of a pharyngeal pouch is just above the crico-pharyngeus, but the fundus compresses the upper oesophagus.*

Inferior constrictor

Crico-pharyngeus

Diverticulum

Oesophagus

therapist and oncologist to plan the optimum treatment. Accurate preoperative staging is important. Radical mutilating surgery is justified if it offers the best chance of cure, or of local control of the disease, but must not be undertaken when it can achieve neither and will merely add to the patient's distress. Postoperatively, the patient will need skilled rehabilitation and speech therapy. Regional centres specializing in this work will achieve better results, and most general ENT surgeons in the UK are no longer performing the occasional major resection for cancer.[10] This work is now totally outside the field of the general surgeon. An isolated general surgeon in a developing country without access to referral facilities is unlikely to be in a position to undertake such an operation, and is even less likely to be able to offer the patient a reasonable expectation of a cure with good rehabilitation.

General surgeons should, however, be aware of the principles of these resections, if only to understand what has been done in the neck of a patient who is subsequently admitted under their care with related or unrelated neck pathology.

LARYNGECTOMY

A horizontal incision is made through skin and platysma. The subsequent dissection will depend on whether the laryngectomy is to be combined with a radical neck dissection. The thyroid lobe on the side of the tumour is commonly removed with the larynx, and the strap muscles on this side are divided at their lower end, and excised as part of the specimen. Thus, the larynx is mobilized laterally by a hemithyroidectomy dissection on one side, and through the plane between the thyroid gland and the trachea on the other. Posteriorly, it must be separated from the oesophagus. Inferiorly, the trachea is transected, and the distal end mobilized so that it can be brought out as an end tracheotomy which is sutured to the skin. Superiorly, the suprahyoid muscles and the stylohyoid ligaments are divided and the hyoid bone is removed with the specimen. Removal of the larynx then leaves an anterior defect in the pharynx which is closed. Various forms of partial laryngectomy with preservation of speech have also been developed.

LARYNGOPHARYNGECTOMY

This more extensive resection is usually performed through an apron or transverse incision. One or both lobes of the thyroid are often included in the specimen, and the resection is commonly combined with a radical cervical lymph node dissection. The tracheostomy is established early in the procedure. The initial dissection is similar to that for a laryngectomy, but laterally the dissection is carried posteriorly, down to the prevertebral fascia, and the pharynx is drawn forwards as part of the resection specimen. Superiorly the resection is above the hyoid, and the base of the tongue is transected leaving a hole into the oral cavity. When the operation is combined with an oesophagectomy, reconstruction is usually with the mobilized stomach or, if this is not possible, with the colon. If the thoracic and distal cervical oesophagus are to be retained, with only the proximal cervical oesophagus included in the resected specimen, a free jejunal flap can be utilized as an alternative for reconstruction. This involves a microvascular anastomosis of the mesenteric pedicle of the free jejunal flap onto the recipient vessels in the neck, and anastomosis of the jejunal tube proximally and distally to bridge the gap from the pharyngeal resection. If microsurgical skill is not available, then a tubularized pectoralis major flap can be used. This flap is a myocutaneous flap with a good blood supply and is illustrated in Figure 10.12, page 188. It has replaced the earlier deltopectoral flap for such reconstructions.

SURGERY OF THE OESOPHAGUS

Surgery of the oesophagus is covered in greater detail in Chapters 16 and 17, which relate to the upper gastrointestinal tract. However, the approach to the cervical oesophagus is described below. Direct surgical access may occasionally be required for an impacted foreign body which cannot be removed endoscopically or, rarely for the repair of trauma which is too severe to be managed conservatively. A pharyngeal pouch lies adjacent to the cervical oesophagus and the same approach is used in that operation.

A cervical oesophageal anastomosis after oesophagectomy is a safer anastomosis if it leaks than one within the thorax, and therefore a more radical oesophagectomy is sometimes preferred in order to bring the anastomosis up into the neck. On other occasions a more proximal tumour itself necessitates a cervical anastomosis.

Oesophagostomy is a permanent or temporary end stoma of the oesophagus. It has a place in a complete oesophageal obstruction, where saliva will pool above the obstruction with threat to the airway, or lead to continual dribbling. A greater role, however, is in those patients who have had a major failure of an oesophageal reconstruction after a resection. In addition to the drainage of the posterior mediastinal sepsis, such patients require an oesophagostomy to divert saliva from the area, and a feeding gastrostomy. A further reconstruction can then be postponed until local conditions in the mediastinum have improved and the patient has recovered good physiological and nutritional status.

An oesophagostomy can also be a temporary solution in a long-segment oesophageal atresia which cannot be reconstructed in the neonatal period. It prevents saliva from entering the bronchial tree and also allows the baby to develop feeding skills while gaining weight on gastrostomy feeding, prior to major reconstructive surgery (see Chapter 17).

THE CERVICAL APPROACH TO THE OESOPHAGUS

A transverse skin crease incision at the anterior border of sternocleidomastoid is made through skin and platysma. The height of this incision will vary according to the level of oesophagus to which access is required, but the level of the cricoid cartilage is most often appropriate. The deep cervical fascia is then incised along the anterior border of sternocleidomastoid, which is retracted laterally. The thyroid is retracted medially and the middle thyroid veins are divided. The carotid sheath is retracted laterally and the inferior thyroid artery ligated and divided. This plane between the thyroid and the carotid sheath takes the surgeon down to the pre-vertebral fascia, and the dissection should be safely lateral to the recurrent laryngeal nerve. The nerve is, however, still in danger in its groove between the trachea and oesophagus, as the oesophagus is mobilized. It is, therefore, safest to identify the recurrent laryngeal nerve as it crosses the medial end of the inferior thyroid artery. Once identified, it can then be followed both up and down.

SURGERY OF THE CAROTID ARTERIES

Carotid trauma is discussed in the trauma section at the beginning of this chapter, but exposure of the carotid vessels and all carotid surgery is covered in Chapters 5 and 6.

ANTERIOR APPROACH TO THE CERVICAL SPINE

The vertebral bodies of the cervical column can be approached anteriorly by using the same dissection as that described above for the oesophagus.

ANTERIOR APPROACH FOR SYMPATHECTOMY

In the past, this was used as a standard approach but has now been generally superseded by minimal access intra-thoracic techniques. The indications for surgery and the extent of ablation of the sympathetic chain are discussed in Chapter 3, page 47.

The cervical approach to the sympathetic chain is initially the exposure of the proximal subclavian artery, as described in Chapter 5, page 90. A transverse incision above the medial third of the clavicle is deepened through platysma, the lateral fibres of sternocleidomastoid are divided, and the external jugular vein ligated and divided. Scalenus anterior is identified as it crosses the operative field to its insertion into the first rib. The phrenic nerve on its anterior surface is retracted and preserved, and the muscle is divided to expose the subclavian artery. The artery can either be depressed downwards, or gently mobilized and retracted upwards by means of a tape passed around it. The supra-pleural membrane is detached from the inner border of the first rib, and the pleura is displaced downwards and laterally to expose the neck of the ribs with the sympathetic chain and ganglia.

THORACIC OUTLET OBSTRUCTION AND CERVICAL RIB SURGERY

Both axillary and cervical approaches can be used for decompression, and the appropriate surgery is discussed in Chapter 6.

REFERENCES

1. Ngakane H, Muckart DJJ, Luvuno FM. Penetrating visceral injuries of the neck: results of a conservative management policy. *Br J Surg* 1990; **77**: 908–10.
2. Lindberg R. Distribution of cervical lymph node metastases from squamous cell carcinoma of the upper respiratory and digestive tracts. *Cancer* 1972; **29**: 1446–9.
3. Crile G. Excision of cancer of the head and neck. *JAMA* 1906; **47**: 1780–6.
4. Kuriakose MA, Hicks WL, Loree TR, *et al.* Risk group-based management of differentiated thyroid carcinoma. *J R Coll Surg Edinb* 2001; **46**: 216–23.
5. *Guidelines for the Management of Thyroid Cancer in Adults*. British Thyroid Association & Royal College of Physicians of London, March 2002.
6. Sivanandan R, Soo KC. Pattern of cervical lymph node metastases from papillary carcinoma of the thyroid. *Br J Surg* 2001; **88**: 1241–4.
7. Moley JF, DeBenedetti MK. Patterns of nodal metastases in palpable medullary thyroid carcinoma: recommendations for extent of node dissection. *Ann Surg* 1999; **229**: 880–7.
8. Rothmund M. A parathyroid adenoma cannot be found during neck exploration of a patient with presumed primary hyperparathyroidism. Clinical dilemma series. *Br J Surg* 1999; **86**: 725–6.
9. Patey DH, Ranger I. Some points in the surgical anatomy of the parotid gland. *Br J Surg* 1957; **45**: 250–8.
10. *Stell and Maran's Head and Neck Surgery*, 4th edn. PM Stell, AGD Maran, J Watkinson (eds). London: Hodder and Stoughton, 2000.

SURGERY OF THE FACE AND JAWS

In the developed world a general surgeon will perform only relatively minor surgery on the face. Facial lacerations will require suturing, and skin lesions will be excised for histology. More major surgery in this area will be passed on to the relevant specialist. Plastic surgeons and ophthalmologists overlap their skills around the orbit. Faciomaxillary, ENT and plastic surgeons frequently work together in the reconstruction required for either a congenital abnormality, or following tissue loss from trauma or the excision of a malignancy. However, some general surgeons will be forced to offer limited surgical services across all these specialities.

WOUNDS

The chief aim in the treatment of all facial wounds is to reduce disfigurement to a minimum. The principles of surgery on the skin are discussed in Chapter 1, and these are of particular importance in the face where a good cosmetic result is so important. Most cases of extensive injury will require the attention of a plastic surgeon who should, if possible, carry out the initial repair. However, if specialist help is not available it is the responsibility of the surgeon carrying out the initial repair to do nothing which will make later reconstruction more difficult. The main concern should be to avoid unnecessary scar formation by careful cleansing of the wound, debridement and accurate repair of the tissues in layers with fine sutures.[1]

Exploration and debridement of the wound

Because of the extensive vascularity of the face, primary suture is usually a safe procedure, even for injuries such as dog bites. Appropriate tetanus and antibiotic prophylaxis should be given for contaminated wounds. Irregular lacerated wounds should be trimmed with a sharp knife or fine scissors. Formal excision of a wound is usually unnecessary, and can result in unjustifiable sacrifice of healthy tissue. It is important, however, to remove all ingrained dirt as only in this way can one avoid leaving disfiguring pigmented scars which are difficult to remove adequately later. Scrubbing with a brush under general anaesthetic may be the only way of doing this effectively, especially for a large area of superficial abrasion with a 'gravel rash'.

Wounds involving deeper structures

Divided facial muscles should be approximated before skin closure. In the case of a wound involving the whole thickness of the lip or cheek, the mucous membrane, muscles and skin should be sutured separately. The mucous membrane is sutured first. In wounds of the eyelid, the tarsal plate must be identified and sutured to reduce the risk of distorting the margins of the eyelids. Careful attention must be paid to the possibility of damage to the canthal ligament and the naso-lacrimal ducts in wounds near the inner canthus, and expert help should be sought if injury to these structures cannot be excluded. Vision in the underlying eye must be checked, and the possibility of a penetrating injury to the eyeball, or into the orbit or cranium, must also be considered.

Damage to the nasolacrimal and parotid ducts, and to branches of the facial nerve, should be suspected in any laceration of the cheek which crosses the path of these structures. The surgeon should be alerted to damage to branches of the facial nerve by partial paralysis of the facial muscles, but this may be difficult to detect when there is significant swelling. Divided branches distal to a perpendicular line drawn down from the lateral canthus rarely need reapproximation as the stump of the nerve tends to re-innervate directly the muscles of facial expression. When a laceration overlies the course of the parotid duct, damage should be actively sought by massaging the parotid gland, and looking for salivary seepage in the wound. If any of these fine structures requires repair, this should ideally be undertaken at the initial operation by someone who is experienced in the use of an operating microscope. It may be impossible to identify and repair fine and complex structures at a secondary operation, and the importance of early involvement of the relevant specialist cannot be over-stressed.

Wounds with skin loss

Since the facial skin is so elastic, skin loss is often more apparent than real, with the wound gaping in a frightening manner due to muscle retraction and oedema. Often it will be found at operation that there is little or no tissue missing once the 'jigsaw puzzle' has been completed. When there is significant tissue loss, skilled reconstruction will be required and plastic surgical expertise should be sought at the primary repair. However, flap repairs should not, in general, be attempted as a primary procedure in a recent facial injury. A full-thickness graft can be applied if conditions are suitable, and even a temporary thin partial-thickness skin graft over a denuded area will reduce contractural scarring. Skin graft 'take' onto denuded bone can be successful if the outer cortical plate of the bone is first perforated. When the whole thickness of the lip, cheek or nose is missing, skin should be united to mucous membrane around the margins of the defect. The elimination of a raw area allows rapid healing with minimal distortion and scarring, and thus facilitates definitive reconstruction.

Skin sutures

Accurate apposition without tension is important, and particular care must be taken at the vermilion border of the lip otherwise an ugly step will be apparent. Fine needles and fine suture material which excite minimal tissue reaction should be used. A 5/0 or 6/0 Prolene is suitable for an interrupted suture, and a 4/0 or 5/0 Prolene for a subcuticular suture. Interrupted sutures should be positioned close to the skin edges to reduce scarring, but they should also approximate the underlying fat (Fig. 10.1) and thus avoid the necessity for additional subcutaneous sutures, which inevitably cause further tissue reaction. If a subcutaneous suture is necessary, it

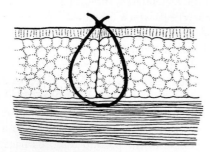

Figure 10.1 *Accurate apposition of skin and subcutaneous fat without tension minimizes scarring. The sutures are placed close to the skin edges.*

should not be closer than 5 mm from the skin. Over-tightening of sutures must be avoided as tissue is strangulated. Interrupted sutures should ideally be removed after 3–5 days to prevent additional scarring from the sutures. The wound, however, should be supported for a further 5–10 days with strips of adhesive skin tape (see Chapter 1).

FRACTURES OF THE FACIAL SKELETON AND THE JAWS

The treatment of these fractures is often complex,[2] and will only be undertaken by general surgeons if they are working in remote areas without access to faciomaxillary expertise.

Fractures of the mandible

Some minor undisplaced fractures only require analgesia, without any fixation. However, in a bilateral fracture, the downward displacement of the anterior fragment may be considerable from the combined forces of gravity and the action of the muscles of the floor of the mouth. The fracture must be reduced accurately, and fixed to allow bony union in a good position to restore dental occlusion. Despite the swelling, there is seldom any impairment of the airway in a conscious patient.

In severe injuries such as those seen from missiles, there may be, in addition to a comminuted fracture of the mandible, fractures of the maxilla and severe soft tissue damage to the face. There may also be associated injury to the pharynx, orbit or brain from the missile.[3] Principles of management of these severe injuries consist of the initial protection of the airway and arrest of haemorrhage. Endotracheal intubation or tracheotomy may be necessary, and crycothyroid puncture may be a temporary life-saving procedure (see also Chapter 9).

RIGID FIXATION

Rigid fixation of a mandibular fracture can be made between the teeth on either side of the fracture to the teeth of the upper jaw. Alternatively, the fracture itself can be exposed for fixation. Any method of direct fixation should remain *in situ* for a minimum of 6 weeks.

Interdental 'eyelet' wiring

This requires healthy stable teeth adjacent to the fracture (Fig. 10.2). An *arch bar* of malleable material can also be fixed by this method against the outer surface of the teeth on either side of the fracture, thus offering some additional support. Although a satisfactory method of stabilizing a dentoalveolar fracture and allowing movement of the jaw, this approach is insufficient fixation for any major mandibular fracture. It is therefore also necessary to wire the lower teeth to the upper teeth to provide adequate stabilization of the fracture. This is, however, at the expense of any jaw move-

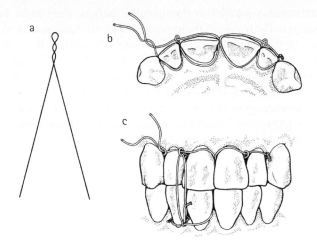

Figure 10.2 *(a) Stainless steel wire (0.4 mm or gauge 26–32) is twisted to make eyelets which can be passed between the teeth. (b) Further wires are linked by passing them through the eyelets. (c) Wires secured to teeth on either side of the fracture can then be linked either between the upper and lower teeth or to a splint.*

ment. Feeding and oral hygiene are difficult but, more importantly, inhalation of vomit can prove fatal. Wire cutters must be immediately available for this emergency.

Open fixation

The main advantage of open fixation is that an accurate reduction can be rigidly supported whilst still allowing the patient jaw movement (Fig. 10.3). Most fractures of the mandible are compound, and the surgical access to the fracture, via the gingivo-labial sulcus, has further potential to contaminate the fracture site with oral bacteria. Despite this, open fixation seldom results in infective complications.

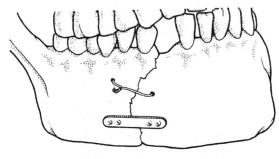

Figure 10.3 *Two methods of open fixation of a mandibular fracture.*

Fractures of the maxilla

Injuries involving the alveolar segment of the maxilla (le Fort 1 fractures) can be stabilized with interdental wiring or a variety of dental splints. Those occurring as part of a complicated middle third facial fracture may be associated with damage to adjacent structures such as the orbit, the nasolacrimal apparatus, the nose and the ethmoid region. An associated fracture of the anterior cranial fossa may be complicated by CSF rhinorrhoea. A general surgeon operating on such an injury can only follow some cardinal principles:

- Adequate exposure in optimum circumstances with a protected airway.
- Recognition that the bony fragments must be reduced and stabilized by wiring, pinning or plating before any soft tissue reconstruction begins.
- In complicated middle third fractures involving the ethmoid region, there may be disruption of the attachments of the medial canthal ligaments. This injury should be repaired primarily by re-attaching the ligament, as secondary revision is fraught with difficulty.
- In patients with combined maxillary and mandibular injuries, the mandible should be reduced and fixed first, and the maxilla subsequently reduced to it, so that antero-posterior projection of the middle third of the face can be restored.

Fractures of the zygoma

These may be easily missed in the presence of severe soft tissue swelling of the face. The zygomatic bone is usually separated from its normal attachments and displaced downwards. The patient may complain of diplopia, sensory change in the distribution of the infra-orbital nerve, or of difficulty in opening the jaw. Examination may reveal a palpable 'step' deformity in the infra-orbital margin, or at the lateral orbital margin in the area of the frontal zygomatic suture. A fracture is best confirmed with an occipito-mental X-ray, but this should be taken at 30 degrees, as those taken at a lesser angle often produce superimposition of the occipital bone over the zygomatic architecture. Zygomatic fractures may occur in isolation, but are often associated with additional damage to the facial skeleton, in particular blowout fractures of the orbital floor. Skilled reduction and fixation is mandatory for a good functional and cosmetic result.[2]

An isolated zygomatic fracture can be levered back into position. A small incision is made in the temporal region inside the hairline and extended down through the temporalis fascia to display the temporalis muscle fibres. An instrument, preferably a Bristow elevator, is then inserted through the incision and directed downwards beneath the zygomatic arch. The elevator is then lifted bodily forwards and outwards, and the zygoma is reduced, usually with an audible click. The technique of using a rolled-up swab as a fulcrum and levering the zygoma back into position exerts considerable pressure on the cranium, and iatrogenic fractures of the temporal bone can occur. If the fracture cannot be reduced or is unstable, an open reduction with exploration of the orbital floor and direct wiring at several sites may be needed.

Fractures of the nasal bones

Nasal fractures are commonly displaced, but this is not always apparent until the swelling subsides. Without reduction, the asymmetry and loss of normal contours can leave a patient with an unacceptable cosmetic result and, in addition, a deviation of the septum can result in an inadequate airway on one side. Reduction of the fracture should be carried out before healing is too advanced, but it is often easier when some of the swelling has subsided. Around 10 days after injury is a satisfactory compromise. After 3 weeks it is normally no longer possible to manipulate the nasal bones.

A post-traumatic septal haematoma should be sought and drained. If it passes undiagnosed it can lead to necrosis of the underlying cartilage and a septal perforation.

INFECTIONS OF THE FACE

Surgical drainage of infections is less often necessary with early access to antibiotic treatment. However, general surgeons practising in areas where many patients are remote from primary healthcare facilities may still have to operate for these conditions.

Soft tissue infections can occasionally lead to major tissue destruction. *Cancrum oris*, which is encountered almost exclusively in malnourished children in the developing world, is a spreading necrotizing synergistic infection. Treatment is with penicillin and metronidazole, nutritional support and the excision of necrotic tissue. The final full-thickness tissue loss extending from the mouth into the cheek will require surgical reconstruction, but should be deferred for 3–6 months.

Infection in the orbit may be secondary to a sinus infection or a penetrating injury. Pus behind the eye is under pressure and the patient has severe pain, proptosis and some unilateral visual impairment. Pus can be drained by an incision in the sclero-tarsal fold. An eye destroyed by pan-ophthalmitis and filled with pus must be excised (see below).

Sinus infections occasionally fail to settle on antibiotic therapy. The sinus is filled with pus which fails to drain through an obstructed outlet, and surgical drainage becomes necessary. The maxillary sinus can be entered trans-nasally and washed out under local anaesthesia. A trochar and cannula is advanced through the bony lateral wall of the nasal cavity under the inferior turbinate.

Infections of dental origin will commonly settle with antibiotic therapy, but if pus has formed then drainage is required. An *alveolar abscess*, around the root of a tooth, subsides rapidly after the offending tooth is extracted. A *subperiosteal abscess* may follow an untreated alveolar abscess. The pus may be on the external or internal surface of the bone and is drained into the mouth by an incision in the muco-periosteum parallel to the alveolar margin. Care must be taken in the region of the lower premolar teeth to avoid damage to the mental nerve. *Ludwig's angina* is a bilateral cellulitis within the submental and submandibular triangles, associated with gross swelling. It is usually secondary to a dental infection. Drainage of pus, or an incision for decompression, may be necessary, and a pre-emptive tracheostomy may have to be considered in such patients. Drainage of the submental space is shown in Figure 10.4.

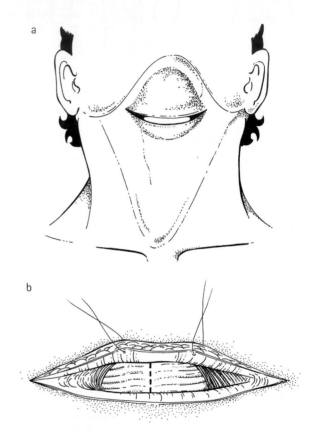

Figure 10.4 *Pus in the submental space may be deep to the mylohyoid muscle. (a) The transverse skin incision; (b) the vertical incision in mylohyoid.*

Osteomyelitis of the jaws is extremely rare in patients who have access to antibiotic treatment for the primary dental or sinus infection. Drainage of pus from the bone, or the removal of sequestra will leave less scarring if it is possible to approach from within the mouth.

A **peritonsillar abscess** (**quinsy**) requires drainage of pus by an incision over the most prominent part of the swelling. Local anaesthesia is safer if only simple general anaesthesia, without airway protection from inhalation, is available. The swelling is first aspirated with a needle to confirm the presence of pus. A mucosal incision is then made, followed by gentle exploration of the abscess cavity with sinus forceps. Any deep incision with a scalpel can result in torrential haemorrhage.

A **retropharyngeal abscess** lies between the pharynx and the vertebral column in the retropharyngeal space, which extends from the base of the skull to the posterior mediastinum. It connects anteriorly with the pre-tracheal space and laterally with the parapharyngeal space. The abscess is visible as a bulging of the posterior oropharynx. In childhood this abscess is seldom tuberculous and can be drained through the mouth; airway protection from inhalation is again crucial. A tuberculous retropharyngeal abscess in an adult, secondary to cervical tuberculosis, is better approached from the neck (see Chapter 9).

Acute mastoiditis which fails to resolve on antibiotic therapy will still occasionally require emergency release of pus from the mastoid cavity in order to prevent intracranial extension of the infection. A postauricular incision is made 2 cm behind the post-aural crease directly onto the bone of the mastoid. The periosteum of the mastoid is elevated until the anterior edge of the mastoid is seen and, superiorly, the elevator should demonstrate the superior wall of the external meatus. Imaginary tangents are drawn from these surfaces and they intersect on the mastoid. The area bounded by these tangents and the external meatus is called Macewan's triangle (Fig. 10.5). Entry into the mastoid should be through this triangle to minimize danger to the facial nerve and the dura. Entry through the bone can be by drill or by chisel. A general surgeon forced to operate on this condition can be content with the release of pus. Further exploration of the mastoid cavity, the underlying dura or of a thrombosed sigmoid sinus is likely to cause more harm than good.

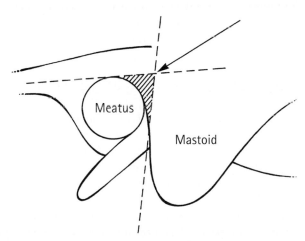

Figure 10.5 *The periosteum is elevated from the bone until the anterior border of the mastoid and superior wall of the meatus can be identified as landmarks. Tangents from these delineates the shaded triangle through which the mastoid cavity can be most safely approached.*

SURGERY AROUND THE EYE

Any surgery around the eye must be undertaken with precision, and the surgeon must be aware of the visual and cosmetic consequences of scarring in this area.

Peri-orbital skin lesions

A general surgeon frequently removes small benign or malignant skin lesions from the peri-orbital skin. He or she must be aware of the nasolacrimal apparatus at the inner canthus and avoid damage, or the patient will be left with a weeping eye. Removal of skin from immediately below the lower lid can drag the lower lid down and cause it to be lifted away from the eyeball, and even to evert. This *ectropion* will result in a watering eye as the inferior punctum is no longer in contact with the eyeball, and the eye is also more vulnerable to injury. This situation can be avoided by a full-thickness graft (see Chapter 1) to the area excised, instead of attempting a primary closure (Fig. 10.6). Referral to an ophthalmologist or a plastic surgeon for the initial surgery should always be considered.

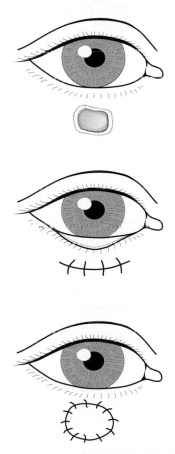

Figure 10.6 *A skin tumour beneath the eye can distort the lower lid if it is excised as an ellipse and closed as a linear wound. A circular excision and a Wolfe graft produces a more satisfactory result.*

External angular dermoids

These are congenital cystic swellings at the superolateral margins of the orbit which enlarge with age. They most often present in early to mid childhood. Excision is usually straightforward, but they may be deeply indented into the outer table of the skull. The occasional dermoid has no bony separation from the dura – a situation of which the surgeon would wish to be aware prior to operation. It is therefore recommended that those which feel fixed to the bone and those which extend under the supra-orbital ridge are examined by preoperative X-ray to confirm an intact inner table of skull. Surgery requires a general anaesthetic with head towelling and a protected airway followed by a careful dissection on the surface of the cyst. The incision should be just below, or occasionally above, and parallel to the eyebrow (Fig. 10.7). The temptation to hide the incision within an eyebrow is mistaken, as hair follicle scarring results in deformity of the eyebrow.

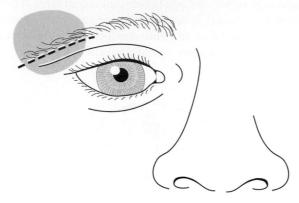

Figure 10.7 *An external angular dermoid is often a deeper lesion than originally appreciated, and excision must be carefully planned.*

Surgery of the eyelids

This fine surgery should normally be passed by a general surgeon to either an ophthalmologist or a plastic surgeon. However, some remote general surgeons may be able to offer some simple but effective surgery on the eyelids which can preserve sight in the underlying eye.[4]

Lid repair after trauma can be successfully achieved by a generalist following general principles of accurate apposition of fine tissues, with particular care to achieve accuracy at the lid margins. The junction between the eyelid skin and the tarsal conjunctiva (the grey line) should be identified and sutured very accurately to avoid a step in the eyelid margin. The tarsal plate is repaired with fine, absorbable sutures placed so that the knots do not irritate the cornea. The skin is then closed with fine, non-absorbable sutures. If, however, a canaliculus is lacerated, repair will be very difficult without the magnification of an operating microscope. When damage is suspected, it is confirmed with a lacrimal probe, and repair is performed around a fine silicone tube passed through the lid punctum, across the divided area in the laceration and on through the distal duct into the nasal cavity. The silicone tube is left *in situ* for 3–6 months.

Tarsorrhaphy is a simple temporary manoeuvre to save an eye as, if an eyelid does not close over an eye during blinking and in sleep, drying and trauma to the cornea follows with impairment of sight. The underlying pathology may be a facial nerve paralysis or a severe proptosis secondary to hyperthyroidism. Occasionally, tissue damage from burns or other trauma in the peri-orbital area can create a similar problem. A more definitive solution to tarsorrhaphy may then be considered later. For example, a patient with a facial nerve palsy may be better served in the long term by the insertion of a gold weight in the upper lid, combined with a procedure to support the lower lid. Tarsorrhaphy consists of the sewing together of the lateral third of the upper and lower eyelids, after an incision has been made along the lid margin, between the eyelashes and the openings of the meibomian glands, to create a raw surface.

Ectropion may simply be the result of senile involution, but when it occurs secondary to infra-orbital scarring the deformity can be corrected by release of the scar tissue followed by full-thickness skin grafting.

Entropion may also occur with senile involution, but in areas of the world where trachoma is endemic it is commonly secondary to conjunctival scarring from this infection. The inverted eyelashes traumatize the cornea. Any infection is first eradicated, after which the entropion can be corrected by excision of the scarred conjunctiva and replacement with a free full-thickness mucosal graft from the mouth. It may also be necessary to divide and evert a deformed inturned tarsal plate. An alternative simpler strategy is a radical excision of the inturned eyelashes without attempts to correct the underlying deformity of the lid. Everting sutures which pass through the skin, tarsal plate and tarsal conjunctiva may be a simple procedure which produces temporary relief of the entropion.

Tumours of the eyelid which involve less than one-quarter of the length of a lid can be excised as a full-thickness wedge, followed by re-constitution of the eyelid.

Surgery within the orbit and of the eyeball

This is an area where a general surgeon without specific training has little to offer. The drainage of intra-orbital pus is described above. Some surgeons may wish to train so as to be able to offer cataract surgery in remote areas, but most other intra-orbital and intra-ocular procedures will probably be impractical in isolated general surgical practice.

Ocular injury can seldom be managed successfully by a generalist. The internal structures may have been disrupted by blunt trauma, or the orbit may have been penetrated. A ruptured eye should be sutured to prevent loss of contents and the collapse which will further disrupt the internal structures.[5] Some useful sight may thus be salvaged. However, an eye injury may occasionally induce a sympathetic ophthalmia in the contralateral eye with loss of sight in this eye as well. The risk of this rare but devastating complication is reduced by early removal of an injured eye. Therefore, if an eye is severely injured and sight already irretrievably lost, procrastination over its removal may be harmful.

Exposure of the posterior sclera is essential when a ruptured globe is suspected, as many ruptures start or extend posteriorly. A 360-degree conjunctival incision is made at the limbus (just outside the corneal–scleral junction) and all four quadrants of the sclera are exposed. A rectus muscle may have to be temporarily detached for access, but is later re-attached with 6/0 absorbable sutures. A scleral wound is sutured with fine interrupted monofilament sutures, and the conjunctiva re-attached at the limbus with fine, absorbable sutures.

Enucleation of an eye can be indicated for an eye destroyed by infection or trauma. The conjunctiva is incised at its junction with the cornea and the plane developed around the eyeball. Each intrinsic muscle is hooked forwards and detached from the globe. One stump should be cut long enough for an artery forceps to be attached for retraction. Finally, the optic nerve is divided, the eye removed, and the conjunctiva closed.

Evisceration is a more minor procedure in which only the contents of the globe are removed. It allows a better cosmetic result as there is some movement of the residual tissue. The cornea is excised and the contents curetted. However, failure to remove all uveal tissue leaves the patient still at risk of sympathetic ophthalmia.

SURGERY AROUND THE MOUTH

This surgery is predominantly the province of the faciomaxillary, plastic and ENT surgeon, although the general surgeon may be involved to a greater or lesser degree dependent on the specialization in his area.

Trauma

Lacerations of the lip can leave an ugly scar with a step at the vermilion border if not apposed accurately. Full-thickness lacerations require separate suturing of the layers. The mucosa is repaired first with absorbable sutures, followed by repair of the orbicularis oris muscle, and finally the lip margin and the skin are closed. Small lacerations confined to the inside of the mouth seldom require sutures. An exception is a full-thickness laceration on the lateral border of the tongue. When a quarter or more of the tongue is divided, the muscle contraction holds the laceration widely open, and a couple of loose absorbable sutures are required for tissue apposition. Deep bites are necessary or the suture will cut through.

Infections and calculi

Infections within the mouth and oropharynx are discussed above.

Salivary calculi are discussed in Chapter 9.

Malignancies

Tumours of the lip can be removed by a wedge incision. On the lower lip up to one-third of the length of the lip can be excised with a satisfactory cosmetic result. The incision must be carefully planned, and the defect is closed as for a full-thickness lip laceration (Fig. 10.8). On the upper lip, however, a wedge excision produces a noticeable asymmetry, and therefore, except for very minor wedge excisions, a flap reconstruction should be considered. Extensive pre-malignant leukoplakia of the lower lip may have to be excised by vermilion advancement (Fig. 10.9). An incision is made just outside the mucocutaneous junction and the mucosa is dissected off the underlying muscle as far as the gingivo-labial sulcus. The leucoplakia is excised, after which the mucous membrane is advanced and re-attached to the skin incision to form a new vermilion border.

Tumours of the buccal mucosa can be simply excised if they are small and confined to the mucosa. They may, however, arise in an area of extensive pre-malignant field change

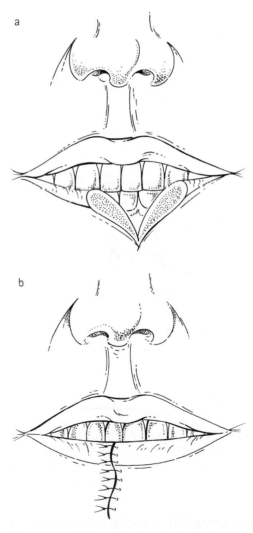

Figure 10.8 *A carefully planned V excision of a lip tumour can give an excellent cosmetic result. (a) The sides of the V are curved to increase the initial depth of the lip and compensate for later contracture of the scar. (b) Alignment of the vermilion edge is crucial for a good cosmetic result.*

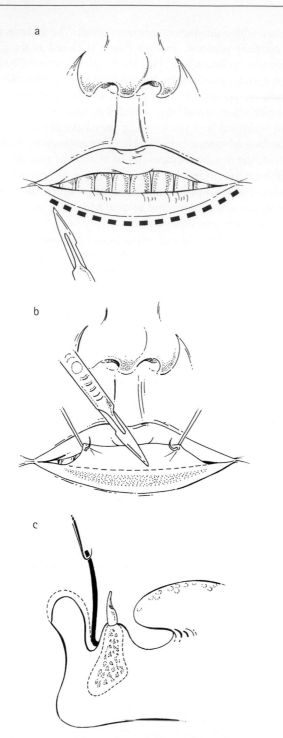

Figure 10.9 *Pre-malignant leukoplakia extending along most of the lower lip can be excised by vermilion advancement. (a) The incision; (b) dissection of the mucosa off the muscle; (c) the dissection continues to the gingivo-labial sulcus.*

in mucosa damaged by carcinogens. Extensive stripping of the abnormal mucosa may then be necessary, after which the defect is covered with a split-thickness skin graft. The graft should be secured to prevent displacement. A 'quilting' technique in which multiple sutures 1 cm apart are placed through the graft to tether it to the underlying muscle is sat-

isfactory. Advanced tumours of the buccal mucosa may require a radical full-thickness excision of the cheek. A myocutaneous flap may then be required for reconstruction (see below). If resection of such tumours involves the parotid duct, then relocation is mandatory if iatrogenic obstructive sialadenitis is to be prevented.

Other intra-oral malignancies can pose major challenges in resection and reconstruction. Small tumours on the tongue or elsewhere in the oral cavity can be excised locally with the removal of 1 cm of macroscopically normal tissue. Unfortunately, isolated generalists are more likely to see patients with advanced invasive malignancies. Not only will they have no faciomaxillary referral possibilities but there may also be no access to radiotherapy or chemotherapy. Curative surgery – or even palliative surgery to gain local control – will have to be very major. For example, a total glossectomy combined with cervical node dissection, and followed by reconstruction with a tunnelled pectoralis flap may be required for an advanced carcinoma of the tongue.[6] A tumour of the floor of the mouth may require resection of part of the mandible en bloc with the tumour and the regional nodes, followed by major soft tissue reconstruction including a vascularized bone graft to replace part of the mandibular arch. The excision of a maxillary tumour will often involve sacrifice of the eye. General surgeons, even if they have the surgical skills to attempt such surgery in unfamiliar surgical territory, are most unlikely, while working in these circumstances, to have the anaesthetic or other facilities available to make such surgery a viable undertaking.

Congenital abnormalities

A **tight frenulum** tethering the tip of the tongue is a common minor abnormality. Frenuloplasty, a simple release of the fibrous band, is all that is sometimes required, but care must be taken not to cut too deep and cause haemorrhage which can threaten the airway. The submandibular duct orifices are also vulnerable to injury. When severe tongue tie exists, early release has been shown to reduce the incidence of mastitis in breastfeeding mothers. Social advantages include the ability to protrude the tongue, whether as an insult or to lick an icecream. Tongue tie is seldom associated with speech difficulties.

Cleft lip and palate deformities are commonly linked, but either may occur in isolation. Early feeding difficulties, due to an inability to suck, are later overshadowed by speech problems from the cleft palate or the cosmetic distress from the cleft lip. Specialist repair undertaken in infancy can offer excellent functional and cosmetic results even with severe variants of the deformity. In areas remote from medical services, most severely affected infants fail to feed and do not survive infancy, but children with milder forms of the abnormality may present in late childhood in the hope that the deformity can be improved.

When no specialist referral is possible a generalist can still improve the cosmetic appearance of a cleft lip. In the milder cases the cleft is commonly unilateral, but with the inevitable associated distortion of the nose (Fig. 10.10a). The repair entails paring the edges of the cleft, lengthening the cleft side of the lip to bring the cupid's bow into a horizontal position, and identification and dissection of the abnormally placed fibres of the orbicularis muscle. These fibres, on either side of the cleft, will be found sweeping upwards and gaining an attachment to the alar base laterally and the base of the columella medially. These bundles must be detached, brought down to a more horizontal position and sutured across the lip to form a new orbicularis oris sphincter.

The first step is to plan accurately, and mark the skin incisions before starting the operation. Three areas of tissue will be excised. These include the two areas above the dotted lines in Figure 10.10a, where the two halves of the cleft upper lip extend up into the nostril. In addition, the small triangle a-b-c is excised. As the lip is pulled over, this triangular defect will allow lengthening of the new midline vermilion border, with localized narrowing of the lip to create a natural indentation, or cupid's bow. The additional full-thickness releasing incision, extending up from point c, is combined with the freeing of the abnormal attachment of the orbicularis muscle fibres to the columella, so that this portion of the lip can be drawn downwards. The extension of the incision under the nostril from point e, combined with the freeing of the orbicularis muscle fibres from the alar base, allows this other half of the lip to be drawn across and down.

As the tissue is drawn into its new position, for the initial approximation of c to d, the releasing incision above c opens up and point e will lie naturally within it. The underlying muscle fibres will also have been carried into a horizontal position and are correctly aligned for the deeper aspects of the repair (Fig. 10.10b). Mucosa, muscle and skin are apposed with fine sutures and, if mobilization has been adequate, there should be no tension. There should also be a significant narrowing of the splayed nostril (Fig. 10.10c).

An isolated generalist may occasionally wish to attempt the repair of a cleft palate, but will require skilled anaesthesia to make this a viable procedure, especially in a young child.[7] Optimum results are obtained with extensive skilled mobilization of tissue, and additional repair of the floor of the nose. A simplified technique consists of the raising of mucoperiosteal flaps off the bony surface of the hard palate. The posterior palatine arteries are identified and preserved (Fig. 10.11a). The soft palate muscles are then detached from their abnormal attachment to the posterior border of the hard palate, and swung medially across the defect and sewn together (Fig. 10.11b). The oral mucosal flaps are then also swung medially over the defect and sutured (Fig. 10.11c).

Reconstruction around the mouth

Myocutaneous flaps are invaluable for reconstruction following tissue loss from trauma, malignancy or necrotizing infection. In the developed world they are exclusively within the practice of plastic or faciomaxillary surgeons, and a wide range of donor flaps exist – especially if expertise in microvascular surgery is available to make free tissue transfer possible (see Chapter 1). Unfortunately, many of the patients requiring reconstructive surgery have been injured in military conflict in regions where the same conflict has disrupted medical services. Resources are limited and even a delayed evacuation for specialist surgery may be impossible. Two simpler flaps are described which may be of use to general surgeons who have no option but to attempt reconstruction themselves.[8] As discussed above, they should not be undertaken as part of the primary procedure in trauma.

A **pectoralis major flap** can be brought up for soft tissue reconstruction of the chin and lower lip. The original injury may have been from a bullet or a landmine explosion, but the wound has healed with major deformity from soft tissue loss. To plan the flap, a line is drawn from the acromion to the xiphisternum. A perpendicular line from the upper end of this line to the midpoint of the clavicle marks the course of

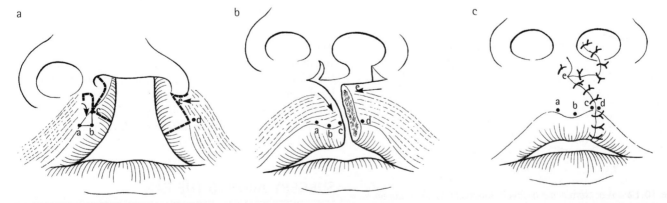

Figure 10.10 *Cleft lip repair. (a) The operation should be planned and the tissues marked before the incisions are made. (b) The incisions have allowed the muscle to be swung down into a horizontal position and the defect can now be closed. (c) A good repair should also correct the alar distortion.*

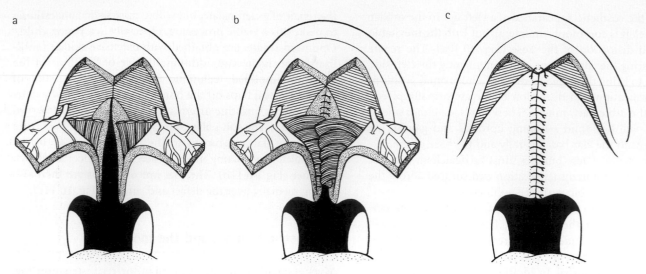

Figure 10.11   *Cleft palate repair. (a) The mucoperiosteal flaps have been raised with preservation of the posterior palatine arteries. The abnormal attachments of the soft palate muscles have been divided. (b) The muscles are then swung medially over the defect and sewn together. (c) The oral mucosal flaps are also apposed in the midline.*

the pectoral branch of the thoraco-acromial artery which supplies the flap. An incision is made around the required island of skin at the lower end of the flap (Fig. 10.12), and this incision is deepened down to the pectoralis major muscle. In the medial portion of the ellipse, the incision is then deepened through the underlying pectoralis muscle to define the area of muscle which is required for the reconstruction. A linear skin incision is then made from the skin island along the axis of the flap. This affords the necessary access for the dissection of the flap pedicle. The plane under the lateral border of pectoralis major is then entered, and the dissection continues on the deep surface of pectoralis major to elevate a muscle pedicle by lifting it progressively off the underlying chest wall. Initially, the muscle pedicle is cut of similar width to the muscle underlying the skin island. The

vascular pedicle, on which the vitality of the graft depends, can then be identified on the under-surface of the muscle as the dissection continues superolaterally. Once the vessels have been identified, the muscle pedicle can be narrowed to reduce its bulk. Finally, the humeral attachment of the muscle pedicle is divided to allow the pedicle to be tunnelled under the skin, but over the clavicle, into the neck. It is then delivered into the defect where it is to be used, either in the neck or lower face.

A **lined forehead flap** can be used to replace full-thickness tissue loss of the cheek. This can be invaluable in reconstruction after cancrum oris or after a full-thickness excision for an invasive carcinoma of the buccal mucosa. The end of the forehead flap is lifted, and a split-thickness skin graft is stitched to the under-surface. The flap is then re-sutured into place in order to give the split skin time to attach (Fig. 10.13a). After 2 weeks the flap can be elevated and swung into position. The split skin graft is sewn to the edges of the mucosal defect and the forehead skin to the defect in the facial skin (Fig. 10.13b). The denuded area of forehead is covered with a temporary partial-thickness graft. After 3 weeks the pedicle is divided, the attachment of the donor tissue to the superolateral edge of the defect is completed, and the remainder of the flap can then be returned to the forehead, removing the temporary split skin graft, which was used as a temporary cover, from this area. Only a small defect remains on one side of the forehead which has already been grafted with split-thickness skin.

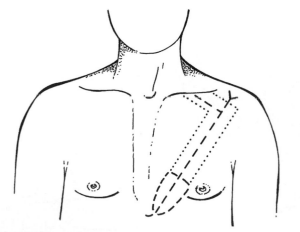

Figure 10.12   *A pectoralis major myocutaneous flap can bring an island of skin to the lower face for reconstruction. It has a more secure blood supply, and reaches further than the alternative fasciocutaneous deltopectoral flap.*

SURGERY AROUND THE EAR

The general surgeon will be restricted to the surgery of the auricle and the external ear.

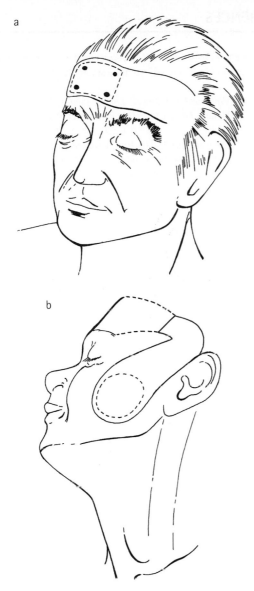

Figure 10.13 *(a) A forehead flap can be swung down for reconstruction of the nose or cheek. The forehead defect can be covered with a partial-thickness skin graft, which would not be suitable for the full-thickness tissue loss in the recipient area. Lining of the undersurface of the flap with split skin, as described in the text, makes this flap suitable for the cheek (b) when buccal mucosa loss must also be replaced.*

Trauma

Haematoma of the auricle should be aspirated on presentation. The skin is lifted away from the normally adherent cartilage by blood clot. Ischaemia from pressure occurs to the underlying cartilage and the clot becomes organized. If no action is taken a 'cauliflower ear' develops. If the haematoma cannot be evacuated with a large-bore needle, then multiple incisions must be made with strict asepsis in order to prevent

perichondritis. Once all clot has been removed, preferably under general anaesthesia, a pressure dressing is applied using cotton wool to fill all the contours of the ear. The ear must be examined daily because further accumulation of fluid will occur for many days. If further fluid accumulates, then two shirt buttons or foam bolsters may be used to act as compression. These are placed on either side of the auricle and sutured together.

Tears from earrings occur when an earring in a pierced ear is forcefully pulled through the tissue. In the acute presentation, the tissue is simply re-approximated. Late presentation is common when the patient discovers that healing has produced an unattractive, bilobed appearance. Reconstruction is simple and usually heals without complication.

Head injuries: blood in the external meatus, in the absence of any obvious superficial injury, is very suspicious of a fracture of the petrous temporal bone, even if basal skull X-rays are not confirmatory. This is a compound fracture with the potential for intracranial infection, but local policies vary as to the use of prophylactic antibiotics in this situation (see also Chapter 8).

Cysts and other benign lesions

Multiple **small sebaceous cysts** around the ear associated with the scarring of acne can be very challenging to excise. Care must be taken to avoid full-thickness 'buttonholing' of the earlobe. Cysts related to the track of an ear piercing are commonly inclusion dermoids and can be excised. Careful preoperative examination is essential to differentiate these from a keloid scar, the excision of which is likely to result in a larger keloid, and should therefore be avoided.

Accessory auricles are most commonly small anterior skin tags with a core of cartilage. Excision is cosmetic and

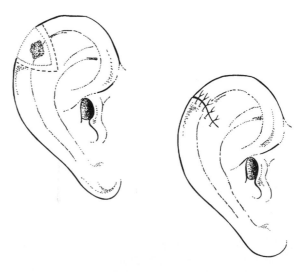

Figure 10.14 *Wedge excision of a tumour of the external ear. The broken line indicates the slightly wider excision of the cartilage.*

should include the core of cartilage which extends deep to the skin.

Tumours of the auricle

There is virtually no mobility of the skin of the external ear on the underlying cartilage, and isolated skin closure after excision of a lesion is seldom possible. A full-thickness skin graft can be used after excision of a centrally placed lesion if underling tissue on which to place a graft has been retained. Tumours at the edge of the external ear can be excised with the underlying cartilage in a full-thickness wedge excision (Fig. 10.14). The V-shaped incision is easy to close, provided that a little more cartilage than skin is excised. Sutures are only required in the skin. Flap reconstruction may give a better cosmetic result when very large excisions are necessary.

REFERENCES

1. *Fundamental Techniques of Plastic Surgery and their Applications*, 10th edn. AD McGregor. Edinburgh: Elsevier Churchill Livingstone, 2000.
2. *Rowe and Williams Maxillofacial Injuries, Volume 1*, 2nd edn. NL Rowe, JL Williams (eds). Edinburgh: Elsevier Churchill Livingstone, 1994.
3. Clarkson P, Wilson THH, Lawrie RS. Treatment of jaw and face casualties in the British Army. *Ann Surg* 1946; **123**: 190–208.
4. *Primary Surgery, Volume I*. M King. Oxford: Oxford University Press, 1990.
5. MacEwen CJ. Ocular injuries – Educational update. *J R Coll Surg Edinb* 1999; **44**: 317–23.
6. *Stell and Maran's Head and Neck Surgery*, 4th edn. PM Stell, AGD Maran, J Watkinson (eds). London: Arnold Publications, 2000.
7. Liu EHC, Richard BM. Drawover anaesthesia for cleft palate and lip surgery in Pokhara, Nepal. *Trop Doct* 2000; **30**: 78–81.
8. *Rowe and Williams Maxillofacial Injuries, Volume 2*, 2nd edn. NL Rowe, JL Williams (eds). Edinburgh: Elsevier Churchill Livingstone, 1994.

11

SPECIAL CONSIDERATIONS IN ABDOMINAL AND GASTROINTESTINAL SURGERY

Intra-abdominal surgery has the potential for major physiological, biochemical and septic complications that are seldom encountered in other areas. The underlying factor is the gastrointestinal tract; both its contents and its function. The details of these considerations are outwith a book on operative surgery, and further reading is essential for optimum preoperative and postoperative management.[1,2] However, an understanding of the issues involved is also essential during the surgery itself. Frequently, there is a choice of surgical solutions to a problem and the surgeon must decide before, or even during, an operation which is the most appropriate. Many factors are important in these decisions, but some general principles which may influence decisions are discussed in this chapter.

FLUID AND ELECTROLYTE DISTURBANCES

Fluid and electrolyte requirements should be considered in two main categories, namely maintenance requirements and replacement of abnormal losses. In Appendix 1, the daily fluid and electrolyte maintenance requirements are given for adults and children. When there is intra-abdominal pathology the situation may be very different as an imbalance develops in the fluid turnover through the gastrointestinal tract. Approximately 6 L of fluid are secreted into the healthy, adult gastrointestinal tract and then re-absorbed each day (Table 11.1). In most abnormal situations secretion continues, even if somewhat reduced, but re-absorption is greatly impaired. The fluid may be lost externally as vomit or nasogastric aspirate, as diarrhoea, or as stoma or fistula effluent. Measurement of these losses in a hospital patient gives a guide to replacement requirements. However, patients with acute intra-abdominal pathology may present to hospital already in a state of advanced dehydration, and fluid and

electrolyte deficits must be addressed prior to surgery. It must be remembered that fluid may also be lost from the circulating volume into the distended gut lumen or into the peritoneal cavity with no external losses apparent. The electrolyte content and acidity of intestinal fluids vary (see Table 11.1), but in general gastrointestinal fluid losses should be replaced with intravenous normal saline with added potassium, in addition to the basic maintenance requirements.[3] At the stage that an ileus is resolving, re-absorption of fluid from the bowel lumen back into the intravascular compartment occurs. If fluid replacement is not cut back at this stage, then fluid overload may occur.

Table 11.1 *Gastrointestinal secretions.*

Secretion(s)	Daily volume (mL)	Na$^+$ (mmol/L)	K$^+$ (mmol/L)
Saliva	1000	10	25
Gastric	1500	60	10
Bile	500	140	5
Pancreatic	500	140	5
Small bowel	3000	140	5
Colonic	Minimal	60	30

The values given are only a guide and have also been approximated for simplicity.

Obstruction

The level of an obstruction, the history of vomiting and the degree of distension are clearly important when considering potential fluid and electrolyte disturbances. In a pyloric or jejunal obstruction, large volumes of fluid are still secreted into the lumen but are not re-absorbed. Fluid is lost as vomit, or aspirate, and distension may be minimal. In contrast, in a distal ileal obstruction distension may be very marked before vomiting commences, and the fluid deficit may again be under-appreciated. A distal large bowel obstruction is often initially incomplete, the absorption of fluid from the gut lumen continues and distension may be minimal until the passage of flatus is also prevented. Vomiting also usually occurs late.

Peritonitis and pancreatitis

The volume of circulating fluid which can be lost into the retroperitoneum, the peritoneal cavity and the oedematous gut wall is often under-estimated in severe intra-abdominal inflammatory conditions.

Fistulae and stomas

Fistula effluent may lead to fluid and electrolyte depletion. A jejunal fistula, or stoma, necessitates intravenous replacement of the large volumes of fluid lost, but a colostomy or colonic fistula should cause minimal disturbance to fluid and electrolyte equilibrium.

VOLUME AND PRESSURE DISTURBANCES

In both mechanical obstruction and ileus, there is distension of the bowel and stasis of gastrointestinal contents. Stasis encourages bacterial overgrowth with the formation of excess gas and resultant increasing distension. The distended gut is increasingly compromised, and both fluid re-absorption and peristaltic function is further impaired. A vicious circle is established (Fig. 11.1), especially as the greater the diameter of the bowel the greater the force of the peristaltic wave required to produce an effective propulsion. This is the situation encountered in a severe postoperative ileus, and the explanation of the dramatic resolution which may occasionally occur following naso-gastric tube deflation.

Gut distension inevitably leads to increases in intraluminal pressure, and also to increases in intra-abdominal pressure and volume. Morbidity is increased.

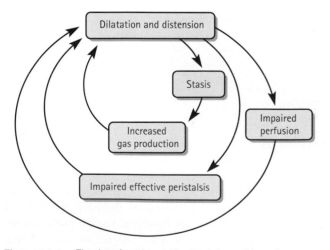

Figure 11.1 *The deteriorating pathophysiology of bowel obstruction.*

Increased intraluminal pressure

Deterioration in gut perfusion occurs in gut distension. As the intraluminal pressure rises it approximates the pressure in the vessels of the bowel wall, and effective perfusion ceases. Gross distension of the large bowel from a distal obstruction with a competent ileocaecal valve causes the caecum to distend more than any other segment. The caecum develops patchy gangrene and finally ruptures. Distension of the whole gut, as seen with a large bowel obstruction and an incompetent ileocaecal valve, is unlikely to cause such an isolated problem. However, the combination of increased intraluminal pressure and the general rise in intra-abdominal pressure impairs gut perfusion. Translocation of gut bacteria through the wall of a compromised bowel ensues with systemic sepsis (see below) if treatment is delayed.

Increased intra-abdominal pressure

Oesophageal reflux may occur from a distended stomach, with resultant oesophagitis. Minor episodes of aspiration may present as inhalation pneumonia. A major vomit may result in the aspiration of a large volume of gastric contents and either sudden death, or severe chemical pneumonitis with the development of an acute respiratory distress syndrome.

Abdominal compartment syndrome is a potential complication of abdominal distension with high intra-abdominal pressure.[4] The mechanism is similar to that of the compartment syndromes in the muscle compartments of the limbs (see Chapter 3). As the pressure rises within the abdomen, the perfusion of all intra-abdominal organs is reduced. Renal and hepatic perfusion are impaired and function deteriorates. Any anastomosis in the relatively ischaemic bowel is more vulnerable, and resolution of ileus is further prolonged but, most importantly, the integrity of the 'gut to circulation interface' is jeopardised. Translocation of endotoxins and bacteria from the gut lumen into the portal circulation ensues, and is an important factor in multiorgan failure. In the most severe forms of abdominal compartment syndrome, the situation is obvious clinically with a grossly distended abdomen, a splinted diaphragm and distended superficial veins in the thigh as venous return through the abdomen becomes impossible. More minor forms, however, may go unrecognized as one of the causes of a deteriorating clinical situation.

Increased intra-abdominal volume

Difficulties with abdominal closure following laparotomy are common when the intra-abdominal volume is increased. Sutures may cut through fascia, and the risk of a burst abdomen or an incisional hernia is increased. The surgeon is also at increased risk of catching a loop of bowel in a suture during closure. If tension cannot be reduced by decompression of bowel, simple primary closure of the abdomen may not be appropriate. Temporary containment of the abdominal viscera, or a laparostomy may have to be considered (see Chapter 12).

Respiratory complications are increased by the mechanical raising and splinting of the diaphragm. In severe cases, blood gas exchange may be inadequate. Even when satisfactory arterial blood gas levels are maintained, the under-ventilation of the lower lobes predisposes to basal pneumonia.

Most of these complications may also result from an increase in intra-abdominal volume and pressure from factors other than mechanical obstruction or ileus. Severe visceral swelling is associated with trauma, pancreatitis or intra-abdominal sepsis. Ascites, blood or packs may be reducing the available intra-abdominal capacity. A similar situation ensues when the abdominal capacity is inadequate to accommodate the normal intra-abdominal contents which are returned to it. These may have been lying free in the amniotic fluid before birth in a baby with a congenital defect of the abdominal wall, or accommodated within a giant hernia.

CONTAMINATION FROM GASTROINTESTINAL CONTENTS

The contents of the gastrointestinal tract are highly damaging to all tissue except the specialized mucosa with which they are normally in contact. The gastrointestinal contents may be released as a consequence of a traumatic, or surgical, breach of the integrity of the gut wall, or the viability of the wall may be damaged by infection or ischaemia. The chemical and enzymatic constituents of gastrointestinal secretions may cause direct tissue damage, but bacterial contamination from intestinal contents is the most important consideration.

- Chemical damage: the acidity of gastric juice released into the peritoneum from a perforated duodenal ulcer causes the severe peritonism and reflex guarding associated with this condition. Sterile bile and small bowel contents are initially less toxic.
- Enzymatic damage: the enzymes within pancreatic secretions are released retroperitoneally in acute pancreatitis, and the profound local and systemic inflammatory response that follows occurs even in the absence of secondary infection.

Bacterial contamination

Gastric acid destroys most ingested bacteria, and the contents of a healthy upper gastrointestinal system are relatively sterile. In achlorhydria or gastric stasis, however, bacterial growth continues in the stomach. The normal small bowel contents are also relatively sterile but, if there is stasis, bacte-

rial overgrowth with faecal organisms occurs rapidly. Bile and pancreatic secretions are also sterile in health, but are often infected in situations where the secretions have escaped their normal confines. In contrast, the faecal material within a normal colon has a large bacterial component. Therefore, although perforation of the gastrointestinal tract at any level may release infection into the peritoneal cavity, or retroperitoneal tissues, colonic perforation is the most serious in this respect.

Necrotic tissue does not maintain its physical integrity, and infarcted gut wall will inevitably perforate with release of the gastrointestinal contents. However, ischaemic but still viable gut also fails as an effective barrier and endotoxins, and finally bacteria, translocate into the circulation. In addition, the damaged ischaemic cells release cytokines and other tissue factors that initiate a cascade of inflammatory responses. The markers of this *systemic inflammatory response syndrome (SIRS)* include the rise of temperature, pulse and leukocyte count, and the later development of a metabolic acidosis. It is these markers which the surgeon is monitoring during a trial of non-operative management. A deterioration in these indices may reflect, under different circumstances, ischaemic bowel, an anastomotic leak or intra-abdominal sepsis.

The bowel may be ischaemic from local occlusion of feeding vessels as in a strangulation, or tissue perfusion may be reduced by increased intra-abdominal pressure. Perfusion is also reduced if a patient is hypotensive. Splanchnic vasoconstriction in shock reduces intestinal perfusion, which may be further jeopardized by the use of some pressor agents (e.g. dobutamine) in attempts to maintain blood pressure and perfusion to other vital organs. In all of these situations a bacteraemia, or frank septicaemia, may occur without any physical breach of the gastrointestinal tract.[5]

A septicaemia with gut organisms after abdominal surgery is always suggestive of an anastomotic leak or non-viable gut. As discussed above, a septicaemia may occur by translocation, but a negative laparotomy may be necessary to exclude a surgically amenable disaster.

Surgery on the gastrointestinal tract is associated with a high incidence of septic complications, as some bacterial contamination of the surgical field is inevitable. Complications may, however, be reduced by mechanical and anti-bacterial measures.

MECHANICAL MEASURES

These include preoperative bowel preparation to empty the colon of faecal contents (see Appendix I) and careful peritoneal toilet if there is contamination. The prevention of spillage of gastrointestinal contents during surgery should also be addressed (see Chapter 13). Instruments and gloves which have been contaminated during an anastomosis should not be used for the abdominal wall closure. These basic precautions, while sometimes carried to extremes in the pre-antibiotic era, are now in danger of being disregarded. Suction drainage of an area where a potentially infected haematoma may develop is a further mechanical measure to reduce sepsis.

ANTIBACTERIAL MEASURES

The most effective measure is prophylactic broad-spectrum systemic antibiotic cover of the operation itself and for the first 24–48 hours afterwards (see Appendix II). This ensures that any intra-abdominal, or wound, collection of fluid or blood has an antibiotic content which will inhibit bacterial growth. Preoperative 'sterilization' of the bowel with oral antibiotics was tried, but largely abandoned as infection with resistant bacteria and yeasts was problematic. However, there has been recent renewed interest in this technique to prevent septic complications in the severely ill patient in intensive care.[6] Methods of replacing the normal gut flora with more harmless bacteria have also been explored.[7]

INTESTINAL FAILURE

Failure of the damaged gastrointestinal system to regulate fluid and electrolyte turnover is immediately apparent. The impaired nutritional function is unfortunately often ignored, despite the recognition, as early as the 1930s, of a higher mortality in malnourished surgical patients.[8] A previously healthy, well-nourished patient, who makes an uncomplicated recovery from intra-abdominal surgery, comes to little harm from a week of starvation. Many patients with intra-abdominal pathology, however, have had either no nutritional intake for several days before their emergency admission, or have a long history of poor intake and weight loss over several months. If a good nutritional intake is then not established by the second postoperative week, a deteriorating clinical picture relating to starvation occurs. This situation should be avoided by commencing *enteral* or *intravenous feeding* before deterioration is evident (see Appendix III), and it is sometimes indicated from the time of surgery.

ENTERAL FEEDING

Enteral feeding is preferable to intravenous feeding and should always be considered, but is, unfortunately, often contraindicated. Enteral feeding has the advantage that the portal circulation is not bypassed, and in addition it preserves the luminal delivery of nutrients to the gut mucosa. This is now known to be important in the prevention of enterocyte and colonocyte dysfunction. The septic complications of intravenous feeding are also avoided. If there is upper gastrointestinal dysfunction, it may still be possible to feed enterally if the feed is delivered more distally. For example, if a prolonged gastric ileus is anticipated a *long double-bore nasogastric tube* can be passed at operation. The surgeon guides the long end through the duodenum into the first loop of jejunum. The shorter end remains in the stomach for

gastric aspiration (Fig. 11.2). Alternatively, a *feeding enterostomy* may be introduced directly into the jejunum at operation.[9] This form of feeding jejunostomy has the advantage of sparing the patient a nasogastric tube solely for the purpose of feeding, but the jejunal puncture and fixation of the jejunum to the abdominal wall have the potential for complications. A needle is introduced obliquely through the jejunal wall through which a catheter is threaded (Fig. 11.3). The needle is withdrawn and a purse-string suture inserted. A similar needle is then used to guide the catheter through the abdominal wall. The jejunum is then fixed to the abdominal wall to prevent kinking.

Enteral feeding should be introduced slowly and increased as tolerated. Long-term gastrostomy feeding may be indi-

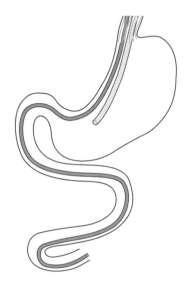

Figure 11.2 *A double-lumen nasogastric tube is placed so that the short tube is in the stomach for gastric aspiration. The longer tube should lie through the duodenum, well into the first loop of jejunum. More proximal positioning will result in reflux of jejunal feed into the stomach.*

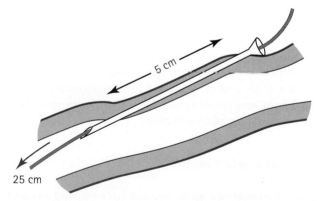

Figure 11.3 *A 7 cm-long, 16-gauge needle is introduced through the jejunal wall so that there is a 5-cm intramural track. A catheter is threaded through the needle and then distally within the lumen for a further 25 cm.*

cated in patients with oesophageal pathology, and also in those patients with dysphagia secondary to neurological disorders. The *feeding gastrostomy tube* can be introduced by the percutaneous endoscopic approach (Fig. 11.4), and can be established in the endoscopy suite under sedation and local anaesthesia. Techniques vary with different devices, but one method is illustrated in Figure 11.4. An open gastrostomy is described in Chapter 13.

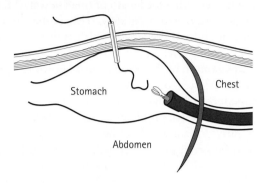

Figure 11.4 *Percutaneous endoscopic gastrostomy (PEG). The gastroscope is used to distend the stomach and elevate it against the anterior abdominal wall. A cannula is introduced into the stomach through a small incision made under local anaesthesia. A thread is then passed through the cannula, gripped through the gastroscope, and delivered out through the mouth where it is attached to the gastrostomy tube which is then gently pulled down into place.*

INTRAVENOUS (PARENTERAL) FEEDING

This is covered in more detail in Appendix III. It is best undertaken through a central venous catheter as the hypertonic solutions cause thromophlebitis in peripheral veins. The placement of subclavian and internal jugular lines is described in Appendix 1. The subclavian line is more comfortable for the conscious patient. Long-term successful intravenous feeding depends on the absence of septic complications. Absolute sterility in the insertion of lines and in their maintenance is essential. A subcutaneous tunnel reduces bacterial contamination (Fig. 11.5).

Temporary intestinal failure

This is common in the patient with a postoperative recovery complicated by sepsis and ileus. Enteral feeding is seldom possible, but after a variable period of intravenous feeding gut function recovers. Ileus often resolves surprisingly quickly after the commencement of intravenous feeding, and the parenteral nutrition may even have initiated the recovery of gut function. It must be remembered that a patient suffering the ill effects of starvation will also have a bowel which is adversely affected by lack of nutrients.

The importance of specific nutrients for intestinal mucosal function has been appreciated only relatively

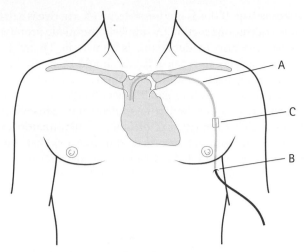

Figure 11.5 *A long-term line with a subcutaneous tunnel has less infective complications. A is the point from which the line is inserted into the subclavian vein (see Appendix I). B is the exit point of the line through the skin after the additional subcutaneous tunnel has been created. At C there is a Dacron cuff on a portion of the line lying in the subcutaneous tunnel. Reaction around this firmly tethers the line in place. When the line is removed, a small incision must be made at this point to release the cuff.*

recently. Short-chain fatty acids are important nutrients for the colonic mucosa. The integrity of gut mucosa has also been shown to be dependent on glutamine, an amino acid which becomes conditionally essential in the critically ill. Reversible loss of function occurs in bowel deprived of luminal nutrients. This may affect the whole gut after a prolonged period of exclusively intravenous nutrition, or affect a segment of bowel from which the intestinal contents have been temporarily diverted.

Prolonged severe postoperative intestinal failure

This usually occurs in association with anastomotic breakdown, fistulae and intra-abdominal collections of intestinal contents and pus. These patients pose major management problems to the surgeon.[10] Initial treatment is resuscitation with correction of fluid and electrolyte imbalance, followed by restitution of body reserves with intravenous feeding. Any intra-abdominal collections of pus, or intestinal fluid must be localized and drained effectively. This can often now be undertaken by percutaneous image-guided techniques, in which a collection is either aspirated, or a drain introduced into it, secured and left *in situ*. However, an open operation may still sometimes be needed. It is then occasionally necessary to leave the abdomen open (laparostomy), either to effect adequate drainage of sepsis, or to prevent high intra-abdominal pressure from closure. Any fistula effluent must be collected in order to prevent damage to the abdominal skin, and this can usually be achieved with skilled application of a stoma bag. If this is not possible, an alternative is a drain on low continuous suction. A simple home-made prototype, favoured by Eric Farquharson, is shown in Figure 11.6. Definitive surgery to repair a fistula should be delayed until the patient's general condition has improved and the fistula has 'matured'. A mature small bowel fistula is one which starts to form a spout similar to an ileostomy. This is a sign that the peritoneal cavity is reforming, as inflammatory exudate and adhesions are absorbed, and indicates that conditions are now favourable for definitive reconstructive surgery to the gastrointestinal tract (see Chapter 22).

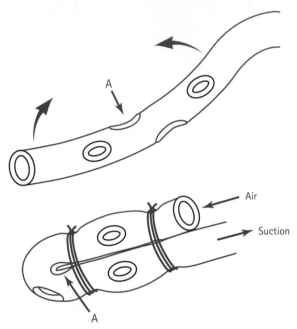

Figure 11.6 *A simple surface drain, constructed from a length of tubing, for the collection of fistula effluent from a deep granulating wound. Hole A allows the tube to be folded without buckling. The air sucked in from the open end prevents blockage of the holes by tissue drawn in by the suction.*

Long-term intestinal failure

A small contingent of patients require long-term nutritional support. The commonest cause of the intestinal failure is a short small bowel following major resection. The surgeon may have had no other option when faced at emergency laparotomy with extensive small bowel infarction. This is discussed further in Chapter 22, but it is most frequently the result of a major vascular occlusion in the superior mesenteric vessels by embolus or thrombus. A small bowel volvulus may also result in extensive infarction, and subsequent resection of a large proportion of the small bowel. The other large group of surgical patients with intestinal failure are those who have severe Crohn's disease and have had multiple resections of severely diseased segments. The surgical management of Crohn's disease is discussed in Chapter 22, but in general resections should always be planned so as to remove

the minimum of normal bowel. However, attempts to avoid further resections in the presence of strictures may be nutritionally counterproductive. A partially obstructed small bowel, proximal to a stricture, becomes dilated with resultant stasis and bacterial overgrowth. This causes mucosal damage which impairs the absorptive capacity of an otherwise normal segment of small bowel.

When a surgeon is planning a major small bowel resection, it is important that the length of small bowel which will be retained is measured accurately. This is the important measurement, and not the length which is to be excised, as the normal small bowel length may vary between 300 and 850 cm. Preservation of the colon is now known to improve nutrition, as well as reducing fluid losses after major small bowel resection. If less than 200 cm of small bowel can be saved, some nutritional problems should be anticipated, but the main early difficulty will be the fluid losses. If less than 100 cm can be saved the patient will need intensive nutritional support, with intravenous feeding during the early months. However, as there is some adaptation of the remaining bowel it may be possible later to wean the patient on to a normal oral intake with supplements. If less than 50 cm can be preserved, the patient will almost certainly need long-term intravenous feeding. If prolonged intravenous feeding is obviously impractical, as in the very elderly patient with major co-morbidity, a resection which leaves only a few centimetres of small bowel merely condemns the patient to a slower and more distressing death than deciding the situation is inoperable, closing the abdomen and giving adequate pain relief. Surgeons practising in areas of the world with limited health resources, and no realistic hope of long-term intensive nutritional support, may have to make a similar decision even in younger, previously fit patients.

Small bowel transplants have been used successfully in occasional patients with irreversible intestinal failure, but these are still in the developmental stage. Rejection is a major problem.

COOPERATION BETWEEN SURGICAL SPECIALISTS IN THE ABDOMEN

Within the abdomen, pathology in one system may result in complications in another. Diverticulitis or colonic cancer may cause a colovesical fistula. An infected aortic graft may present with an aorto-duodenal fistula and gastrointestinal haemorrhage. Similarly, the surgery of one system may cause complications in another. Surgery on the uterus or bowel may damage a ureter, and surgery on the aorta may render the colon ischaemic. Radiotherapy to one organ may damage another. Cooperation between surgical specialists is required both for these problems, and for the extensive radical surgery sometimes indicated for advanced malignancy.

In reconstructive urological surgery small bowel is required as a urothelial substitute, and the general surgeon may be involved in these operations, or in the complications of such procedures. Small bowel is of great value within the abdomen and pelvis for reconstruction. Its excellent blood supply allows a segment to be isolated on its vascular pedicle, and the techniques are described in Chapter 21. The stomach or colon may be mobilized into the chest, or even up into the neck, to replace the oesophagus, and the general surgeon may be working with the thoracic or ENT surgeons.

COOPERATION WITH NON-SURGICAL INTERVENTIONALISTS

Historically, many intra-abdominal problems could only be managed by open surgery. Today, many such problems are also amenable to intervention by endoscopic or radiological techniques, and cooperation between surgeons and non-surgical interventionists is of particular importance. Haemorrhage from a duodenal ulcer can frequently be arrested at gastroscopy by a range of techniques, including the injection of adrenaline around the bleeding vessel, and most large bowel polyps can be removed at colonoscopy. Stones in the common bile duct can be removed at endoscopic retrograde cholangiopancreatography (ERCP) and sphincterotomy. Malignant obstructions of the cardia, pylorus and colon can be relieved by endoluminal stenting by endoscopist or radiologist, as can malignant jaundice by stenting of the bile ducts.

Localized intra-abdominal collections can be drained percutaneously by either ultrasound or computed tomography-guided percutaneous aspiration. A drain can also be accurately sited and secured under image control. Nephrostomy drainage of an obstructed kidney is now routinely established using a similar technique. Embolization of a bleeding vessel may be preferable to surgery and has been used in angiodysplastic colonic bleeding, secondary haemorrhage after radical gastrectomy, and in liver and pelvic haemorrhage from major trauma. Embolization may also be used to reduce the vascularity of a renal tumour, or to obliterate a varicocele. Further endovascular intra-abdominal procedures performed by radiologists include stenting of the aorta and renal arteries for aneurysmal disease and stenosis respectively, and the placement of inferior vena caval filters for the prevention of pulmonary emboli. When a portocaval shunt is indicated for portal hypertension, this can be performed by the endovascular TIPSS (transhepatic insertion of a portosystemic shunt) procedure and an open operation avoided. Lumbar sympathectomy is now seldom performed as an open operation, but rather as a percutaneous image-guided injection procedure.

Alternatives to surgical intervention are discussed where relevant throughout the text. The choice of method is often more dependent on the availability of equipment and the individual skills of the surgeon, radiologist and endoscopist than on the pathology itself.

REFERENCES

1. *Clinical Surgery in General*, 4th edn. RM Kirk, WJ Ribbans. Edinburgh: Elsevier Churchill Livingstone, 2003.
2. *Essential Surgical Practice*, 4th edn. A Cuschieri, R Steele, A Moossa. London: Hodder Arnold, 2001.
3. Karanjia ND, Walker A, Rees M. Fluids and electrolytes in surgery. *Surgery* 1992; **10**: 121–8.
4. Schein M, Ivatury R. Intra-abdominal hypertension and the abdominal compartment syndrome. Leading article. *Br J Surg* 1998; **85**: 1027–8.
5. MacFie J. Bacterial translocation in surgical patients. *Ann R Coll Surg Engl* 1997; **79**: 183–9.
6. D'Amico R, Pifferi S, Leonetti C, *et al.* Effectiveness of prophylaxis in critically ill adult patients: systematic review of randomised controlled trials. *Br Med J* 1998; **316**: 1975–85.
7. Oláh A, Belágyi T, Issekutz Á, *et al.* Randomised clinical trial of specific lactobacillus and fibre supplement to early enteral nutrition in patients with acute pancreatitis. *Br J Surg* 2002; **89**: 1103–7.
8. Studley HO. Percentage of weight loss: a basic indicator of surgical risk in patients with chronic peptic ulcer. *JAMA* 1936; **106**: 458–60.
9. Sarr MG. Appropriate use, complications and advantages demonstrated in 500 consecutive needle catheter jejunostomies. *Br J Surg* 1999; **86**: 557–61.
10. Scott NA, Leinhardt DJ, O'Hanrahan T, *et al.* Spectrum of intestinal failure in a specialised unit. *Lancet* 1991; **337**: 471–3.

12

SURGICAL ACCESS TO THE ABDOMEN AND SURGERY OF THE ABDOMINAL WALL

Access through the abdominal wall for open surgery must be made through an incision of sufficient length to allow the surgeon a good view of the operating field, and to permit the entry of hands and instruments. An exception is an operation on a mobile structure which can be delivered through a small wound, and the surgery performed outside the abdomen (e.g. appendicectomy).

In laparoscopic surgery, the surgeon's hands remain outside the abdomen, while a gas-filled space is created into which the camera and instruments are inserted. Good views and operating conditions can be obtained for deep set structures which would require large incisions for safe conventional surgery to be performed. Laparoscopic surgery is still advancing, and with refinement of both skills and equipment an increasing number of procedures will become feasible. A compromise between laparoscopic and open techniques may be beneficial. For example, after a laparoscopic dissection a small incision may be employed for the delivery of an intact specimen. A small incision may also be used to exteriorize the bowel for an intestinal anastomosis. A hand port is another development in laparoscopic surgery which combines the advantages of the superior laparoscopic visualization with the facility for manual palpation and retraction.

Other minimal access techniques have evolved. Endoscopy is no longer a purely diagnostic tool, and is now used for a range of 'surgical procedures' within the abdomen. Endoscopic techniques are not within the remit of this book, but they are mentioned in the text where they offer a reasonable alternative to open or laparoscopic surgery.

GENERAL TECHNIQUES

Patient position

For most abdominal procedures the patient is supine. The general considerations are similar for all surgery and are discussed in Appendix II. It is frequently helpful to roll the patient to one side or the other, or to tilt the table head-up or -down for part of the operation. This should be anticipated in the initial positioning of the patient, who must also be secure in the new position with pressure points protected. If there is any likelihood of dissection being required in the pelvis the legs should be elevated, and suitably supported as shown in Figure 12.1. Simple straps are suitable for a short operation, but the pressure points are inadequately protected and the hips are too acutely flexed for this position to be suitable for a more lengthy procedure. A 'legs-up' position allows access to the perineum for surgery, and there is room for an assistant to stand between the legs. For loin and thoraco-abdominal incisions the patient may be in a full or partially lateral position. Lateral flexion of the patient will then increase the access between the ribs, and between the costal margin and the iliac crest. This can be achieved by angulation of the upper and lower portions of the operating table, or simply with the placement of a sandbag (Fig. 12.2).

Anaesthesia and relaxant

An intra-abdominal operation requires relaxation of the abdominal musculature in addition to anaesthesia. When a muscle relaxant is used in combination with a general

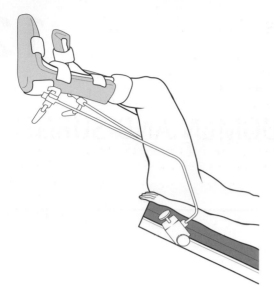

Figure 12.1 *The Lloyd Davis position which is suitable for prolonged surgery. The perineum is accessible and an assistant can stand between the patient's legs. The Trendelenberg head-down tilt improves pelvic access as mobile abdominal contents fall out of the pelvis.*

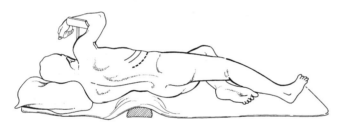

Figure 12.2 *Patients placed in a lateral position require support for the upper arm. They are more stable if one leg is flexed and one bent, but will still require restraints to prevent rolling. Lateral flexion induced by angulation between the two portions of the table increases loin access. If the operating table does not 'break', a similar position can be simply achieved with a sandbag.*

anaesthetic, the patient must be ventilated. A spinal or epidural anaesthetic can provide good operative conditions for a lower abdominal laparotomy. The patient is conscious and able to breathe spontaneously, but the abdominal muscles are relaxed. This approach is less suitable for an upper abdominal laparotomy. Epidurals are also frequently used as an adjunct to a general anaesthetic, and are then continued for postoperative pain relief. Local infiltrative anaesthesia does not provide muscle relaxation, and often gives poor anaesthesia of the parietal peritoneum. However, this can be overcome by combining local infiltration with blockade of intercostal nerves as they emerge from under the costal margin. Although such local anaesthetic techniques may occasionally be useful, it must be remembered that the success of major intra-abdominal surgery, especially in the ill or elderly

patient, is heavily dependent on the intensive intraoperative management of the patient by the anaesthetist.

Urinary catheterization

For most major intra-abdominal surgery the anaesthetist will wish the patient to be catheterized so that intraoperative urine output can be measured. Surgical access to the pelvis is hampered by a bladder which is filling during the operation, and is another indication for catheterization. Urinary catheter drainage, once established, is usually continued postoperatively as it is easier for the patient during the first few days after major surgery. In addition, any elderly male patient who has had pelvic surgery, and any patient who is receiving epidural postoperative pain relief, will almost certainly develop urinary retention if not catheterized.

Gastric aspiration

Intraoperative gastric distension may limit surgical access in the upper abdomen, and a nasogastric tube, inserted by the anaesthetist before surgery is commenced, can be helpful. If a prolonged ileus, or a delay in gastric emptying, is predicted, the tube is left *in situ* for continued aspiration during the postoperative period.

ANATOMY OF THE ABDOMINAL WALL

Muscles

The muscles of the anterior abdominal wall are the external oblique, the internal oblique, the transversus abdominis, and the rectus abdominis. (The pyramidales muscles are frequently absent and are of no surgical importance.) In general, the first three of these have attachments to the lower ribs and the iliac crest. The second and third muscles also arise from the lumbar fascia. As they traverse the front of the abdomen they become aponeurotic, and are inserted mainly into the *linea alba*, a band of fibrous tissue extending in the midline from the xiphoid process to the pubis. Before they reach the linea alba they combine to form a sheath for the rectus muscle. Above the umbilicus the linea alba is 1–2 cm wide, but in its lower part it is much narrower.

- *External oblique* runs mainly downwards, forwards and medially, but its upper fibres are nearly horizontal. Its lower fibres, inserting into the iliac crest, are nearly vertical. Its lower free border forms the *inguinal ligament* which stretches from the anterior superior iliac spine to the pubic tubercle.
- *Internal oblique* runs mainly in a slightly upward and medial direction, but its lowest fibres, which descend to the pubis, are almost vertical.

- *Transversus abdominis* is the deepest muscle, and runs mainly horizontally, although its lowest fibres run downwards along with those of internal oblique as the conjoint tendon. Its deep surface is lined by transversalis fascia; between this and the peritoneum there is a layer of extraperitoneal fat of variable thickness.
- *Rectus abdominis* lies alongside the linea alba, stretching from the front of the pubis inferiorly to the xiphoid process and beyond to the 5th, 6th and 7th costal cartilages. Its substance is traversed by three horizontal *tendinous intersections,* one opposite the umbilicus, another near the xiphoid, and a third midway between these.

RECTUS SHEATH

This is formed by the aponeuroses of external oblique, internal oblique and the transversus abdominis, the last two of which are arranged in a somewhat complicated manner (Fig. 12.3).

The *anterior sheath* is complete from rib margin to pubis. In its upper three-quarters it is formed by external oblique and by the anterior lamina of internal oblique. In the lower one-quarter it is formed by all three aponeuroses. It is adherent to the tendinous intersections of the rectus muscle.

The *posterior sheath* is complete only as far down as a point midway between umbilicus and pubis, where it ends as a free border, the *arcuate line.* Below this level the sheath is deficient, the rectus being separated from the peritoneum by transversalis fascia alone. The posterior sheath is formed by the posterior lamina of internal oblique fused with transversus. Some fleshy fibres of transversus appear in the upper part of the posterior sheath. The tendinous intersections do not extend to the posterior surface of the rectus abdominis.

Vessels

The *inferior epigastric vessels* are of considerable surgical significance. The artery, arising from the external iliac, passes medial to the deep inguinal ring as it runs upwards and medially on the deep aspect of the abdominal wall musculature and enters the rectus sheath. The companion vein joins the external iliac vein. The smaller *superior epigastric artery* is a terminal branch of the internal thoracic artery and enters the sheath from under the costal margin. The two vessels have anastomotic connections within the belly of the muscle. It is this vascular arrangement which enables the surgeon to use the rectus muscle as a reconstructive flap which can be swung cranially or caudally.

Nerves

The nerves of the abdominal wall are the *lower five intercostal,* the *subcostal,* the *iliohypogastric* and the *ilioinguinal.* They run an oblique course in the abdominal wall, lying mainly between transversus and internal oblique. All except for the last two enter the rectus sheath and pierce the rectus to end as cutaneous branches.

INCISIONS FOR ABDOMINAL SURGERY

Many approaches to the abdomen are suitable (Fig. 12.4), and the choice of incision is mainly related to the access required. The surgical indications for each incision and their execution are discussed individually below, but the technique for opening the peritoneum is similar in all incisions and therefore considered first.

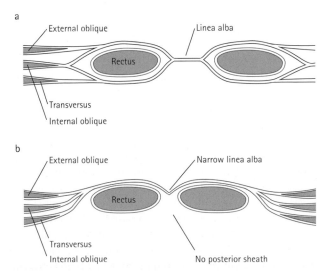

Figure 12.3 *The rectus sheath is formed from the aponeuroses of external oblique, internal oblique and transversus. (a) A transverse section of the sheath above the arcuate line; (b) a transverse section of the sheath below the arcuate line.*

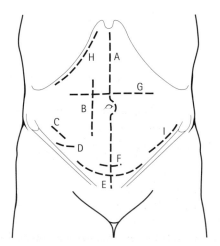

Figure 12.4 *A selection of common abdominal incisions.*
A *midline;* B *paramedian;* C *gridiron;* D *Lanz;* E *Pfannenstiel;*
F *suprapubic;* G *transverse upper abdominal;* H *subcostal 'Kocher';*
I *oblique iliac muscle-cutting.*

Opening the peritoneum

The utmost care must be taken to ensure that no underlying viscus is injured during incision of the peritoneum. Except at the umbilical cicatrix and at surgical scars, the peritoneum is separated from the abdominal wall by a variable layer of extraperitoneal fat. When the peritoneum has been exposed, a small bite is taken with artery forceps, and is lifted forwards. It is an advantage to do this during expiration, when the viscera tend to fall away from the abdominal wall. The fold which is lifted up may be given a gentle shake to dislodge any adherent structure, or it may be pinched between finger and thumb so that its thickness can be estimated. A second artery forceps is then applied alongside the first, and the fold is carefully incised (Fig. 12.5). If an opening is not immediately apparent the forceps should be taken off and re-applied. As soon as the peritoneum is breached, air enters and a space is created between the parietal peritoneum and the intraperitoneal structures. When the initial opening has been made it is enlarged – usually by cutting with scissors or diathermy

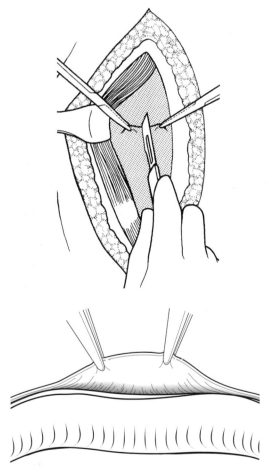

Figure 12.5 *The initial incision through the parietal peritoneum is inherently dangerous as the peritoneal cavity is only a potential space until air can enter. The creation of a peritoneal fold between two forceps is a time-honoured manoeuvre to exclude bowel from this incision.*

under direct vision. If the under-surface of the peritoneum is not visible, a finger should be inserted to check that no bowel is adherent to the peritoneum in the line of the incision. Particular care must be taken in opening an old incision, as the abdominal wall musculature and peritoneum are adherent and often fused into a single layer of fibrous scar to which loops of small bowel may be adherent. Even with great care inadvertent enterotomy may occur and greatly increases morbidity.[1]

Midline incisions

Midline incisions provide good access to the whole abdomen. The linea alba may be divided from xiphisternum to symphysis pubis, although commonly a shorter incision is made and only extended if necessary. A large xiphisternum can be excised if it is restricting access. Troublesome bleeding may then occur from the terminal branches of the internal thoracic artery, which will require diathermy coagulation. The main disadvantage of a midline incision is that it crosses the natural crease lines of the skin and a hypertrophic scar is common, especially in young children. In addition to the cosmetic issues, the thickening and shortening of the scar at the waist crease may be irritated by clothes. The umbilicus presents an additional cosmetic challenge. A straight incision through the umbilicus is favoured by some surgeons, but most prefer to curve the incision around it, taking care to cut the skin perpendicular on the curve. Forceps placed on the umbilical skin, retracting it to one side and holding the skin taut while the skin incision is made, may be helpful. An alternative is to make the whole skin incision paramedian, followed by a midline incision through the linea alba.

The incision is deepened through the subcutaneous fat, either with a scalpel or with diathermy, and any bleeding vessels controlled, until the linea alba is exposed throughout the length of the incision. At the umbilical cicatrix the peritoneum is in close apposition to the linea alba, and this is often the easiest and safest place to gain access to the peritoneal cavity. Two forceps are applied to the linea alba, one either side of the midline, and it is lifted upwards while the fascia is carefully incised. If this incision does not enter the peritoneal cavity the peritoneum is incised separately. The linea alba above and below the umbilicus is separated from the peritoneum by a significant layer of extraperitoneal fat and may be divided without immediate entry through the parietal peritoneum, which is then incised as a separate layer.

As the incision is extended it is possible, if exactly in the midline, to encounter no muscle fibres. Below the arcuate line however, the linea alba is narrow and there is no posterior sheath. In addition, pyramidalis may be obvious. In this area visible muscle fibres do not indicate that the incision has strayed from the midline. The rectus muscles may be separated right down to the symphysis pubis, but care must be taken in extending the peritoneal division down to this level or an inadvertent incision may be made into the bladder. The peritoneal incision must therefore be deviated laterally if further low division is required for access. In the upper abdomen there is a significant pad of extraperitoneal fat which extends a few centimetres either side of the midline. Some surgeons therefore prefer to divide the peritoneum lateral to this. The fold of the falciform ligament extending from the liver to the anterior abdominal wall may cause some confusion, and it may need to be divided for access. Vessels running within the ligament can cause troublesome bleeding if not secured.

Suprapubic incisions are transverse skin incisions placed just above the pubis. The incision through the abdominal wall, however, is a lower abdominal midline incision. The skin and subcutaneous tissue are reflected up, off the anterior rectus sheath, and the remainder of the incision is then vertical. The skin incision lies in, or parallel to, a deep skin crease, in contrast to a midline skin incision which crosses it. If access is required to the prostate or bladder the peritoneum is left intact after separation of the recti and the pre peritoneal space is developed distally.

Closure of a midline incision is perfectly adequate in a single layer (mass closure), with a continuous suture. The peritoneum may be included in the closure, but this is not essential as it will appose naturally when the fascia is closed. The suture material must retain tensile strength until the healing fascial scar has developed its own. Thus, either a non-absorbable material should be used, or an absorbable material which loses its tensile strength slowly. A strong (gauge 1 or 0) monofilament nylon or polydioxanone (PDS) suture is therefore suitable. Closure is started at one end and a knot formed. If the first stitch is inserted from under the fascia, the knot will lie deep to the fascia. Each suture should be placed so that it lies no more than 1 cm advanced from the previous suture and the needle should be inserted 1 cm from the cut edge (Fig. 12.6). If the incision has entered the rectus sheath, the anterior sheath may retract, and great care must be taken to include it in the sutures as this is the most important layer for the strength of the wound. The temptation to pull the suture tight must be resisted as this strangulates the tissue. The suture should only be as tight as is required to hold the edges in apposition. If these rules are followed, the total length of suture material used will be at least three times the length of the incision. Two or three lengths of suture will be required for a long midline incision. An Aberdeen knot (see Chapter 1) may be used to tie the suture at the end of a continuous suture, but a more satisfactory method is to start a second suture from the opposite end and tie the two ends together where they meet. A non-absorbable knot outside the fascia can be troublesome in a thin patient. Again it is possible, by finishing the suture on the inside, to tie a knot which will lie under the fascia. Alternatively, the cut ends of a knot should be passed under an adjacent suture to hold it lying flat.

The midline incision only became universally popular with the development of inert non-absorbable suture mate-

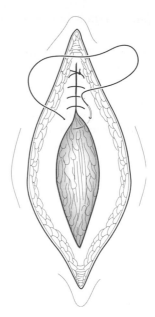

Figure 12.6 *Wound dehiscence and incisional herniae can be largely avoided by meticulous closure of the abdominal wall. The sutures must not be pulled tight. They must be suitably spaced at a maximum of 1 cm apart. Each tissue bite must be of adequate strength, and the suture should be introduced about 1 cm from the cut edge.*

rial such as nylon, and slowly absorbable synthetic material such as PDS. Silk was never popular for abdominal wall closure after gastrointestinal surgery since, if a wound infection developed, healing did not occur until all infected braided suture material was removed. Catgut was in general use for abdominal closure but, as it lost its tensile strength within two weeks, burst abdomens and incisional herniae were a relatively common complication with midline wounds. Paramedian incisions were favoured for their additional strength. However, it should be remembered that incisional herniae are still more common following midline than following paramedian incisions, even when modern suture materials are used.[2]

Paramedian incisions

These provide broadly similar access to midline incisions, but they are no longer in regular use. They were favoured for their additional strength when catgut was the suture material for abdominal wall closure. The paramedian skin incision avoids the challenges posed by the umbilicus, and is deepened down to the fascia of the anterior layer of the rectus sheath. This is incised in line with the skin incision to expose the rectus muscle, which is displaced laterally preserving its innervation. The muscle must be released from the sheath where it is tethered at the tendinous intersections. The posterior sheath is exposed and then divided in line with the anterior incision and the peritoneum is opened as described above.

Closure of a paramedian incision is undertaken in two layers. After the posterior sheath has been repaired, the rectus muscle is released back into its original position before the anterior sheath is sutured. The muscle lies between the two suture lines and may give some strength to the closure (Fig. 12.7). The additional tension sutures in this old illustration underlines the concern over dehiscence when catgut was in routine use.

Appendix muscle-splitting incisions

These provide limited access, but sufficient for an appendicectomy as the appendix and part of the caecum can be delivered out through the incision. The gridiron and Lanz incisions (see Fig. 12.4) differ in their skin alignment, but the deeper aspects of the incisions are similar. The external oblique aponeurosis is divided in line with its fibres to expose the fleshy internal oblique. Internal oblique and the underlying transversus are split in line with their fibres by blunt dissection (Fig. 12.8). Retraction displays the peritoneum which is entered as described above. If more extensive access becomes necessary, the incision may be extended upwards and laterally by converting it to a muscle-cutting incision and dividing internal oblique and transversus in line with the external oblique division. Alternatively, medial access can be increased by dividing the lateral edge of the rectus sheath.

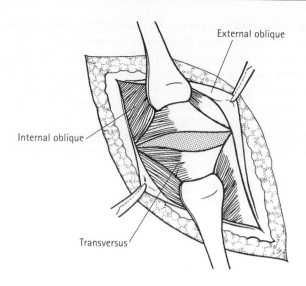

Figure 12.8 *An appendix muscle-splitting incision. The external oblique aponeurosis has been split in line with its fibres. The internal oblique and transversus are split between muscle bellies in a more or less transverse direction, and held apart by retractors to expose transversalis fascia and peritoneum.*

This allows wider separation of the internal oblique and transversus muscles, and the rectus muscle can be displaced medially (Fig. 12.9).

Closure of appendix incisions is performed in layers. The peritoneum is closed first with a continuous absorbable suture. One or two loose absorbable sutures appose the muscles, and finally the external oblique is closed with a continuous or interrupted absorbable suture (Fig. 12.10). Even when catgut was routinely used for these wounds incisional herniae were very rare.

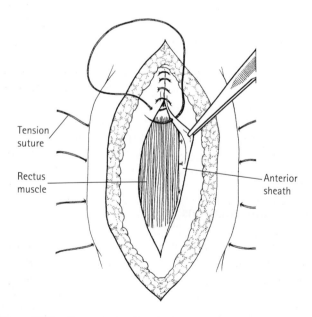

Figure 12.7 *The posterior sheath of this paramedian incision has been closed and the rectus muscle returned to the neutral position where it will lie between the two suture lines, giving support to the catgut closure. Note the additional 'tension sutures'; this was another feature of abdominal wound closure prior to the availability of modern suture materials.*

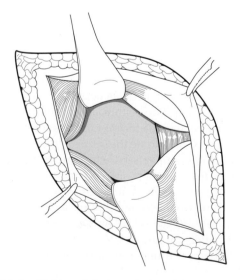

Figure 12.9 *Division of the lateral edge of the rectus sheath may be a useful manoeuvre to enlarge an appendix incision.*

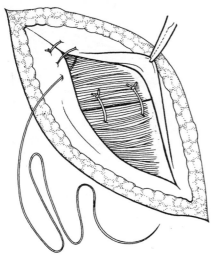

Figure 12.10 *Closure of an appendix incision is in layers. The muscle sutures must be loose in order to avoid tissue strangulation.*

Pfannenstiel incisions

Pfannenstiel incisions also avoid the division of muscle. The scar is less obtrusive than the alternative lower abdominal midline incision, but at the cost of altered sensation of the lower abdominal skin. These incisions afford good access to the bladder, prostate and female reproductive organs, and are extensively used by gynaecologists. However, they are less suitable for rectal surgery as the splenic flexure will frequently have to be mobilized before an anastomosis can be performed, and access for this manoeuvre is very limited. The skin incision is a curved transverse incision, convex downwards, centred a few centimetres above the pubis. The abdominal muscles are not divided transversely. The anterior layer of the rectus sheath alone is divided in line with the skin incision, dissected off the rectus muscle, and sheath and skin are reflected upwards (Fig. 12.11). The rectus muscles

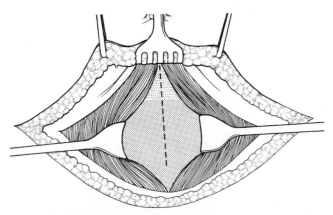

Figure 12.11 *A Pfannenstiel incision. The anterior rectus sheath is divided transversely and elevated with the skin. The recti are separated and the abdomen entered vertically.*

are separated in the midline and retracted to expose the transversalis fascia and the peritoneum (above the arcuate line there will also be posterior rectus sheath).

Closure of Pfannenstiel incisions is in layers, and particular care must be taken over the fascial closure at the upper extremity or an incisional hernia may develop at the umbilicus.

Muscle–cutting incisions

These can be adapted to provide the access required, and may be either transverse or oblique. The fascia and muscles are generally divided in line with the skin incision. Diathermy division of the muscle bellies reduces blood loss from small vessels, but larger vessels require individual ligation. Retraction of the divided muscle fibres is seldom a problem except when the lower rectus muscle is cut transversely. Rectus muscle retraction in the upper abdomen is prevented by the muscle's tendinous intersections, which are attached to the rectus sheath. After division of the abdominal muscles in line with the skin incision, the peritoneum is picked up, incised and the peritoneal cavity entered as described above.

A **long transverse muscle-cutting** incision, either just above or below the umbilicus, provides good access to most of the abdomen. Access however is partially dependent on patient build, and this incision generally allows better access in those with a short wide abdomen and a wide costal angle (see Fig. 12.4). A transverse incision divides the abdominal skin in line with the skin creases and gives a good cosmetic scar. The postoperative pain is restricted to fewer dermatomes, and in particular the avoidance of an upper abdominal wound results in better respiratory effort during the early postoperative period. Access to the oesophageal hiatus and the pelvis is however usually inferior to that obtained with a long midline incision.

In *infants*, transverse incisions are preferable to midline incisions. The abdominal muscle bulk is small, the abdomen is short and wide and the costal angle is obtuse, allowing easy access to the diaphragm. The pelvis is poorly developed in infancy, and pelvic access is not made any more difficult by a transverse approach. A transverse scar is cosmetically superior in the infant and child, especially as a vertical scar forms a 'contracture' as the child grows. In neonatal abdominal surgery the vessels associated with the placenta may still be patent and require formal ligation. The umbilical vein lies in the midline above the umbilicus, initially between the linea alba and the peritoneum before turning deep to run towards the liver in the free edge of the falciform ligament. The umbilical arteries lie either side of the midline below the umbilicus and converge towards the umbilicus from their origin from the internal iliac arteries. They lie between the peritoneum and the abdominal wall muscles.

Oblique subcostal muscle-cutting incisions provide good access to the upper abdomen. A right subcostal (Kocher) incision can be used for liver and biliary surgery, and a left subcostal for splenic surgery. The angulation of the incision overcomes the limitations imposed by a narrow costal angle, but several abdominal nerves are divided. A bilateral subcostal incision – sometimes described as a chevron or rooftop incision – is in essence a modification of a transverse incision which gives excellent access to the upper abdomen, though many of the advantages of a transverse incision at the level of the umbilicus are lost.

Oblique iliac fossa muscle-cutting incisions are useful for access to the sigmoid colon and the ureter. They are similar to the appendix incisions except that no attempt is made to separate the internal oblique and transversus muscles in the line of their fibres. The muscles are cut in the same axis as the incision of external oblique. If access to the retroperitoneal organs is desired the peritoneum is not opened, but swept medially.

Loin incisions

A loin incision is often just a more posterior variety of the oblique muscle-cutting incision. At the posterior end of the incision latissimus dorsi, serratus posterior inferior and quadratus lumborum replace the external and internal oblique muscles of the more anterior incision (Fig. 12.12). All muscles are divided in line with the skin incision. The incision may be positioned to be subcostal, or over and in line with the 10th to 12th ribs. If the incision is *subcostal*, posterior division of the renal fascia gives access to the retroperitoneal fat (Fig. 12.13) and the peritoneum is swept away anteriorly. A higher incision gives better access to the kidney or adrenal. A *supracostal* incision along the superior border of the 10th, 11th or 12th rib will usually allow good renal access. Alternatively, the incision may be through the bed of the lowest palpable rib – the 12th, or the 11th if the

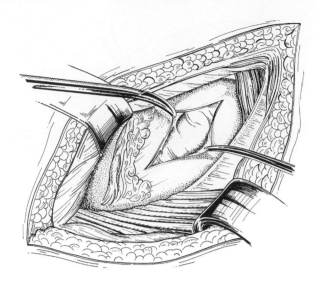

Figure 12.13 *The renal fascia is incised posteriorly so that it is not confused with the peritoneum, which is swept away anteriorly as the perinephric fat is entered.*

12th is rudimentary. The periosteum over the rib is exposed and incised. The rib is freed sub-periosteally, and then divided near its angle and the anterior part removed. Incision of the bed of the rib gives access into the retroperitoneal space. If the incision is at the level of the 10th rib, access can be increased by conversion to a *posterior thoraco-abdominal incision*. The thoracic component of the incision is deepened and the pleura opened. The diaphragm is incised in line with the incision.

A further alternative in the loin is the **lumbotomy**, in which a vertical incision is made from the lowest rib to the iliac crest along the lateral border of sacrospinalis, and deepened through muscles and fascia into the retroperitoneal space (Fig. 12.14).

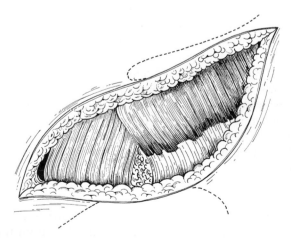

Figure 12.12 *The oblique loin incision exposes the external oblique muscle anteriorly and the latissimus dorsi posteriorly. These are divided in line with the skin incision to expose the second layer of musculature, the division of which exposes the renal fascia.*

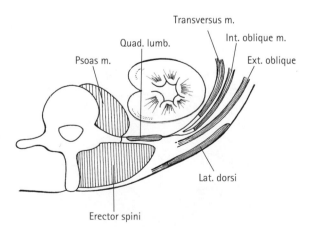

Figure 12.14 *The lumbotomy incision. The vertical incision through latissimus dorsi exposes the free posterior edge of external oblique. This is retracted forwards to expose the fused layers of the lumbodorsal fascia. Division of this layer exposes the renal fascia.*

Closure of all muscle-cutting incisions is usually in two layers, using a continuous suture. The inner layer consists of peritoneum, transversalis fascia, transversus and internal oblique muscles – or the more posterior equivalents – along with the posterior rectus sheath. Most surgeons prefer to use an absorbable suture for this layer. The outer layer consists of external oblique and the anterior rectus sheath, and normally incorporates a variable portion of the rectus muscle. This layer should be closed either with non-absorbable material or with an absorbable suture which retains tensile strength for several weeks. The covering fascia of the muscles has more strength than the muscle fibres and should always be included in the bites. Sutures must not be over-tightened or muscle strangulation occurs.

Anterior thoraco–abdominal incisions

These incisions provide simultaneous access to the abdomen and chest by division of the costal margin (Fig. 12.15), and can be used for access to the lower oesophagus or liver. Division of the costal margin impairs postoperative respiratory function, and this incision is now often avoided in favour of a trans-diaphragmatic or transhiatal approach (see Chapters 7 and 16). Thoraco-abdominal incisions extend obliquely upwards and laterally from a point midway between the umbilicus and xiphisternum to cross the costal margin and continue along the 8th interspace. The abdominal portion of the incision is an oblique, muscle-cutting incision. Alternatively, an initial midline incision can be extended laterally across the costal margin. Entry into the chest may be through an intercostal space or through the base of a rib after resection (see Chapter 7).

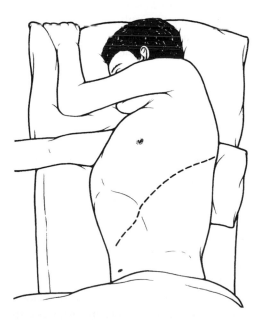

Figure 12.15 *Thoraco-abdominal incisions give good simultaneous access to chest and abdomen, but division of the costal margin carries significant morbidity.*

The diaphragm can be divided radially from the costal margin towards the hiatus to produce a single abdominothoracic cavity. Alternatively, it can be divided circumferentially 2 cm in from the chest wall – thereby preserving its innervation and leaving a cuff of diaphragm for re-attachment. This incision allows simultaneous access to both chest and abdomen, but these remain as two separate body cavities.

Closure of thoraco-abdominal incisions must include careful attention to diaphragmatic closure in order to prevent an iatrogenic diaphragmatic hernia. The use of a chest drain is usually indicated.

LAPAROSCOPIC ACCESS

Intraperitoneal laparoscopic surgery

This approach depends first on the safe establishment of access to the peritoneal cavity. A pneumoperitoneum creates the space within which the surgeon works with high-quality visualization from a light source and a video camera. Initially, blind puncture with a Veress needle through the linea alba was the favoured technique, but this has been increasingly abandoned as it carries a risk of damage to the bowel, and in slim patients major injuries to the aorta and iliac vessels have been reported. It is safer to establish initial access under direct vision.[3] The first port is most commonly established at the umbilicus, where a 1- to 2-cm incision in the umbilical pit allows the linea alba to be picked up with two artery forceps. The peritoneum is then opened by the same technique that is used for an open laparotomy. The pneumoperitoneum is created through this opening by gas insufflation and, once established, the camera is inserted. Insertion of the subsequent ports is much safer as the abdominal wall is lifted forwards away from the bowel by the pneumoperitoneum and, in addition, the point of the trocar can be viewed from within as it pierces the parietal peritoneum. On each occasion a small skin incision is made prior to the introduction of the trocar.

The position of subsequent ports depends not only on the surgery to be performed but also on the preference of the surgeon. Instruments which are introduced through the ports should ideally converge in the surgical field at an angle of between 60 and 90 degrees to ensure maximum manoeuvrability. Ports which are positioned too close to each other will result in the intraperitoneal portions of the trocars clashing during manipulation of the instruments. In an adult abdomen this is unlikely to be a problem if the ports are never established less than 15 cm apart. For some procedures three ports are sufficient, but more commonly four ports are used of which two are 5 mm and two are 11 mm. At the end of the procedure the smaller port sites require only skin closure, but fascial closure of the larger port sites is recommended to prevent herniation.

Extraperitoneal laparoscopic surgery

This approach relies on the creation of a space outside the peritoneal cavity, although direct gas insufflation creates a disappointingly small space for the surgeon. The gas tracks over a wide field and fails to disrupt the tough fibromuscular septa within the fat.

The introduction of a balloon technique to create a larger, more localized space, allowed the development of a minimal access approach as an alternative to open surgery for most retroperitoneal structures.[4] The surgery is, however, technically demanding and good results will only be achieved by those surgeons with a special interest.

An initial 1- to 2-cm skin incision is made in the lumbar, iliac, infra-umbilical or suprapubic position. It is deepened through the abdominal wall by a combination of sharp and blunt dissection. The deflated balloon with catheter is then introduced along the track into the extraperitoneal fat. Inflation of the balloon creates the space for surgery. A transparent balloon into which the laparoscope is passed is an adaptation which allows the work space to be formed under direct vision.

COMPLICATIONS FROM ABDOMINAL WOUNDS

Wound infections

Wound infections after gastrointestinal surgery have been reduced by the administration of prophylactic antibiotics. When there is an established infection, it will occasionally settle with antibiotic therapy, but frequently there is an infected haematoma which requires drainage. If the infected collection is subcutaneous, the skin scar can be disrupted easily, and virtually painlessly, at this early stage of healing. The wound must be opened over a sufficient length so that there is no residual infection deep to intact skin. Re-suturing is sometimes considered once the wound is clean, but is seldom necessary as the open wound heals surprisingly quickly. A wide skin scar can be revised if the final appearance is unsatisfactory.

Deep wound infections within the abdominal muscles often require formal re-exploration for drainage of pus. Systemic antibiotics are indicated and the surgeon must be alert to the dangers of a necrotizing infection in the abdominal wall (see Chapter 3). Occasionally, what appears initially to be a simple wound infection quickly declares itself as an intestinal cutaneous fistula as intestinal contents drain through the wound. This may have occurred secondary to an anastomotic breakdown, or from damage to a loop of bowel during the dissection or the abdominal closure. If there is no evidence of generalized peritonitis, exploration and repair should be delayed; the surgical management of such fistulae is discussed in Chapter 22.

Burst abdomen

Although a burst abdomen or complete abdominal dehiscence is now fortunately a rare complication, it was relatively common when laparotomy wounds were closed with catgut. It is now almost exclusively an indication of faulty technique. A poorly tied knot may have slipped, or the knot may have damaged the suture material, which subsequently fractured. The suture may have been pulled too tight and cut through the tissue, or the suture may have been carelessly sited and the fascia not included in the bites. The patient is usually making slow progress with a prolonged ileus. At around 7–10 days postoperatively, leakage of clear or serosanguineous fluid from the wound is the first ominous sign of incipient dehiscence. The fluid is from within the peritoneal cavity, and leaks because the deep layers of the wound have already separated. Often it is the removal of the skin sutures which allows the dehiscence to manifest and loops of bowel are extruded. Treatment consists of protection of the exposed bowel during a short period of fluid and electrolyte resuscitation. The patient should be returned to the operating theatre as soon as possible for secondary closure of the abdomen. Abdominal compartment syndrome may be of concern and, in exceptional circumstances, it may be preferable to manage the situation with temporary abdominal containment, or to leave the abdomen open as a laparostomy.

Incisional herniae

Incisional herniae may become apparent during the early months after surgery when there has almost certainly been some deep wound dehiscence in the postoperative period. A poor-quality scar, as a result of a wound infection or faulty closure technique may disrupt later however, and both morbid obesity and chronic cough greatly increase the risk.

TEMPORARY ABDOMINAL CONTAINMENT AND LAPAROSTOMY

Occasionally, it is impossible to close the abdomen due to a temporary increase in volume of the abdominal contents. The problem may be due to oedematous bowel or a retroperitoneal haematoma, or there may be packs to control bleeding which have reduced the available intra-abdominal capacity. Abdominal closure under tension should not be attempted as the sutures may cut through such that wound dehiscence is likely. Alternatively, if the wound closure does remain sound the increased pressure embarrasses respiratory function and intra-abdominal perfusion (see Chapter 11). A permanent mesh may be considered, but this may be unnecessary for a temporary situation, or contraindicated due to sepsis. A temporary container for the viscera can be constructed by sewing an intravenous fluid bag to the edges of the laparotomy wound[5] and the closure delayed for up to a week.

Gross intraperitoneal sepsis and fistulae may make any attempt to close an abdomen impossible. Consequently, the abdomen can be left open for several weeks while the sepsis is controlled, though such patients will require intensive care and often also respiratory support. When the abdomen is left open in this fashion it is described as a *laparostomy*.

ABDOMINAL WALL HAEMATOMA

Spontaneous rupture of an inferior epigastric artery results in a rectus sheath haematoma, and patients receiving anticoagulants are at increased risk of this condition. The tender abdominal mass can cause diagnostic confusion. Surgery is seldom indicated as there is a tamponade effect on the vessel from the blood clot. However, absorption of clotting factors within the haematoma may cause further derangements in blood clotting, with an ensuing 'vicious circle'. Anticoagulation will require to be reversed, clotting monitored, and consideration given as to whether to evacuate the haematoma or to treat the patient conservatively.

RECTUS ABDOMINIS FLAPS

The rectus abdominis myocutaneous flap is a versatile tool for reconstruction of the breast, chest wall and perineum.[6] The muscle can be used on its own, or with an ellipse of overlying anterior rectus sheath and abdominal skin to replace perineal or breast skin loss. The skin paddle, if required, is incised first. For perineal or sternal reconstruction, a vertical skin paddle is frequently used, and the flap is described as a vertical rectus abdominis myocutaneous (**VRAM**) flap. For breast reconstruction, a transverse skin paddle is preferred, and the flap is described as a **TRAM** flap. The muscle above and below the skin paddle is then exposed by a paramedian incision through the anterior rectus sheath. The whole muscle can be used, or only part of its width. The muscle is freed from the sheath at its tendinous intersections.

If the muscle is to be rotated into the pelvis, both the insertion and the origin of the muscle are divided, but great care must be taken to preserve the deep inferior epigastric vessels entering the muscle from below. For breast reconstruction the flap may be pedicled up on the superior epigastric pedicle. However, this artery, which is the continuation of the internal thoracic artery, is relatively small and the blood supply more precarious. For this reason, and to avoid the epigastric bulge caused by the tunnelling of the pedicle, a free TRAM flap is preferred by some breast surgeons. It is raised on the larger deep inferior epigastric artery and a microvascular anastomosis performed onto an artery in the axilla, or onto the internal thoracic vessels.

A transverse skin paddle can also be raised as a free flap, leaving the entire muscle behind. The small perforating vessels, on which the skin perfusion depends, are traced through the muscle to the main artery. This requires training, skill and magnification. The flap is described as a deep inferior epigastric artery perforator (**DIEP**) flap.

ABDOMINAL WALL HERNIAE

Spontaneous herniae of the abdominal wall occur most frequently in the midline and in the groin. Incisional herniae may develop in any surgical scar, and thus are also common in the midline. The surgical management of groin herniae, both inguinal and femoral, is discussed in Chapter 24, while hiatus herniae are discussed in Chapter 17. The surgical issues, and the repair, of the other spontaneous and incisional abdominal wall herniae are very similar, and are therefore considered together.

Most herniae have a sac of parietal peritoneum into which any mobile intraperitoneal structure may herniate. Some small herniae – of which epigastric are the commonest examples – initially have no sac and consist solely of extraperitoneal fat. They only acquire a sac if the herniae later enlarge. Many large herniae have both a sac and a significant extraperitoneal component, which may consist solely of extraperitoneal fat, but may also include a partially extraperitoneal viscus such as the bladder, caecum or sigmoid colon. These *sliding herniae* are particularly common in the groin (see Chapter 24).

A patient may request the repair of a hernia for either comfort or cosmesis, or a surgeon may recommend repair because of the risk of strangulation. As many patients are elderly or unfit, and somewhat reluctant to have unnecessary surgery, the surgeon must consider the risks in each individual case.

A hernia is said to be *strangulated* when the tissue which has herniated is constricted in such a way as to diminish its blood supply. The constriction may be from the edges of the fascial defect, in which circumstances any extraperitoneal tissue is also vulnerable. More often, the constriction is from the narrow neck of the peritoneal sac. A third point of potential constriction is by the neck of a peritoneal loculus within a sac. This most often occurs in a multiloculated para-umbilical hernia. The risk of strangulation is greatest in narrow-necked sacs and these herniae are usually difficult to reduce. The danger associated with strangulation is dependent on the tissue involved. A strangulated knuckle of extraperitoneal or omental fat is relatively harmless compared with an infarcted knuckle of small bowel or colon. Strangulated herniae with gut ischaemia or infarction are discussed in Chapter 22.

Elective abdominal wall hernia repair

Before surgery on any abdominal wall hernia it is helpful to mark on the skin the exact position and size of the defect and, in addition, the perimeter of the swelling when the hernia is at its maximum size. These marks can serve as a useful guide during the dissection. A linear incision is suitable unless the hernia is large with stretched overlying skin, when an elliptical excision to remove redundant skin is preferable. The subcutaneous fat is incised until the peritoneum of the sac, or its covering of extraperitoneal fat or thinned fascia, is encountered. The plane is then developed between this and the surrounding subcutaneous fat. This plane will lead to the edges of the fascial defect which can then be defined. It is helpful at this stage to clear the subcutaneous fat off the fascia for a few centimetres around the defect to aid the subsequent repair (Fig. 12.16). If there is stretched fascia over the hernia this is divided at the junction with the healthy tissue at the edge of the defect. If the sac is still complete it should be opened at this stage unless it is wide-necked and the surgeon is sure it is not multiloculated. Any intraperitoneal viscus adherent to the sac is freed and returned into the abdomen, and it may be necessary to enlarge a small defect to achieve this. The redundant sac is excised and the abdominal defect is closed with interrupted or continuous sutures, a non-absorbable variety being preferable. There is often no plane between the peritoneum and the abdominal fascia, and both layers may be closed together. If, however, the peritoneum separates from the abdominal wall musculature it may be closed as a separate layer. If the edges of the defect cannot be apposed without tension a mesh should be used (see below). Any significant dead space in the subcutaneous fat should be obliterated with sutures. A subcutaneous vacuum drain should be considered.

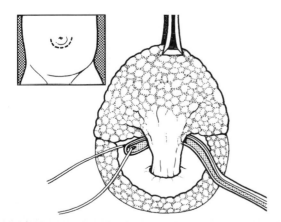

Figure 12.16 *The fascia around the defect has been cleared of fat in preparation for the repair. The fascial covering of the sac of this umbilical hernia is divided at its junction with the linea alba.*

Epigastric hernia

These midline herniae occur between the umbilicus and the xiphisternum. They occur at all ages, and are also seen in infancy. A supra-umbilical (or low epigastric) hernia in infancy must be differentiated from a true umbilical hernia as spontaneous closure of the low epigastric hernia will not occur. Epigastric herniae are often no more than a small protrusion of extraperitoneal fat through a defect in the linea alba, but larger herniae may contain a peritoneal sac. These small herniae are often irreducible as the knuckle of fat is trapped by the edges of a very small defect in the fascia. Repair is through a vertical or transverse incision. The fatty protrusion, and sac if present, are ligated and excised; the defect in the linea alba is then closed by one or more sutures.

Umbilical hernia

A true umbilical hernia occurs through a circular defect at the umbilical cicatrix, and causes a symmetrical protrusion of the umbilical skin. They are common in infancy and reduce easily. If ignored, many congenital umbilical herniae close spontaneously, and this is a safe policy as strangulation is very uncommon in children. Those still present at the age of four years are unlikely to close and will require surgical repair. A similar hernia is seen in many women in late pregnancy and may disappear after delivery. A small irreducible umbilical hernia is often encountered as an incidental finding in an overweight man. These are plugged with omentum and, although there may be no immediate concern, there is a long-term risk of strangulation and surgery should be considered.

Repair can be performed through an inconspicuous, small curved incision at the inferior edge of the umbilicus. The subcutaneous fat is divided to expose the linea alba and the medial edge of the rectus sheath on either side. The hernial sac protrudes through a circular opening in the midline, towards the apex of the umbilicus and is covered by a condensation of fascia that is continuous with the linea alba (see Fig. 12.16). The junction of fascia and linea alba is defined, and forceps passed round above the umbilicus to provide traction. The hernial sac rarely contains viscera but should nevertheless be opened with care. To achieve this, the fascia over the inferior half of the neck of the sac is first divided to expose the underlying peritoneum which, in turn, is opened and the interior of the sac inspected. Adherent omentum is released. The neck of the sac is then transected, leaving a circular defect in the linea alba and peritoneum, which can be closed in one layer in a transverse manner, although some surgeons prefer to overlap the edges. A long-acting absorbable suture such as Vicryl or PDS is suitable in children, although most surgeons would prefer a non-absorbable suture repair in an adult. After repair, the final cosmetic appearance can be improved by fixing the apex of the umbilicus to the linea alba with a subcutaneous stitch to invert the umbilical cicatrix. The sac may be left *in situ* on the under surface of the umbilical skin as it is densely adherent. Sometimes a narrow-necked large sac will continue to evert the umbilicus, and this should be partially excised to allow flattening of the skin. If there is excessive redundant skin, this can be excised.

Para–umbilical hernia

These herniae are common in parous, obese, middle-aged and elderly women. As the risk of strangulation is high, surgery should usually be recommended. They occur most frequently through the linea alba just above the umbilicus, and are clinically differentiated from an umbilical hernia in that they displace the umbilicus by their asymmetrical protrusion but do not evert and stretch the umbilical skin unless they become very large. However, at operation some are found to be large, true umbilical herniae and the umbilical skin has merely migrated distally with age, giving the appearance of a supra-umbilical swelling. Others are a compound defect in the fascia. The peritoneal sac is often irregular and loculated. Bowel may be trapped and strangulated within loculi, even though the linea alba fascial defect feels large and unlikely to cause trouble. Even in the presence of strangulation, the significance of the hernia may be overlooked as the cause of the intra-abdominal symptoms as the bulk of the hernia is soft and reducible.

Repair is through a transverse incision over the hernia just above the umbilicus, although it is sometimes preferable to make an elliptical excision to excise the redundant skin and even the umbilicus itself (Fig. 12.17). The dissection down to the fascial defect and the clearing of fat off the surrounding fascia is performed in standard fashion. The sac and stretched fascia are excised at the edge of the defect. Even in a small wide-necked sac it is important to open the sac, free the omentum and bowel from loculi within it and excise the irregular peritoneum of the sac. If the abdominal wall defect is simply closed over a loculated sac, although the hernia has been repaired, the loculi remain as an area where bowel can be trapped and become strangulated. Not infrequently these herniae consist of two adjacent defects with a narrow intervening strip of intact linea alba. This should be divided to create one defect before repair. The peritoneum may be closed as a separate layer or together with the fascia. Extension of the defect laterally aids closure, which is performed with interrupted non-absorbable sutures in a transverse direction, unless a longitudinal repair will result in less tension. Some surgeons prefer an overlapping Mayo repair (Fig. 12.18). If the edges do not come together without tension, a mesh repair should be considered (see below). The umbilicus is a potentially infected site, and antibiotic cover should be considered in all repairs; it is certainly mandatory if a mesh is to be used.

A form of para-umbilical hernia is also reported in young children. These occur through a transverse elliptical defect in the linea alba just above the umbilicus. Strangulation is uncommon, but repair should be recommended as they do not close spontaneously.

Intermuscular hernia

The most common of these relatively rare herniae is the *Spigelian hernia*. Herniation occurs only through the inner

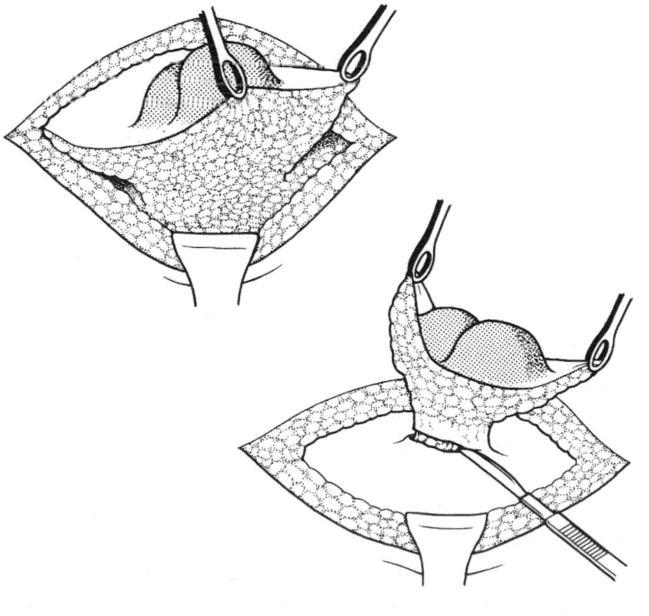

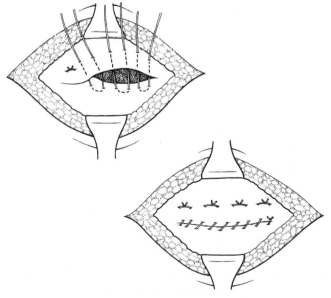

Figure 12.17 *The stretched ellipse of skin, overlying this para-umbilical hernia and adherent to the fundus of the sac, will be excised. The sac is entered at the junction of the fascia and the stretched coverings at the neck of the sac.*

Figure 12.18 *An overlapping Mayo repair is favoured by some surgeons for the repair of umbilical and para-umbilical herniae. It must be remembered, however, that if an overlap produces tension the repair will be less, and not more, robust.*

layer of abdominal musculature, and the sac enlarges in the plane between the layers of the abdominal wall. Diagnosis may be difficult as the hernia only produces a diffuse bulge, often in an obese abdomen, and the defect itself is seldom palpable. In a classical Spigelian hernia the neck of the sac is through a defect at the lateral edge of the rectus sheath at the level of the arcuate line, but other sites of herniation also occur. Even if an open repair is planned an initial laparoscopy is sometimes helpful, both to confirm the diagnosis and to identify the site of the defect over which the incision should be centred.

Lumbar hernia

These may arise spontaneously or as an incisional hernia after surgery. Complications are rare and surgery is seldom indicated.

Inguinal and femoral herniae

These are the most common of all abdominal wall herniae, and their surgical repair is described in the section on groin surgery (Chapter 24).

Obturator, gluteal and sciatic herniae

These herniae are all exceedingly rare. A palpable external swelling is even rarer, so diagnosis is usually at laparotomy for small bowel obstruction when a loop of bowel is found to be trapped within a sac. Repair of these defects is therefore from within the abdomen after reduction of the hernial contents. It is occasionally difficult to deliver strangulated bowel from the obturator canal at laparotomy, and the sac can be approached from below by an additional vertical incision, 2 cm medial to the femoral vessels. The sac lies deep to adductor longus and pectineus. Closure of an obturator defect is difficult, and the obturator vessels and nerve are easily injured by sutures. A simple safe technique consists of inversion and ligation of the sac, followed by incision of the peritoneum over the pecten pubis. The peritoneum is elevated to expose the obturator canal and a mesh placed in a retroperitoneal position covering the canal.[7] The mesh is secured superiorly to the pectineal ligament and medially to fascia over the pubis before the peritoneum is replaced and sutured (Fig. 12.19).

Incisional hernia

The aetiology of these herniae has already been discussed. Easily reducible wide-necked defects may often be ignored. Some form of elasticated support for comfort is often all that a patient wishes, but if repair is planned it is important to decide whether only part of the wound, or the whole wound, needs to be explored. If there is more than one area

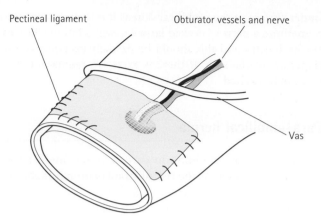

Figure 12.19 *The mesh lies in a pre-peritoneal position covering the obturator canal. Suture fixation is only to the pectineal ligament and the fascia of the pubis and injury to vital structures can be avoided.*

of herniation it is usually advisable to repair the whole wound. Accurate preoperative skin marking of the extent of the palpable sac and the fascial defect is helpful. Access is via the original scar, and excision of the scarred skin gives a better cosmetic result. The sac is defined and the plane around it followed to identify the defect. Before repair, the edges of the defect must be defined by incising the junction of normal fascia with the attenuated fascial covering of the sac.

A shallow peritoneal protrusion from most of a scar need not be opened and to do so unnecessarily merely increases the risk of small bowel injury, and of ileus. Therefore, if the peritoneum can be freed from the under-surface of the abdominal wall it can be left intact, and the fascia repaired over it. A peritoneal sac through a narrow defect should be excised, and the peritoneum should also be opened if there is any concern that a wide-necked sac could be loculated. More often, the peritoneum has to be opened because it cannot be separated from the abdominal wall, but this has the advantage that the surgeon has the opportunity to palpate the under-surface of the adjacent scar for weak areas which need to be repaired at the same operation.

If the peritoneum has been opened it may either be closed separately or with the abdominal wall repair. The edges of the abdominal wall defect are excised so that there is a freshly cut edge of healthy tissue for closure. The suture technique used is similar to that for any abdominal wall closure as described above, but particular care must be taken to encompass healthy fascia in the suture bites. A non-absorbable continuous suture is suitable. If the abdominal wall has retracted laterally and there is any tension, then a mesh or other technique should be used. There is also increasing evidence that some form of mesh repair may be the better option, even when the surgeon is confident that satisfactory tension-free apposition of the fascia can be achieved by using a simple suture technique.[8] An on-lay mesh, placed over the closed fascia and secured to it with sutures, is the simplest technique. However, any superficial wound infection is likely to result in a chronic infection in the mesh. Vacuum drainage of the subcutaneous fat to prevent postoperative haematoma collection and prophylactic antibiotics will reduce the incidence of this complication.

Frequently the fascial edges of an incisional hernia do not appose without tension. Several techniques which mobilize the abdominal wall fascia to close large defects have been described. For example, longitudinal incisions may be made through the lateral side of the anterior rectus sheath which is then elevated off the muscle, folded medially and sutured in the midline.[9] A mesh overlay can be used in addition to ensure extra strength to this repair. This is an operation which, although attractive in theory, is disappointingly difficult to execute satisfactorily, especially when there is extensive abdominal scarring. Most surgeons, however, when faced with this problem would use mesh to bridge the defect in the abdominal fascia, as described below.

Parastomal hernia

When a colostomy or ileostomy is performed there is a potential channel for herniation beside the bowel. These parastomal herniae are difficult to repair, and the stoma has often to be re-sited through another area of abdominal wall. These procedures are discussed further in Chapter 21.

MESH IN ABDOMINAL WALL REPAIR

The development of inert meshes, such as monofilament polypropylene, has greatly simplified the treatment of most difficult herniae. A mesh may be used over or under a simple repair to provide additional strength. The mesh must be placed so that it is in contact with normal tissue for some distance on either side of the closure, and a few sutures are then used to prevent it becoming displaced in the immediate postoperative period. Ultimately, the mesh becomes incorporated into the tissues and adds greatly to the strength of the final scar.

Alternatively, a mesh may be used to bridge a defect in the abdominal wall which cannot be closed without unacceptable tension. The defect may be a large hernia, a congenital abnormality, or represent a portion of the abdominal wall lost through trauma, or excised for malignancy. The ideal position for such a mesh is between the closed peritoneum and the abdominal wall, where intra-abdominal pressure pushes it against the muscles and fascia, and the peritoneum separates it from the bowel (Fig. 12.20). This is only possible if the peritoneum can be separated from the overlying muscles and sufficient peritoneum from the sac can be saved to allow peritoneal closure. Unfortunately, this situation is often unattainable and the mesh has to replace both the peri-

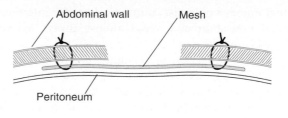

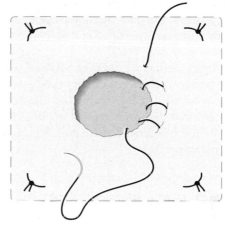

Figure 12.20 *The ideal position for a mesh is between the closed peritoneum and the partially deficient abdominal wall. The mesh should be considerably larger than the defect so that there is overlap with strong healthy tissue. Four sutures will prevent the mesh edges from rolling, after which the edge of the abdominal defect is sewn to the top surface of the mesh, with care being taken to avoid injury to any underlying bowel.*

toneum and the fascia of the defect. In this position a mesh may be in direct contact with bowel, if omentum cannot be placed between. Although there are concerns that this might increase the risk of fistula formation and mesh infections, the results of recent studies have suggested that these fears may be unfounded.[10]

A mesh should be several centimetres larger than the defect it will replace, as it is only in the areas of overlap that it can be incorporated into tissue and provide any inherent strength. An extraperitoneal or an intraperitoneal mesh first requires four sutures (as shown in Fig. 12.20) to prevent any rolling of the edges of the mesh. The edges of the fascial defect are then sewn with a continuous non-absorbable suture down onto the top surface of the mesh, with care being taken to prevent injury to any underlying viscus.

Any implanted mesh may become infected. The infection is difficult to eradicate as bacteria may be in a protected environment where there is poor antibiotic penetration, and in spaces too small to allow access to neutrophils. Recent advances in mesh material and pore size have improved this problem, but the surgeon should still be very wary of using a mesh in any potentially infective situation, and antibiotic cover is always recommended. A vacuum drain in the subcutaneous fat reduces the risk of a haematoma as a potential culture medium for infection. An infected non-absorbable mesh almost always has to be removed completely.

Smooth inert patches of expanded polytetrafluoroethylene (ePTFE), marketed as 'Gore-Tex', are an alternative to polypropylene meshes. The reduction in fibrosis may decrease bowel complications when the mesh has to be in direct contact with the bowel, but the poor tissue in-growth inevitably results in a weak attachment of the patch to the abdominal wall and a greater risk of recurrence. Compound meshes with an inner layer of ePTFE and an outer layer of polypropylene may have a role.

Inert collagen meshes are a recent advance, which can be used in the presence of infection. They can be of great value in bridging a fascial defect left when an infected mesh has had to be removed. However, as this material is extremely expensive, its use is limited to situations where other techniques are inappropriate.

ABDOMINAL WALL RECONSTRUCTION WITH FLAPS

As discussed above, non-absorbable mesh reconstruction may be inadvisable if there is sepsis, whether associated with fistulae, chronic infection in the mesh of a previous repair or a primary infective cause for the loss of the abdominal wall. A mesh repair is also inappropriate if skin loss is such that healthy skin cover of the mesh is not possible. In these situations a distant fasciocutaneous flap (see Chapter 1) can provide healthy tissue for reconstruction. Tensor fascia lata flaps with, or without, prior tissue expansion have proved versatile in most situations.[11]

CONGENITAL ABDOMINAL WALL PROBLEMS

Umbilical hernia

This common condition is often appropriately managed by general surgeons with a paediatric interest, and the surgery is described above. However, a general surgeon should only operate on the conditions outlined below if no referral is possible.

Exomphalos

This is a herniation of abdominal viscera through an abdominal wall defect into the base of the umbilical cord. The visceral contents are contained by a semi-transparent covering made up of peritoneum and amniotic membrane. The condition is arbitrarily divided into *minor* and *major* depending on whether the defect is smaller or larger than 5 cm. The contents of an exomphalos vary from a few coils of ileum to most of the abdominal viscera including liver, spleen, stomach, small bowel and colon. Mal-rotation is common, remnants of vitello-intestinal duct may persist, and there is an increased incidence of diaphragmatic hernia. In two-thirds of babies there is an associated congenital abnormality. The magnitude of the surgical challenge therefore varies enormously. A minor defect with only a small visceral protrusion can be easily repaired. The sac is excised at the junction of membrane and skin, and the umbilical vessels and urachus identified and ligated. The bowel is inspected for any other abnormality, returned to the abdomen, and a simple sutured repair performed. A major defect, with considerable visceral protrusion, may be impossible to approximate immediately. Surgical options include closing the defect with skin alone and repairing the inevitable incisional hernia at a later date, or a staged repair using a temporary prosthesis. A pouch of Dacron-reinforced silastic sheet is sutured to the defect and repair attempted 10 days later. Historically, an alternative non-operative management was to await spontaneous epithelialization of an intact exomphalos, and to delay definitive management of the abdominal wall defect. The application of mercurochrome to dry and toughen the sac is, however, inadvisable as absorption of mercury will occur.

Gastroschisis

This condition is often misdiagnosed as a ruptured exomphalos, but is a separate entity. The gut has herniated through a defect adjacent to, and usually to the right of, the umbilicus, but the bowel lies free as there is no covering membrane. The prolapse is normally limited to the midgut which is oedematous, apparently short, and covered with a fibrinous exudate. The incidence of associated anomalies is small. There is no alternative to surgery as the bowel is exposed, but temporarily covering the extruded bowel with 'cling film' reduces heat and fluid loss during transfer to a specialist centre. At operation the abdominal wall defect is enlarged, the bowel is returned to the abdominal cavity and the defect is repaired, if this is possible without undue tension. If the tension is too great, then placing the bowel in a temporary prosthetic sac sutured to the abdominal wall allows the oedema to settle, and 10 days later either repair can be achieved, or a second smaller bag can be sutured in place.

Persistent urachus or vitello-intestinal duct

Partial persistence of these structures is common; as an upward extension to the bladder, or as a Meckel's diverticulum. More complete failure of involution results in a fistulous communication, and umbilical discharge of urine or gastrointestinal contents. Surgical excision of the fistula should be undertaken. A transverse incision lateral to the umbilicus provides good access for either condition. A urachus is traced to the bladder, divided and the bladder repaired. Coexistent bladder outlet obstruction should be excluded by a cystogram before surgery; the contrast is introduced into the bladder through a catheter inserted at the umbilicus. A vitello-intestinal duct is traced to the ileum and excised.

Ectopic bladder

Major failure of development of the lower abdominal wall results in a widely separated symphysis pubis, and the trigone of the bladder lies exposed on the surface with visible ureteric orifices. In male infants the penis is epispadic and even rudimentary. Reconstruction requires specialist surgery.

Congenital diaphragmatic hernia

These are more common on the left, and much of the gut is often lying within the chest. Presentation is usually with respiratory distress, and the diagnosis is confirmed by a chest X-ray. Although the surgery itself is straightforward, referral to a major paediatric centre is essential as, even after surgery, many babies still require intensive respiratory support. The presentation with respiratory distress is related more to the hypoplastic lungs associated with this condition than to the displaced bowel lying in the chest. It is for this reason that those babies who present with respiratory difficulties at birth have a much worse prognosis than those in whom presentation is delayed until some hours later. Nasogastric aspiration is mandatory during transfer to a specialist centre, as a dilated stomach in the left chest further compromises gas exchange.

At operation, which is performed via a transverse upper abdominal approach, the abdominal viscera are delivered from the thorax. The diaphragmatic defect is closed with interrupted non-absorbable sutures or, if the defect is too large, a mesh is used to bridge the defect.

Minor variants of the condition may present in late childhood and in adult life, and their management is discussed in Chapter 17.

REFERENCES

1. Van der Krabben AA, Dijkstra FR, Nieuwenhuijzen M, et al. Morbidity and mortality of inadvertent enterotomy during adhesiotomy. Br J Surg 2000; 87: 467–71.
2. Cox PJ, Ausobsky JR, Ellis H, et al. Towards no incisional hernias: lateral paramedian versus midline incisions. J R Soc Med 1986; 79: 711–12.
3. Bonjer HJ, Hazebroek EJ, Kazemier G, et al. Open versus closed establishment of pneumoperitoneum in laparoscopic surgery. Review. Br J Surg 1997; 84: 599–602.
4. Extraperitoneal laparoscopic surgery. C Eden. Oxford: Blackwell Science, 1997.
5. Ghimenton F, Thomson SR, Muckart DJJ, et al. Abdominal content containment: practicalities and outcome. Br J Surg 2000; 87: 106–9.
6. Radice E, Nelson H, Mercill S, et al. Primary myocutaneous flap closure following resection of locally advanced pelvic malignancies. Br J Surg 1999; 86: 349–54.
7. Lobo DN, Clarke DJ, Barlow AP. Obturator hernia: a new technique for repair. J R Coll Surg Edinb 1998; 43: 33–4.
8. Cassar K, Munro A. Surgical treatment of incisional hernia. Review. Br J Surg 2002; 89: 534–45.
9. Whiteley MS, Ray-Chaudhuri SB, Galland RB. Combined fascia and mesh closure of large incisional hernias. J R Coll Surg Edinb 1998; 43: 29–30.
10. Vrijland WW, Jeekel J, Steyerberg FW, et al. Intraperitoneal polypropylene mesh repair of incisional hernia is not associated with enterocutaneous fistula. Br J Surg 2000; 87: 348–52.
11. Mathes SJ, Steinwald PM, Foster RD, et al. Complex abdominal wall reconstruction: a comparison of flap and mesh closure. Ann Surg 2000; 232: 586–96.

13

GENERAL TECHNIQUES IN ABDOMINAL AND GASTROINTESTINAL SURGERY

PROBLEMS OF ACCESS

Optimal surgery depends on two separate skills. The first is clinical judgement, and is extremely important in all surgery. It includes the decision whether to operate or not, the timing of surgery, the choice of which operation to perform, and the preoperative and postoperative management of the patient. The second skill is the technical ability to perform the surgery. In many situations, an operation is technically demanding through difficulties of access, and this is particularly so in intra-abdominal surgery. In some areas access is inherently difficult, whereas in others certain manoeuvres make the surgery immediately easier.

Difficult access can often be improved by either tilting or rolling the table. The bowel can be made to fall away from the operative field, and gravity can also be utilized to increase potential spaces, for example between the diaphragm and liver.

Abdominal wall access

The choice of abdominal incision is important. An inadequate incision is the commonest cause of operative difficulty (see Chapter 12). The abdominal muscles must be relaxed, both to reduce intra-abdominal pressure and to allow retraction of the abdominal wall. A self-retaining retractor is useful in major intra-abdominal surgery as it frees the assistant for the more precise and dynamic retraction in the area of dissection (Fig. 13.1). A self-retaining retractor makes access more difficult to the lateral aspects of the anterior abdominal wall, and the release of any adhesions in this area should be completed before the retractor is positioned. Traditionally,

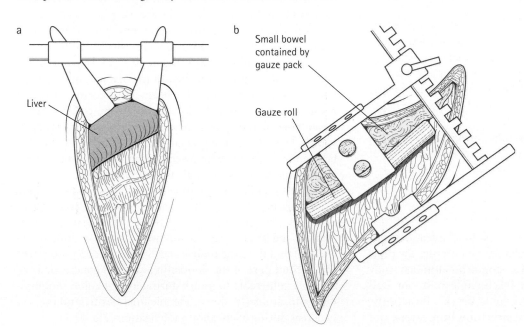

Figure 13.1 *(a) Mechanical fixed retraction to a horizontal bar attached to the operating table lifts the costal margin upwards and cranially, increasing sub-diaphragmatic access. (b) The deep self-retaining 'Finochetti' retractor is holding the wound edges apart and is also holding the small bowel out of the pelvis. The small bowel has been wrapped in a large gauze pack, and a gauze roll has been placed along the left side of the mesenteric root.*

a — Liver

b — Small bowel contained by gauze pack — Gauze roll

the wound edges are protected from the retractor by large swabs but, more importantly, care must be taken not to catch a loop of small bowel. It is also easy to damage the abdominal or chest wall skin in the ratchet mechanism of a retractor.

Bowel distension

Grossly distended gut reduces intra-abdominal access. Hence, deflation may be required before any dissection can be undertaken safely (see below).

Adhesions

Intraperitoneal adhesions may severely limit access within the abdomen. Thus, the release of these adhesions is often necessary before the planned surgery can proceed, and this may greatly increase the duration of an operation.[1] Adhesions are commonly the result of previous surgery, but they may also follow an intraperitoneal infective process, or closed blunt trauma. Adhesions of small bowel to the anterior abdominal wall beneath an old scar are particularly dangerous as it is easy to damage the bowel on the initial entry into the peritoneal cavity. Small bowel adhesions in the pelvis, to the site of previous gynaecological surgery or pelvic infection, can also be difficult to release safely. Gentle traction will usually show the plane which requires division, either between the bowel loops, or between bowel and the abdominal wall. Blunt dissection should be avoided as a dense adhesion has a tensile strength greater than that of bowel and intestinal tears will occur. Sharp dissection with scissors is safer than diathermy, which may burn the bowel wall. Adhesions between loops of small bowel which are causing folds rather than kinks may be safely left undisturbed. Band adhesions, around which bowel loops could twist, should be divided even if division is not required for access.

If an injury to the bowel occurs during dissection, the segment should be examined carefully for any mucosal breach which will require repair. A seromuscular tear may be ignored, but it is often thought to be safer to support the thin intact mucosa with a partial-thickness seromuscular suture. If any repair is deemed advisable it should not be deferred as it may be subsequently overlooked.

Various products are currently bring evaluated in attempts to reduce adhesions, though convincing evidence of their efficacy has not yet been established.

Mobilization of viscera

Even in the absence of adhesions, access to all intra-abdominal viscera is not secured immediately on entering the peritoneal cavity. For example, the stomach, although fully clothed in peritoneum, has an inaccessible posterior wall until entry has been gained into the lesser sac. Posteriorly, fully and partially retroperitoneal structures lie in layers, and access to the more posterior structures must await mobilization of the more anterior. There are three retroperitoneal planes in which the surgeon can dissect to achieve this mobilization. The first plane is behind the colon and in front of the duodenum. The second plane is behind the duodenum, pancreas and spleen but in front of the kidneys, ureters and gonadal vessels. The third plane is behind the kidneys. The anatomy of the posterior abdominal planes and of the lesser sac, and the concept of discrete retroperitoneal mesenteries can all be appreciated more readily from an embryological viewpoint.

Surgical embryology of the abdomen

Access within the abdomen is complicated by the intrauterine folding of the gastrointestinal tract, and some understanding of abdominal embryology is essential for the surgeon.[2] In early intra-uterine life the entire gastrointestinal tract is a simple tube which is suspended from a midline dorsal mesentery. The blood supply is from the three midline visceral arteries to the fore, mid and hind gut. These persist in adult life as the coeliac axis, the superior mesenteric artery and the inferior mesenteric artery, all arising in the midline from the front of the aorta.

The small bowel persists into adult life on a mesentery orientated approximately in the midline. The large bowel, however, rotates in an anti-clockwise direction, and the mesenteries of the ascending and descending colon then merge with the retroperitoneal tissue. The two layers of peritoneum in contact are absorbed. It is relatively easy to appreciate this arrangement as there is an areolar plane which can be dissected with precision between the 'mesentery' of the ascending or descending colon and the truly retroperitoneal structures. If the ascending or descending colon is lifted forwards, a white line is visible on the peritoneum a few centimetres lateral to the colon. The areolar plane is entered by division of the peritoneum along this line, and the incision is continued around the colonic flexures. Access to the splenic flexure may be difficult, as it lies higher and deeper than the hepatic flexure, and is attached to the diaphragm by a peritoneal fold, the phrenocolic ligament. Excessive traction must be avoided or adhesions between the colon and the lower pole of the spleen may be disrupted with resultant splenic tears. Once the areolar plane behind the colon has been entered, it can be followed to the midline and the colon is once again on its original midline mesentery. This is an important mobilization manoeuvre which is the first step in a radical hemicolectomy. It also allows operative access to the posterior retroperitoneal structures. This first posterior plane is relatively easy to follow, and when difficulty is encountered the surgeon has usually strayed too posteriorly. The second part of the duodenum and the pancreatic head are thus vulnerable to injury during a right colon mobilization, and, similarly, the duodenojejunal flexure and body of pancreas during a left colon mobilization (Fig. 13.2).

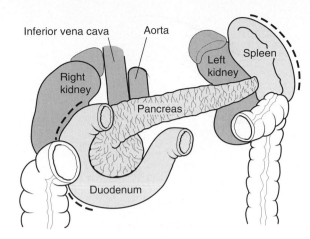

Figure 13.2 *The embryological folding of the gut produces layers of mainly retroperitoneal organs which can be separated along areolar planes. The anterior layer consists of colon. The middle layer, of pancreas, duodenum and spleen, can be mobilized forwards by peritoneal incisions in the positions marked by the dotted lines. The posterior layer is made up of the kidneys, adrenals, aorta and vena cava.*

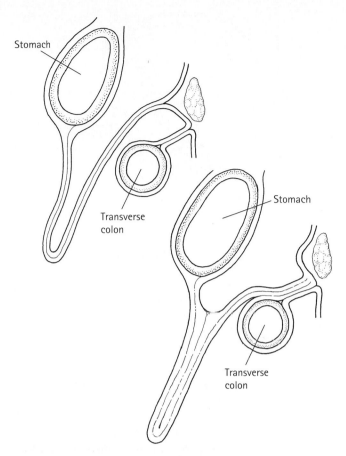

Figure 13.3 *The developmental rotation and differential growth of the gut results in complicated upper abdominal anatomy. The greater omentum with the transverse colon effectively divides the abdomen into a supra-colic and an infra-colic compartment.*

In the *pelvis*, a similar merging of tissue occurs between the mesorectum and the tissue of the pelvic wall. Again, there is a discrete plane of areolar tissue between the structures of the hindgut and the other structures in the pelvis. Fusion of the peritoneum in the depths of the rectovaginal, or rectovesical, pouch forms Denonvillier's fascia, which is an important anatomical landmark in radical surgery of the rectum.

In the *upper abdomen* the developmental rotation of the foregut is more complicated (Fig. 13.3). Subsequent fusion of folds also complicates the anatomy around the transverse colon. The stomach originates as a dilatation of the foregut, with a dorsal and ventral mesentery. The dorsal aspect of the stomach grows more rapidly than the ventral aspect, forcing the distal stomach and duodenum upwards and to the right. The ventral mesentery becomes the lesser omentum and the dorsal mesentery the greater omentum. The duodenum also rotates to the right, and its right side loses its peritoneal covering as it fuses with the retroperitoneal tissue. There is a plane here which can be developed in the manoeuvre entitled '*Kocherization of the duodenum*'. An incision of the peritoneum outside the lateral border of the second part of the duodenum allows the duodenum and the head of the pancreas to be lifted forwards off the right kidney and inferior vena cava (IVC). The equivalent plane on the left is behind the spleen and tail of the pancreas. It is entered by division of the peritoneum lateral to the spleen (see Fig. 13.2); this is the second posterior plane.

The adult anatomy of the upper gastrointestinal tract is shown in Figure 13.4. The *lesser sac* forms behind the stomach as it rotates, the anterior wall of the sac being composed mainly of the posterior wall (the original right wall) of the stomach. It is in communication with the rest of the peri-

toneal cavity – the *greater sac* – but, due to differential growth, only by the small communication deep to the free edge of the lesser omentum. Lesser sac access is necessary for many upper gastrointestinal and hepatobiliary operations. The natural communication between the greater and lesser sacs cannot be enlarged as the common bile duct, portal vein and hepatic artery run in the free edge of the lesser omentum, and the other boundaries of the channel are the IVC, the duodenum and the liver. The lesser sac may be entered through the lesser omentum away from the structures in the free edge, but access is limited. Entry below the greater curve of the stomach, through the gastrocolic part of the greater omentum, is satisfactory, but multiple ligations of gastric or omental branches of the gastro-epiploic arcade are required and devitalization of the omentum may occur. Access through the transverse mesocolon risks injury to middle colic vessels, although a relatively avascular window to the left of these vessels can be utilized. The best access can be obtained by separating the natural plane between the greater omentum and the anterior surface of the transverse colon. Once the plane has been identified it can be followed to right and left for a considerable distance, providing extensive

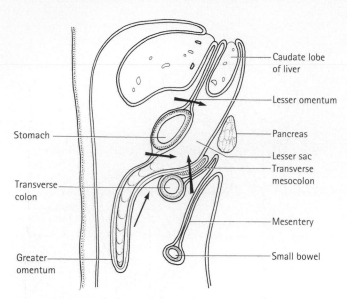

Figure 13.4   *A diagrammatic sagittal section through the abdomen to show the disposition of the omentum and lesser sac. Arrows indicate routes of access into the lesser sac.*

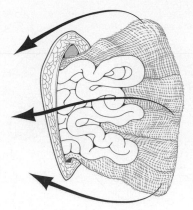

Figure 13.5   *A large pack is tucked into the left side of the mesenteric root. It is folded over the small bowel, which can then be retained in the right half of the abdomen by the method shown in* Figure 13.1(b).

access to the lesser sac. Only occasional small vessels cross the plane and require ligation. This plane is continuous around the colonic flexures with the plane which is developed to mobilize the ascending and descending colon.

Access to major vessels for vascular control is more fully addressed in Chapter 5. In general, however, the infra-renal aorta may be approached by swinging the transverse colon up and the small bowel to the patient's right. The posterior peritoneum is opened to the left of the fourth part of the duodenum. The IVC is exposed by Kocherization of the duodenum but access to the intrahepatic IVC requires full mobilization of the right half of the liver. The third posterior plane behind the kidneys may be valuable for access to the posterior aspect of the intra-abdominal aorta or IVC.

Bowel containment

Mobile bowel falls naturally into any intraperitoneal space in which the surgeon is working, and must be restrained out of the surgical field. One solution is to deliver the bowel outside the abdomen and to place it in a bowel bag of a synthetic material which prevents fluid loss from the surface. Postoperative ileus may be less of a problem if the bowel can be 'packed away' within the abdomen. For example, if a left hemicolectomy is planned, the small bowel is delivered externally over the right abdominal wall. A large pack soaked in saline is then tucked into the mesenteric root from the left and the small bowel swung back on top of it. The remainder of the pack is then folded over the small bowel and used to retain it under the right side of the abdominal incision (Fig. 13.5). A 20-cm (8-inch) gauze roll can then be placed to the left of the wrapped bowel along the mesenteric root, and a

deep self-retaining wound retractor opened so that the blade on the right wound edge pushes on the roll and the small bowel is held securely within the right half of the abdomen (see Fig. 13.1b).

Removal of debris and blood, fluid and smoke of diathermy

These must be removed from the operative field so that a clear view is maintained. Mechanical suction is satisfactory except when there is solid matter. Blood clots and solid faecal material will block a sucker, and it is preferable to remove them with a swab. The suction end may have a single terminal opening, allowing accurate clearance of a defined area. A clear view of the sucker tip is essential as, if the single suction hole is occluded against tissue, damage can occur as the tissue is sucked into the device. Alternatively, a guard with multiple holes is screwed over the sucker. This is a safer instrument because if one hole is occluded against the bowel wall the remaining open channels continue to draw in fluid, or air. This prevents the suction from drawing in tissue. It is therefore safe to pass a guarded sucker amongst small bowel loops to aspirate fluid or blood. Gentleness is still essential to avoid injury, but the surgeon does not need to be able to see the end of the instrument.

GENERAL PRINCIPLES OF INTRA-ABDOMINAL SURGERY

Swab counts

In intra-abdominal surgery it is easy to leave a swab undetected within the peritoneal cavity. It is therefore essential to check the number of swabs and instruments, and to account for all, before closing the peritoneum. If a swab is still missing after re-checking the peritoneal cavity, the surgeon must not assume that it is lost somewhere else in the operating theatre before an abdominal X-ray has proved that it is not within the patient.

Principle of general laparotomy

When a limited access abdominal incision has been made it is not possible to check the whole abdomen for other pathology, but those areas which are accessible can still be examined. After the removal of a normal appendix it is usually possible to check at least the terminal ileum and the right ovary for an alternative pathology, without enlarging the incision. Laparoscopic surgery has the advantage of allowing a full inspection of the abdomen, but without the benefit of palpation. When a major abdominal incision has been made, the opportunity to check for another obvious intra-abdominal pathology should not be missed. It is a good discipline to do this immediately on opening the abdomen or it may be forgotten later. Mobilization of organs or entry into the lesser sac is only required if there is a specific concern which justifies it. On first opening the abdomen through a midline incision, the greater omentum or small bowel presents. The small bowel can be followed proximally to the duodenojejunal junction and distally to the ileocaecal valve, for inspection and palpation throughout its length. Gentle traction on the greater omentum brings the anterior surface of the stomach into view. The antrum, pylorus and the first part of duodenum can be inspected, but the incision may not allow a view of the fundus. A hand can be introduced up over the front of the stomach and the whole stomach palpated. A hand into the right hypochondrium can palpate the liver and the gallbladder. If the greater omentum is lifted, the transverse colon is visible on the under surface and can be followed by palpation laterally to both flexures. The hepatic flexure, ascending colon and caecum are easily palpated. The splenic flexure is deeper and difficult to palpate without mobilization. In addition, splenic injury should be avoided. The descending and sigmoid colon are then palpated, followed by examination of the pelvis. Only the upper rectum is accessible to palpation, but the uterus, ovaries and fallopian tubes can be adequately examined.

Retroperitoneal structures should also be palpated. The kidneys are deep to the colonic flexures, and are firm and relatively easily palpated through overlying structures. The pancreas can be palpated through the lesser omentum or through the transverse mesocolon, but only gross pathology will be detected unless the lesser sac is opened.

This general examination of the intra-abdominal contents is an important part of any laparotomy when the pathology is still in doubt, and when a surgeon has to operate in the absence of any preoperative endoscopy or imaging. It assumes lesser importance when a patient has been extensively investigated preoperatively, especially as CT or MRI scans can detect liver, pancreatic or renal pathology which

may not be possible to feel at laparotomy. A CT scan is particularly valuable for retroperitoneal structures and solid organs. Preoperative endoscopy, or barium studies, may detect gastroduodenal and colonic pathology which the surgeon cannot palpate. However, the principles of the 'general laparotomy' should not be abandoned. Even if the patient has undergone extensive preoperative imaging, there are some pathologies (e.g. peritoneal malignant deposits) which, although easily visualized and palpated, are difficult to demonstrate with sophisticated imaging, and may be unsuspected before the abdomen is opened.

Dissection

Much of the dissection within the abdomen consists of finding developmental areolar planes or the planes between adhesions. During dissection, the tissues must be held on stretch and the areolar tissue is divided by sharp dissection or diathermy. Diathermy has the added advantage of reducing minor bleeding, but also has a greater potential for damage, especially in the hands of the inexperienced. Diathermy may also cause thermal damage to a structure which initially displays no visible injury. It is therefore safer to use sharp dissection with scissors when dissecting close to bowel wall, a major vessel or a ureter. Blunt dissection may result in tears in the bowel, liver or spleen, and should be avoided as much as possible. In addition, fine structures such as autonomic nerves lie adjacent to the planes, and although they can be preserved with careful sharp dissection they are almost invariably torn in blunt dissection.

Prevention of spillage of gastrointestinal contents

Gastrointestinal surgery is associated with a high risk of septic complications. Antibiotic prophylaxis and preoperative mechanical bowel preparation reduce the problem (see Chapter 11 and Appendices I and II), but every effort should still be made to prevent contamination of the peritoneal cavity with gastrointestinal contents. Preoperative bowel preparation achieves an empty large bowel, whilst a short preoperative fast provides a relatively empty proximal gastrointestinal tract. In emergency surgery there is no opportunity to achieve an empty bowel, and if the surgery is for obstruction then the potential for peritoneal contamination is further increased. Gastric and upper jejunal deflation can, however, be achieved using nasogastric tube aspiration.

Deflation may be necessary early in a laparotomy if distended obstructed bowel is impeding access for safe dissection. Occasionally, deflation is necessary to permit abdominal closure. However, when a resection is planned, deflation is most often undertaken at the time of the resection. A sucker is introduced through the initial incision into the lumen, and the lumen emptied before proceeding further. The surgeon can milk small bowel contents into the segment into which a sucker has been introduced, or back into the stomach from where they can be aspirated via a nasogastric tube (see Fig. 22.3, page 412).

Distended small bowel may also be deflated by the introduction of a needle, attached to suction, obliquely through the wall of the distended bowel. This technique, while excellent for gas or thin fluids, is unsuitable for thicker contents. Alternatively, the whole sucker is introduced through a small enterotomy into the bowel lumen. Before making the incision, a purse-string suture should be placed which can be tightened immediately on introduction of the sucker to prevent leakage. After removal of the sucker the suture is tightened and tied to close the enterotomy. This is a safer technique in the small bowel than in the colon. An obstructed distended colon has solid matter which blocks suction tubing, and the only satisfactory solution may be *on-table lavage*, which is described in Chapter 22.

If spillage is likely from an opened lumen, then non-crushing occlusion clamps may be placed proximally and distally to isolate the area of bowel to be opened from inflow of gastrointestinal contents until the breach is closed or the anastomosis is complete (Fig. 13.6). However, this has the disadvantage of compromising the blood supply which may be critical to the healing of the anastomosis.

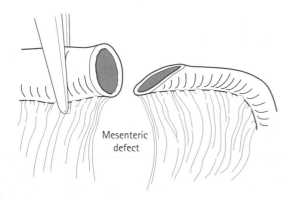

Mesenteric defect

Figure 13.6   *The anastomotic diameter can be increased by oblique division of the bowel. The mesenteric border should be longer than the anti-mesenteric to ensure good blood supply. A longitudinal incision or 'cut-back' at the anti-mesenteric border produces the same effect. A soft occlusion clamp has been used to prevent spillage of intestinal contents. After completion of the anastomosis the mesenteric defect should be closed.*

Gastrotomies, enterotomies and colotomies

These terms describe simple incisions into the lumen of the gastrointestinal tract. The incisions are closed with a similar technique to a sutured anastomosis, and are described below.

Gastrostomies, enterostomies and colostomies

These terms indicate the establishment of a connection from the lumen of the gastrointestinal tract to the abdominal wall

skin. Those in which a mucocutaneous anastomosis, or stoma, is formed are described in Chapter 21. A connection can also be established by a tube secured into the lumen.

- Gastrostomy: a tube gastrostomy may be fashioned when the abdomen is already open. A balloon catheter is introduced through the anterior abdominal wall in a position against which the stomach can lie without tension. A small incision is then made in the anterior stomach wall inside a purse-string suture, the catheter is introduced, and the suture snugged around the catheter. The anterior wall of the stomach should then be fixed to the anterior abdominal wall to prevent dragging, to eliminate a length of intraperitoneal catheter around which bowel could twist and to minimize the consequences of any minor leakage. More often, a gastrostomy is achieved by a non-operative percutaneous endoscopic gastrostomy (PEG) method (see Chapter 11).
- Enterostomy: a fine-bore tube enterostomy can be used for enteral feeding; the technique for this is described in Chapter 11.
- Caecostomy: a tube caecostomy is established by a similar technique to that used for an open gastroscopy. It is occasionally indicated for a dilated caecum, and is discussed in more detail in Chapter 22.

ANASTOMOTIC TECHNIQUE

The basic principles of this procedure are similar whether the surgery is to close a simple incision into the gastrointestinal lumen or to create an anastomosis. A simple opening into a lumen may be made to retrieve a gallstone from the common bile duct, or a foreign body from the stomach which cannot be retrieved endoscopically. The duodenum may have been opened to gain access to the ampulla, or to oversew a bleeding ulcer. An incision may have been made accidentally into the small bowel during the dissection of adhesions. A clean incision is simply sutured, as in the construction of an anastomosis. Care must be taken not to narrow a small diameter lumen however, and it is therefore sometimes appropriate to close a short longitudinal incision transversely, provided that this does not put tension on the closure. More often, a lumen is opened prior to a resection or bypass, and the anastomosis is then performed to restore gastrointestinal continuity.

An anastomosis may be either end-to-end (Fig. 13.7), end-to-side (see Fig. 21.15, page 391) or side-to-side (see Fig. 13.11). It may be created between two segments of bowel, or between small bowel and another viscus; for example, the stomach, pancreas or bile duct. It may even be between an isolated loop of small bowel and the bladder. Individual circumstances and techniques are described in the relevant sections, but the principles are universal, whether the anastomosis is hand-sutured or stapled, and whether it is performed at laparotomy or laparoscopy.

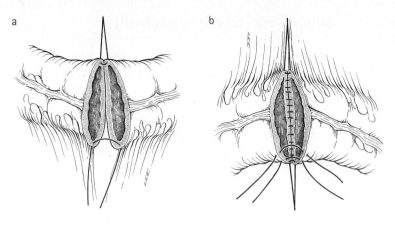

Figure 13.7 *An end-to-end small bowel anastomosis with a single layer of interrupted extra-mucosal sutures. (a) The first two sutures are placed at the mesenteric and the anti-mesenteric borders, and used as stay sutures; (b) half of the anastomosis is completed, and the bowel has been turned over to suture the second half.*

BLOOD SUPPLY

For sound healing, the perfusion of both sides of an anastomosis must be good. It may be possible to see the vessels in the mesentery, or in an obese patient to feel for their pulsation, in order to choose a site for the resection where the blood supply of the divided bowel will be optimal. The viability of the ends must be confirmed before commencing the anastomosis. The mucosa should be pink, and the bleeding from cut submucosal vessels should be bright red. (This sign is lost if the bowel is divided by diathermy.) If an artery close to the bowel wall at the level of the anastomosis is divided before ligation, pulsatile arterial bleeding from the cut end is an extra reassurance. In general, the blood supply of the colon is more precarious than that of the small bowel and stomach. A dusky grey pink mucosa and bleeding which is the dark ooze of venous back-bleeding are indications that the circulation is inadequate for an anastomosis. The ends must then be resected back to healthy, well-perfused tissue. In a side-to-side anastomotic bypass, blood supply is unlikely to be of concern.

TENSION

The two sides of the anastomosis must lie easily together, without tension. Any anastomosis created under tension will be under greater tension 48 hours later as inflammatory swelling and postoperative ileus develop. Such an anastomosis is under great danger of disruption. The surgeon must also take into account increased tension caused by changes in body position. The filling of the stomach or the bladder will also change the alignment and the tension of an anastomosis to these organs. If the tension is not acceptable, then further mobilization of the ends, without causing damage to the blood supply, is required. If this cannot be achieved, a more sophisticated method of restoring continuity is required.

ANASTOMOTIC DIAMETER

An end-to-end anastomosis inevitably reduces the lumen at the site of the anastomosis, whether hand-sutured or stapled. Temporarily, the lumen is further narrowed by postoperative oedema, and if it becomes obstructed then the risk of anastomotic breakdown is increased. This problem is greater if the lumen is of small diameter or the luminal contents are viscous. The traditional sutured two-layer anastomotic technique – which is now seldom used for intestinal end-to-end anastomoses – narrowed an anastomosis significantly as the suture line was invaginated (Fig. 13.8). Paediatric surgeons changed to a single-layer technique before the general surgeons, as the narrowing was more critical in the narrow

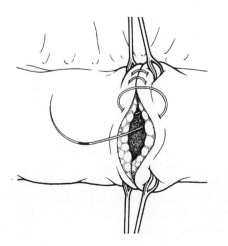
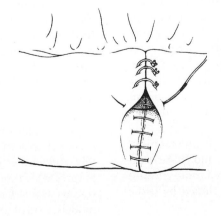

Figure 13.8 *The classic two-layer anastomosis is now seldom employed for an end-to-end anastomosis.*

lumen of the neonatal bowel. A side-to-side anastomosis can be fashioned with whatever anastomotic diameter the surgeon chooses. A hand-sewn, end-to-end anastomosis may be enlarged by an oblique division of the ends, or an enlargement created by cutting back on the anti-mesenteric border. This is also a useful manoeuvre if the diameter of the two ends are significantly disparate (see Fig. 13.6). Temporary intubation of an anastomosis may be protective and is sometimes used for the bile and pancreatic ducts, and for the ureter.

MESENTERY

On completion of an anastomosis there is usually a mesenteric defect which is a potential site for an 'internal hernia'. Small bowel may pass through this, with resultant volvulus or strangulation, and these defects should be closed (see Fig. 13.6). The suture material and method of closure are not important, but care must be taken to avoid injury to mesenteric vessels. A stitch which only picks up the peritoneum of the mesentery is safest.

DRAINS

A surgeon may be concerned over an anastomosis because of a marginally adequate blood supply, or minimal tension. There may have been peritonitis at the time of surgery, or the patient's general condition may be poor. The surgeon considers 'protecting' the vulnerable anastomosis with a drain. However, sutures or staples can hold non-viable tissue in position and delay a leak for 1–2 weeks. The drain would have to remain *in situ* for 2 weeks to be of any value in this situation, and there is some concern that a drain in contact with an anastomosis for this time could in itself cause damage. Pancreatic anastomoses are, however, particularly prone to delayed leaks and, therefore, are commonly drained and the drain left *in situ* until this period of danger is passed. In low rectal anastomoses, although a leak is normally delayed, the cause of a leak may occasionally be an infected haematoma which has collected in the 'dead space' of the emptied pelvis during the 48 hours after surgery. A short-term pelvic suction drain is therefore often employed to prevent this collection and to protect the anastomosis.

The commonest manifestation of an anastomotic leak from an intraperitoneal anastomosis is a generalized peritonitis. An intraperitoneal drain is of little protection against this. There are some instances, however, where a drain may be of value. For example, many sound urological anastomoses leak a considerable volume of urine during the first 72 hours, but then seal and heal satisfactorily. These anastomoses are therefore normally drained, whether they are extraperitoneal or intraperitoneal.

Low-pressure suction is preferable to high-pressure suction, which may draw tissue into the drain and cause damage. In addition, low-pressure suction is often more effective as the drain holes are less likely to be occluded by tissue drawn into them.

Sutured end-to-end anastomosis

This versatile anastomosis is illustrated for small bowel (see Fig. 13.7). Mobility makes the surgery technically easy, the blood supply is good and breakdown uncommon and, therefore, a small bowel anastomosis is often the first which a trainee surgeon performs. As discussed already, the two ends must have a good blood supply and be able to be brought together easily without tension. Discrepancies in diameter between the ends can be adjusted by the spacing of sutures as the bowel wall is elastic. Alternatively, the smaller end can be cut at the anti-mesenteric border to equalize the diameter (see Fig. 13.6). Care should be taken over orientation, because if there is ample mobility then one end can be inadvertently rotated. The anastomosis should be undertaken without fear of spillage of contents during the procedure, and an occlusion clamp may be necessary. Minor bleeding points in the submucosa can be ignored. Precise coagulation diathermy will arrest the more troublesome bleeding points, but many surgeons prefer to divide the bowel with diathermy to avoid this problem.

SUTURE MATERIAL

The choice of suture material is often dependent only on the preference of the surgeon, but in some instances it is important. Non-absorbable silk sutures were found in late anastomotic ulcers in the stomach, and within calculi which formed postoperatively in the biliary and urinary tracts. Traditionally, catgut was used in these areas, but silk was still preferred for the more vulnerable colonic anastomoses where the accelerated breakdown of catgut exposed to faecal organisms was considered a possible cause of anastomotic breakdown. Silk has been implicated as a contributory risk factor for recurrent Crohn's disease at the anastomotic site, and is generally better avoided in the surgery of inflammatory bowel disease. Synthetic absorbable materials (e.g. Vicryl) retain strength for longer than catgut and are suitable in most situations.

TECHNIQUE

A single layer of interrupted extramucosal sutures is now favoured by the majority of surgeons. A continuous suture acts like a drawstring, and will tend to narrow the lumen, especially in the early phase, when postoperative swelling further tightens the suture. In addition, a continuous suture reduces the blood supply to the cut ends; this is disadvantageous except in very vascular areas where a haemostatic suture may be beneficial. Sutures which include the mucosa have no advantage other than haemostasis. They do not add significantly to the strength of the anastomosis, nor do they improve apposition as the mucosa lies in apposition after accurately placed extra-mucosal sutures. Mucosa heals rapidly, and a watertight seal will have formed within 24 hours. Sutures which include the mucosa merely delay this by the trauma and ischaemia that they cause, and in experimental models, a small mucosal ulcer can be seen at each suture site.

Historically, when two layers of sutures were used routinely, it was believed that the second seromuscular layer was important to invaginate and bury the mucosa of the cut ends (see Fig. 13.8). This does not confer any benefit and causes narrowing and greater tissue strangulation.

The first two sutures are placed to unite the two ends at the mesenteric and the anti-mesenteric borders, and they divide the anastomosis into two equal sections. These sutures are tied, the ends left long and held in artery forceps (Fig. 13.7a). Each suture should start on the outside and emerge between the mucosa and the muscularis mucosa. It is important to include the muscularis mucosa, which is visible as a white line, as it has significant strength. These layers are distinct and mobile on each other if the bowel has been cut with scissors or a scalpel. Diathermy division of the bowel to some extent 'fuses' the layers, and the anatomy of the layers may be less distinct. The ideal size of the suture bite may be difficult to judge. A larger bite has less danger of cutting out, but creates a larger bulk of potentially strangulated tissue to narrow the lumen. In the adult small bowel a reasonable compromise is to introduce the suture 0.5 cm from the cut end. The suture is then introduced into the other cut bowel end between the muscularis mucosa and the mucosa and brought out through the peritoneal surface (0.5 cm from the cut end). Care must be taken as the throws on the knot are tightened to prevent the whole suture tightening and strangulating the tissue. The spacing of sutures is difficult to judge, and the temptation to place them very close, in anticipation of the dilatation of postoperative ileus, should be resisted. The additional compromise to the blood supply outweighs any benefits of an apparently more watertight early closure. In an adult small bowel, sutures separated by 0.5 cm is a satisfactory compromise. Subsequent sutures are placed until half of the anastomosis is complete. The bowel is then turned over and the other half of the anastomosis completed (Fig. 13.7b).

In most other situations access is less ideal, and it is important to complete the back of the anastomosis first. A similar technique to that described above can be employed if the surgeon starts at the back corner which is furthest away, and this first suture is left long as a stay suture. This suture makes the placement of the next suture easier, and it is possible to continue along the back wall of the anastomosis until the back corner nearest the surgeon is reached. This last suture is also left long as a stay suture (Fig. 13.9a). The front wall is then anastomosed. Another alternative is to introduce the sutures along the back wall of the anastomosis from within the bowel lumen (Fig. 13.9b). These sutures have knots in the submucosal plane, which in theory is less than ideal but in practice is satisfactory. In a difficult anastomosis, where access is very restricted, sutures may be *railroaded* into position. The two ends are only apposed after all sutures are in place (Fig. 13.10). Many of these problems, which are encountered particularly in oesophageal and rectal anastomoses, can be overcome by use of a circular stapling device.

In some structures, such as the common bile duct, a separate mobile mucosa may not be apparent. The interrupted

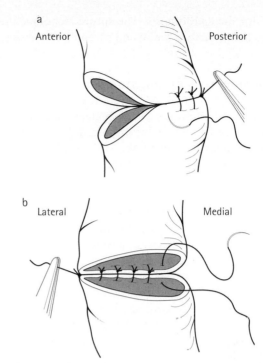

Figure 13.9 *(a) The back wall of a colorectal anastomosis sutured from behind. All knots are on the serosal surface; (b) an alternative is to place the back wall sutures from within the lumen. The knots will lie in the submucosal plane.*

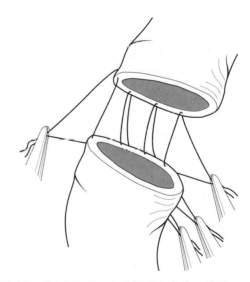

Figure 13.10 *The sutures are all in place before the two ends are apposed. This 'railroad' technique is useful where access is very restricted.*

sutures should then be placed full thickness if it is not practical to exclude the mucosa.

An **end-to-side sutured anastomosis** is merely an adaptation of the end-to-end technique. An incision is made in the side of the viscus to which the end is to be joined. The length of the incision should be such that there are two equal 'lumens' for the anastomosis. The suture technique used is similar to that described for an end-to-end anastomosis.

Sutured side-to-side anastomosis

This is a useful anastomosis when a segment of gastrointestinal tract is to be left *in situ*, but bypassed. It may be undertaken in a similar fashion to the end-to-side anastomosis described above and constructed with a single layer of interrupted sutures. If, however, both sides of the anastomosis have a rich blood supply, making haemostasis of the cut ends important, a continuous suture technique has advantages. A second suture layer also adds stability to the anastomosis, and there need be no concern in a wide side-to-side anastomosis that a two-layer continuous technique will significantly narrow the anastomotic diameter. This is a method commonly employed in anastomoses between the stomach and small bowel. A standard, hand-sewn technique for gastroenterostomy, or enteroenterostomy, is described below.

Most surgeons use clamps for this operation, in order to steady the gut, control haemorrhage and to prevent the escape of contents, but others prefer to rely on a skilled assistant. The clamps must be of the light *occlusion* type, which will cause the minimum trauma to the segment of each viscus included in the clamp. An 8- or 9-cm portion should be held within the clamp for a gastroenterostomy, but for an enteroenterostomy about half of this length will suffice. A swab is lain underneath to absorb any spillage, and the two clamps are approximated. They are secured either with a locking device, or are tied together (Fig. 13.11). The outer suture is a continuous seromuscular suture, and the inner suture is an 'all-layer' continuous suture. This is achieved by four separate suturing manoeuvres.

Posterior seromuscular suture: this is a continuous absorbable suture which does not include the mucosa, and which unites the adjacent surfaces of gut. A short end is retained in forceps at the start of this layer and, at completion, the suture is retained for later use as the anterior seromuscular suture. The suture is tied to the loop of the last stitch at the end of the posterior seromuscular layer. This locks the continuous suture, and also provides a loop of suture material which can be held in artery forceps as a stay suture to steady the anastomosis when the clamps are removed. The lumen of each segment is now opened, within the limits of the posterior seromuscular suture, by an incision parallel to the suture line and approximately 5 mm from it (Fig. 13.11a). The incision for a gastroenterostomy will therefore be about 5–6 cm. In the first instance, the incision should be made through the serosal and muscular coats only; the mucosa is then picked up with forceps and incised separately. If diathermy is used for the incision, care must be taken to avoid injury to the opposite mucosal layer. On occasions when no clamps are employed, a sucker should be introduced through the initial mucosal incision to remove contents and to prevent spillage.

Posterior all-layer suture: the suture begins at one extremity of the incisions and unites the posterior cut edges, traversing all coats of the gut. The first stitch should enter the lumen lateral to the end of one incision and, after ligation, the end of the suture is held in forceps (Fig. 13.12). An ordinary over-and-over continuous suture is employed, but, after every five or six stitches, a lock-stitch may be inserted to prevent a possible purse-string effect as the suture is

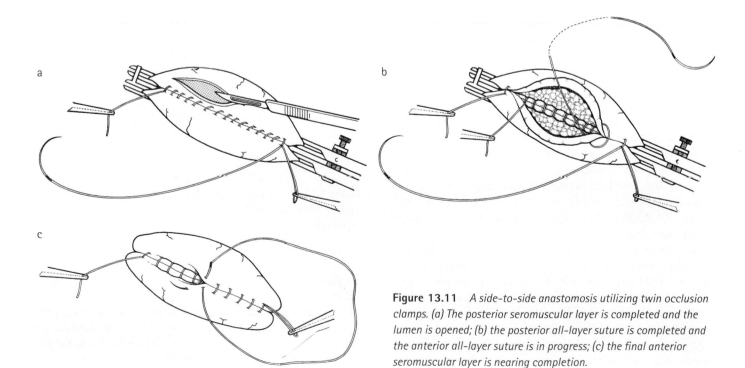

a

b

c

Figure 13.11   *A side-to-side anastomosis utilizing twin occlusion clamps. (a) The posterior seromuscular layer is completed and the lumen is opened; (b) the posterior all-layer suture is completed and the anterior all-layer suture is in progress; (c) the final anterior seromuscular layer is nearing completion.*

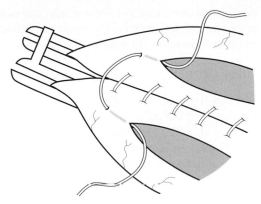

Figure 13.12 *The first suture should enter the lumen lateral to the end of the enterotomy incision. At the other end, care must again be taken to place the suture beyond the extremity of the incision.*

tightened. When the other extremity of the incision is reached, the suture is carried round the corner and continued in the reverse direction as the anterior all-layer suture. Particular care must be taken when turning the corner to ensure that an all-layer suture is again placed beyond the extremity of the incision.

Anterior all-layer suture: this begins as a continuation of the posterior layer, the needle passing from one lumen to the other as before, except that the wall of each gut edge must be traversed separately (see Fig. 13.11b). As the suture is tightened, the mucosa is inverted by the loop of thread which has been inserted. Any tendency to eversion can be overcome by the assistant gently pressing on the cut edges with forceps as the suture is tightened. The suture is continued in this manner, to complete the junction of the cut edges of gut. The suture is tied to the original end which was held in forceps at the start of the posterior all layer suture. The anastomosis should now be watertight and the clamps are removed.

Anterior seromuscular layer: this begins as a continuation of the posterior seromuscular suture, and on completion is tied to the end that was held in forceps at the start of the procedure (see Fig. 13.11c).

Numerous minor modifications of this technique are in common use.

MECHANICAL STAPLING DEVICES WITHIN THE ABDOMEN

In recent years, mechanical stapling devices have improved and become more versatile, so that many surgeons now use them routinely as an alternative to a sutured technique.[3] In many situations the main advantage is speed, whilst the disadvantage is cost. However, a hand-sewn anastomosis can be very difficult when access is severely limited, and it is in these circumstances that mechanical stapling devices have major advantages. One or more rows, or circles, of staples holds the

tissue in apposition. When the device is employed from outside the bowel lumen, the mucosa is held in apposition and an eversion closure of the bowel wall is produced (Fig. 13.13). When the device is employed from within the lumen, the serosa is held in apposition, with an inversion anastomosis (Figs. 13.14 and 13.15). Initial theoretical concerns that healing would be poor when either intact mucosa, or intact serosa, were apposed have proved to be unfounded. An additional theoretical objection to an everted stapled anastomosis is that it leaves mucosa exposed to the peritoneal cavity. This was against all the early surgical principles of anasto-

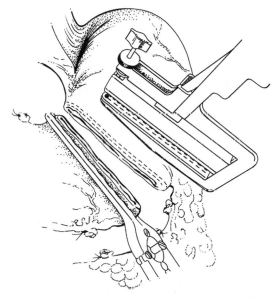

Figure 13.13 *A crushing clamp temporarily seals the distal stomach, which will be removed in this partial gastrectomy. The proximal stomach has been sealed with a double row of staples delivered from a linear stapling device. The stomach has been divided between the two sealed lines.*

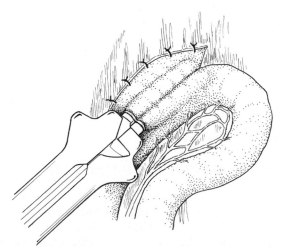

Figure 13.14 *A linear cutting stapling device, with one blade in the stomach and one in the jejunum, can be used to create a stapled gastro-enterostomy. The two small incisions for the insertion of the blades must then be closed.*

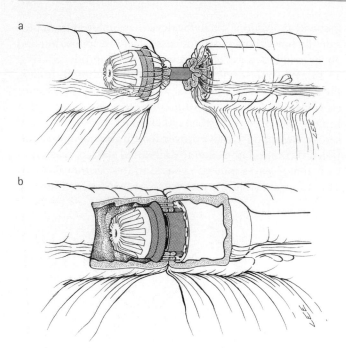

Figure 13.15   *An anastomosis with a circular stapling device. (a) The two parts of the stapling device are initially separate. Each is inserted and the bowel ends drawn over the area through which the staples are fired. The two parts of the device are locked together; (b) the parts of the device are approximated. Firing delivers two circles of staples and excises, with a circular blade, all excess tissue inside the circles of staples.*

motic technique. In general, little difference has been found in numerous studies comparing outcome in stapled versus hand-sewn anastomoses. Stapling devices can be divided broadly into linear and circular instruments, and into those that incorporate a cutting action, and those that do not.

Linear staplers

These staplers deliver several rows of parallel staples, and may in addition have a cutting mechanism between the rows of staples. The staple line is commonly either in line with, or at right-angles to, the handle of the instrument, but other angulations are also available. Preference for each type is dependent on the challenges of access (see Figs. 13.13 and 13.14).

LINEAR STAPLERS WITHOUT A CUTTING BLADE

When fired from outside the bowel, two parallel rows of staples appose the mucosa and close the lumen, but the tissue is not divided (Fig. 13.13). These staplers can be used, for example, to reduce the size of the available stomach in a gastropexy for morbid obesity, and to close the rectum below a tumour during an anterior resection. A linear stapler, fired with one blade inserted into an intermittently retracting ileostomy, will hold the serosal surfaces of the spout apposed

and prevents retraction. A simple linear stapler can easily be mistaken for one which also cuts between the staple line, and care must be taken to select the appropriate instrument.

LINEAR STAPLERS WITH A CUTTING BLADE

These extremely useful instruments deliver four rows of parallel staples and cut between the middle two staple lines. They may be used for dividing bowel and sealing both ends. They are particularly useful when one end is to be brought out as a terminal stoma, as abdominal wall contamination is minimized and the bulk of a clamp is avoided. The distal divided end is also already closed and can simply be dropped back into the peritoneal cavity. The duodenal division in a gastrectomy is another application of this technique. Many surgeons opt for an additional seromuscular suture both to bury the exposed mucosa, and to provide additional security to the closure of a stapled stump left *in situ*.

If the two blades of the stapler are placed in different segments of gut, firing the device creates an anastomosis (Fig. 13.14). There is, however, still the necessity to close the defects through which the blades have been introduced. These stapling devices are used extensively in gastric anastomoses, and for creating ileal and colonic pouches. Further details of their use in these situations are described in the relevant sections.

Small linear stapling devices with a cutting blade can secure and divide a blood vessel, and have a particular role in laparoscopic surgery. Ligation, or transfixion ligation, is suitable for most vessels which have to be divided at open surgery. Some short wide vessels cannot be secured in this fashion, and a sutured closure of the short stump of such a vessel is technically demanding if access is restricted. These small linear stapling devices have thus proved extremely useful in this situation and are used, for example, for the division of the hepatic veins in hepatectomy.

Circular stapling devices

These are the instruments which revolutionized the challenges in low rectal and in oesophageal anastomoses. The instrument can be separated into two portions which are later locked together. In a classical end-to-end low colorectal anastomosis, the smaller portion (or head) of the instrument is inserted through the cut end of the mobilized descending colon, which is drawn over the instrument with a purse-string suture so that only the locking mechanism protrudes. The larger main instrument is then introduced through the anus. The distal bowel wall must also be drawn securely over the portion of the device from which the staples are fired. If the rectal stump has been closed by staples, the spike of the locking device has simply to pierce the closed stump. Alternatively, a purse-string suture is inserted into the open end of the distal rectum and drawn around the locking device. It is important that the bites of any purse-string are not too large, and that any excess tissue has been cleared off the gut which overlaps the ends, as otherwise satisfactory approximation of the two ends is prevented (Fig. 13.15a). Staples which are fired through too great a bulk of tissue will be insecure. A monofilament non-absorbable suture which slides atraumatically through the tissue is most suitable for this purse-string. The two spikes are locked and the ends apposed (Fig. 13.15b). The device is then 'fired'. This delivers two circles of staples to form the anastomosis. A circular blade amputates the excess tissue within the staple line as two 'doughnut' rings. The stapling device can then be removed. The head has to traverse the anastomosis, and with some instruments the head flips into a vertical plane to ease removal.

There are many possible variations of the above procedure when access to an orifice is not possible, or when an end-to-side anastomosis is favoured. The main instrument may be introduced through a separate incision in the lumen (Fig. 13.16). Alternatively, the main instrument, or the head, may be introduced through an open cut end (Fig. 13.17). The opening for the introduction of the main instrument cannot be closed until after completion of the circular anastomosis, and the surgeon must consider whether access for this closure will still be possible.

A circular stapling device may also be used to transect and re-anastomose an intact segment of the gastrointestinal tract. The instrument is introduced locked but separated so that tissue can be drawn between the two halves before they are screwed together. The instrument is fired and a single 'doughnut' of tissue is excised, and continuity is restored by a circular stapled anastomosis. This technique can be used for oesophageal transection for oesophageal varices (Fig. 13.16). The tissue is invaginated by an external ligature around the oesophagus (see Chapter 20). A similar principle is utilized in a stapled haemorrhoidectomy, wherein a circumferential suture, confined to the mucosa, is inserted per anum, and used to draw the mucosa and submucosal haemorrhoidal plexus into a specially adapted circular stapling device (see Chapter 23).

LAPAROSCOPIC PRINCIPLES

Laparoscopic surgical skills are very different from those used in open surgery, and at the start of the laparoscopic era general surgeons embarking on laparoscopic surgery had unacceptably high rates of major complications. An initial patient enthusiasm for smaller scars and faster recovery quickly turned to a climate of suspicion and litigation. It was realized that any surgeon, whether already experienced in open surgery or a trainee, required specific training in laparoscopic skills. National audits were commenced,[4,5] and structured training programmes and simulated workshops were established. Many surgeons, however, find laparoscopic techniques difficult and elect to restrict their practice to open surgery. There are only a few operations in which a laparo-

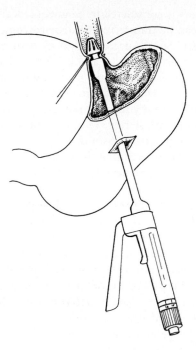

Figure 13.16 *The circular stapler has been introduced through a separate gastrotomy to perform an oesophageal transection and re-anastomosis for varices.*

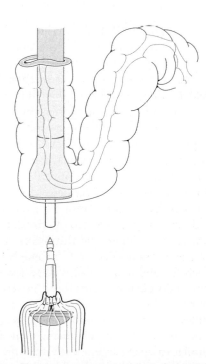

Figure 13.17 *The circular stapling device has been introduced through the open end of the colon for a side-to-end anastomosis onto the top of the rectum. Access to the open end of the colon to close it may, however, be difficult.*

scopic approach is considered to be unequivocally superior, and patients can be transferred to a laparoscopic enthusiast for this surgery. Some surgeons elect to perform much of their surgery laparoscopically, and it is likely that only they will achieve good results from the more complex procedures. Those operations in which a laparoscopic approach is preferable are described in the relevant sections, but basic laparoscopic techniques must first be appreciated theoretically,[6] and in simulated practical sessions.

It must be remembered that the goals in surgery, and the fundamental surgical principals, are the same whether the operation is performed by an open or a minimal access technique. The threshold for surgery may be lower for a laparoscopic procedure as it is rightly viewed as less invasive, but this must not be carried to extremes. Postoperative pain is less, ileus is shortened and respiratory function is better than after open surgery. However, a general anaesthetic is still required and the procedure often takes longer. A routine manoeuvre in an open operation may be difficult to achieve laparoscopically, and it is then sometimes omitted for this reason alone. Surgeons must be honest with themselves over this as it is tempting instead to justify the omission by altering the perceived indications. This situation occurred in the changing indications for intraoperative imaging in the early laparoscopic cholecystectomy practice. A dissection may be more difficult laparoscopically, but any compromise in the dissection of a malignancy is likely to outweigh any short-term benefit from a minimal access operation.

ACCESS

Problems in access are very different in laparoscopic surgery. The positioning of ports is as important in laparoscopic surgery as the choice of the optimum incision in open surgery (see Chapter 12). The view that the surgeon has of the operative field is often superior to that obtained at open surgery, but the manipulation of tissue is more difficult. In general, a laparoscopic approach is more suitable for surgery where access to only one or two quadrants is required.

Retraction of the abdominal wall is achieved by the pneumoperitoneum, which lifts the abdominal wall away from the intraperitoneal structures. The increased intra-abdominal pressure has both cardiac and respiratory effects. In addition, carbon dioxide absorption into the circulation must be eliminated through the lungs, and this places an additional respiratory burden. These effects can be avoided by a technique in which the abdominal wall is lifted away mechanically from the abdominal contents, but this has not found general favour.

All principles to achieve intra-abdominal access by division of adhesions and the development of embryological planes are similar to open surgery, even if the methods are a little different. Intra-abdominal mechanical retraction of structures is more difficult, and more use is made of patient positioning to keep small bowel out of the operative field by gravity.

DISSECTION

Laparoscopic dissection is performed by holding tissue on stretch, and dividing areolar planes in a similar fashion to open surgery. A variety of blunt graspers have been designed for the retraction of tissue. A monopolar diathermy hook and scissors are the standard instruments for dissection. Meticulous haemostasis is essential or visualization rapidly deteriorates. Irrigation of the surgical field will clear small adherent blood clots, but irrigation fluid will then pool in dependent areas of the intraperitoneal space and can be challenging to aspirate.

SUTURES AND LIGATURES

To insert a suture, or to tie a knot, is technically challenging laparoscopically. Greater use is therefore made of clips and stapling devices. Pre-tied sutures in which a loose noose is passed over a structure such as the appendix, and then tightened, can be of great value in some circumstances but have limited application. The suture material for these nooses is important as it must swell in contact with body fluid so that the knot does not slip after it has been tightened. A knot can be tied laparoscopically with two instruments. The technique is similar to that described in Chapter 1 for the instrument tie in open surgery. However, as this is a relatively difficult manoeuvre laparoscopically, diathermy or clips are usually preferred for securing small vessels, and clips or stapling devices for larger vessels.

Many sophisticated mechanical stapling instruments have been introduced for minimal access surgery. They are used for anastomoses, and also for the control and division of larger vessels for which a simple clip would be inadequate. A large proportion of this sophisticated laparoscopic equipment can only be used once, which makes the cost of a laparoscopic operation often significantly higher than that of an open procedure. There are few surgeons who can practice surgery free of all financial constraints. Therefore, when there is only a marginal benefit from a minimal access operation, financial considerations have limited the expansion of laparoscopic techniques.

SPECIMEN RETRIEVAL

An appendix, or a gallbladder, can be retrieved through an 11-mm port, but a bulky specimen may require a small laparotomy incision for delivery. The morbidity from the wound may still be significantly reduced, as the wound is smaller than for open surgery, and can often be made in the lower abdomen, thereby minimizing postoperative respiratory complications. When a specimen is retrieved through a port site, or the smallest laparotomy incision through which it can be extracted, there is a risk of wound contamination by the specimen. Although a wound infection is a significant consideration when removing an infected appendix or gallbladder, the danger of wound contamination by malignant cells when removing a malignancy should be a much more major concern. Retrieval of a specimen within a waterproof bag will protect the port site or mini-laparotomy wound edges. In some situations a specimen may even be broken up within such a bag to facilitate removal from the abdomen. However, the surgeon must remain alert to the dangers of spillage, and be aware that histological examination and staging of a specimen which is no longer intact may be more difficult (see also Chapter 15).

ANASTOMOSES

All the same principles of accurate apposition without tension of well-vascularized ends applies, whether surgery is undertaken by an open or laparoscopic route. It is sometimes possible to combine open and laparoscopic techniques, as a *laparoscopic assisted operation*, to avoid an intracorporeal anastomosis. The dissection for mobilization is performed laparoscopically, and the specimen is then delivered through a small incision and the anastomosis constructed outside the abdomen. When an intracorporeal anastomosis is unavoidable, a specially adapted mechanical stapling device is normally employed, and a hand-sewn laparoscopic anastomosis avoided as suture manipulation is both time-consuming and technically demanding.

REFERENCES

1. Coleman MG, McLain AD, Moran BJ. Impact of previous surgery on time taken for incision and division of adhesions during laparotomy. *Dis Colon Rectum* 2000; **43**: 1297–9.
2. *Last's Anatomy*, 10th edn. CS Sinnatamby. Edinburgh: Elsevier, 1999.
3. Moran BJ. Stapled instruments for intestinal anastomosis in colorectal surgery. Review. *Br J Surg* 1996; **83**: 902–9.
4. Fullarton GM, Bell G. Prospective audit of the introduction of laparoscopic cholecystectomy in the west of Scotland. West of Scotland Laparoscopic Cholecystectomy Audit Group. *Gut* 1994; **35**: 1121–6.
5. Dunn D, Nair R, Fowler S, *et al*. Laparoscopic cholecystectomy in England and Wales: results of an audit by the Royal College of Surgeons of England. *Ann R Coll Surg Engl* 1994; **76**: 269–75.
6. *Laparoscopic Surgery of the Abdomen*. BV MacFadyen, ME Arregui, S Eubanks, JH Peters, NJ Soper. Berlin: Springer-Verlag, 2003.

14

EMERGENCY LAPAROTOMY

INTRODUCTION

An *exploratory laparotomy* is carried out in conditions where the need for an operation is recognized but where a definitive diagnosis cannot be made until the abdomen is opened. Whenever possible, however, an attempt should be made to arrive at an accurate, or at least a provisional, diagnosis before surgery. This not only allows the surgeon to plan the optimum surgical approach to the problem, but may also indicate an intra-abdominal pathology which would be more satisfactorily managed by non-operative means.

Most exploratory laparotomies are performed in the emergency situation, where the value of exhaustive investigations has to be balanced against any deterioration which may occur in the patient's general condition during the inevitable delay. A short delay, during which both active resuscitation and preliminary investigations are performed, is however usually beneficial as surgery on severely shocked or septic patients carries a high mortality. Intensive preoperative resuscitation has the potential to improve physiological status, and reduce the risk of perioperative death, but unfortunately deterioration can also occur. Cardiovascular stability, and adequate tissue perfusion, may not be attainable in the presence of continuing haemorrhage, and as total blood loss rises, coagulopathy may develop. Tissue already compromised by strangulation, or excessive dilatation, may infarct with resultant perforation and sepsis, and absorption of toxic products from any dead tissue will also continue (see Chapter 11). The timing of surgery is therefore very important. The surgeon, aware of the deteriorating intra-abdominal situation, is often impatient to operate on a patient unfit for major intervention. The anaesthetist, in contrast, may strive too long to optimize a patient preoperatively in situations where deterioration is inevitable until the underlying pathology has been addressed by urgent surgery. Any apparent conflict of interest between anaesthetist and surgeon needs discussion and compromise. An adequate level of postoperative care must be planned for such cases.

An emergency laparotomy may be required for major, or persistent, intra-abdominal haemorrhage, whether spontaneous or as a sequel to abdominal trauma. It is also necessary for any traumatic, infective or ischaemic condition in which the integrity of the gastrointestinal wall as a barrier is threatened, or has already been breached. The surgery of intestinal obstruction is covered in more detail in Chapter 22, but the initial management of the obstruction is conservative unless the gut wall is threatened by ischaemia. Similarly, infective intra-abdominal pathologies, in the absence of any threat to gastrointestinal integrity, can often be successfully managed conservatively with antibiotic therapy. Inflammation will resolve and even small collections of pus can be re-absorbed. Larger collections or pus must be drained, but a laparotomy can be avoided in many situations by the use of image-guided percutaneous drainage techniques.

EMERGENCY LAPAROTOMY FOR NON-TRAUMATIC HAEMORRHAGE

Immediate intervention is indicated for massive intra-abdominal haemorrhage which may be intraluminal, but more often is intraperitoneal or retroperitoneal. Surgery is required in parallel with the continuing resuscitation, as any delay is detrimental when the requirement for blood replacement is massive and continuous. *Urgent* intervention is indicated in some instances for continuing, or recurrent, smaller bleeds. Preliminary investigations may have already defined the problem.

Spontaneous intraperitoneal and extraperitoneal haemorrhage

A shocked hypovolaemic patient without a history of trauma, or external blood loss, may have had a massive spontaneous intraperitoneal bleed. The most likely underlying pathology will depend on the age and sex of the patient. Ruptured ectopic pregnancies (see Chapter 26) and ruptured abdominal aortic aneurysms (see Chapter 6) account for the majority of cases. Rarer causes include haemorrhage from a liver tumour, rupture of a splenic artery aneurysm, and the spontaneous rupture of a spleen, rendered more fragile by glandular fever, malaria or adjacent pancreatitis. In some situations the bleeding initially may be contained retroperitoneally. The patient remains haemodynamically stable for a variable period before free haemorrhage into the peritoneal cavity ensues. If the diagnosis is in doubt, a computed tomography (CT) scan is helpful, but the delay for imaging is contraindicated in the unstable patient, and the surgeon must proceed directly to laparotomy without the benefit of confirmatory diagnostic evidence. The abdomen is opened through a generous midline incision, and the surgery is then that of the underlying condition, as discussed in the relevant chapters. However, the first duty of the surgeon is to arrest the bleeding by a clamp, digital pressure or packing to allow the anaesthetist to stabilize the patient. Clean intraperitoneal blood may be filtered and used as an auto-transfusion (see Appendix II). Unfortunately, unless this is a procedure in common use in an operating theatre, attempts to institute it in an occasional emergency usually fail.

Many elderly patients on long-term anticoagulation are at risk of a spontaneous intra-abdominal haemorrhage. Presentations vary, but are seldom sudden or dramatic. The patient is more often anaemic than profoundly shocked. The haemorrhage is usually within the mesentery, the anterior abdominal wall or retroperitoneum, where the expanding haematoma produces pressure effects and pain. The haematoma also activates and consumes clotting factors, and causes further derangements of coagulation. Haemorrhage may have commenced with the International Normalized Ratio (INR) just above the therapeutic range of 2.5–3.5, but this continues to rise, and levels as high as 8 or above are not uncommon in these circumstances. The first priority is to restore blood clotting by reversal of anticoagulation (see Appendix I), and no surgical intervention may be necessary. If there is a large haematoma evacuation may be justified, especially as normal coagulation may be difficult to achieve with the haematoma *in situ*, but this surgery must be covered with a fresh-frozen plasma infusion.

Postoperative haemorrhage

PRIMARY HAEMORRHAGE

Primary haemorrhage during the first 24 hours after abdominal surgery may be dramatic and sudden, indicating the failure of a ligature on a major vessel, and immediate re-laparotomy is indicated. More often, only a small vessel is involved but if bleeding continues then surgical intervention may have to be considered. Clotting abnormalities should be checked, and corrected, and it should be remembered that a large haematoma will derange the clotting factors. If bleeding continues, re-exploration is indicated. Often a haematoma is found, and evacuated, but no bleeding vessel, or persistent haemorrhage, can be identified. The abdomen is closed with a suction drain to the area from which the haematoma was evacuated, and further haemorrhage seldom ensues. If an actively bleeding vessel is identified, it is ligated but occasionally, although significant persistent bleeding is found, it is not possible to identify or ligate specific bleeding points. In this situation packing with large gauze swabs, which are removed at a second laparotomy around 48–72 hours later, is often effective.

SECONDARY HAEMORRHAGE

Secondary haemorrhage, which most commonly occurs at around 10 days after surgery, is very difficult to deal with satisfactorily at reoperation. It may occur in the pelvis after rectal surgery, or from the posterior wall of the lesser sac, either as a complication of pancreatitis or after gastric surgery. It is associated with infection, and the tissue is friable. Sutures and ligatures tear through the tissue, and packing is normally the only practical operative manoeuvre. Ligation of a major feeding vessel at some distance from the bleeding point may be successful but, if interventional angiography facilities are available, selective embolization offers a better alternative to surgical ligation.

Haemorrhage into the lumen of the gastrointestinal tract

Occasionally, the surgeon is forced to operate for massive and continuous intraluminal blood loss without the benefit of preoperative endoscopy, but more often the surgery can be delayed for full resuscitation, and endoscopic and radiological investigations. The surgical management of upper gastrointestinal haemorrhage is discussed in Chapter 17, and that of lower gastrointestinal haemorrhage in Chapter 22.

Gynaecological and obstetric haemorrhage

For details, see Chapter 26.

EMERGENCY LAPAROTOMY FOR PERITONITIS

The decision to operate on a patient with an acute abdomen and suspected peritonitis is always based on a range of clinical, haematological and biochemical factors, supported by increasingly sophisticated imaging. Often, however, the clinical examination of the abdomen is still one of the most sensitive diagnostic tools. Inflammation of the parietal peritoneum triggers the tenderness and the reflex guarding of peritonism. The clinical signs may be elicited over the whole anterior abdominal wall, suggesting a generalized peritonitis, or they may be restricted to one quadrant of the abdomen, suggesting a localized peritonitis. The clinical diagnosis is not always easy. Some patients have referred pain and reflex guarding from supradiaphragmatic, scrotal or retroperitoneal pathology. Basal pneumonia, myocardial infarction and testicular torsion can all mimic a surgical abdomen. Retroperitoneal pathology, including an infected or obstructed urinary system, pancreatitis, and the distension of retroperitoneal tissues from the initial contained rupture of an aortic aneurysm, can also cause diagnostic confusion.

Some intra-abdominal pathologies, such as biliary colic and the capsular distension of a congested liver, can produce signs of peritonism in the absence of peritoneal inflammation. It must also be remembered that some medical pathologies, including sickle cell crises and porphyria, can produce abdominal pain and confusing clinical signs. Ketoacidosis in diabetic patients may present with an apparent surgical abdomen, and this is a particularly common presentation in children. The root pain from shingles precedes the vesicular rash; this is unilateral and localized but may cause diagnostic confusion.

Additionally, not every patient with peritoneal irritation has an intra-abdominal pathology for which surgery is indicated.

Generalized signs of peritonitis

When the signs of peritoneal irritation extend over the whole abdominal wall, this usually indicates the presence of either free intraperitoneal pus or gastrointestinal contents, or alternatively, multiple loops of ischaemic or infarcted bowel. When there are signs of generalized peritonitis an emergency laparotomy is usually indicated, but the surgeon must first consider the other conditions which may mimic peritoneal inflammation, in addition to those causes of general peritoneal inflammation for which surgery is not indicated. Pancreatitis should be excluded when the aetiology of peritonitis is in doubt. A serum amylase measurement, which can normally be available within 1 hour, may prevent an unnecessary laparotomy. The inflammation from a severe gastrointestinal infection may cause a generalized peritoneal reaction. *Campylobacter* is the micro-organism which most often causes confusion with an acute abdomen in the UK. The other conditions outlined above which can mimic peritoneal irritation should also be considered.

When a decision to operate has been made there is often still only the incomplete diagnosis of 'acute abdomen'. Surgical delay for intensive preoperative resuscitation should be considered in all very ill patients, but the 'window of opportunity' must not be missed, and delay beyond 4 hours is usually counterproductive.

Surgical access
Palpation of the relaxed abdomen, once the patient has been anaesthetized, may reveal a mass which was not previously apparent. This may help to elucidate the diagnosis, and indi-

cate the most appropriate surgical approach. A midline incision, which can be extended either up or down as necessary, is the most versatile when the underlying pathology is still obscure. However, if a perforated appendix is strongly suspected as the cause of the generalized peritonitis, it is reasonable to make a small appendix incision. If the diagnosis is wrong it may be possible to deal with the problem by a limited muscle-cutting extension, but more often it is safer to close the initial incision and make a separate midline laparotomy. Some surgeons favour an initial laparoscopy for diagnostic purposes, after which access can be converted to the appropriate abdominal incision if pathology is identified which would be better managed by an open approach.

Ischaemic or infarcted tissue
If ischaemic gut is encountered on opening the abdomen, a mechanical cause of strangulation, by internal herniation or volvulus, should be sought. Mechanical release of a restriction, or the untwisting of a mesentery, restores the circulation and the viability of the segment can be confirmed. However, the restoration of circulation to infarcted tissue should be avoided if at all possible, as the products of the dead tissue, when released into the circulation, will cause further systemic insult. Infarcted tissue must be resected and the surgeon may have to proceed with a small or large bowel resection, a cholecystectomy, gastrectomy or oophorectomy, as described in the following chapters. On occasion, ischaemic but non-infarcted bowel is encountered due to a mesenteric vascular thrombus or embolus, and restoration of perfusion may still be an option (see Chapters 6 and 22). Unfortunately however, the ischaemic damage from mesenteric vascular accidents is usually already irreversible at the time of laparotomy. The ischaemia associated with a severe intramural infective process rapidly progresses to infarction and is irreversible. Ischaemia from a severe intramural vasculitic process usually follows a similar course.

Purulent peritonitis
If free intraperitoneal pus or gastrointestinal contents are encountered, they should be removed from the peritoneal cavity by suction, and the cause located. This is usually obvious, and the surgical options for the various pathologies are discussed in the following chapters. If the cause of the peritonitis is not immediately apparent, the colour, odour and consistency of the pus can give helpful clues. Thin, bile-stained pus suggests an upper gastrointestinal perforation, while faeculent pus suggests a colonic perforation. Gastric acid induces an intense peritoneal reaction, even before any secondary infection develops, and at laparotomy for a perforated duodenal ulcer the peritoneal fluid may not be purulent. Perforation can occur into the lesser sac, and a generalized peritonitis then only follows as the contamination spreads. This must be remembered when no gastrointestinal perforation can be found. A perforation into the lesser sac can only be excluded if the lesser sac is opened (see Fig. 13.4, page 220). When there is pelvic pus, the underlying pathology may be difficult to determine as any

structure lying within it will be secondarily inflamed. The pus from a ruptured diverticular abscess may thus be erroneously ascribed to infection of the appendix or fallopian tube. If a generalized, or pelvic, peritonitis from salpingitis is discovered, the pus should be removed by suction and the patient treated with antibiotics. A tubo-ovarian abscess or an underlying septic abortion, however, will require further intervention. Gynaecological pathology, which can present as an emergency leading to a laparotomy by a general surgeon, is discussed further in Chapter 26.

Occasionally, no cause for a purulent peritonitis can be found. In these circumstances all the surgeon can do is to be sure that no pathology has been missed, remove all pus by suction and send a pus sample for culture. The peritoneal cavity should be washed out with saline, or with an antibiotic wash (e.g. tetracycline, 1 g/L saline). The abdomen is closed, and broad-spectrum antibiotics continued until the sensitivities of the causative organisms are known. *Primary tuberculous, streptococcal* and *pneumococcal peritonitis* are now rare in the developed world, although primary peritonitis is a recognized complication in patients undergoing peritoneal dialysis.

- In *acute tuberculous peritonitis* the peritoneal exudate is clear and straw-coloured. In addition, tuberculous nodules and lymphadenopathy are apparent. If tuberculosis is suspected, tissue samples should be taken for histology.
- In *chronic tuberculous peritonitis* the laparotomy has usually been undertaken for small bowel obstruction, and multiple adhesions rather than exudate predominate.
- The fluid in *streptococcal peritonitis* is turbid and may be blood-stained.
- In *pneumococcal peritonitis* the pus is thick and greenish yellow.

Occasionally, although the preoperative diagnosis of peritonitis is not upheld at laparotomy, the correct diagnosis is immediately obvious. The enlarged lymph nodes of mesenteric adenitis may be easily palpable, Henoch–Schonlein purpurae may be visible on the serosa of the bowel, or patches of saponification indicating acute pancreatitis may be apparent in the omental fat. No operative procedure is helpful, and the abdomen is simply closed. When no intraperitoneal pathology is apparent the surgeon must reconsider the other conditions which can mimic the surgical abdomen.

POSTOPERATIVE PERITONITIS

This is difficult to diagnose, as local symptoms and signs are masked by the recent laparotomy. In addition – and especially in the elderly – the systemic toxicity can take the form of general cardiac and respiratory problems, with associated neurological deterioration, and the underlying surgical cause is easily missed. The time since surgery, and the nature of that surgery, provide some indication of the most likely underlying pathology. Infarction of a major segment of the gastrointestinal tract, or pancreatitis, usually present early, whereas an anastomotic dehiscence most often occurs between the 7th and 14th days after surgery. An anastomotic leak at some sites can be confirmed by a water-soluble contrast study, and the management is almost invariably operative. The surgery of anastomotic dehiscence is discussed further in the following chapters. In general, however, repair of a delayed anastomotic leak is seldom practical, and the emergency surgery consists of drainage, and some form of diversion of the gastrointestinal contents, so that further contamination of the peritoneal cavity is prevented.

THE ACUTE ABDOMEN IN INTENSIVE CARE

The critically ill patient in intensive care poses difficult decisions for the surgeon when an intra-abdominal catastrophe is suspected. Diagnosis is not straightforward as these patients are often on mechanical ventilation, sedated, and receiving inotropic support. Any clinical abdominal signs are masked and the systemic signs of the systemic inflammatory response syndrome (SIRS) are modified, or suppressed, by intensive management.

The patient who has had recent trauma, or abdominal surgery, is at increased risk of an intra-abdominal complication. Previously unsuspected blunt abdominal injury may have occurred in addition to the major neurological, or thoracic, trauma for which the patient is receiving treatment. The left colon may become ischaemic following abdominal aortic surgery, or an anastomosis may have leaked after gastrointestinal surgery. Postoperative haemorrhage is difficult to diagnose in patients who are cardiovascularly unstable from multiple causes. There may be a cardiogenic, or a septicaemic, component to the hypotension. In addition, fluid shifts and the haemodilution of over-hydration make the interpretation of hypovolaemia, or of a falling haemoglobin, difficult. A return to the operating theatre for a repeat laparotomy adds little to the total physiological insult in a severely ill patient on ventilatory support, and more is lost by delaying a second look than in performing an unnecessary further procedure.

Intra-abdominal surgical complications are increasingly recognized in the non-surgical ITU patient. Mesenteric vascular thrombosis is common. Immunosuppressed patients receiving cytotoxic chemotherapy may develop right-sided neutropaenic colitis necessitating a right hemicolectomy. Acalculus cholecystitis, which usually requires an emergency cholecystectomy, is a common cause of an acute abdomen in a patient in intensive care, and is not related to recent abdominal surgery. Primary peritonitis, as a complication of peritoneal dialysis, is treated conservatively unless there is evidence of another intra-abdominal pathology requiring surgical intervention.

Localized signs of peritonitis

A more confident provisional diagnosis is possible when there are signs of peritoneal inflammation restricted to one quadrant of the abdomen, and the surgeon is able to be more selective in proceeding to laparotomy. Urgent intervention is indicated if the integrity of the gastrointestinal wall is threatened, whether the underlying pathology is infective or ischaemic.

INFECTIVE PATHOLOGY

The history, and the localized signs, may suggest an infective inflammatory process in the gallbladder, the fallopian tubes, the appendix or in a segment of sigmoid diverticular disease. All of these conditions may settle spontaneously, or respond to antibiotic therapy. Early surgery is indicated in those conditions which carry a high risk of progression to peritoneal contamination with gastrointestinal contents or faecal pus. Thus, the management of appendicitis is operative, and that of salpingitis conservative. Cholecystitis and colonic diverticulitis will usually settle on conservative management with antibiotics. If, however, deterioration on medical management is occurring the surgeon must not forget the potential for rupture and generalized peritonitis. Emergency cholecystectomy and sigmoid colectomy are described in the relevant chapters.

ISCHAEMIA

If the peritonism is of ischaemic origin, then intervention before infarction, perforation or systemic sepsis is the over-riding surgical concern. Localized peritonism, in association with a small bowel obstruction, usually suggests an ischaemic loop of small bowel and is an indication to abandon conservative management in favour of a laparotomy. In a large bowel obstruction, or an exacerbation of pan-proctocolitis, right iliac fossa peritonism indicates compromised caecal perfusion, impending caecal rupture and the need for emergency surgery. However, any inflammatory process involving the full thickness of the bowel wall can induce peritonism from direct involvement of the peritoneum in the inflammation. A segment of Crohn's disease, causing both an obstruction and local peritonism, can be difficult to differentiate preoperatively from a strangulated loop of bowel. Other non-ischaemic full-thickness inflammatory conditions of the bowel, including tuberculosis, typhoid fever and amoebic dysentery, pose similar difficulties with interpretation of signs, as local peritonism may indicate neither ischaemia nor incipient perforation. However, some unnecessary laparotomies may still have to be performed to prevent the serious implications of undue delay when a surgical complication of an inflammatory pathology is missed.

INTRAOPERATIVE DILEMMAS IN THE ACUTE ABDOMEN

The surgeon may find unexpected surgical pathology on opening the abdomen, but if this requires operative intervention then there is simply a change of plan. The incision can be enlarged or, if an initial appendix incision is obviously unsuitable, a separate midline incision is performed. Specialist surgical help may have to be sought and the anaesthetist may require additional monitoring facilities, or blood for transfusion. However, for many surgical conditions there are a variety of operative solutions. In the emergency situation the ideal surgical procedure may be contraindicated by the poor condition of the patient, or the lack of specialist expertise or facilities, and considerable surgical judgement is required. The situation may be further complicated if a malignancy is the primary pathology. If the tumour is still potentially resectable, the emergency surgery must not jeopardise the chances of cure. Conversely, optimal palliation must be considered when a surgical complication of an advanced malignancy is encountered (see Chapter 15).

Some intraoperative dilemmas are related to the realization that the operation was not indicated. If a surgeon opens an abdomen and finds a non-surgical pathology, such as mesenteric adenitis or salpingitis, the abdomen is simply closed, and the patient managed conservatively. More problematic, however, are the situations which might have been managed by a period of initial conservative treatment so that emergency surgery could have been avoided, and now the abdomen has been opened. If *cholecystitis* is found unexpectedly at laparotomy, a cholecystectomy is justified even for a mildly inflamed gallbladder in order to avoid later interval surgery. When an initial appendicectomy incision has been made, the decision is less straightforward. A short segment of severely inflamed *Crohn's disease* should be resected, but the decision is more difficult in extensive disease. If *diverticulitis* is encountered unexpectedly, the decision whether to proceed with a major resection is difficult if the condition is relatively mild. If the left iliac fossa is merely drained, the abdomen closed and the patient treated conservatively, a minority will return for emergency surgery during the same hospital admission. These patients would have been served better by a resection at the initial laparotomy. However, if instead a difficult sigmoid resection is performed on unprepared bowel, in a patient whose diverticulitis would have settled on conservative treatment, this decision may also have been sub-optimal. An emergency colectomy carries greater morbidity, a higher chance of a stoma and, if an underlying cancer was present, a reduced chance of a curative resection. The surgical management of diverticular disease is discussed further in Chapter 22. Intraoperative decisions have to be made on a variety of factors, including the general condition of the patient and the experience of the surgeon.

SURGERY FOR THE DRAINAGE OF LOCALIZED PUS

Localized intra-abdominal pus may be either intraperitoneal or retroperitoneal, or trapped within organs. Small collections of pus may be absorbed, and effective antibiotics have increased the potential for conservative management. Any significant collection still requires drainage as it must be remembered that antibiotics cannot penetrate into an abscess cavity.

Intraperitoneal pus

Localized collections of pus may occur around any intra-abdominal infective pathology which has been walled off from the general peritoneal cavity by omentum, or loops of bowel. This is encountered in appendicular and diverticular abscesses, the surgical management of which is discussed in Chapters 21 and 22. Any minor leak of gastrointestinal contents, secondary to a perforation or anastomotic failure, may become walled off in a similar manner. Localized collections of pus can also persist after the resolution of a generalized peritonitis, and are classically encountered in the pelvis and subphrenic space. Infected haematomas following intra-abdominal surgery are another source of intra-abdominal abscesses. In the pre-antibiotic era, localized intra-abdominal pus was both a common and life-threatening condition that was treated by urgent surgical drainage. Prophylactic antibiotic cover for gastrointestinal surgery, and full antibiotic courses when there is established infection, have greatly reduced this complication.

A patient with suspected intra-abdominal infection is treated initially with intravenous antibiotics. If improvement and resolution does not follow, an ultrasound or CT scan may demonstrate the presence and site of a collection. Image-guided percutaneous drainage of the collection is now preferred to open exploration in most circumstances, and can be employed for pelvic, subphrenic and localized intraperitoneal abscesses. If this facility is not available however, open surgical drainage may still be required.

PELVIC ABSCESS

A pelvic collection can sometimes be confirmed clinically by a palpable boggy swelling in the rectovesical pouch on digital examination. Those abscesses which can be felt in this way will usually drain spontaneously per rectum, or per vaginum. This may be the safest management, as surgical drainage, either per rectum or at a laparotomy, can endanger friable, inflamed small bowel loops in the pelvis. Percutaneous image-guided drainage is increasingly employed for those abscesses in which imminent spontaneous discharge seems unlikely.

SUBPHRENIC ABSCESS

Harmless spontaneous drainage of subphrenic pus does not occur. More frequently, the abscess persists with general systemic toxicity, but occasionally drainage occurs spontaneously through the diaphragm into the lung. Before sophisticated imaging, subphrenic abscesses were difficult to diagnose and greatly feared as a surgical complication with a high mortality. Hiccoughs, a high right hemidiaphragm and right basal lung signs increased suspicion, but diagnosis was frequently based on the maxim, 'Pus somewhere, pus nowhere else, pus under the diaphragm.' The classic air fluid level was unfortunately seldom present. The abscesses were described as anterior and posterior, and were also divided into true subphrenic, and subhepatic, collections. Traditionally, attempts were made to drain subphrenic collections without entry into the peritoneal cavity as this was believed to be safer. The surgical approaches for these procedures are now only of historical interest as, if open drainage is indicated, an approach via an upper midline laparotomy incision is now recommended. This allows access to both the suprahepatic and subhepatic spaces bilaterally, and often there is more than one collection. In addition, a subphrenic abscess may be the result of an anastomotic leak after upper gastrointestinal or biliary surgery. If the peritoneum is opened an anastomosis can be inspected and, if disrupted, decisions taken on the optimal management of the complication which has caused the abscess.

Retroperitoneal pus

A perinephric abscess may be secondary to an infected kidney, but may also occur as a primary blood-borne staphylococcal infection. Similarly, a psoas abscess may be secondary to a posterior colonic perforation, or a vertebral osteomyelitis, but may also be a primary myositis. A loin, or anterolateral extraperitoneal, approach will be suitable for drainage of the pus. Infected retroperitoneal and lesser sac collections associated with pancreatitis are considered in Chapter 19.

Pus trapped within intra-abdominal organs

The surgical management of abscesses in the pancreas and liver are discussed in Chapters 19 and 20. In general, however, these abscesses require urgent, rather than emergency, management. Emergency intervention is required for pus trapped within an obstructed hollow viscus. An empyema of the gallbladder and a pyometrium are examples, but the greatest danger is from infection in an obstructed biliary system or kidney.

Cholangitis is often initially diagnosed as a cholecystitis, and treatment initiated with antibiotics and general resuscitative measures. The swinging fever, severe toxicity and deepening jaundice alerts the surgeon to the more serious diagnosis. Ultrasound imaging may show a stone impacted in the common bile duct. Emergency drainage of the biliary tree is essential, and may be achieved by endoscopic sphincterotomy to allow the impacted stone to pass. If this is not available, then open or laparoscopic exploration of the common bile duct to allow free drainage of bile is mandatory (see Chapter 18).

Pyonephrosis also requires urgent drainage of the obstructed hydronephrotic renal pelvis. The underlying pathology may be a mechanical obstruction from a ureteric calculus, or a functional obstruction from a congenital abnormality of the pelvi-ureteric junction. The situation is usually managed by image-guided percutaneous drainage of the dilated renal pelvis. If radiological skills are not available, the urologist may be able to pass a ureteric stent past the obstruction at cystoscopy. A general surgeon, without urological training, who is faced with this problem may be forced to operate directly on the ureter to remove the calculus, or on the renal pelvis to establish nephrostomy drainage (see Chapter 25).

ABDOMINAL TRAUMA: GENERAL PRINCIPLES

Abdominal trauma may occur as a result of either blunt or penetrative injury. Many patients have associated chest, skeletal and head injuries, and cooperation with all specialists involved is essential. Assessment, and initial management, along the principles of the Advanced Trauma Life Support system (ATLS) is important, and should ensure that other relevant injuries are not overlooked.[1]

- *Blunt trauma* includes direct blows, crushing injuries, blast and deceleration forces. Any intraperitoneal organ may be ruptured without superficial evidence of trauma. The history of the mechanism of injury is important in predicting the likely pattern of internal damage.
- *Penetrating trauma* includes knife and bullet wounds and, again, the pattern of damage varies with the object which has penetrated the abdomen. In gunshot injuries, the velocity of a bullet is also important (see Chapter 3). The abdominal cavity is most frequently breached from an external wound in the anterior abdominal wall, but entry into the peritoneal cavity and damage to intra-abdominal organs can also occur from penetrating wounds in the thorax, the loin, the buttock or the perineum.

Surgery for abdominal trauma is indicated for suspected breaches in the gastrointestinal tract and for continuing haemorrhage. Less commonly an intra-abdominal vascular injury may present with distal ischaemia (Fig. 14.1).

Assessment of the need for laparotomy

An immediate laparotomy may be required for massive intra-abdominal haemorrhage. However, in most instances the urgency is less acute, and unless any delay is obviously detrimental, initial stabilization and evaluation is beneficial. In addition, in many patients it may not be clear initially whether a laparotomy is indicated, or not. The traditional teaching was that all penetrating trauma of the abdomen should be explored, whereas blunt injury could be observed

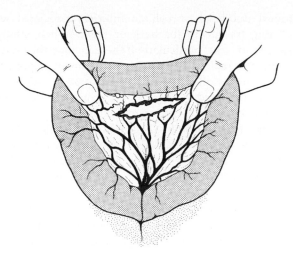

Figure 14.1 *This mesenteric tear will result in an ischaemic segment of small bowel.*

as the incidence of bowel injury was much lower. A patient with a blunt injury was observed, and a laparotomy performed if there was any evidence of peritonitis or intraperitoneal bleeding. It is known, however, that many injuries to the liver, spleen and kidney may bleed significantly initially and then stop and that no surgical intervention is required.[2–4] Experience from the USA and South Africa, where there is a heavy burden of penetrating abdominal trauma, has shown repeatedly that an expectant policy may also be safe in penetrating trauma with a reduction in unnecessary laparotomies.[5] Although an expectant policy may be safe in a stab wound – especially if there is doubt as to whether the peritoneum has even been breached – most surgeons believe that in gunshot wounds exploration is safer as the risk of injury to a hollow viscus is significantly higher.[6]

During the period of active observation further assessment and treatment are continued. Blood and fluid replacement must be adequate for good tissue perfusion, but aggressive over-perfusion must be avoided as it may be a factor in encouraging injuries to re-bleed.[7] A major pelvic fracture, with opening of the pelvic ring, can be associated with massive pelvic venous bleeding. The first line of management is external stabilization of the pelvic fracture to prevent further opening of the ring and to compress the torn pelvic veins, and not an early laparotomy (see Fig. 4.7, page 56).

The decision to proceed to laparotomy following abdominal trauma is based on clinical judgement, often supplemented by imaging and peritoneal lavage.

CLINICAL ASSESSMENT

Laparotomy is indicated for suspicion of injury to a hollow viscus. A clinical assessment of peritoneal irritation, and the signs of SIRS (see Chapter 11), are often more accurate in assessing an injury to the gut than sophisticated imaging. However, early clinical signs may be minimal in retroperitoneal duodenal or colonic injuries, associated with penetrating trauma to the back or flank. When multiple injuries are present, particularly if these include the head or chest and the patient is receiving ventilatory support, the clinical picture is often misleading. In these situations it is often safer to proceed to a laparotomy on a lower level of suspicion than to continue with an expectant policy.

Laparotomy may also be required for continuing haemorrhage but, as bleeding will frequently cease spontaneously, selected patients can be managed conservatively. The total estimated blood loss, and the rate and pattern of bleeding, are all important in the decision regarding laparotomy. Repeated episodes of bleeding, with temporary haemodynamic instability, are more worrying than a slower continuous haemorrhage. The organ injured, and the severity of that injury shown on imaging, may be a more important indicator for the need for intervention than the total blood loss.

IMAGING

Imaging procedures include the following:

- *Plain abdominal* and *chest X-rays* provide some limited information. Fractures of the lower ribs show that there has been an injury which has the potential to damage the liver or spleen, while pelvic fractures indicate potential injury to pelvic organs. Obliteration of a psoas shadow, and fractures of the bodies, or transverse processes, of the upper lumbar vertebrae are markers of significant retroperitoneal trauma. The X-ray may show a diaphragmatic rupture, or it may demonstrate free intraperitoneal or retroperitoneal gas, thus confirming a breach in the gastrointestinal tract.
- An *intravenous urogram* (IVU) provides some assessment of the severity of the damage to a kidney, but more importantly confirms both the presence and the function of the contralateral kidney.
- *CT scanning* is of limited value in excluding a bowel injury, but is an excellent modality for imaging solid organs and the retroperitoneum. If performed with contrast, it can give valuable information not only on the anatomical damage to the liver, spleen, kidney or pancreas, but also information on renal function, major vessel damage and the presence of arterial bleeding into a haematoma. It is therefore a more valuable imaging modality than an IVU in renal trauma. The initial and serial CT appearance of solid organ damage is an increasingly useful predictor of the untreated outcome of an injury, and thus influences the balance between laparotomy and continued conservative management. It may also indicate situations where it is possible to stop the haemorrhage by selective embolization, and avoid surgical intervention. Embolization occludes the vessels at the site of haemorrhage, whereas surgical ligation of the main feeding artery does not take into account any additional collateral inflow.

PERITONEAL LAVAGE

This investigation has been given a high profile in ATLS courses, despite the limited information it provides. Initial descriptions were of blind needle puncture of the peritoneum but, as there is potential for injuring loops of bowel, a small open incision under local anaesthesia is now preferred. This makes the procedure more invasive, more difficult in the obese, and less applicable in a child who may not tolerate it under local anaesthesia. More information will be obtained by a laparoscopy which in turn is even more invasive. The concept of peritoneal lavage overlooks the potential for bleeding to be self-limiting, and many surgeons believe it leads to unnecessary intervention if laparotomy automatically follows a 'positive' test for red blood cells (RBCs). A 'positive' test for white blood cells (WBCs) is more significant as it indicates peritoneal contamination from damage to the gastrointestinal tract.

The patient should already have a nasogastric tube and urinary catheter *in situ* before a diagnostic peritoneal lavage is undertaken. A 5-cm vertical incision is made under local anaesthetic, centred one-third of the way from umbilicus to xiphisternum, and is deepened down to peritoneum, which is then incised under direct vision. A dialysis catheter is inserted and 10 mL/kg body weight of warmed normal saline (to a maximum of 1 L) is run into the peritoneal cavity. After 5–10 minutes the lavage solution is drained and examined microscopically.

A 'positive' result is:

- RBCs > 100 000 per mL; or
- WBCs > 500 per mL.

Gut contents visible on microscopy, or a Gram stain which demonstrates bacteria, also demonstrate a breach of the gastrointestinal tract.

LAPAROTOMY FOR TRAUMA

Significant intra-abdominal trauma can sometimes be managed more appropriately in a non-operative manner. These situations are outlined in the discussion below of the operative management of injuries to specific organs. In cases where the surgeon decides on an emergency laparotomy, consideration must be given to other potential injuries. For example, an apparently minor chest injury with an undetected small pneumothorax, may convert to a tension pneumothorax from the positive-pressure ventilation during a laparotomy. A chest drain should be inserted prior to induction of anaesthesia if this is felt to be a risk. An associated head injury must not be overlooked, and neurological monitoring will be difficult during anaesthesia. If a cervical spine injury cannot be excluded, the neck must be adequately immobilized during the laparotomy.

A midline incision is the most appropriate in almost every circumstance in which an emergency laparotomy is indicated. Blood, or intestinal contents, may be encountered on opening the peritoneum, but a 'clean' peritoneal cavity does not exclude a significant injury. A perforation can easily be missed, and a careful inspection of the whole gastrointestinal tract is essential. A large collection of blood usually indicates damage to the spleen or liver, or to a vessel in the mesentery or omentum. The first priority is haemorrhage control, followed by a thorough exploration to evaluate other injuries.

Injuries to the spleen

Minor injuries to the spleen were often not diagnosed before sophisticated imaging. Many healed without complication, but the occasional delayed splenic rupture occurred. Selected minor splenic injuries, diagnosed on CT in haemodynamically stable patients, can be managed conservatively. An emergency splenectomy is indicated if a major hilar laceration or a totally disrupted spleen is demonstrated, as even if bleeding has temporarily abated, significant further bleeding is almost inevitable. Minor subcapsular haematomata, and peripheral lacerations, can be managed conservatively if bleeding is not excessive (Fig. 14.2).

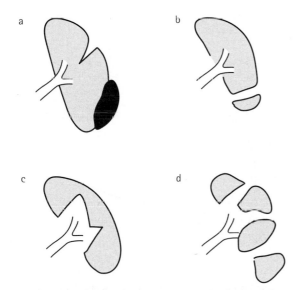

Figure 14.2 *Varieties of splenic injury which may be diagnosed preoperatively on CT scans. (a) A subcapsular haematoma and a peripheral laceration, both of which may heal without intervention. (b) An avulsion of a small portion of one pole; this injury is also compatible with splenic preservation. (c) A hilar laceration, which will almost certainly bleed again. (d) A fragmented spleen.*

Surgical approach
Before the start of an emergency laparotomy the splenic injury may have been confirmed, or the diagnosis may only be of intraperitoneal haemorrhage. If major bleeding is continuing, rapid delivery of the spleen is essential. The left peritoneal leaf of the lienorenal ligament is incised, or broken with a finger (see Fig. 19.12a, page 355), the spleen dislocated forwards and its vascular pedicle compressed between finger

and thumb. This is safer than immediate clamping, which can injure the tail of the pancreas. When haemorrhage is under control, the tail of pancreas is separated from the hilar vessels, and the splenic artery and vein clamped and ligated separately (see Fig. 19.12b, see page 355). Care must also be taken not to injure the splenic flexure of the colon. Elective splenectomy is discussed in Chapter 19, and the emergency splenectomy differs only in the need to control haemorrhage rapidly.

Occasionally, a relatively minor splenic injury is encountered, which has not bled significantly, or has ceased to bleed and was not in fact the indication for the laparotomy. Splenic preservation should then be considered, especially in a child. It will however be more difficult to monitor re-bleeding in the early postoperative period than when an initial decision was made to manage the injury conservatively. Various splenorrhaphy techniques, which can save more severely injured bleeding spleens, have been developed,[8] but opinion is divided over the wisdom of the more aggressive attempts at spleen preservation. However, most surgeons feel it is appropriate to seal a peripheral laceration, or an area of surface oozing, with argon beamer coagulation, or by the application of a surface agent such as fibrin glue. More aggressive repair techniques include the suturing of a laceration, or encasement of the spleen with an absorbable mesh. The spleen must be formally mobilized before any repair can be undertaken, and great care must be taken to avoid further injury. A partial splenectomy is sometimes possible, consisting of excision of the damaged upper or lower pole, after formal ligation of the segmental vessels to the damaged portion.

Injuries to the liver

Haemorrhage from a liver laceration is often self-limiting, and uncomplicated healing can occur even in relatively major liver trauma. Intervention is indicated when haemorrhage is excessive, fails to cease spontaneously, or a CT scan demonstrates an expanding central haematoma with arterial bleeding. This latter injury is unsuitable for conservative management, even if the patient is haemodynamically stable, as the expanding haematoma continues to destroy the surrounding normal liver, and eventually ruptures intraperitoneally. Arterial embolization should be considered for deep-seated arterial bleeding, and the patient should be transferred, if at all possible, to a specialist liver surgery centre.

Surgical approach
When a surgeon performing a laparotomy for trauma encounters massive haemorrhage from the liver it should be temporarily packed, or manually compressed while the extent of the damage is assessed. The bleeding can be reduced by using the Pringle manoeuvre, in which a non-crushing clamp is placed across the free edge of the lesser omentum, occluding inflow from the hepatic artery and portal vein. This should not be left *in situ* for more than 1 hour. Continuing bleeding suggests an aberrant hepatic artery. It

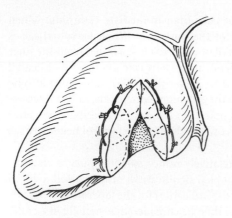
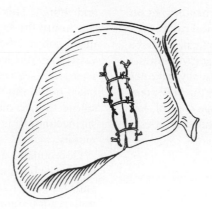

Figure 14.3 *Deep mattress sutures were traditionally used first to compress the edges of the laceration and arrest the haemorrhage, and then further sutures opposed the edges. The sutures cut through the liver parenchyma, but this was overcome by buttressing the sutures over omental fat and taking generous bites of liver substance. More precise techniques have superseded this method in almost all circumstances.*

should be sought in the lesser omentum, where it arises from the left gastric artery, and it is also then temporarily occluded. Temporary aortic control above the coeliac trunk is occasionally necessary. If major haemorrhage continues from behind the liver, avulsion of hepatic veins from the inferior vena cava (IVC) is likely. Access is limited, and repair of these injuries is extremely difficult. A major resection may even be necessary before there is sufficient access for any venous repair. Temporary clamping of the IVC, above and below the liver, or temporary venous shunts, have been attempted. A Foley catheter passed up into the right atrium can secure superior control. The chance of a successful outcome with such heroic manoeuvres is remote even in expert hands, and, as judicious packing has been successful even in these major venous injuries, it is usually the best initial strategy. However, if bleeding cannot be adequately controlled, any window of haemodynamic stability should be used to transfer the patient to a specialized liver unit.

Usually, however, the measures described above provide temporary control of bleeding. Ideally, if the patient becomes more stable, the surgeon may then be able to mobilize the liver by division of the falciform, coronary and triangular ligaments. The liver can then be rotated into the wound, fully examined, and a decision taken regarding surgical intervention or more formal packing. An individual bleeding vessel in a laceration can be ligated, and a surface small vessel ooze can be treated by coagulation with diathermy or an argon beamer. Alternatively, fibrin glue can be used. These techniques are discussed in more detail in Chapter 20. Deep sutures in the liver to compress a bleeding laceration are not now recommended as they cause parenchymal strangulation, but may still occasionally have a place (Fig. 14.3). Formal packing of the liver is regaining favour as the sole measure necessary to control haemorrhage in many injuries. Packing is designed to compress a laceration and should therefore be around the liver (Fig. 14.4), and not into the laceration itself. Ideally, the liver should be the 'filling' of a sandwich with the packs, placed behind and in front, representing the 'bread'. Packs within a laceration are not recommended as they are liable to cause extension of a tear. (However, balloon catheters have been used effectively to tamponade the depths of a bleeding stab or low-velocity bul-

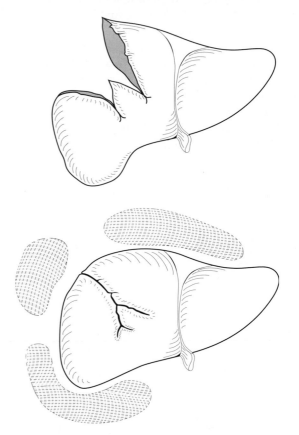

Figure 14.4 *Packs should be placed around the liver to close and compress a laceration. Packing into a laceration causes further damage.*

let track.) Packing has been found to be effective even in severe injuries involving the hepatic veins. Excessive packing may compress the vena cava and, except with a severe posterior injury, care must be taken to avoid this, otherwise venous return is compromised leading to hypotension and peripheral engorgement. The packs should be removed at a second laparotomy at 24–48 hours, but this may be delayed longer if the clotting, or platelets, are still severely deranged.

Arterial bleeding cannot be controlled by packs. Accessible arteries can be ligated, but haemorrhage from an artery deep within the liver parenchyma may be inaccessible without a major resection. There may be no surface laceration, or bleeding from a laceration may have ceased following packing, or the placement of sutures to oppose the superficial portion of the laceration. The expanding haematoma will destroy surrounding normal liver. If this situation is diagnosed on a preoperative CT scan, selective embolization can be most effective. Occasionally, selective hepatic artery ligation may be justified for arterial bleeding which cannot be stopped by other means. This measure is a last resort, but may prepare the situation to allow referral to an experienced surgeon to perform a resection.

Major liver resection for trauma is sometimes indicated, and is described in Chapter 20. It may be an anatomical resection, or a resection dictated by the planes of the injury, removing only devitalized tissue and ligating bleeding vessels. Any emergency resection carries a high mortality except in expert hands, and therefore packing is now considered the first line in treatment. This may be all that is surgically required, or it may be a holding measure to allow transfer of the patient to a specialized liver unit.[9]

On many occasions the surgeon has proceeded to a laparotomy because of other injuries, and a relatively minor liver injury is an additional finding. It can be very difficult to know how aggressive to be in the operative management of an injury which, if it had occurred in isolation, would have been suitable for a conservative approach. Small non-bleeding lacerations can be ignored.

Late complications of liver trauma include liver abscesses, parenchymal necrosis, bile leaks, haemobilia and arterioportal fistulae. These are discussed further in Chapter 20.

Injuries to the kidney

Blunt and penetrating injuries can both cause renal contusion and parenchymal lacerations. Most renal injuries can be managed conservatively, and useful function of even severely damaged kidneys can be regained spontaneously. A cortical laceration will form a perinephric haematoma (Fig. 14.5a), and a medullary laceration will bleed into the renal pelvis with resultant haematuria (Fig. 14.5b). A full-thickness laceration will show on imaging with extravasation of contrast medium (Fig. 14.5c). A non-functioning kidney suggests severe fragmentation, or central renal vessel damage. Even these severe injuries can be treated conservatively if the patient is haemodynamically stable, as the haematoma has a tamponade effect. Angiography of a non-functioning kidney will clarify the extent of the damage further but, as the kidneys can withstand ischaemia for only 15 minutes, little is to be gained by exploring vascular pedicle injuries with a view to restoring renal perfusion.

Attempts to repair an injured kidney in an emergency setting are often unsuccessful, even when undertaken by an experienced urologist. A nephrectomy, which might have been avoided, becomes inevitable as the surgical exploration releases the tamponade and repair of the renal damage becomes essential to arrest the haemorrhage. The treatment is therefore conservative unless an early nephrectomy is essential for severe haemorrhage with haemodynamic instability. The situation must, however, be monitored as a delayed nephrectomy, or an attempt at repair a few days after the injury, may become unavoidable if a falling haemoglobin and serial CT scans indicate an expanding haematoma and continuing haemorrhage. Specialist urological opinion should therefore be sought early, and long-term follow-up is also essential as many patients develop hypertension.

Surgical approach

Massive renal haemorrhage may necessitate an emergency nephrectomy, and is often, in reality, the control of the torn renal artery and vein in a partially avulsed kidney. An abdominal approach in trauma is therefore preferable to a loin approach, even when no associated intraperitoneal damage needs to be excluded. Vascular clamps must be available before the haematoma is entered and any remaining tamponade lost. While haemorrhage is temporarily controlled, an on-table IVU is required to check for function in the contralateral kidney, if this has not been assessed preoperatively.

It may be possible to arrest continuing haemorrhage from a deep laceration, or to preserve some functioning tissue with a partial nephrectomy (see Chapter 25). This can be technically challenging, and a general surgeon, forced to operate on the kidney in an emergency, is more likely to have to proceed

a
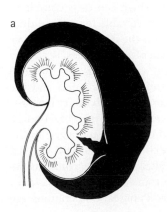

b
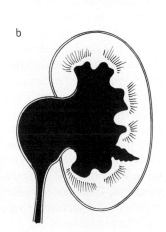

c
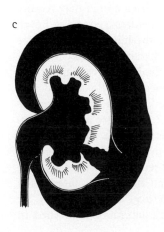

Figure 14.5 *(a) A cortical tear with the resultant perinephric haematoma which tamponades the injury; (b) a medullary tear will lead to haematuria; (c) gross leakage of contrast material on imaging indicates at least one full-thickness laceration, but also confirms that the kidney is still functioning.*

to nephrectomy. A significant renal injury in a solitary kidney therefore requires urgent specialist urological involvement, particularly if surgical intervention appears likely.

Not infrequently, the laparotomy has been performed for another indication, and a perirenal haematoma is encountered. Exploration of this terminates the tamponade effect, and a kidney, which might have regained useful function, has to be removed. Unless the haematoma is actively expanding, or there is massive bleeding into the peritoneal cavity, the injured kidney should be left undisturbed. This would appear to be true even in the management of renal gunshot wounds.[10]

Injury to major vessels

Lacerations of the aorta and IVC require temporary vascular clamps and vascular repair. Massive pelvic haemorrhage can be reduced by ligation of the internal iliac artery on the affected side, but this is less effective than embolization. Temporary clamps on the infrarenal aorta, or on the supradiaphragmatic aorta, may be valuable as a temporary measure to control haemorrhage. Other possibilities include intraluminal balloon catheters and temporary shunts. A non-expanding retroperitoneal haematoma can usually be left undisturbed if it is the result of blunt trauma, the distal flow is normal, and it is not adjacent to a major artery, or the pancreas. An expanding pulsatile haematoma, or one associated with penetrating trauma, requires exploration. Proximal and distal control must be secured before exploration. The surgical approaches and the repair of visceral and renal vessels, the aorta and the IVC are discussed in Chapters 5 and 6. A right or left medial visceral rotation technique should be remembered as a useful manoeuvre when access is required for an injury to the posterior aspect of the aorta or IVC.

Injuries to the stomach and small bowel

The whole small bowel, and its mesentery, must be inspected. Mesenteric tears should be repaired, and bleeding mesenteric vessels ligated. A mesenteric laceration is the commonest cause of intraperitoneal blood if the spleen and liver are intact. A large mesenteric haematoma may require gentle evacuation, and ligation of the damaged vessel. Bowel may have been devascularized by the initial laceration (see Fig. 14.1), but the surgeon must take care not to cause further damage to mesenteric vessels during evacuation of a haematoma, or in the repair of a mesenteric hole. Any devascularized bowel must be resected, and lacerations in the small bowel, or stomach, require repair. Care must be taken not to miss a posterior injury to the stomach, which will only be evident when the lesser sac is opened, or a tear at the duodenojejunal flexure, which is well recognized in deceleration injuries. Primary closure of clean holes with interrupted extramucosal sutures is satisfactory. Resection may be advisable when there are multiple lacerations confined to one segment of the gut, or when lacerations are associated with extensive bruising.

Injuries to the duodenum and pancreas

These injuries may occur separately, but are often combined injuries and may even be associated with major vessel damage. An upper midline retroperitoneal haematoma suggests significant damage, and should usually be explored. The need for urgent vascular control of the IVC or aorta should be anticipated, and vascular clamps should be available before any haematoma is opened. Full mobilization of the duodenum is essential before it can be adequately assessed or repaired.

Isolated duodenal injury

Many clean duodenal lacerations can simply be sutured, but more severe injuries may require complex reconstructive procedures.[11] Even after full mobilization, repair of the second part of the duodenum is not possible if there is any significant tissue loss, or contusion. A gastroenterostomy diversion, even with occlusion of the pylorus, will only divert gastric secretions. Bile and pancreatic juice will continue to enter the damaged segment. A Foley catheter can be inserted through the duodenal defect, and once a mature fistula track has been established it can be removed and spontaneous closure of the fistula anticipated. Alternatively, a Roux-en-Y loop can be brought up and sewn to the edges of the defect (Fig. 14.6a). A surgical solution for severe damage to the duodenum above the ampulla is illustrated in Figure 14.6b, and an option when the injury is below the ampulla is shown in Figure 14.6c. A feeding jejunostomy may be extremely useful postoperatively, and should be established at the initial emergency laparotomy.

Isolated pancreatic injury

When an isolated pancreatic injury is suspected and the pancreatic haematoma has been explored, the area of damage should be drained. If the main pancreatic duct has been transected, an external fistula will result. Although this is a controlled situation in which a stable patient can be transferred at a later date to a surgeon with pancreatic expertise, two alternatives offer a definitive solution at the initial laparotomy.[12] A distal pancreatectomy, which is usually combined with a splenectomy, is therefore preferable for a distal duct transection, and a Roux loop, with the open end sewn over the disrupted duct within the head of the pancreas, is a better alternative for a proximal duct transection. Fortunately, many pancreatic blunt injuries occur in isolation and the diagnosis is delayed. The most common such injury is a pancreatic transection over the convexity of the vertebral bodies. The diagnosis may be suspected clinically, and a rise in the blood amylase level supports the clinical diagnosis. A delayed CT scan, performed a few days after the injury, confirms the diagnosis. It is then possible to transfer such patients to an experienced pancreatic surgeon. Pancreatic operations are described in Chapter 19.

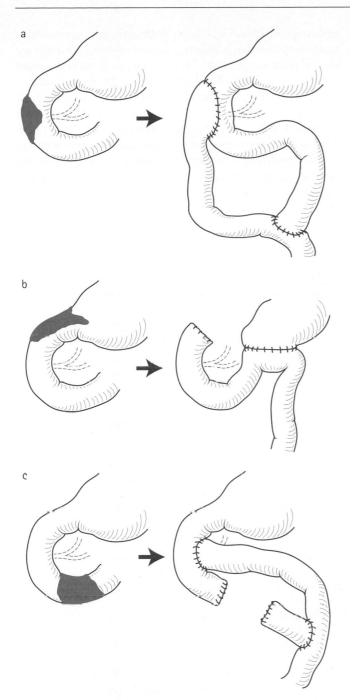

Figure 14.6 *Mobility of the duodenum is very limited, and primary repair may be impossible if there is any tissue loss. (a) A Roux-en-Y loop has been brought up and anastomosed to the edges of a peri-ampullary defect in the second part of the duodenum. (b) An injury proximal to the ampulla can be treated by antrectomy and closure of the proximal duodenum, followed by restoration of continuity with a gastroenterostomy. (c) A transection injury distal to the ampulla can be treated by closure of the ends and drainage of the duodenum by a Roux-en-Y loop.*

Combined injuries

Patients with a very severe injury to the pancreatic head and duodenum occasionally require a pancreaticoduodenectomy, but in an emergency this carries a high mortality even in expert hands. A Roux loop for drainage of the pancreas combined with diversion of gastric secretions away from the duodenum is a safer alternative. Severe pancreaticoduodenal injury may be associated with additional damage to the bile ducts, portal vein or mesenteric root, and survival from such injuries is unlikely.

Injuries to the colon

Colonic injury may be immediately apparent on opening the peritoneum. It is important to remember that a penetrating wound, or a rupture of the colon from a blunt injury, may also occur retroperitoneally, where the consequences of faecal contamination are equally devastating. If there is any likelihood of this the colon must be fully mobilized and inspected. Traditional military teaching was that all colonic injuries should be exteriorized, and primary repair not attempted.[13] However, this is no longer considered necessary, and primary repair, whether by a sutured closure or a resection with primary anastomosis, is now recommended. It has been shown to be safe even in unfavourable circumstances,[14] but some caution should remain regarding left-sided colonic trauma. The peritoneal cavity is cleaned of all contaminants and washed with saline, or an antibiotic wash. Broad-spectrum systemic antibiotics are given and continued postoperatively. On-table colonic lavage (see Fig. 22.4, page 415) may reduce the risk of anastomotic leakage, and the advisability of a temporary proximal loop stoma should be considered if the surgeon has any concern over an anastomosis, or a sutured laceration, in the large bowel (see Chapters 21 and 22).

Injuries to the rectum

The rectum may be injured in a major crushing injury of the pelvis. Damage more often occurs from penetrating lower abdominal injuries, or from perineal impalement. In the latter, the direction and depth of impalement will determine whether the rectal injury is retroperitoneal or intraperitoneal, and also whether any additional damage has been sustained to the bladder, membranous urethra or intra-abdominal structures. When there are signs of peritonitis after a perineal impalement, a laparotomy should be performed, as this has the advantage of excluding additional injuries to the bladder, or to loops of small bowel. The rectum is then mobilized by division of the pelvic peritoneal reflections to open the retro-rectal space. In the absence of peritonism, or evidence of bladder damage, a perineal wound can be explored initially from below, with the patient in the prone jack-knife position.

A rectal laceration should be repaired if this is possible. When a perineal wound is found to enter the rectum, additional abdominal access for rectal mobilization should always be considered, but despite a combined approach from the abdomen and perineum, access for repair may not be practical for a rectal injury below the peritoneal reflection. Occasionally, an injury to the rectum is suspected but cannot be identified, and there is continuing doubt as to whether significant injury has been sustained, or not. If after exploration, there is any suspicion of an unconfirmed rectal injury, an injury has been visualized but cannot be satisfactorily repaired, or even if a laceration has been identified and sutured, the rectum should be defunctioned during healing (see Chapter 21), and a drain should be left in the retrorectal space. Maximal defunctioning will be achieved by an end (rather than a loop) colostomy, and this may be preferable when there is a severely injured rectum. The sigmoid loop is divided and the rectum washed out through the distal cut end. The proximal sigmoid cut end is brought out as a temporary end colostomy. The distal end is closed and fixed to the lower end of the abdominal closure where it can be easily identified at the subsequent operation to restore continuity.

Injuries to the bladder

An intraperitoneal bladder tear is sutured in two layers with absorbable material and a urethral catheter left *in situ* on free drainage for 10 days. Extraperitoneal bladder tears and urethral injuries are discussed further in Chapters 24 and 25.

Injuries to the diaphragm

Rupture of the diaphragm can occur with blunt trauma. Penetrating injuries to the abdomen or chest may also lacerate the diaphragm, and the incidence may be as high as 15 per cent in lower chest stab wounds. The injury is easily missed, and presentation may be years later in a patient who never came to surgery at the time of trauma. When an emergency laparotomy for trauma is undertaken, the diaphragm should be checked and any laceration carefully sutured (see also Chapter 7).

Massive intra-abdominal trauma

Occasionally, an immediate laparotomy is necessary in parallel with intensive resuscitation, and the surgeon is faced with exsanguinating haemorrhage, widespread massive injury and gross peritoneal soiling. In addition, there may be retroperitoneal and mesenteric haematomata of doubtful significance. The patient is probably hypothermic, acidotic and coagulopathic. Once active haemorrhage is controlled, a temporary solution is prudent. Gastrointestinal contents are cleared from the peritoneal cavity, and any areas of damaged leaking gut simply isolated with staples. The abdominal wall fascia is left open, but the skin is closed if this is possible. If the tension is too great, due to haematoma or liver packs, a temporary containment should be used (see Chapter 12). The patient is transferred to intensive care with the intention to perform definitive surgery in 6 to 48 hours when his or her general condition has improved.[15] Sophisticated imaging will be difficult to perform during this period but, from the initial laparotomy, problems will be anticipated for which the assistance of a particular specialist might be needed.

REFERENCES

1. Advanced trauma life support (ATLS) course manual.
2. Carrillo EH, Platz A, Miller FB, *et al*. Non-operative management of blunt hepatic trauma. Review. *Br J Surg* 1998; **85**: 461–8.
3. Konstantakos AK, Barnoski AL, Plaisier BR, *et al*. Optimising the management of blunt splenic injury in adults and children. *Surgery* 1999; **126**: 805–13.
4. Morrow JW, Mendez R. Renal trauma. *J Urol* 1970; **104**: 649–53.
5. Shaftan GW. Indications for operation in abdominal trauma. *Am J Surg* 1960; **99**: 657–64.
6. Saadia R, Degiannis E. Non-operative treatment of abdominal gunshot wounds. Review. *Br J Surg* 2000; **87**: 393–7.
7. Bickell WH, Wall MJ, Pepe PE, *et al*. Immediate versus delayed fluid resuscitation for hypotensive patients with penetrating torso injuries. *N Engl J Med* 1994; **331**: 1105–9.
8. Feliciano DV, Spjut-Patrinely V, Burch JM, *et al*. Splenorrhaphy; the alternative. *Ann Surg* 1990; **211**: 569–81.
9. Parks RW, Chrysos E, Diamond T. Management of liver trauma. Review. *Br J Surg* 1999; **86**: 1121–35.
10. Velhamos GC, Demetriades D, Cornwell EE, *et al*. Selective management of renal gunshot wounds. *Br J Surg* 1998; **85**: 1121–4.
11. Degiannis E, Boffard K. Duodenal injuries. Review. *Br J Surg* 2000; **87**: 1473–9.
12. Johnson CD. Pancreatic trauma. Leading article. *Br J Surg* 1995; **82**: 1153–4.
13. Edwards DP, Galbraith KA. Colostomy in conflict; military colonic surgery. Leading article. *Ann R Coll Surg Engl* 1997; **79**: 243–4.
14. Kamwendo NY, Modiba MCM, Matlala NS, *et al*. Randomized clinical trial to determine if delay from time of penetrating colonic injury precludes primary repair. *Br J Surg* 2002; **89**: 993–8.
15. Hirshberg A, Mattox KL. 'Damage control' in trauma surgery. Leading article. *Br J Surg* 1993; **80**: 1501–2.

SURGERY OF INTRA-ABDOMINAL MALIGNANCY

The surgery of intra-abdominal malignancy forms a large proportion of the workload of a gastrointestinal surgeon. Almost without exception, the only single intervention which can offer a patient the chance of a cure is a well-performed operative resection. However, the need for surgical intervention to establish the diagnosis has diminished with improvements in endoscopic and radiological technology, and palliative intervention is now shared with radiologists, radiotherapists and oncologists. When a curative resection is possible, it is therefore of the utmost importance that a surgeon does not jeopardize the possibility of cure by inadequate or poorly planned surgery. When cure is no longer possible, radical surgery sometimes still offers the best palliation, but the surgeon must avoid inappropriate radical surgery. A simpler operative procedure may be as effective in relieving symptoms, and in other situations surgery may have no place. Surgeons must understand the methods of spread, and the natural history of, the various intra-abdominal malignancies if they are to make the best operative decisions.

ADENOCARCINOMA OF THE GASTROINTESTINAL TRACT

This is the commonest intra-abdominal malignancy. The mode of tumour spread, and therefore the principles underlying a radical resection, are similar throughout the gastrointestinal tract. However, the importance of the various modes of spread show regional variation along the gastrointestinal tract and influence surgical strategy.

SUBMUCOSAL EXTENSION

Submucosal extension of malignant cells beyond the macroscopic edge of a tumour has long been recognized,[1] and is a major problem in upper gastrointestinal tract tumours. In oesophageal cancer, involved resection margins are not uncommon even with a macroscopic clearance of 5 cm.[2] Multifocal field change is another problem in oesophageal malignancy,[3] and it may be difficult to differentiate from submucosal spread (Fig. 15.1). In colonic cancer, despite early research suggesting significant intramural extension, the macroscopically normal mucosa a few millimetres beyond a tumour is almost invariably free of malignant cells.[4]

DIRECT INVASION

Direct invasion by a tumour to involve adjacent structures classifies it as a locally advanced (T4) tumour, but this is not always associated with metastatic spread. There may be no lymphatic, or blood-borne metastases, and cure by radical surgery is still possible. Preoperative radiotherapy improves the chance of a curative resection in some T4 rectal cancers (see Chapter 22). The tumour must not be 'ruptured' at operation, and therefore any involved structures must be removed en bloc (Fig. 15.2). For instance, the rectum can be excised

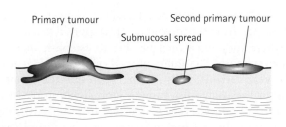

Figure 15.1 *Some carcinomas spread along the submucosal plane. Multifocal primary tumours can also arise within areas of pre-malignant field change. In both situations a wide clearance of the macroscopic primary tumour is necessary to ensure tumour-free resection margins.*

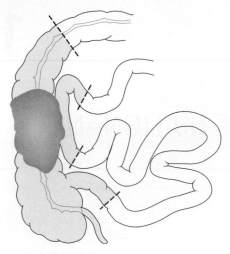

Figure 15.2 *A radical resection of this ascending colon cancer requires an en bloc excision of the adherent loop of small bowel with the primary tumour. An additional small bowel anastomosis will be required.*

with a seminal vesicle or a cuff of vagina. A colonic tumour can be excised with an adherent disc of anterior abdominal wall, the dome of the bladder or a loop of small bowel. This is more often appropriate in lower rather than in upper gastrointestinal tract tumours. In the latter case a locally advanced tumour is rare in the absence of dissemination.

It is often difficult at operation to distinguish between malignant infiltration by a tumour and an inflammatory adhesive reaction to a tumour. Differentiation can only be made on histological examination, and the surgeon therefore has no option but to assume that the adhesion represents malignant infiltration if curative surgery is to be attempted. Inflammation, with desmoplastic fibrosis, will be the explanation in around 50 per cent of such cases.

Direct invasion along perineural planes is increasingly recognized as a separate phenomenon from lymphatic spread. It is seen particularly in pancreaticobiliary tumours, and carries a poor prognosis.[5]

Metastases

In order for metastases to be established, viable tumour cells must be shed from the tumour and transported to a new host site, where they must then be able to establish their own microcirculation. The ability of shed cells to implant at new sites is very variable. Cells may be taken into the lymphatic system or they may form tumour emboli within blood vessels. In addition, cells may be released from the surface of a tumour into the gut lumen or into the peritoneal cavity. Shedding of viable tumour cells occurs spontaneously, but it may also occur during surgery, especially if the dissection enters the primary tumour or transects the lymphatic drainage channels. This 'infective' capacity of tumour cells has long been recognized.[6]

TUMOUR SPILLAGE

Intraluminal spread

Intraluminal seeding of tumour cells has been reported in haemorrhoidal wounds in the presence of a colorectal carcinoma.[7] It has also been shown to occur from an oesophageal tumour to the anterior abdominal wall around the placement of a gastrostomy tube.[8] The anastomotic suture line recurrences in colorectal cancer surgery reflect both this phenomenon and the ingrowth of inadequately excised lymph node disease. Intraluminal cytotoxic washes are used perioperatively to prevent intraluminal seeding.

Transcoelomic spread

This is a frequent mode of spread in gastric cancer, but is less frequent in colonic cancer. It can occur in any cancer which has breached the serosa and then sheds cells intraperitoneally. Viable tumour cells may also be spilled at the time of surgery from intraluminal spillage, tumour rupture during dissection or transection of involved lymphatic channels. Meticulous surgical technique is therefore important, and can be combined with tumoricidal peritoneal washes. Even washes with water will cause osmotic disruption and cell death. Serosal seeding may occur on any peritoneal surface, but the ovary is a particularly fertile site for implantation. Tumour cells will also implant preferentially in areas of peritoneal damage, and this may explain some local anastomotic recurrences and laparoscopic port site metastases.

Macroscopic seedlings at the time of surgery virtually preclude a curative resection. In upper gastrointestinal malignancy, where other modalities often offer better palliation than surgery, metastases should, if possible, be diagnosed preoperatively. Small peritoneal deposits are not easily detected by computed tomography (CT) scans or other imaging, and a laparoscopy before resectional surgery may avoid an unnecessary laparotomy. In colonic malignancy a resection is usually still the best palliation, so little is gained by the addition of a routine preoperative laparoscopy.

The fear of *microscopic peritoneal deposits* has encouraged surgeons to consider intraperitoneal chemotherapy at the time of surgery, and this will almost certainly offer a chance of cure to an occasional patient.[9] The great majority, however, will be treated unnecessarily as they are either already cured, or are already incurable from distant metastases at the time of surgery. The increased morbidity and mortality associated with perioperative intraperitoneal chemotherapy makes it unsuitable for general use.

LYMPHATIC SPREAD

Metastases occur in the mesenteric lymph nodes of the gut along the lymphatic drainage channels of the tumour. Lymphatic drainage follows the arterial vascular system (Figs. 15.3 and 15.4), and metastases usually occur in an orderly pattern, with involvement first of the nodes adjacent to the organ, followed by those close to the roots of the three visceral arteries, and finally in the pre-aortic nodes. All radi-

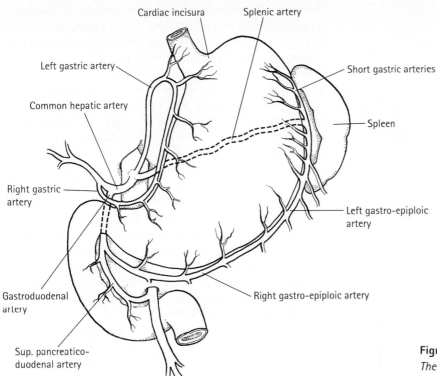

Figure 15.3   *The arterial anatomy of the stomach. The lymphatic drainage channels follow the arteries (see Fig. 15.5).*

cal carcinoma surgery aims to remove the lymphatic drainage of a tumour en bloc with the tumour itself. Even if the nodes are macroscopically normal, they may contain microscopic deposits. En bloc resection is important as dissection across lymphatic channels may spill viable tumour

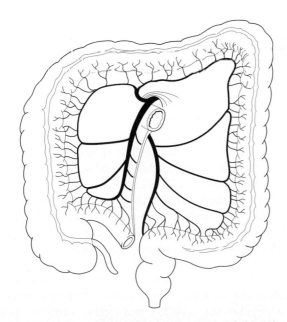

Figure 15.4   *The lymphatic drainage of the colon follows the arteries. A radical lymphadenectomy can therefore be planned on the basis of the arterial anatomy. The arterial division then dictates the length of bowel which will have to be excised.*

cells into the peritoneal cavity. The radicality of lymph node resection varies, and the decision is difficult when increased radicality is known to result in higher operative morbidity or mortality – especially in tumours where the surgeon is aware that in most patients greater radicality is either unnecessary or fruitless.

Gastric cancer metastasizes to the lymph nodes along the four gastric arteries, and then to the pre-aortic nodes. The lymphatic drainage has been extensively mapped and the nodes divided into separate groups (Fig. 15.5). The traditional radical gastrectomy did not include all these groups of lymph nodes, and it was initially hoped to improve the cure rates by a more radical lymphadenectomy. Previously, a more radical lymphadenectomy had only been carried out for clinically involved nodes, in situations where it was already too late to attempt a cure. It has now been established that, in the absence of liver secondaries, peritoneal seedling or pre-aortic enlarged nodes, a more radical lymphadenectomy may increase cure rates of the disease, but at the expense of a higher perioperative mortality from the more extensive surgery.[10] Early mucosal T1-stage cancers diagnosed on endoscopy pose further problems. In those in which lymph node metastases are very unlikely, a local excision either without lymphadenectomy or with only excision of the nodes adjacent to the stomach wall close to the tumour may be all that is required. These issues are discussed further in Chapters 16 and 17.

Oesophageal cancer drains to cervical and coeliac nodes in addition to thoracic nodes. Radical resections include the dissection and en bloc excision of these drainage nodes.

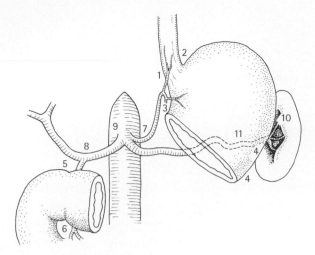

Figure 15.5   *Gastric lymph nodes have been mapped and numbered. Nodes 1–6 are in the greater and lesser omentum, adjacent to the stomach wall, alongside the arterial arcades. Nodes 7–11 are along the more proximal course of the gastric and gastro-epiploic arteries which are now retroperitoneal in position. Nodes 12–16, which are not shown in this diagram, lie either outside the main lymphatic drainage pathways of the stomach or, in the pathway but proximal to the coeliac root.*

There is, however, no containing mesentery and no apparent 'tumour package'. Local extension and distant metastases also occur early.

Pancreatic cancer drains directly to retroperitoneal nodes, but this tumour also metastasizes early both to the liver and within the peritoneal cavity. These metastases and direct extension into the portal vein, or mesenteric vessels, are usually more important limiting factors to a radical curative resection than lymph node metastases. *Primary liver tumours* spread by infiltration along planes within the liver, and lymphatic spread is not a major consideration.

In *rectal and colonic cancer*, lymphadenectomy decisions are fairly easily made as removal of the whole of the mesenteric drainage area as far as the mesenteric root adds little to the morbidity and much to the cure rates (see Fig. 15.4). The removal of pre-aortic nodes is usually considered fruitless if they are involved – and pointless if they are not – although it is still possible that there could be a marginal gain in those patients with only microscopic involvement.

Squamous cell carcinoma of the anal canal drains to the inguinal nodes, in addition to some drainage to the nodes along the inferior mesenteric artery. Treatment of this malignancy is no longer primarily surgical (see Chapter 23).

HAEMATOGENOUS SPREAD

Portal vein dissemination
The portal vein is the main route for the haematogenous spread of all gastrointestinal carcinomas within the portal venous drainage system. (The intrathoracic oesophagus and lower anal canal also drain directly into the systemic system.)

Extra-mural invasion of veins by tumour is sometimes reported by the pathologist, and this in general is an indicator of a poor prognosis. Primary and secondary tumours in the liver can invade branches of the portal vein and spread to other sites within the liver by this route.

Secondary deposits in the liver can occur early in the growth of a carcinoma, and many patients with an apparently normal liver at the time of surgery are shown subsequently to have already had micro-metastases. This was the basis of the trial in which 5-fluorouracil (5-FU) was administered via the portal vein for 7 days immediately after surgery.[11] A catheter is introduced at the time of surgery into the portal venous system through the obliterated umbilical vein, which lies in the free edge of the falciform ligament. If this cannot be cannulated, then alternative access is possible via a gastro-epiploic vein, or a small bowel mesenteric vein. Only a small benefit was shown, similar to that reported from the more conventional postoperative chemotherapy regimens.

Patterns of liver metastases vary among different tumours. Multiple tiny seedlings throughout the liver are clearly unsuitable for surgical removal. Colonic tumours often produce only a few secondaries in the liver and surgical excision, if technically feasible, should always be considered as cure is still possible. Although this has been known for some years,[12] many patients who would be suitable are never referred for assessment.

Systemic blood-borne dissemination
Systemic metastases most often occur as part of a generalized dissemination of tumour in a patient who already has intraperitoneal, retroperitoneal and liver secondaries. Isolated secondaries do, however, occur in such sites as the brain and lungs.

CARCINOID TUMOURS

Carcinoid tumours arise from the enterochromaffin cells which are present throughout the gastrointestinal tract, and may be either benign or malignant. A small benign carcinoid is most often encountered in an appendix which has been removed due to appendicitis. The tumour, rather than a faecolith, has obstructed the lumen and initiated the appendicitis. A small bowel carcinoid may cause obstructive symptoms, and at surgery will be excised as a possible small bowel carcinoma. These tumours are frequently multiple and the whole small bowel must be carefully examined. Malignant carcinoid tumours have a pattern of spread similar to that of gastrointestinal carcinomas, but they are slower-growing and a patient with metastatic carcinoid may remain in reasonable health for some years. Carcinoid tumours secrete 5-hydroxytryptamine (5HT) and other related active compounds which are metabolized in the liver. When the systemic levels of these active compounds rise and the symptoms of 'carcinoid syndrome' develop, it indicates that the tumour is draining directly into the systemic circulation.

Thus, it usually indicates liver metastases draining into the hepatic veins, but the liver can also be bypassed when there are tumour deposits in the retroperitoneal nodes. The flushing, diarrhoea and bronchoconstriction of the carcinoid syndrome can be controlled with octreotide (which blocks 5HT release), but the resection of liver secondaries should also be considered, especially as this is one of the few situations where even partial removal of liver secondaries may lead to a significant improvement in symptoms and prognosis.[13]

OTHER HORMONE-PRODUCING INTRA-ABDOMINAL TUMOURS

This group includes all the relatively rare tumours which present almost exclusively as a result of their biochemical activity, and the physiological effects which they engender. They are often only a few centimetres in diameter, frequently multiple, and may be either benign or malignant. Many patients have a familial endocrine disorder. The diagnosis and localization of these tumours has become increasingly sophisticated and outwith the scope of an operative general surgical textbook.[14] Insulinomas and gastrinomas may require pancreatic resection, and adrenal tumours an adrenalectomy (see Chapter 19).

PSEUDOMYXOMA PERITONEI

This rare tumour produces a peritoneal cavity filled with mucoid jelly. The visceral and parietal peritoneal surfaces have adherent tumour consisting of cysts of trapped jelly, and tumour masses form in the omentum, around the spleen and in the pelvis. Classical pseudomyxoma is a mucinous adenoma, or low-grade mucus-producing adenocarcinoma, which is locally 'malignant' on the peritoneal surface but does not have the ability to metastasize. The commonest site of origin is from an adenoma of the appendix, and it is only after rupture that peritoneal dissemination occurs.[15] In women, many cases are incorrectly classified as ovarian cancers as large deposits grow on the ovaries, and there can also be confusion with frankly malignant mucinous adenocarcinomas of the colon. Worthwhile long-term palliation, and even cure, is possible with an extensive peritonectomy and intraperitoneal chemotherapy.

The surgery is specialized, and involves a radical omentectomy, inside the gastro-epiploic arcade, and extensive stripping of involved parietal and visceral peritoneum by diathermy dissection, combined with the excision, if necessary, of extensively encased organs such as spleen, gallbladder, stomach and segments of colon. Fortunately, the small bowel and its mesentery is relatively spared. Specialized centres have been established for the surgical management of these tumours, and referral is indicated. If this tumour is suspected at laparotomy, histology should be obtained,

preferably by an omental biopsy. Any partial debulking procedure, or hysterectomy, should be avoided as the tumour will seed onto any raw, non-peritonealized surfaces exposed by the surgery. The resultant encasement of vital structures, such as ureters, makes subsequent complete cytoreduction more hazardous. Primary peritoneal mesothelioma poses similar surgical challenges, but the prognosis is worse.

INTRA-ABDOMINAL SARCOMAS

Gastrointestinal stromal tumours (GISTs)

These mesenchymal tumours can occur throughout the gastrointestinal tract, and were previously classified as leiomyomas and leiomyosarcomas. Their clinical behaviour is very varied, but they should all be regarded as potentially malignant. The gastrointestinal stromal sarcomas (GISSs), in common with other sarcomas, recur locally if the margins of excision have been inadequate. They metastasize via the bloodstream but, as lymphatic spread is not an issue, surgery is focused on wide local excision rather than lymphadenectomy. Chemotherapy has little to offer, and radiotherapy can seldom be deployed without unacceptable toxicity at dosages which might be curative. An increased understanding of their origins, probably from pacemaker cells of the gut, has led to the development of Imatinib (a tyrosine kinase inhibitor) as an effective treatment for irresectable disease.

Retroperitoneal sarcomas

These are generally more aggressively malignant than GISSs. They present late as there is no early obstruction or gastrointestinal haemorrhage. Surgical excision is often combined with radiotherapy, which can be focused to give adequate doses to the tumour while avoiding excessive exposure to the small bowel.

Desmoids

Desmoid tumours are a borderline malignant soft-tissue tumour which can occur both in the abdominal wall and intra-abdominally. They are common in patients with familial adenomatous polyposis. Desmoid tumours do not metastasize but are locally aggressive, with a propensity for recurrence after resection. The more common abdominal wall tumours are seldom life-threatening, but the intra-abdominal lesions, which are most often located within the mesentery, may cause small bowel complications. Management decisions are difficult as the proximity of the tumours to mesenteric vessels renders surgical excision technically difficult, with a high morbidity and mortality.[16] The natural history of the lesion, if left *in situ*, is very variable and may be modified by the administration of tamoxifen, non-steroidal anti-inflammatory agents or cytotoxic chemotherapy. These tumours are best managed in specialized centres.

LYMPHOMA

Lymphoma can occur within any mesenteric or retroperitoneal lymph node. In addition, a lymphoma can arise from the lymphoid tissue in the gut wall, classically producing a thickened area of small bowel which may ulcerate or obstruct. A lymphoma may also form the apex of an intussusception. Although the definitive treatment is medical, the initial surgical presentation with a mechanical complication, haemorrhage or inflammation often necessitates a resection, which also provides the tissue for histological diagnosis.

UROLOGICAL MALIGNANCY

The treatment of urological malignancies is discussed briefly in Chapter 25. Hypernephroma is the commonest renal tumour, and should be considered preoperatively in the differential diagnosis of an intra-abdominal mass. Malignant spread is both by local extension and haematogenous metastases. Local extension into the peritoneum is uncommon. Carcinoma of the prostate and bladder seldom cause generalized intra-abdominal problems, and symptoms are commonly restricted to the urological system. Most patients with advanced disease die either from uraemia caused by ureteric obstruction, or from distant metastases. However, a locally aggressive urological malignancy can produce a similar appalling fistulous situation in the pelvis as a rectal carcinoma which has invaded the prostate or bladder. If careful assessment indicates a tumour which has not metastasized, a radical pelvic exenteration with faecal and urinary stomas may be indicated. More often, only palliation of the obstruction, or of the recto-vesical fistula, is possible. A colostomy to divert the faecal stream improves the urinary symptoms considerably. Radiotherapy may offer additional palliation to those patients with a longer life expectancy.

GYNAECOLOGICAL MALIGNANCY

Carcinoma of the cervix and uterus have little impact on the practice of general surgeons, although they may be involved in an extensive pelvic clearance for a locally advanced tumour. Ovarian carcinoma, in contrast, produces an intraperitoneal mass to which bowel can adhere. It also spreads trans-coelomically to form deposits throughout the peritoneal cavity. These deposits result in an omental 'cake' of tumour and malignant adhesions between loops of bowel, and the patient may present with a small bowel obstruction, ascites or an intra-abdominal mass. Surgical treatment is dis-

cussed further in Chapter 26, but the surgery is again influenced by the behaviour of the tumour. In contrast to most other widespread intra-abdominal malignancies, good palliation can be achieved with chemotherapy. This is more effective if the tumour burden has been reduced, and therefore a debulking procedure should be attempted. Gynaecologists generally recommend a total hysterectomy with bilateral salpingo-oophorectomy and an infracolic omentectomy.

It must also be remembered that an ovarian mass and extensive intraperitoneal deposits are not diagnostic of ovarian malignancy. Any tumour cells which have seeded trans-coelomically will thrive on the surface of the well-vascularized ovary, and may be encountered in the absence of other macroscopic intraperitoneal deposits. Large, and often bilateral, secondary tumour masses in the ovary associated with gastric cancer were first described by Krukenberg in 1896. Tumour cells can also reach the ovary through the bloodstream, and similar, apparently isolated, ovarian secondaries are occasionally seen in metastatic breast carcinoma. It is the routine practice of some surgeons to remove the ovaries prophylactically during the course of any laparotomy for malignancy in a post-menopausal woman. This will avoid the possible necessity of a later operation for a symptomatic ovarian secondary, but it is unlikely that many additional cures will be achieved by this policy. A bilateral oophorectomy will also protect the patient from a primary ovarian cancer in the future, and an argument could therefore be made for routinely removing post-menopausal ovaries at any laparotomy. Patient attitudes to this are very varied, and preoperative discussion is imperative.

PELVIC NODE MALIGNANCY

Presentation may be with iliac fossa pain or a palpable mass. Alternatively, encasement of the common iliac vein with resultant obstruction from compression, or distortion, will cause lower-limb swelling from venous obstruction. The inguinal nodes, draining the lower limb and perineum, are continuous with the external iliac chain at the ilio-inguinal ligament. The internal iliac nodes drain the prostate, bladder and uterus (Fig. 15.6). A malignant mass of iliac nodes may represent a primary lymphoma, or it may be the presentation of an occult malignancy within the drainage area. A malignant melanoma or a prostatic carcinoma are probably the most likely cancers to present in this way, although lymph node metastases in this site may occur with any intra-abdominal or pelvic malignancy. Occasionally, no primary lesion can be identified, a lymphoma is suspected and a tissue diagnosis is required. A CT-guided biopsy will be sufficient to diagnose a secondary malignancy, but the core of tissue obtained is usually inadequate to confirm a lymphoma, or to differentiate between the different varieties. The surgical approach for an open biopsy is via a left iliac fossa muscle-cutting incision, staying extraperitoneal and sweeping the

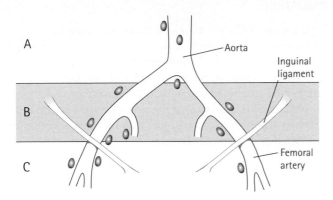

Figure 15.6 *The para-aortic nodes (A) drain the two iliac chains (B). The uterus, prostate and bladder drain to the internal iliac nodes. The external iliac nodes are an extension of the inguinal chain (C) which drains the lower limb and perineum.*

peritoneum medially. Great care must be taken as the matted nodes lie in close proximity to the iliac vessels, and the anatomy may be both obscured and distorted. A laparoscopic biopsy is another possibility.

A *radical lymphadenectomy* of the pelvic nodes may be performed as part of a potentially curative resection for urological, testicular or gynaecological malignancy. In rectal cancer, spread to these nodes is an indication of advanced disease, and little is gained by radical excision. The iliac nodes, as an extension of the inguinal chain, are sometimes excised as part of a radical groin dissection for melanoma or penile cancer, and this operation is described in Chapter 24. Palliative excision of symptomatic nodal involvement is seldom indicated, or indeed possible. Radiotherapy or chemotherapy may be appropriate, depending on the primary pathology, and consideration should be given to the possibility of relieving venous obstruction by intraluminal vascular stenting.

PREOPERATIVE INVESTIGATION AND STAGING OF TUMOURS

Recently, the preoperative imaging of tumours has assumed increasing importance. Previously, a laparotomy was often the only means of establishing the diagnosis and of assessing the resectability of a tumour. When a curative resection was not possible, a palliative resection or surgical bypass offered the best alternative. The diagnosis, and the potential for a curative resection, can now often be established before surgery. Management decisions can be taken before a laparotomy, and in advanced malignancy alternative palliative measures considered. Endoscopic stenting of malignant obstructions has continued to evolve and now offers superior palliation to surgery in many situations.

Carcinomas of the oesophagus, stomach and pancreas metastasize early, and life expectancy with metastatic disease is short. Endoscopic stenting of the oesophagus, pylorus or

common bile duct have proved to be comparable with, or superior to, surgical bypass or palliative resection in most situations. Control of the local obstructive symptoms is maintained until the patient dies of distant metastases. Preoperative assessment of upper gastrointestinal or hepatobiliary malignancy is therefore very important as unnecessary laparotomies can be avoided. However, temporary preoperative stenting of a potentially curative malignancy of the biliary system should be avoided as it will commonly introduce infection.

In colorectal cancer a patient with known metastatic disease is often better served by resection of the primary lesion. Life expectancy is longer, and severe local symptoms are difficult to control. If the primary tumour is left *in situ* luminal loss of blood and mucus will continue, involved adherent bowel loops may obstruct, and rectal cancer has the potential to invade the bladder or pelvic side wall nerves with severe symptoms. However, colonic stenting can be used to relieve obstruction and is an excellent palliative measure when life expectancy is short and the risk of a major operation high.

Preoperative sophisticated imaging, which can accurately stage a malignancy, has enabled a more coordinated, multimodality approach to be taken to cancer treatment. Preoperative radiotherapy, chemotherapy or chemoradiotherapy are increasingly used to 'down-size' and 'down-stage' tumours before surgery. Surgery may then be delayed for several months to obtain the maximum benefit from this treatment, and repeat imaging can monitor the response. Some locally advanced malignancies become resectable and potentially curable with this approach, which has been employed most frequently in oesophageal and rectal cancer. A similar benefit with preoperative chemotherapy has been found with some initially inoperable liver secondaries.

INTRAOPERATIVE DILEMMAS IN ABDOMINAL MALIGNANCY

The acute abdomen and curable malignancy

Many malignancies present as an acute problem, and a laparotomy may have been performed as an emergency for obstruction, perforation or haemorrhage arising as a complication of the tumour. Alternatively, the inflammation around a tumour may have been misinterpreted as a minor benign condition such as an appendicitis. If a potentially curative radical resection is possible, it should ideally be undertaken at this laparotomy. If this is not appropriate due to the patient's poor general state, the surgeon's inexperience, or other factors, it is important that the emergency surgery does not jeopardise the possibility of subsequent cure. A temporary solution such as a defunctioning stoma may be sufficient to treat the emergency presentation, and definitive surgery can be performed under more ideal circumstances at a later date.

Inoperable malignancy

When, at laparotomy either in an emergency or an elective setting, an incurable malignancy is encountered, the surgeon must first decide if any operative procedure will offer palliation. An estimation of the patient's life expectancy, and the quality of remaining life, will be as valuable in this decision as an assessment of surgical feasibility. Resection of an obstructing primary tumour may still be the best palliative option, but alternatives such as bypass should be considered. The additional distress of a stoma during the final few months of life should be avoided if there is any alternative. A gastrostomy, however, may save the patient from prolonged nasogastric tube drainage, and should be considered. Occasionally, no useful surgical procedure is possible. There may be multiple levels of obstruction from intraperitoneal malignant dissemination. The risk of anastomotic dehiscence is increased in advanced malignancy, and the risk of enterocutaneous fistulae should temper surgical over-enthusiasm in this situation.

Tumour biopsy for histology is important, and an omental deposit is often the easiest to excise. A diagnosis of carcinoid, lymphoma, metastatic breast or gynaecological cancer, or even pseudomyxoma will radically change both the management and the prognosis. It must also be remembered that not all liver secondaries are incurable and the biopsy of liver metastases, although widely practised, can result in needle tract seeding and should be avoided.[17]

Probable, but unconfirmed, malignant pathology

Even in elective surgery there may be no absolute proof of malignancy, despite a high level of suspicion and extensive preoperative investigations. In this situation the surgeon will have to proceed to a radical dissection to avoid an oncologically inadequate operation, but in the knowledge that in perhaps 30 per cent of cases the final histology will prove to be benign, and the extent of the surgery unnecessarily radical. Circumscribed pancreatic cancers can be difficult to differentiate from benign lesions, and a hilar cholangiocarcinoma may be indistinguishable from sclerosing cholangitis. The differentiation of sigmoid cancer from diverticular disease can pose similar difficulty.

LAPAROSCOPIC SURGERY IN ABDOMINAL MALIGNANCY

DIAGNOSIS

Laparoscopy is the most accurate tool for the detection of peritoneal seedlings, and is well established as one of the modalities for staging a tumour. Laparoscopic staging can be enhanced by the use of an intra-abdominal laparoscopic ultrasound probe.

PALLIATION

Laparoscopic biliary bypass of a pancreatic malignancy is an alternative to an endoscopic stent in a patient with a longer life expectancy. It has the potential to offer better palliation than a stent, which may require replacement, and the operation can be combined with a gastric drainage procedure as a prophylactic measure against the possibility of a later duodenal obstruction from an enlarging tumour. Recovery is faster compared to an open procedure.

RADICAL LAPAROSCOPIC RESECTION IN MALIGNANCY

The dissection for the radical excision of a malignancy may be performed laparoscopically, but a separate small incision is usually required for specimen retrieval. Early experience with laparoscopic resections for malignancy revealed an unacceptably high port site recurrence rate, which was occurring even in potentially curative situations.[18] Peritoneal trauma at port sites, offering a particularly favourable environment for implantation, could not be the only explanation as open surgery for malignancy is not generally associated with abdominal wound recurrence. The possibility that the environment at laparoscopic surgery enhances the ability of free tumour cells to implant has been extensively explored. The effects of positive-pressure ventilation and carbon dioxide have been implicated, and intraperitoneal immune function has been shown to be suppressed.[19] However, increased contamination of the peritoneal cavity, or the port site wounds, by tumour cells during a laparoscopic resection remained the most likely explanation. This implied either a higher rate of tumour rupture, or lymphatic transection, during the dissection, or port site contamination during delivery of the specimen, and there were concerns that a good oncological operation was more difficult to perform laparoscopically. Local contamination of port sites will obviously occur if the tumour ruptures on delivery, but a tumour which has breached the serosa may also contaminate the wound as it is drawn through a port site, or the small incision made for specimen retrieval. The use of cell-proof retrieval bags in which the specimen is isolated before delivery should avoid this source of contamination. It is also possible to cut up a tumour within such a bag so that a separate incision is unnecessary and it can be removed through a port site. However, histological orientation will be more difficult and the surgeon must beware of compromising potential cancer cure for mainly short-term or cosmetic advantages.

As port site recurrences became a considerable concern, following the early laparoscopic colonic resections for potentially curative tumours, national guidelines were introduced recommending that laparoscopic colorectal resections for malignancies should only be performed within trials until the situation was clarified. Although follow-up is not yet complete from these studies, it would now appear that these guidelines can start to be relaxed. Port site metastases have become rare. In skilled hands, the dissection can be performed to the same standard as in an open operation, and abdominal wall contamination, as the specimen is delivered, is preventable.

REFERENCES

1. Handley WS. The surgery of the lymphatic system. Hunterian lecture. *Br Med J* 1910; **i**: 922–8.

2. Lam KY, Ma LT, Wong J. Measurement of extent of spread of oesophageal squamous carcinoma by serial sectioning. *J Clin Pathol* 1996; **49**: 124–9.

3. Maeta M, Kondo A, Shibata S, *et al*. Esophageal cancer associated with multiple cancerous lesions: clinicopathological comparisons between multiple primary and intramural metastatic lesions. *Gastroent Jpn* 1993; **28**: 187–92.

4. Williams NS, Dixon MF, Johnston D. Reappraisal of the 5 centimetre rule of distal excision for carcinoma of the rectum: a study of distal intramural spread and of patients' survival. *Br J Surg* 1983; **70**: 150–4.

5. Nagakawa T, Mori K, Nakano T, *et al*. Perineural invasion of carcinoma of the pancreas and biliary tract. *Br J Surg* 1993; **80**: 619–21.

6. Ryall C. Cancer infection and cancer recurrence: a danger to avoid in cancer operations. *Lancet* 1907; **ii**; 1311–16.

7. Killingback M, Wilson E, Hughes ESR. Anal metastases from carcinoma of the rectum and colon. *Austr NZ J Surg* 1965; **34**: 178–87.

8. Becker G, Hess CF, Grund KE, *et al*. Abdominal wall metastasis following percutaneous endoscopic gastrostomy. *Supp Care Cancer* 1995; **3**: 313–16.

9. Yu W, Whang I, Suh I, *et al*. Prospective randomised trial of early postoperative intraperitoneal chemotherapy as an adjuvant to resectable gastric cancer. *Ann Surg* 1998; **228**: 347–54.

10. Bonenkamp JJ, Songun I, Hermans J, *et al*. Randomised comparison of morbidity after D1 and D2 dissection for gastric cancer in 996 Dutch patients. *Lancet* 1995; **345**: 745–8.

11. Fielding LP, Hittinger R, Grace RH, *et al*. Randomised controlled trial of adjuvant chemotherapy by portal-vein perfusion after curative resection for colorectal adenocarcinoma. *Lancet* 1992; **340**: 502–6.

12. Scheele J, Stang R, Altendorf-Hofmann A, *et al*. Resection of colorectal liver metastases. *World J Surg* 1995; **19**: 59–71.

13. Dejong CHC, Parks RW, Currie E, *et al*. Treatment of hepatic metastases of neuroendocrine malignancies: a 10-year experience. *J R Coll Surg Edinb* 2002; **47**: 495–9.

14. *Endocrine Surgery: A Companion to Specialist Surgical Practice*, 2nd edn. JR Farndon (ed.). Philadelphia: Elsevier, 2001.

15. Esquivel J, Sugarbaker PH. Clinical presentation of the pseudomyxoma peritonei syndrome. *Br J Surg* 2000; **87**: 1414–18.

16. Smith AJ, Lewis JI, Merchant NB, *et al*. Surgical management of intra-abdominal desmoid tumours. *Br J Surg* 2000; **87**: 608–13.

17. Ohlsson B, Nilsson J, Stenram U, *et al*. Percutaneous fine-needle aspiration cytology in the diagnosis and management of liver tumours. *Br J Surg* 2002; **89**: 757–62.

18. Wexner SD, Cohen SM. Port site metastases after laparoscopic colorectal surgery for cure of malignancy. Review. *Br J Surg* 1995; **82**: 295–8.

19. Gupta A, Watson DI. Effect of laparoscopy on immune function. Review. *Br J Surg* 2001; **88**: 1296–306.

16

CLASSIC OPERATIONS ON THE UPPER GASTROINTESTINAL TRACT

OLIVER McANENA AND MYLES JOYCE

During recent years, the approach to upper gastrointestinal surgery has changed greatly, as advances in the understanding of some pathologies, combined with advances in pharmacology, have led to a number of conditions no longer being managed routinely from a surgical standpoint. In addition, malignancy can be more accurately staged preoperatively such that surgery, when it offers no benefit, can be avoided entirely. In the developed world, the use of interventional endoscopy and radiology has also led to the removal of many operations from the routine practice of many surgeons. In contrast, technical advances in surgical practice, and in particular minimal access techniques, have led to surgery being a better alternative to conservative management for some conditions. In addition, improvements in anaesthesia and critical care, combined with advances in operative techniques, have reduced the mortality and morbidity of the more major surgical procedures.

Many standard operations are described in this chapter. Some of these, although seldom required nowadays in the United Kingdom, may still be of value to surgeons practising in less well-developed areas. The surgical options in the management of upper gastrointestinal disease will be discussed in Chapter 17.

ANATOMY

Oesophagus

The oesophagus is an epithelial lined muscular tube which lies mainly in the superior and posterior mediastina. It commences in the neck as a continuation of the pharynx, with its upper end encircled by the cricopharyngeal sphincter. The bodies of the cervical vertebrae lie posterior to the oesophagus, and the trachea lies immediately anteriorly. The recurrent laryngeal nerves lie in the groove between the oesophagus and trachea. In its intrathoracic course, the oesophagus is related anteriorly to the trachea, the right pulmonary artery and the pericardium in succession. Throughout its course it lies on the bodies of the thoracic vertebrae. It passes through the diaphragm in a hiatal sling formed mainly by the fibres of the right crus. Its final 2 cm is as an intraperitoneal organ before it terminates at the *cardia*, or gastro-oesophageal junction. Gastro-oesophageal reflux is prevented by a functional lower oesophageal sphincter, which is dependent more on the distal portion of the oesophagus lying intra-abdominally, and the angle at which it enters the stomach, than any anatomical sphincter at the cardia. The vagus nerves form a plexus on either side of the oesophagus, but at the level of the hiatus the left vagus lies anteriorly and the right vagus posteriorly. The epithelial lining is squamous, except for the distal 2 cm where there is a variable transition zone to gastric mucosa.

ARTERIAL SUPPLY

The arterial supply of the oesophagus is from the inferior thyroid artery from above, the left gastric and inferior phrenic arteries from below, and in its middle portion it is also supplied by bronchial arteries and small branches directly from the aorta. There is an extensive anastomosis between the arteries in the muscular and submucosal layers of the oesophageal wall. A *submucosal venous plexus* connects with that of the stomach and becomes varicose in portal hypertension, allowing portal venous blood to pass via the azygos vein to the superior vena cava.

LYMPHATIC DRAINAGE

There is an extensive lymphatic plexus in the submucosal layer of the oesophageal wall. This connects with another extensive para-oesophageal plexus, where lymph from the entire length of the oesophagus can mix before finally draining to cervical, thoracic and abdominal lymph nodes. Lymphatic drainage then follows the arterial supply.

Stomach

The stomach is divided, mainly for descriptive purposes, into three major zones (Fig. 16.1). The fundus lies above the gastro-oesophageal junction. The angle of His is the acute angle between the fundus and the oesophagus. The body is below the gastro-oesophageal junction and is limited distally by the incisura angularis, a somewhat variable angulation of the lesser curve. The antrum is the portion of stomach distal to the incisura and extends to the pylorus. The pyloric sphincter is a condensation of the circular muscle of the stomach.

The stomach is completely invested in peritoneum, except for a small area posteriorly just below the cardia. The peritoneum covering the anterior and posterior walls of the stomach meet at the lesser curve and pass upwards as the lesser omentum, or gastrohepatic ligament, to the porta hepatis and a fissure on the posterior aspect of the liver. At the greater curve the peritoneal layers meet to form the greater omentum, and the gastrosplenic and gastrophrenic ligaments. These peritoneal folds around the stomach, and the subsequent division of the peritoneal cavity into a greater and lesser sac (see Fig. 13.4, page 220), are easier to understand from an embryological viewpoint (see Fig. 13.3, page 219). As they are important to all surgeons operating within the abdomen, this topic was covered in Chapter 13. The

mucosa of the body and fundus of the stomach contains *parietal cells* which secrete acid, and *chief cells* which secrete pepsinogen. The mucosa of the antrum contains *G cells* which secrete the hormone gastrin, which stimulates the parietal cells to secrete acid.

ARTERIAL SUPPLY

The arterial supply of the stomach is almost exclusively from the coeliac axis, which arises from the aorta behind the lesser sac. The branches to the stomach enter the extremities of the lesser and greater omentum to form two arterial arcades which lie between the peritoneal folds, 1–2 cm from the stomach wall. Multiple branches from these arcades to the lesser and greater curve of the stomach supply it with its rich blood supply (Fig. 16.2). The gastric arcade, within the lesser omentum, is formed by the descending branch of the left gastric artery and the right gastric branch of the common hepatic artery. The gastroepiploic arcade, within the greater omentum, is formed by the right gastroepiploic branch of the gastroduodenal artery and the left gastroepiploic branch of the splenic artery. In addition, the upper part of the greater curvature receives some four or five short gastric arteries from the splenic artery, or one of its terminal branches. It is this rich anastomotic blood supply from several arteries converging from different directions which makes much of gastric surgery possible. There are also collateral anastomoses, both with branches of the superior mesenteric artery supplying the duodenum, and with the aortic branches supplying the oesophagus. For this reason, gastric ischaemia in occlusive vascular disease is very uncommon, even when the coeliac axis is completely occluded. The venous drainage of the stomach is into the portal system, except for the alternative systemic route via the submucosal venous plexus, across the gastro-oesophageal junction, and into the azygos vein.

LYMPHATIC DRAINAGE

The lymphatic drainage of the stomach follows its arterial supply, in a similar fashion to the pattern encountered throughout the gastrointestinal tract (see Chapter 15). The main lymphatic channels are therefore initially along the gastric and gastroepiploic arterial arcades, and the perigastric lymph nodes lie alongside the vessels. The lymphatics then accompany the main arteries supplying the stomach to their origin from the aorta. Further nodes lie alongside the retroperitoneal routes of these arteries, and the lymph finally drains into the pre-aortic nodes. There are anastomotic lymphatic channels which form a similar function to arterial collaterals, and become of greater importance when the main channels are blocked by tumour. Knowledge of the lymphatic drainage of the stomach has important implications for the staging and treatment of gastric cancer. Nodes have been named and numbered. They have also been divided into 'tiers' of lymph nodes to which gastric cancer may

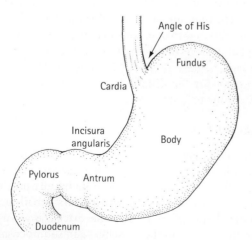

Figure 16.1 *The stomach.*

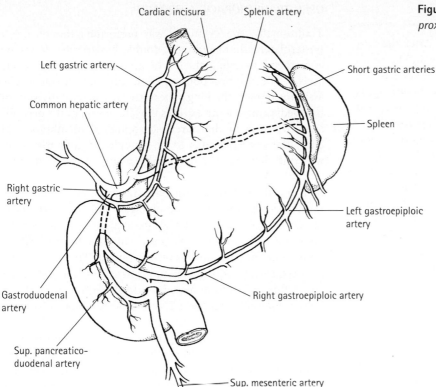

Figure 16.2   *Arterial supply of the stomach and proximal duodenum.*

spread in a progressive fashion. As a simplification this can be viewed as:

- 1st tier – (N1) – perigastric nodes closest to the tumour.
- 2nd tier – (N2) – further more distant perigastric nodes, and nodes along the course of the main artery which supplies the area of stomach from which the tumour has arisen.
- 3rd tier – (N3) – nodes outside these main pathways.

Resections can now be planned to excise all N1 nodes, or to excise all N1 and N2 nodes, or even to include some N3 nodes. However, this is complicated by the different lymphatic drainage in different areas of the stomach, and an N1 node for a pyloric cancer will be an N2 node for a cancer at the cardia. Gastric lymphadenectomy is discussed in more detail in the sections on gastric cancer, both later in this chapter and in Chapter 17.

NERVE SUPPLY

The stomach has both sympathetic and parasympathetic innervation, the latter being provided by the vagus nerves. Shortly after emerging from the oesophageal hiatus the anterior vagus gives off hepatobiliary fibres, and the posterior vagus a branch to the coeliac plexus. There are also branches to the cardia. The main trunks continue as the anterior and posterior nerves of Latarjet (Fig. 16.3). The nerves of Latarjet supply multiple further branches to the body of the stomach, with each branch passing into the stomach wall close to a vascular pedicle. These fibres are motor to the upper stom-

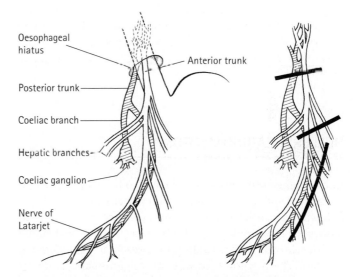

Figure 16.3   *Vagal innervation of the stomach. The three bars indicate the level of transection in truncal vagotomy, selective vagotomy and highly selective vagotomy.*

ach but, more importantly, stimulate the secretion of acid by the parietal cells. They are divided in the operation of highly selective vagotomy. The nerves of Latarjet continue towards the antrum, to end in a configuration known as the 'crow's foot' which innervates the myenteric plexus of the antrum. The terminal crow's foot is preserved in a highly selective vagotomy as it is a motor nerve to the pylorus from the anterior vagus, on which effective gastric emptying depends.

Duodenum

The duodenum commences at the pylorus. After the first 2–3 cm it loses much of its peritoneal covering and becomes a retroperitoneal, relatively fixed segment of the small bowel until the duodenojejunal flexure where the bowel again becomes mobile on a mesentery. The duodenum is curled around the head of the pancreas so that its *first part* lies horizontally above it, the *second part* vertically to its right, and the *third part* horizontally below it. The *fourth part* then ascends to the left of the aorta. The bile and pancreatic ducts enter the concave medial wall of the second part at the *ampulla of Vater*. The duodenum is intimately related to the hilum of the right kidney, the hepatic flexure of the colon and the aorta, in addition to the pancreas. It thus forms a landmark during many intra-abdominal dissections, and must often be mobilized during pancreaticobiliary, renal and aortic surgery (see Fig. 13.2, page 219).

ARTERIAL SUPPLY

The duodenum is supplied from both the coeliac axis and the superior mesenteric artery (see Fig. 16.2). The superior pancreaticoduodenal artery, the inflow of which is from the coeliac axis, and the inferior pancreaticoduodenal branch of the superior mesenteric artery form an arcade around the head of the pancreas. Most of the arterial supply of the duodenum is from this arcade, although there are additional branches which cross the pylorus, to the first part of the duodenum, from the gastric and gastro-epiploic arteries.

HELLER'S CARDIOMYOTOMY

If the diagnosis of achalasia is correct, more than 90 per cent of patients will have a significant improvement in dysphagia following a cardiomyotomy. The operative principle is to reduce the lower oesophageal sphincter pressure by dividing the muscle wall, while avoiding any breach of the underlying mucosa. The myotomy consists of longitudinal division of the muscle fibres of the lower oesophagus, and should extend across the gastro-oesophageal junction for 1–2 cm to ensure the division of all constricting muscle fibres. Most centres, when considering surgical intervention for achalasia, will nowadays use a minimally invasive thoracoscopic or laparoscopic approach.

Preoperative management prior to a Heller's cardiomyotomy includes the insertion of a wide-bore nasogastric tube, but removal of solid food retained in the dilated oesophagus is still difficult. The anaesthetist should be aware of the aspiration risk during induction and protect the airway appropriately. Broad-spectrum antibiotic prophylaxis is usually recommended on induction.

OPEN TRANSTHORACIC APPROACH

Traditionally, the myotomy was performed though a left posterolateral thoracotomy. A double-lumen tube allows the anaesthetist to deflate the left lung, improving intrathoracic access. The inferior pulmonary ligament is divided. The assistant retracts the lung superiorly, and careful division of the mediastinal pleura exposes the lateral wall of the oesophagus. Division of the phreno-oesophageal membrane will allow the gastric fundus to be brought up into the chest, with the division of some short gastric vessels if there is undue tension during gastric mobilization. The oesophageal fat pad is then removed. An extensive myotomy is then performed across the gastro-oesophageal junction, extending proximally for 6–8 cm. Careful lateral dissection through the myotomy incision allows the muscle fibres to be lifted off the underlying mucosa, and lets them retract. This manoeuvre may reduce subsequent stricture formation. Thereafter, an anti-reflux procedure may be added; either a modified Belsey fundoplication or a Dor partial fundoplication (see below).

However, many surgeons questioned the need for such an extensive proximal myotomy in classical achalasia, as the principal dysfunction is across the gastro-oesophageal junction and lower oesophagus. A more limited myotomy can be performed from the abdomen, and the thoracic approach is now mainly reserved for the motility disorders involving the whole oesophagus where a more extensive myotomy is needed.

Laparoscopic Heller's cardiomyotomy

Some surgeons favour the views provided from operating on the patient's left side. The present authors' preference is for the patient to be placed in a lithotomy position, allowing the surgeon to operate from between the legs, using a port placement as shown in Figure 16.4a. The first camera port is inserted midway between the umbilicus and xiphisternum, using an open Hasson's technique, thereby creating a pneumoperitoneum to 15 mmHg using CO_2 insufflation. An angled 30-degree lens is used for the procedure. A non-traumatic liver fan-type retractor is inserted through the right hypochondrial port to elevate the left lobe of the liver and allow visualization of the gastro-oesophageal junction. A Babcock forceps placed through the left inferior port allows the stomach to be retracted inferiorly and laterally, putting the gastrohepatic ligament on stretch. It is important to avoid tearing the stomach with excess traction. The thin, transparent, gastrohepatic ligament is then divided using diathermy (or ultrasonic) dissection via the left hypochondrial port. This should be a bloodless dissection, and usually commences superior to the hepatic branches of the vagus nerve. These vagal fibres innervate the gallbladder and liver, with proponents of preservation citing increased gallbladder stasis and cholelithiasis when they are divided. However, if they interfere with access then they may have to be sacrificed.

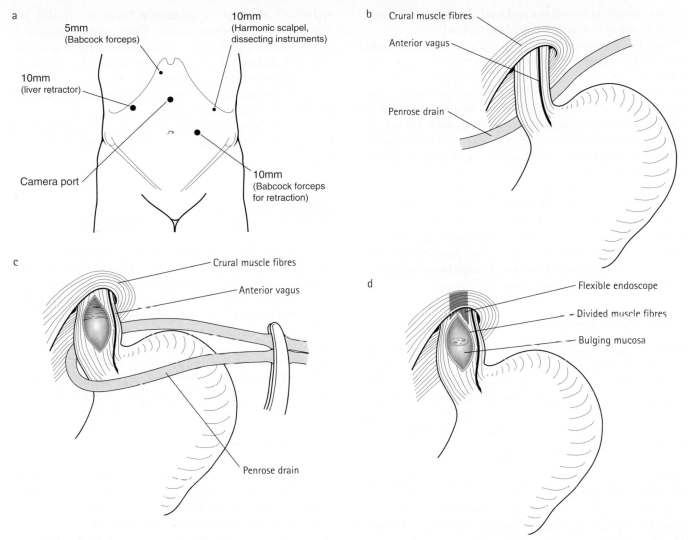

Figure 16.4 *Heller's cardiomyotomy. (a) Port positions for a laparoscopic Heller's cardiomyotomy or a Nissen fundoplication. (b) The vulnerable position of the anterior vagus nerve. (c) Division of the longitudinal muscle fibres and the underlying circular muscle fibres to expose the mucosa. (d) Air insufflation via the flexible endoscope to confirm integrity of the mucosa following completion of the myotomy.*

Occasionally, an aberrant left hepatic artery is encountered in this plane and can be safely divided.[1]

As the dissection continues, the right sling of the diaphragmatic crus is exposed. If the achalasia segment is extensive, further oesophageal mobilization as for a laparoscopic fundoplication may be required.

A flexible endoscope is inserted to facilitate the myotomy. It is imperative that the anterior vagus nerve is identified and isolated prior to myotomy (Fig. 16.4b). The nerve usually lies in close approximation to the anterior oesophagus, in contrast to the posterior vagus nerve which lies more freely in the posterior oesophageal plane. The myotomy is commenced 1–2 cm distal to the gastro-oesophageal junction using coagulating shears or hook dissection. However, these techniques carry the inherent risk of thermal injury to the underlying mucosa, particularly in the presence of fibrosis, and thus many surgeons favour scissors alone for this part of the procedure. The dissection may be commenced more distally if there is oesophageal scarring secondary to previous treatment such as pneumatic dilatation or the use of botulinum toxin.

The anterior longitudinal muscle fibres are divided, exposing the underlying circular fibres. The circular fibres can then be elevated off the submucosa and divided (Fig. 16.4c). The flexible endoscope is used to transilluminate the working field, reducing the potential for mucosal breach. The myotomy is extended proximally for 4–6 cm, at which stage the dilated proximal portion of oesophagus should have been reached. Incomplete myotomy is a common cause of failure following a Heller's procedure. Bleeding from the anterior oesophageal wall is usually self-limiting, and excessive blind use of diathermy should be avoided.

When the myotomy is complete, saline is injected around the working field and air insufflated via the endoscope (Fig. 16.4d). The presence of bubbles, as from a punctured tyre, indicates a mucosal breach requiring immediate repair. The defect may be closed by laparoscopic suturing, but if it is more extensive it requires conversion to an open procedure. When there has been any concern, water-soluble contrast studies help to confirm oesophageal integrity prior to allowing oral intake.

The decision to include a fundoplication is taken on a case-by-case basis. If the peri-hiatal dissection is minimal, a fundoplication is generally not required. If there has been an oesophageal mucosal injury, then a Dor partial anterior fundoplication provides good mucosal protection (see below). Here, the anterior fundus is anchored to the free edges of the myotomy in addition to the hiatus.

THORACOSCOPIC APPROACH

The thoracoscopic approach to a cardiomyotomy may be performed through the left or right thoracic cavity, and is usually reserved for cases where a more extensive myotomy is indicated. The general principles of video-assisted thoracoscopic surgery were covered in Chapter 7. Underlying lung disease, with associated pleural adhesions, increases the risk of this approach. Damage to lung parenchyma can occur during port insertion, despite the use of double-lumen tubes, as adhesions can prevent the lung from collapsing. The first port, which will be used for the camera, is placed inferior to the tip of the scapula through the sixth intercostal space. If the lung is not fully collapsed, then insufflation with CO_2 to a maximum pressure of approximately 5 mmHg, creating a low-pressure pneumothorax, may be helpful. If there is any cardiorespiratory disturbance during the procedure then the CO_2 is released immediately. The videoscope allows the working ports to be inserted under direct vision. These ports are placed at positions which allow the surgeon easy, unrestricted movement. The positions chosen vary between surgeons, but the present authors favour two further ports anterior to the mid-axillary line through the fifth and seventh intercostal spaces. A fourth port can then be inserted more anteriorly through the sixth intercostal space, and this can be used by the assistant to retract the lung. If the patient has underlying cardiorespiratory disease and tolerates single-lung ventilation poorly, the collapsed lung may be inflated periodically throughout the procedure.

The operation then proceeds in a similar fashion to the open thoracotomy approach described above. When an extensive myotomy is indicated, it can be extended from the diaphragm to the level where the oesophagus is crossed by the aorta or azygos vein. A right-sided approach has the advantage that the azygos vein can be divided if further proximal extension of the myotomy is required. Care must be taken not to damage the vagi. As in the laparoscopic approach, the longitudinal muscle fibres are divided followed by the underlying circular fibres until the mucosa is seen to bulge. The flexible endoscope facilitates this dissection and reduces the potential for mucosal perforation. When the myotomy is completed the edges of the muscle fibres are dissected off the mucosa to minimize subsequent scarring and stricture formation.

Again, at the end of the procedure an air-insufflation test is performed, and a chest drain inserted prior to lung re-inflation.

ANTI-REFLUX SURGERY

The majority of surgeons now perform anti-reflux procedures using a minimally invasive laparosopic approach. Improvements in pharmacological and endoscopic treatment, combined with the development of minimally invasive surgical techniques, have greatly improved the management of benign conditions affecting the oesophagus and gastro-oesophageal junction. Previously, patients required an extensive upper abdominal, or thoracotomy, incision as the cardia is relatively inaccessible at open surgery. These incisions in themselves carried significant morbidity, but when the morbidity of surgery can be kept to a minimum a definitive surgical solution may be a better option than long-term medical management.

Although the open operations are described only briefly, all surgeons, despite being proficient in laparoscopic techniques, must be familiar with the steps required for open surgery. On occasion conversion to an open approach is necessary in the presence of uncontrolled bleeding or distorted anatomy. Sometimes, if the patient has had previous upper abdominal or gastric surgery with extensive adhesions, an open approach should be considered from the outset.

The principles of anti-reflux surgery irrespective of the technique used include:

- Restoration of an intra-abdominal portion of oesophagus to maintain a pressure differential between the thoracic and abdominal oesophagus.
- Creation of a loose wrap around the gastro-oesophageal junction to restore the mechanical effect of the oesophagogastric junction.
- Reduction of any hiatus hernia and approximation of the crural fibres to narrow the oesophageal hiatus.
- Identification and management of any associated anatomical abnormalities such as a shortened oesophagus.

Open surgery

A great variety of different operations have been developed over the years for the treatment of gastro-oesophageal reflux.

Some operations were performed through a laparotomy incision, and others through a thoracotomy, or a left thoraco-abdominal, incision. Some of the procedures could be undertaken, with only minor modifications, from a variety of approaches. A few of these operations have been adapted to make them suitable for laparoscopic practice, while others have remained as alternative open procedures to be considered in particular circumstances.

BELSEY MARK IV

This refers to the fourth modification of the operation initially described by Allison. It is a partial anterior wrap, which is undertaken through a left sixth intercostal space postero-lateral thoracotomy. The oesophagus is mobilized from the level of the aortic arch to the cardia, thus freeing it from its diaphragmatic attachments. It may be necessary to divide the superior and inferior bronchial arteries and the oesophageal branches of the distal descending thoracic aorta. The gastric fundus is plicated to the lower 4 cm of the oesophagus for 270 degrees anteriorly and laterally, while leaving the posterior quarter of the oesophagus and the posterior vagus nerve undisturbed. The repair is carried out in two layers. The first layer of sutures attaches the gastric fundus to the lower 2 cm of oesophagus, and the second layer includes bites of the oesophagus, the fundus of the stomach and the tendinous portion of the diaphragm (Fig. 16.5). The posterior segment of oesophagus not included in the wrap is buttressed against the hiatus. Sutures are placed posteriorly in the crural opening to narrow the hiatus. Nowadays, this operation is rarely performed.

COLLIS GASTROPLASTY

This operation was initially undertaken through a thoraco-abdominal incision, but nowadays it is principally performed using a transthoracic approach. It is designed to give a tension-free repair for patients with a hiatus hernia, in

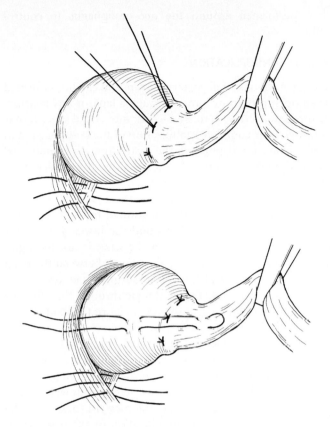

Figure 16.5 *Belsey mark IV procedure.*

combination with a shortened oesophagus. The technique consists of isolating the upper part of the lesser curve in the form of a tube in continuity with the oesophagus. The distal end of this tube can then be considered as the new gastro-oesophageal junction. This oesophageal-lengthening technique allows several centimetres of the neo-oesophagus to lie below the diaphragm (Fig. 16.6). An anti-reflux procedure is

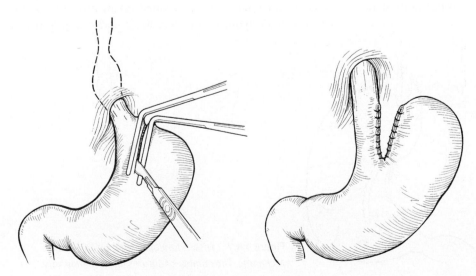

Figure 16.6 *A Collis gastroplasty.*

then performed around the neo-oesophagus to control reflux.

NISSEN FUNDOPLICATION

This operation is a full posterior wrap, and can be performed as an open procedure either through a laparotomy incision, or through a left posterolateral sixth intercostal space thoracotomy. After complete mobilization of the oesophagus and cardia from the diaphragm, the gastric fundus is mobilized by dividing the short gastric arteries along the greater curve and the upper branches of the left gastric artery in the gastro-hepatic ligament. The fundus of the stomach is passed behind the oesophagus and then sutured to itself anteriorly forming a 360-degree wrap around the lower 4 cm of the oesophagus. It is important that the wrap is not too tight, and it should be possible to pass a finger between the wrap and the anterior oesophagus. Some surgeons favoured creating the wrap with a 40 Fr size Bougie through the cardia to prevent over-tightening, as shown in Figure 16.7. Sutures are then placed in the crura to narrow the hiatus.

A thoracotomy incision is generally preferred when the gastro-oesophageal junction is lying intrathoracically with a shortened oesophagus. If access through the stretched hiatus is insufficient, a diaphragmatic incision allowed simultaneous exposure of the upper abdomen. In these cases the key to success is adequate mobilization of the oesophagus from the diaphragm to the aortic arch, in addition to mobilization of the cardia and fundus as described above, with particular care being taken to free the cardia from the diaphragm. The division of the short gastric vessels allows the body and fundus of the stomach to be brought into the chest. The fundoplication is performed in the chest and is then returned in the abdomen. The hiatal defect is narrowed by tying the crural sutures, which were inserted prior to the creation of the wrap.

Laparoscopic Nissen fundoplication

The basic principles of the operation are similar to those of an open Nissen procedure.

Operative procedure

A similar placement of ports to that employed for a laparoscopic Heller's procedure is suitable (see Fig. 16.4a, page 261). The surgeon stands between the patient's legs, while the first assistant stands to the right of the patient, operating the camera with the right hand. A liver retractor is inserted through the right hypochondrial port, allowing elevation of the left lobe of the liver with the assistant's left hand. The second assistant is placed on the left-hand side, primarily for stomach retraction using a Babcock forceps inserted through the left inferior port.

The present authors favour the harmonic coagulation shears for dissection. This uses high-frequency mechanical vibrations in the ultrasonic range to fragment tissues, and can seal vessels up to 5 mm in diameter. Whilst it generates heat, it is generally accepted that the zone of thermal energy produced is considerably less than with monopolar or even bipolar electrocautery, unless applied for prolonged periods. Additionally, less smoke and steam are generated, both of which can impair visibility during a laparoscopic procedure.

The liver retractor allows access and visualization of the working field. A Babcock forceps is placed on the stomach and retracted inferiorly and laterally. This places the gastro-hepatic ligament on stretch. This tissue is usually avascular, and is divided distal to the hepatic branch of the vagus nerve up to the level of the right diaphragmatic crus. However, these vagal fibres are sacrificed if they limit visualization of the oesophageal hiatus. An aberrant left hepatic artery may be encountered in this region. Most surgeons are nervous about dividing this vessel because of the potential risk of hepatic ischaemia. However, no adverse hepatic effects have been reported in a series of over 50 patients in whom an aberrant left hepatic artery was divided.[1] It may be ligated with standard clips or sealed with the harmonic shears. It is important to remember the proximity of the inferior vena cava, lying between the caudate lobe and the right crus, as injury to this vessel can result in catastrophic haemorrhage.

Having identified the right crus, the phreno-oesophageal ligament overlying the distal oesophagus and gastro-oesophageal junction is then divided, taking care not to damage the underlying oesophagus or anterior vagus nerve.

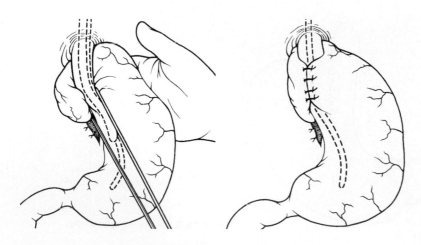

Figure 16.7 *Nissen fundoplication using an open technique. The number of sutures inserted may vary.*

Caudal traction on the fundus will help to identify the distal oesophagus. Careful dissection will expose the posterior vagus nerve which must be preserved and the confluence of the crural muscles fibres behind the oesophagus. If the gastro-oesophageal fat pad is large it is excised. The gastric fundus is then retracted to the patient's right, and the upper short gastric vessels are divided to allow complete fundal mobilization, and access to the fibres of the left crural sling. This allows the creation of a space between the crural fibres and the posterior aspect of the oesophagus. On returning to the right side, the posterior oesophageal window is easily opened with minimal dissection. In general, there is no need to use a Penrose drain for retraction.

The gastric fundus is then pulled gently through the posterior oesophageal window using the *shoe-shine* technique. This consists of placing a Babcock forceps on the gastric fundus as it emerges from the posterior oesophageal window, and a second forceps on the splenic side. Gentle traction back and forth between the forceps allows emergence of the wrap without tearing. Some surgeons favour the use of a roticulator, but the present authors feel that if this is required then the oesophageal window has been inadequately mobilized, and tension on the wrap may ensue. Tension may increase the risk of wrap disruption and post-operative dysphagia.

Two 2/0 non-absorbable sutures are used to plicate the gastric wrap. One of these sutures incorporates the muscular coat of the intra-abdominal oesophagus (Fig. 16.8a), reducing the potential for wrap slippage. The crural fibres are then approximated using two to three 2/0 non-absorbable sutures to narrow the oesophageal hiatus (Fig. 16.8b). This also reduces the likelihood of intrathoracic migration of the wrap. While it may increase the incidence of postoperative dysphagia, this is usually transient. If the dysphagia persists, then a crural stitch may be removed laparoscopically.

The insertion of a Bougie is not favoured by these authors either during or after the procedure, mainly because of the significant risk of perforation. Postoperatively, patients can return to a soft diet within 24 hours.

THORACOSCOPIC FUNDOPLICATION

Thoracoscopic access is established as described for a thoracoscopic cardiomyotomy. This approach may be chosen if the oesophagogastric junction is lying intrathoracically. The oesophagus requires extensive mobilization, as discussed above for the open transthoracic Nissen procedure. Particular care must be taken to free the cardia from the diaphragm. Thereafter, division of the short gastric vessels will allow the body and fundus of the stomach to be brought into the chest for the fundoplication. After completion it is placed in the abdomen, and the hiatal defect is narrowed by tying the crural sutures, which were inserted prior to the creation of the wrap.

INTRAOPERATIVE COMPLICATIONS

Intraoperatively, there is potential for splenic injury in addition to gastric or oesophageal perforation. The incidence of perforation is reported as 1 per cent, and it carries a significant risk of morbidity and mortality, particularly if not recognized at the time of injury. The mechanism may involve a tear from excessive traction during the dissection, or a delayed necrotic injury due to thermal energy. It is believed that the use of ultrasonic coagulation shears may reduce the potential for thermal injury. Intraoperative insertion of a Bougie or nasogastric tube has also been reported as a possible cause of perforation. Occasionally a suture, if under excessive tension, can cut through the gastric or oesophageal tissue, leaving a perforation. If recognized intraoperatively, the perforation can be repaired. For anterior oesophageal perforations, interrupted sutures may be inserted laparoscopically, but posterior perforations, due to difficulty of access, usually require conversion to an open procedure. Gastric perforations can be closed using an endoscopic gastrointestinal stapling device.

POSTOPERATIVE COMPLICATIONS

Dysphagia

In most scenarios, any postoperative dysphagia after Nissen fundoplication is transient and settles within a few days, but if it persists and is disabling, then a check endoscopy is performed. The oesophageal lumen may be compromised due to excessive closure of the hiatal opening, a tight wrap or inadequate mobilization of the gastric fundus associated with failure to divide the short gastric vessels. If the endo-

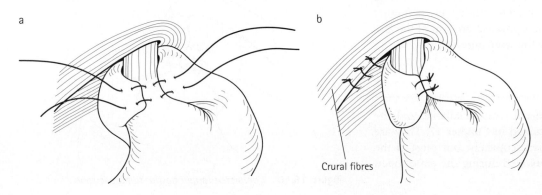

a   b

Crural fibres

Figure 16.8 *Nissen fundoplication. (a) When creating the wrap, one of the sutures must incorporate the abdominal oesophagus to prevent wrap migration. (b) Closure of the hiatal defect by approximation of the crural fibres.*

scope passes freely to the stomach, dilation is carried out with care, and this usually gives a good functional result. Most patients will respond to dilatation, although a small number will require reoperation. If endoscopy identifies complete obstruction of the distal oesophageal lumen, the patient is re-laparoscoped and the wrap assessed. Usually, the upper stitch on the crural fibres is the offending agent and when it is removed the endoscope passes freely. Very occasionally the full Nissen wrap has to be converted to a partial wrap.

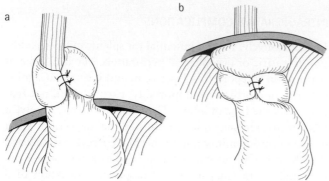

Figure 16.9 *Wrap migration. (a) Up through the hiatus into the chest. (b) Down around the stomach.*

Wrap migration

Herniation of the fundoplication through the hiatal opening into the chest is a cause of failure (Fig. 16.9a). The patient may complain of sudden onset of epigastric or substernal pain rather than reflux symptoms. This may occur due to inadequate closure of the crural defect at the time of repair. However, it is important when closing the defect to balance adequate closure against the risk of strangulation and dysphagia. Many surgeons insert a stitch to anchor the distal oesophagus and prevent migration and rotation of the wrap. Other risk factors thought to contribute to intra-thoracic migration include an early return to strenuous exercise and postoperative vomiting. Patients with a very large hiatal opening may also be at increased risk. In many cases, failure to recognize a shortened oesophagus is a significant cause. This iatrogenic para-oesophageal herniation represents a surgical emergency as the herniated fundus can strangulate, and it must be repaired as soon as the patient is stabilized.

Occasionally, the wrap may slip down the stomach (Fig. 16.9b). To counteract the potential for this problem, it must be ensured that the sutures incorporate a portion of the distal oesophagus when suturing the wrap anteriorly.

Partial wraps

There is a wide variety of partial wraps available, and the indications for them are discussed in Chapter 17. They are now generally performed laparoscopically, but most of the original procedures were developed during the era of open surgery.

TOUPET FUNDOPLICATION

The Toupet procedure is the most commonly used laparoscopic partial fundoplication. It is a partial posterior wrap, and the initial steps are similar to that for a laparoscopic Nissen's fundoplication. Again, the short gastric vessels are divided, facilitating fundal mobilization. The posterior oesophageal window is created and the gastric fundus eased through using the 'shoe-shine' technique. The right leading limb of the fundus is then sutured to the right anterior aspect of the oesophagus, taking care not to damage or incorporate the anterior vagus nerve in the stitch. The lateral left aspect of the fundus is then sutured to the anterolateral aspect of the oesophagus (Fig. 16.10). The fundus may be further sutured to the crura to prevent wrap rotation.

The Toupet partial fundoplication is associated with a lower incidence of dysphagia in comparison to a complete wrap. However, it is also associated with a higher incidence of failure to control reflux symptoms. Nonetheless, it has a role in a carefully selected subset of patients.

DOR FUNDOPLICATION

This is a partial anterior fundoplication which can be used to provide good mucosal protection after a cardiomyotomy. The fundus is brought up anterior to the oesophagus and sutured to its right and left sides. Other anterior partial fundoplications have also been described, and these include a variable proportion of the oesophageal circumference in the wrap. The original Belsey Mark IV is an anterior partial fundoplication.

HILL'S GASTROPEXY

This procedure is more of a gastropexy than a fundoplication, as the oesophagogastric junction is fixed with sutures to the arcuate ligament as it arches over the aorta (Fig. 16.11). However, postoperative endoscopy suggests that it is effective as a form of fundoplication.

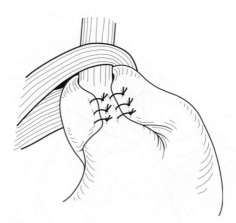

Figure 16.10 *Completed Toupet partial fundoplication.*

NISSEN–ROSETTI PROCEDURE

This is another variation of fundoplication, and consists of a smaller wrap with the fundus brought posterior to the oesophagus, but sutured to the anterior portion of the lesser curvature only. This operation does not require division of the short gastric vessels, but is thought to be associated with a greater incidence of postoperative dysphagia.

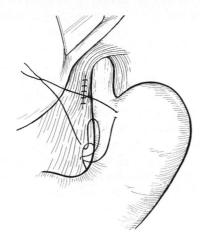

Figure 16.11 *Hill's gastropexy.*

VAGOTOMY

Vagotomy in its three forms – truncal, selective and highly selective – abolishes vagal stimulation of the parietal cell mass and reduces the output of gastric acid. For many years, these operations were important in securing the healing of peptic ulcers, and this role is discussed in more depth in Chapter 17. The *truncal vagotomy* is the simplest to perform, but the side effects of extensive vagal denervation of the fore and midgut stimulated attempts at selective denervation. A *selective vagotomy* preserves the vagal hepatic branches and the vagal branches to the coeliac ganglion. However, although some advantages over a truncal vagotomy are claimed, gastric emptying is still impaired. Truncal and selective vagotomies should therefore be combined with a gastric drainage operation. The *highly selective vagotomy* preserves antral and pyloric motor function. It can be performed without a drainage procedure and has minimal side effects, but it is associated with a higher incidence of ulcer recurrence.

Truncal vagotomy

A truncal vagotomy denervates the whole stomach, and must be combined with a gastric drainage procedure such as a pyloroplasty, or a gastrojejunostomy. It also denervates the gallbladder, and this leads to motility problems and predisposes to gallstone formation. The high incidence of diarrhoea following a truncal vagotomy is at least partly attributed to denervation of the small intestine.

Operative procedure

Abdominal access is via an upper midline laparotomy incision. Access to the abdominal oesophagus can be improved by the use of fixed retraction under the sternum to Goligher-type bars or to an Omnitract system. A head-up tilt of the table by 15–25 degrees will also help.

The falciform ligament and any adhesions are divided. Gentle traction is then applied to the anterior wall of the stomach, which delivers it out of the wound. The abdominal oesophagus is identified by palpating the nasogastric tube between the finger and thumb of the right hand. The peritoneum overlying the distal oesophagus is incised, and the oesophagus is mobilized by gentle blunt dissection between finger and thumb. The oesophagus is encircled by a Penrose drain, traction on which will aid in identification and isolation of the vagi. In over 80 per cent of cases a single anterior, and a single posterior, vagal trunk are present, but two anterior trunks are present in 15 per cent of subjects and two posterior trunks occur in 1 per cent. The anterior vagal trunk, or trunks, are usually easily visualized at this stage, but if not they can be readily palpated as taut bands. They can either be divided between ligatures or clipped, divided and then ligated. Some surgeons recommend that a 2-cm segment is removed and sent for histological examination to confirm that the nerve has been correctly identified. The posterior vagal trunk is found between the right crus and the oesophagus, and is similarly divided. It may give off some proximal branches to the gastric fundus, which must also be identified and divided.

Selective vagotomy

A selective vagotomy denervates the whole stomach while preserving the hepatic and coeliac branches of the vagal trunks. The patient again requires a gastric drainage procedure such as a gastrojejunostomy or pyloroplasty.

Operative procedure

The initial steps of the operation are similar to those of a truncal vagotomy. The anterior vagal trunk and its hepatic branches are identified and encircled with loops. Stretching the gastrohepatic ligament aids in their identification. Having identified the origin of the hepatic branches, the anterior vagus and all its branches distal to this point are divided (see Fig. 16.3). The neurovascular bundles are divided en bloc. The posterior vagal trunk and the origin of its coeliac branch are similarly identified. Thereafter, all tissue between these nerves and the lesser curvature is divided. The branches to the cardia from the vagi proximal to the coeliac and hepatic branches must also be identified and divided.

Highly selective vagotomy

In a highly selective vagotomy the aim is to denervate the parietal cell mass of the fundus and body of the stomach, whilst preserving motor innervation of the antrum through intact nerves of Latarjet (see Fig. 16.3). The coeliac and hepatic branches of the vagi are also preserved. There is no need for a gastric drainage procedure, and the incidence of post-vagotomy problems, including diarrhoea and cholelithiasis, are also significantly reduced. However, there is a higher incidence of ulcer recurrence, and this is discussed further in Chapter 17.

Operative procedure

This operation takes significantly longer to perform than a truncal vagotomy, and it must be performed meticulously or the results will be disappointing. The areas of failure were extensively explored.[2] Good access is essential. In addition to the measures taken to display the abdominal oesophagus for a truncal vagotomy, the left lobe of the liver should be mobilized by division of the left triangular ligament so that it can be retracted inferiorly. However, care must be taken not to release this too far and damage a phrenic, or even an hepatic, vein.

The anterior nerve of Latarjet can usually be seen clearly, some 1–2 cm from the lesser curve of the stomach. As it approaches the antrum it fans out into several branches, the appearance of which is described as the 'crow's foot'.

Some surgeons recommend division of the gastrocolic omentum outside the gastroepiploic arcade as the first step of the operation. This early access into the lesser sac can make the downward retraction of the stomach easier while the surgeon dissects the branches of the anterior nerve of Latarjet. It

then also allows the stomach to be elevated, providing access to the posterior leaf of the lesser omentum and the posterior nerve of Latarjet. Other surgeons prefer to dissect the posterior nerve from the front, and the final release of any adhesions crossing the lesser sac can be performed through the opening in the lesser omentum. An opening into the lesser sac to the right of the nerves of Latarjet is also helpful for retraction of the vagi to the right during the dissection (Fig. 16.12a).

The anterior leaf of the lesser omentum is incised close to the lesser curve and to the left of the crow's foot. The dissection continues along the lesser curve towards the cardia. The nerves enter the stomach with the vessels, and each neurovascular bundle is divided and secured. This may be done by division between ligatures, or by clipping, dividing and tying. Clips and heat-bonding techniques are further options. However, the dissection is within the gastric arterial arcade, directly on the wall of the lesser curve. Surgeons should be aware of the rare, but well-documented, complication of lesser curve necrosis. Although this can occur independently of the method employed, thermal damage to the stomach wall must be avoided. The dissection and ligation continues along the lesser curve and finally inclines across the front of the cardia to the left of the gastro-oesophageal junction (Fig. 16.12b). A middle layer of small blood vessels and nerves must then be divided before the posterior layer is dissected.

The branches of the posterior nerve of Latarjet are divided close to the lesser curvature by a similar serial division of neurovascular bundles (Fig. 16.12b). This dissection can be

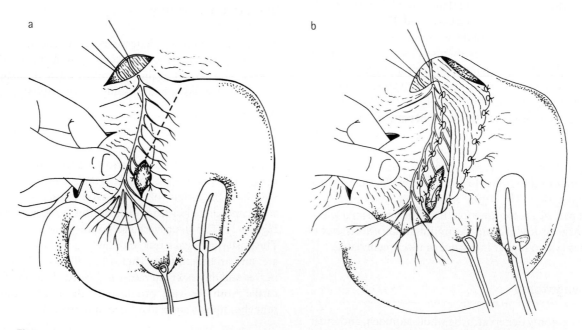

Figure 16.12 *Highly selective vagotomy. (a) The anterior nerve of Latarjet has been demonstrated by retracting the stomach down and to the left. The incision has been started in the anterior leaf of the lesser omentum, and will be continued as shown by the dotted line. The additional opening through the lesser omentum allows a sling to be passed around the vagi for retraction, or it can be used to facilitate manual retraction, as shown. (b) The division of the neurovascular bundles in the anterior leaf of the lesser omentum has been completed, and the incision has been carried over the front of the cardia. The posterior leaf division has been commenced from in front.*

approached posteriorly via the lesser sac, or anteriorly as discussed above. The gastro-oesophageal junction is then cleared. At this stage, a sling around the oesophagus retracting it to the left, and a second sling around the vagus nerves, retracting them to the right, is helpful as the dissection is continued up the oesophagus. Around 7–8 cm of the lower oesophagus should be cleared to ensure that there are no residual vagal fibres passing downwards on the wall of the oesophagus towards the stomach. Failure to complete this part of the dissection is a major cause of incomplete parietal cell vagotomy. When the oesophagus has been cleared, the dissection continues toward the fundus as far as the first short gastric vessels, dividing all the peritoneum passing from fundus to diaphragm. This peritoneal fold may contain vagal fibres, including the 'criminal' nerve of Grassi. Any congenital adhesions crossing the lesser sac to the stomach should also be divided as they may occasionally contain vagal nerve fibres.

Finally, attention is turned to the crow's foot. If the whole of it is left intact, the most distal parietal cells may still be innervated. It is recommended that only about 5–6 cm of antrum should remain innervated, and this usually necessitates sacrifice of the proximal one to two divisions of the crow's foot.

Although the highly selective vagotomy has produced excellent results for some surgeons, others had a high incidence of recurrent ulcer. When it was a common procedure, either a Burge or a Grassi intra-operative test was often used to ensure that the parietal cell mass was completely denervated.[3] However, many surgeons found they could achieve good results by adhering to the details of the dissection outlined above.

Posterior truncal vagotomy with anterior seromyotomy

This is a simpler and quicker operation than a highly selective vagotomy, and it compares favourably as regards parietal cell vagal denervation.[4] A gastric drainage procedure is not required. A posterior truncal vagotomy is completed as described above, after which an anterior seromyotomy is performed by dividing the seromuscular layers of the anterior stomach wall, taking care not to breach the gastric mucosa. Small vessels are coagulated. The seromyotomy follows the lesser curvature at a distance of 2 cm from it, starting at the angle of His and extending to approximately 5 cm from the pylorus. On completion, air is insufflated via the nasograstic tube to help identify any perforations. The edges of the seromyotomy can be oversewn with a continuous running suture for haemostasis.

Laparoscopic vagotomy

A laparoscopic approach is eminently suitable for all forms of vagotomy. Truncal vagotomy may also be performed via a thoracoscopic route. It is interesting that vagotomy was initially performed at thoracotomy, and it was only the later development of a transabdominal approach that established its role in ulcer surgery.[5] Surgeons who perform laparoscopic anti-reflux procedures regularly find that familiarity with the relevant anatomy and dissection planes ensures that the learning curve is minimal. However, a steep decline in the number of vagotomies performed has occurred during the laparoscopic era, with the result that laparoscopic vagotomy has not become a common procedure. It must be remembered that the indications for performing a laparoscopic vagotomy are similar to that for an open vagotomy. This is discussed in Chapter 17.

The principles of vagotomy are the same, whether an open or a minimal access approach is employed. Laparoscopic and thoracoscopic access, and dissection around the proximal stomach, cardia and oesophagus, are described above in the section on gastro-oesophageal reflux surgery.

GASTRIC DRAINAGE PROCEDURES

Gastric drainage is required in a wide range of scenarios. For example, there may be a mechanical obstruction of the pylorus or duodenum, or the distal stomach may have been resected or excluded. The operation may also be performed to aid gastric drainage after a vagotomy.

Gastrostomy

A gastrostomy is only suitable as a temporary form of gastric drainage. A tube gastrostomy is occasionally established at the time of surgery as an alternative to nasogastric aspiration. It may be more comfortable than a nasogastric tube, and is associated with fewer respiratory complications. The technique is described in Chapter 13. More often, a gastrostomy is required not for drainage but for enteral feeding, and endoscopic insertion is usually more appropriate in these circumstances (see Chapter 11).

Pyloroplasty

This is most frequently performed in combination with a vagotomy, and improves gastric drainage by destroying the sphincter effect of the pylorus. The prelude to any type of pyloroplasty is adequate mobilization of the second part of the duodenum by full Kocherization.

HEINEKE–MIKULICZ OPERATION

This operation has undergone several modifications since its original description, but is in essence a longitudinal incision across the pylorus which is then closed transversely. Two deep stay sutures are inserted 1 cm apart in the anterior aspect of the pyloric ring. A 6-cm longitudinal incision is then made between the sutures into the lumen. Traction on

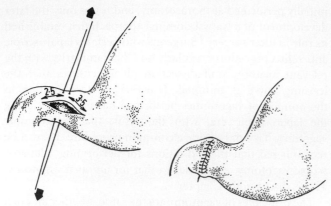

Figure 16.13   *Heineke–Mikulicz pyloroplasty.*

the stay sutures converts the longitudinal incision to a diamond-shaped opening, which is closed transversely using a single layer of interrupted absorbable sutures such as 3/0 polydioxanone (PDS) (Fig. 16.13). Further layers of sutures, as originally described, are no longer recommended as they narrow the pyloric channel. The pyloroplasty may then be buttressed with omentum. This operation is not feasible if the pylorus is grossly thickened or scarred.

FINNEY'S PYLOROPLASTY

Although often described as a pyloroplasty, this operation is really a gastroduodenostomy (Fig. 16.14). Its only advantage over a Heineke–Mickulicz operation is that it is still a

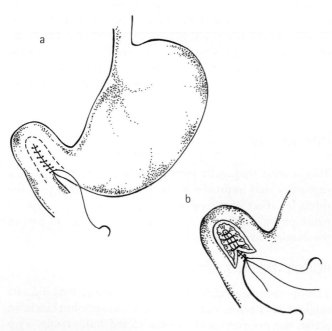

Figure 16.14   *Finney gastroduodenostomy. (a) A posterior seromuscular suture is inserted before an inverted U-shaped incision is made. (b) The posterior all coat suture has been started.*

possible option in situations where scarring is more severe. However, in these circumstances most surgeons would opt for a gastroenterostomy.

PYLORIC DILATATION AND PYLOROMYOTOMY

The pyloric sphincter mechanism can also be overcome by *pyloric dilatation*, which is now sometimes used as a substitute for pyloroplasty when a vagotomy is performed laparoscopically. A *pyloromyotomy*, in which the muscle is incised longitudinally but the mucosa is preserved intact, is the standard treatment for a congenital pyloric stenosis, and is described in Chapter 17. It is also one option employed to improve drainage from the intrathoracic gastric conduit used for reconstruction after oesophagectomy.

Gastrojejunostomy

A gastrojejunostomy involves the anastomosis of a loop of proximal jejunum to the stomach. This may be used as a drainage procedure in conjunction with a vagotomy, or as a bypass for a gastric outlet or duodenal obstruction. The most frequent causes of obstruction are malignancy and chronic peptic ulcer disease. When the distal stomach and pylorus have been excised, and an anastomosis to the duodenum as a Billroth I reconstruction is not possible, a loop of jejunum is brought up for a Billroth II, or Polya, reconstruction. This anastomosis is in essence another form of gastroenterostomy.

Operative procedure

The anastomosis is a side-to-side anastomosis between a dependent portion of the stomach and the proximal jejunum. The opening in the stomach can be either horizontal, oblique or vertical, and according to the direction of the jejunal loop may be described as isoperistaltic or antiperistaltic. There appears to be no specific advantage in one configuration over another. The anastomosis can be in front of the transverse colon, when it is described as an anterior or antecolic gastroenterostomy, or behind the transverse colon when it is described as a posterior or retrocolic gastroenterostomy (Fig. 16.15).

Posterior (retrocolic) anastomosis The omentum and transverse colon are lifted up, and the duodenojejunal flexure and the first jejunal loop are identified. The anastomosis can usually be made to the segment between 10 and 20 cm from the duodenojejunal flexure, but it must reach the stomach without tension. A window is created in the transverse mesocolon in the avascular plane, usually to the left of the middle colic vessels, taking care not to damage them. A dependent part of the gastric antrum is then brought through the mesocolic window using atraumatic Babcock forceps (Fig. 16.15a).

In recent years there has been a shift towards the use of intestinal stapling devices for the anastomoses as they offer a reduction in operative time. However, for many surgeons

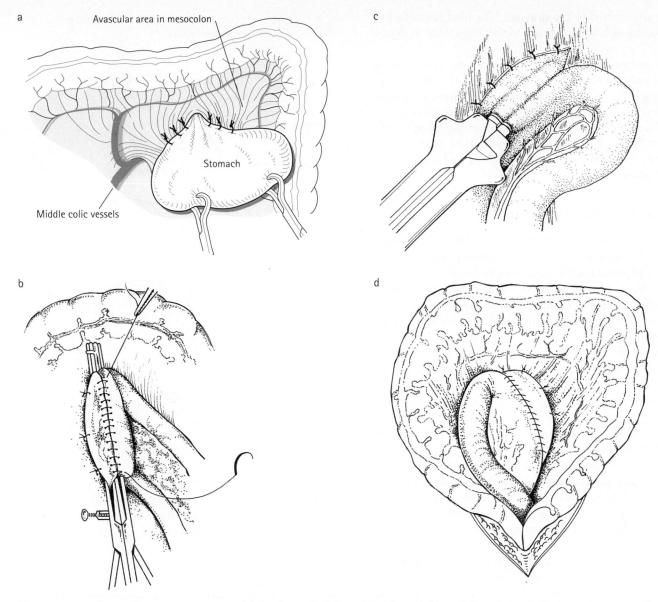

Figure 16.15 *Retrocolic gastroenterostomy. (a) Gentle manipulation of the stomach through the window in the transverse mesocolon using atraumatic Babcock forceps. (b) The classical hand sewn anastomosis. (c) The alternative stapled anastomosis. (d) A completed oblique isoperistaltic anastomosis lying below the transverse mesocolon, and the mesocolic window has been closed.*

the cost implications of a stapled anastomosis are a major consideration. Irrespective of the technique used, the principles that ensure a successful outcome include a good vascular supply to the segments being approximated, no distal obstruction and a tension-free anastomosis. These principles were explored more fully in Chapter 13. The classic two-layer, hand-sewn, side-to-side anastomosis suitable for a gastroenterostomy was described in detail in Chapter 13, and illustrated in Figures 13.11 and 13.12. The alternative stapled anastomosis using a linear cutting stapling device is also described in Chapter 13. In a retrocolic anastomosis, whether a stapled or a hand-sewn technique is used, the margins of the defect in the mesocolon are sutured

to the stomach in order to prevent herniation of the small intestine through the mesocolic window (Stammers' hernia).

In obese patients with a short thick mesocolon and a relatively fixed stomach, a conventional hand-sewn posterior gastroenterostomy can prove difficult. In this event, the gastrocolic ligament can be divided to gain access to the lesser sac, and the selected loop of jejunum can then be drawn upwards, through a window in the transverse mesocolon. Anastomotic clamps can then be applied and the anastomosis performed with relative ease above the transverse colon. On completion, the anastomosis is drawn down, through the window in the mesocolon, and the edges of the mesocolic window are sutured to the stomach. The final alignment of the anastomosis is thus identical to that illustrated in Figure 16.15d.

Gastric emptying after a gastroenterostomy is sometimes very delayed (see Gastroparesis in Chapter 17). With long-standing gastric outlet obstruction, an element of gastric atony develops, and there may also be obstruction of the stoma from oedema. If this complication has been anticipated and a fine-bore transanastomotic tube inserted (see Chapter 11), enteral feeding can be maintained while awaiting resolution.

LAPAROSCOPIC GASTROENTEROSTOMY

A laparoscopic gastrojejunostomy is quite feasible, although an antecolic approach is usually favoured for technical reasons. The present authors use an open Hasson's technique to insert the camera port at the umbilicus and create a pneumoperitoneum to 15 mmHg using CO_2 insufflation. As for all laparoscopic surgery, particular care should be taken when inserting ports, especially if there is a history of previous surgery with associated adhesions. A full laparoscopic examination of the abdominal cavity is performed. The other working ports are placed in accordance with the surgeon's preference, but in general a 10-mm port is used in the left hypochondrium and a 5-mm port at the xiphisternum. Additional working ports can be inserted if required at any stage.

The segment of jejunum to be used is identified, and stay sutures are then inserted. A straight needle is inserted percutaneously and directed through the jejunum and the stomach, close to the intended gastrotomy and enterotomy sites. The needle is then exteriorized again under direct vision. This suture approximates the stomach and duodenum. A second stay suture may be inserted in a similar fashion just beyond the far end of the intended anastomosis (Fig. 16.16a). These sutures provide control of the segments being united and also allow them to be elevated, thereby improving access and reducing spillage. The stomach and the antimesenteric border of the jejunum are then opened using laparoscopic diathermy scissors, or an ultrasonic scalpel (Fig. 16.16a). A Babcock forceps, inserted through the 5-mm port, provides control, and the laparoscopic scissors are inserted through the 10-mm port. The length of these enterotomies should only be sufficient to accommodate the stapling device. A laparoscopic intestinal stapling device is then inserted through the 10-mm port, and a limb is manoeuvred through each of the enterotomies. The device is then closed and fired (Fig. 16.16b). It is important to check that the hilt of the endoscopic gastrointestinal anastomotic stapling device is snug to the enterotomies before firing to ensure an adequate opening. The enterotomies themselves may be closed using a second fire of the device, or by laparoscopic suturing. Care must be taken to avoid narrowing the opening at this stage. The stay sutures are removed and the stomach insufflated via the nasogastric tube to look for any leakage. The greater

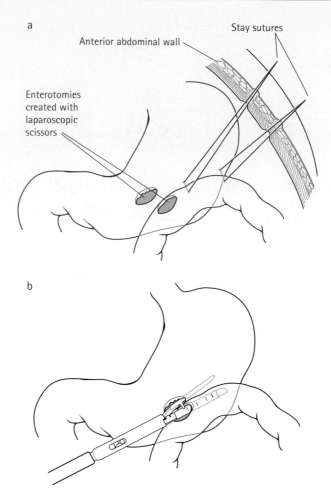

Figure 16.16 *Laparoscopic gastrojejunostomy. (a) Stay sutures are inserted prior to the creation of the enterotomies. (b) Insertion of the endoscopic gastrointestinal stapling device through the enterotomy openings.*

omentum can be placed over the anastomosis. There is usually no indication for a drain.

ROUX LOOP

An alternative form of gastroenterostomy is the anastomosis of a Roux-en-Y loop of jejunum to the stomach, as an end-to-side anastomosis rather than the classical side-to-side gastroenterostomy. This is a particularly appropriate method of gastric drainage when there is only a small residual proximal stomach remnant. It is also used in the reconstruction after a Whipple's pancreatectomy (see Chapter 19).

GASTRECTOMY

Gastrectomies are classified in three different ways which, at the outset, can be confusing.

1. Gastrectomies can be classified according to the amount of stomach that is excised; a total or a partial

gastrectomy. A partial gastrectomy can be a proximal partial gastrectomy, when it is usually combined with a distal oesophagectomy. More often, a partial gastrectomy is a distal partial gastrectomy, and these can be subdivided into an antrectomy, in which only the gastric antrum is removed, the standard partial gastrectomy in which around half the stomach is excised, and a subtotal gastrectomy.

2. As an alternative, gastrectomies can be classified according to the method of reconstruction. After a distal partial gastrectomy, the remaining stomach can be anastomosed to the mobilized duodenum, and is described as a Billroth I gastrectomy (Fig. 16.17a). If instead the duodenum is closed and the first loop of jejunum is brought up for the anastomosis, this is described as a Billroth II, or a Polya, gastrectomy (Fig. 16.17b). Although the two operations were initially considered slightly different, the names are now usually used synonymously. A further alternative reconstruction is with a Roux-en-Y loop, as illustrated in Figure 16.17c.

3. The third classification is related to the radicality of the lymphadenectomy that is combined with the gastrectomy. A D0 gastrectomy is an excision inside the gastric and gastroepiploic arcades and no lymph nodes are removed with the stomach, a D1 gastrectomy includes only the N1 nodes, and a D2 gastrectomy also includes the N2 nodes.

Billroth I gastrectomy for benign disease

Professor Hans Theodore Billroth described his first gastric resection for malignancy in 1881. A Billroth I gastrectomy describes the removal of a distal gastric segment, followed by primary anastomosis with preservation of duodenal integrity. Nowadays, the classic Billroth I gastrectomy is an operation which is almost entirely reserved for benign pathology, as in the standard operation only a very limited lymphadenectomy is achieved. Surprisingly however, this method of reconstruction is still possible after a radical partial gastrectomy and lymphadenectomy as there has been extensive mobilization.[6] The advantage of a Billroth I gastrectomy over a Billroth II procedure is the maintenance of the physiological and anatomical gastroduodenal pathway. Thus, it offers a lower incidence of post-gastrectomy syndromes, minimal disturbance of pancreatic function, and a possible lower incidence of late development of carcinoma in the stomach remnant.

Operative procedure

The abdomen is usually opened by a midline laparotomy incision, though some surgeons prefer a right paramedian or a bilateral subcostal incision. A Balfour retractor should provide adequate access, but for very obese patients Goligher-type bars or an Omnitract retractor system may improve access. The stomach and greater omentum are

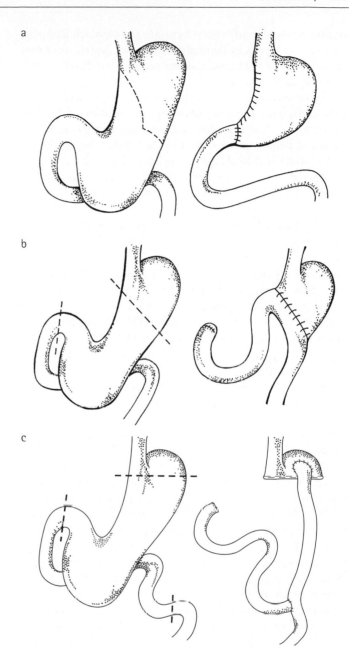

Figure 16.17 *Diagrammatic representation of modes of reconstruction after partial gastrectomy. (a) Billroth I. (b) Billroth II or Polya. (c) Roux-en-Y loop.*

drawn out of the wound and retracted inferiorly by the assistant.

Starting close to the pylorus, the greater omentum is detached from the stomach. With benign disease the plane of dissection may be between the stomach and the gastro-epiploic vessels, with ligation of only the gastric branches of the arcade (Fig. 16.18a). Preservation of the gastroepiploic vessels provides additional blood supply, ensuring a healthy anastomosis. (In carcinoma, the greater omentum is removed en bloc with the stomach.) The dissection along the greater curve may require ligation of the lower short gastric vessels. Avascular adhesions between the stomach and pancreas are divided. Occasionally, a posterior gastric ulcer may extend into the pancreas, and this requires careful dissection ensuring haemostasis.

The lesser omentum is then incised in its avascular plane outside the gastric arcade, allowing identification of the right gastric artery. The right gastric artery may be represented by a leash of vessels rather than a single trunk, whereas the left gastric artery is almost always represented by a single, usually substantial, vessel. The right gastric artery is ligated and divided. Division of the lesser omentum continues parallel with the lesser curvature. In benign disease the descending branch of the left gastric artery can usually be preserved, so that the gastric remnant receives additional blood supply from the proximal portion of the left gastric artery. The stomach is lifted forwards and the inferior border of the first part of the duodenum is separated from the pancreas, carefully dissecting and ligating small vessels.

Kocherization of the duodenum will facilitate the anastomosis and reduce tension at the suture line. The duodenum beyond the proposed resection line must be inspected to ensure that it is healthy and of sufficient calibre for the gastroduodenal anastomosis. The duodenum is then divided between two non-crushing clamps (Fig. 16.18a), or with a linear cutting stapling device.

The line for the gastric resection is determined and the stomach divided using a linear stapler (Fig. 16.18b). This may require to be fired twice to divide the whole way across. Many surgeons elect to oversew the staple line in order to ensure haemostasis. A clamp is then applied at an angle to the original stapled closure at the greater curvature and a segment removed to correspond to the duodenal lumen (Fig. 16.18c). For those surgeons working with financial restrictions that make stapling devices impractical, these two manoeuvres can be performed by applying clamps at an angle to each other. The stomach is divided close to the clamps with a scalpel. The lower clamp encloses a portion of the gastric lumen suitable in size for the anastomosis, whilst the transected stomach held in the upper clamp is closed in two layers to create a new 'lesser curve' (Fig. 16.17a).

Provided that the greater curvature has been adequately mobilized, the gastric remnant can be brought to the duodenum and anastomosed without tension. Stay sutures are inserted into the tissues that are to be approximated. Either a single- or a two-layer anastomotic technique is suitable. When a two-layer technique is used, the outer layer usually consists of interrupted seromuscular sutures, and this posterior outer layer is placed first. The posterior wall is then completed by an all-layer continuous suture. This suture is continued forwards as the all-layer suture of the anterior aspect of the anastomosis, before the final anterior interrupted seromuscular sutures are placed. In a one-layer technique only the continuous all-layer suture is employed, and the outer interrupted seromuscular sutures are omitted. Particular care must be taken with suture placement at the

'angle of sorrow', the lesser curve of the anastomosis, which is especially prone to leakage.

Alternatively the anastomosis may be performed using an end-to-end anastomotic (EEA) circular stapler (Fig. 16.18d). The stapler head is inserted into the duodenum and secured using a purse-string suture. The stapler is inserted into the stomach through a small incision at a more proximal site. The spike of the locking device is brought out distally, avoiding the staple or suture line of the distal stomach. The two portions of the stapling device are locked into place, approximated, and the staples fired. The gastrotomy used to introduce the circular stapler is then closed by elevating it between Babcock forceps and firing a linear stapler. Alternatively, the defect can be sutured. To confirm duodenal integrity some saline is instilled around the anastomotic site, a non-crushing clamp is placed distal to the duodenum and the duodenum inflated with air via the nasogastric tube. An absence of bubbles helps to confirm integrity. The principal aim of achieving a good outcome for a Billroth I gastrectomy is a tension-free anastomosis with a good blood supply.

There is usually no indication for a drain. The nasogastric tube is left *in situ* until gastric function returns. It is used to aspirate gastric secretions and will also help to detect postoperative intraluminal bleeding. Gastric emptying can be slow to recover, either from gastric paresis, or oedema at the site of the anastomosis. For this reason, a feeding jejunostomy tube, inserted at the time of surgery, is very useful following most upper gastrointestinal surgery that involves the formation of an anastomosis as it facilitates enteral access for feeding.

Billroth II (Polya) gastrectomy

Many different types and variations of this gastrectomy have been described, but a Billroth II essentially involves a distal gastric resection, with closure of the duodenal stump, and restoration of intestinal continuity by a gastrojejunostomy. The basic Polya gastrectomy was first described in 1911. Since then surgeons have opted for longer loops of jejunum, with some favouring an antecolic anastomosis and others a retrocolic anastomosis. While the Billroth II reconstruction is associated with a higher incidence of reflux gastritis and dumping syndrome than Billroth I, it offers an alternative in any situation where a Billroth I is not technically possible due to excess tension at the anastomotic site. In a patient with cancer, a Billroth II allows radical margins of tumour clearance without concerns regarding tension on the anastomosis.

Operative procedure
In benign disease, the incisions for the operation, and mobilization of the stomach, are similar to that described for a Billroth I gastrectomy. However, a smaller gastric remnant is often left as it need not reach the duodenum for reconstruction. The greater omentum is more often included in the

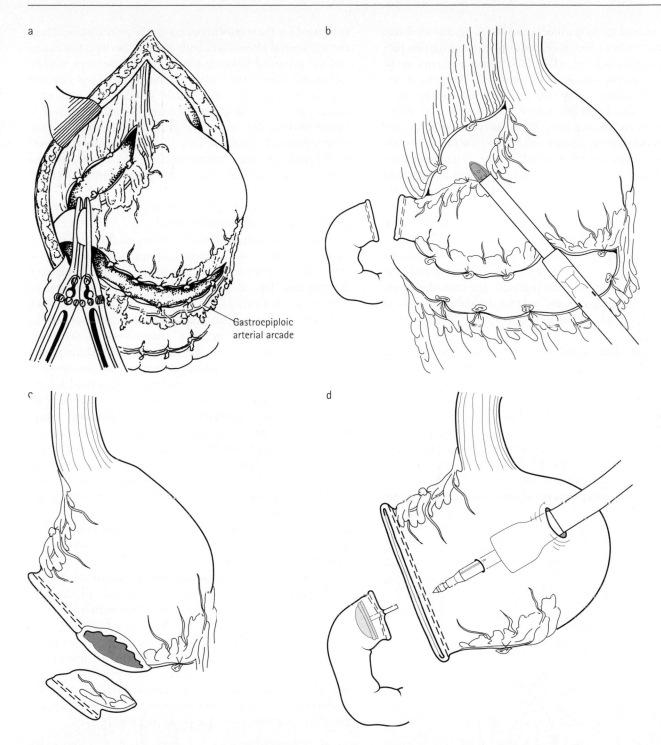

Figure 16.18   *Billroth I gastrectomy. (a) The greater curve has been mobilized inside the gastroepiploic arcade, and the lesser curve outside the gastric arcade. The duodenum is divided with a stapling device or between clamps. (b) The stomach is divided with a linear cutting stapling device. (c) A wedge at the greater curve is excised for the anastomosis. (d) A stapled alternative to the traditional hand-sewn Billroth I anastomosis. It is advisable to oversew all staple lines to ensure haemostasis.*

resected specimen, and the descending branches of the left gastric vessels are seldom preserved. They must be identified and ligated with care. At this stage, the zone of demarcation between ischaemic and well perfused stomach acts as a guide when deciding the level for the gastric transection.

The duodenum is then Kocherized. The stomach is lifted forwards, allowing the inferior border of the first part of the duodenum to be separated from the underlying pancreas. Caution is advised at this stage or troublesome bleeding can ensue. Occasionally, the duodenum may be adherent to the pancreas secondary to an ulcer, and must be dissected free under direct vision. Once the inferior portion of the first part of the duodenum is freed, a GIA 60 is passed posterior to the duodenum and the duodenum transected. The rows of staples on the duodenal stump may then be reinforced by a continuous absorbable seromuscular suture (e.g. 3/0 PDS), which buries the suture line. Those surgeons who do not have access to stapling devices will have to use one of the traditional techniques for duodenal closure. The duodenum can be divided between two straight crushing clamps, and the distal end closed with two layers of absorbable sutures. This can be difficult when there is inflammation or scarring, and the first layer of sutures must be placed before the clamp is removed. The old 'sewing machine' stitch for the first layer may be useful when the duodenal stump is short and difficult to invaginate (Fig. 16.19). Occasionally, it is not possible to close the duodenal stump; this is usually the case when there is a very large duodenal ulcer, and this difficulty is discussed further in Chapter 17, with two solutions illustrated in Figure 17.4.

Transection of the duodenum allows the stomach to be elevated, providing access to the left gastric artery as it reaches the lesser curvature just below the gastro-oesophageal junction. When operating on patients for carcinoma, the artery can be divided at its origin to increase the radicality of the lymphadenectomy. The blood supply to the gastric remnant is then solely from the left gastroepiploic and short gastric arteries. Both the lesser and greater curvature should be free of omentum at the site selected for transection. The next stage depends on whether stapling devices are

to be used for the transection, and for the anastomosis. There are still several alternatives with stapling devices. For example, the proximal stomach can be divided between a distal clamp and a proximal linear horizontal stapling device (see Fig. 13.13, page 227), or it can be divided and both ends sealed using a linear cutting stapling device, as shown in Figure 16.18b. The staple line is then oversewn to ensure haemostasis. The proximal loop of jejunum is then brought up through the transverse mesocolon, and a gastrojejunostomy can be fashioned using an intestinal stapling device as described in Chapter 13 (Fig. 13.14). Alternatively, a portion of the staple line at the greater curve can be trimmed and a hand-sewn anastomosis constructed.

When no stapling devices are employed, the stomach and duodenum are divided between clamps. It is customary to insert the posterior seromuscular suture before the stomach is transected (Fig. 16.20a). A crushing clamp is then applied to the stomach 1 cm distal to the suture line, and the stomach is divided with a scalpel, flush along the underside of the crushing clamp. A hand-sewn anastomosis is then performed using locking twin clamps in a similar fashion to that described for a standard gastroenterostomy in Chapter 13. If the whole width of the transected stomach is used for the anastomosis, this results in a very wide outflow channel from the stomach with a probable increased incidence of 'dumping'. A narrower stoma can be created by restricting the jejunal incision to 3–4 cm, and using only that portion of stomach that is opposite this incision for the anastomosis. The remainder of the gastric transection is closed (Fig. 16.20b). After completion of the gastroenterostomy the anastomosis is drawn through the defect in the transverse mesocolon, the margins of which are attached to the wall of the gastric remnant with interrupted sutures placed about 1 cm above the suture line.

The Roux-en-Y gastrojejunostomy is an alternative technique to restore gastrointestinal continuity. Elevation of the transverse colon in a cephalad direction with head-down tilt will help to identify the duodenojejunal junction. The first suitable loop of jejunum is divided distal to the duodenojejunal junction. The distal divided end of jejunum is anastomosed to the stomach using an end-to side or side-to-side anastomosis. The proximal end is then anastomosed 40–50 cm downstream, thus providing an outflow pathway for biliary contents (see Chapter 21 and Fig. 16.17c).

RADICAL GASTRECTOMIES

Although the Billroth I and II gastrectomies were originally designed as operations for gastric cancer, it is now customary to perform a more radical local, and lymphatic, clearance of the tumour in potentially curative situations. The principle of operative intervention for gastric cancer is to achieve complete resection of the primary tumour with an en bloc regional lymphadenectomy. Gastric cancer has a high

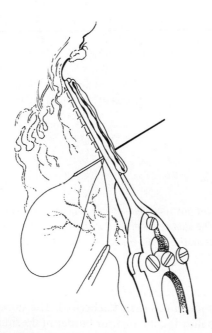

Figure 16.19 *The 'sewing machine' stitch can still be a useful suture for the closure of a difficult duodenal stump when no stapling devices are available.*

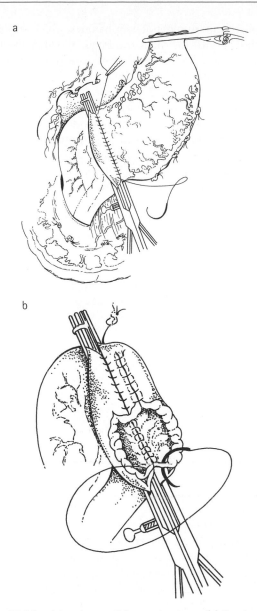

Figure 16.20 *A hand-sewn Polya gastrectomy. (a) The duodenum has been divided between clamps and the stomach elevated so that the posterior seromuscular layer of the gastrojejunal anastomosis can be completed before the clamp is applied to the proximal limit of the gastric dissection. The full width of the stomach, and the jejunal loop, are held in twin occlusion clamps. (b) The appropriate-sized opening is made in the jejunal loop opposite the greater curve, and only this portion of the divided stomach is used for the anastomosis. The remainder of the transected stomach has been closed. The all-coat posterior layer of the anastomosis has been completed and will be continued round anteriorly. The additional seromuscular suturing of the jejunal loop to stomach protects the anastomosis from distraction forces.*

propensity for regional lymphatic spread, and clearing the nodal basins will reduce the incidence of locoregional recurrence. The extent of the lymph node clearance is important, with many Japanese studies reporting improved survival figures attributed in part to extensive nodal dissection. This is

discussed further in Chapter 17. In addition, pathological staging is more likely to be inaccurate if less than 15 lymph nodes are available for histological analysis.[7] Radical gastrectomies are technically challenging operations that require extensive surgical experience, and a knowledge of gastric anatomy and of the multiple lymph-bearing regions.[6,8]

Total gastrectomy with Roux-en-Y reconstruction for gastric cancer

A total gastrectomy may be indicated when the extent, or location, of the primary tumour is such that adequate margins of resection (i.e. 4–6 cm) are not possible by a subtotal gastrectomy. This particularly occurs with proximal gastric tumours and extensive lesions, including linitis plastica. The principle of gastric cancer surgery is to obtain macroscopic and microscopic clearance (R_0 resection), and this should not be compromised by performing a subtotal gastrectomy when a total gastrectomy is indicated.

Preoperative management
Preoperative evaluation requires thorough assessment of a patient's cardiac, respiratory and nutritional status (see Appendix I). Cardiorespiratory co-morbidity is particularly important when the lesion is in the gastric cardia, or near the gastro-oesophageal junction, as radical excision may necessitate a thoracic incision. Preoperative staging (as discussed in Chapter 17) is very important so that surgery can be avoided in those for whom it can offer no benefit.

Operative procedure
Operative access is obtained via an upper midline, or bilateral subcostal 'roof-top' incision. A *left thoraco-abdominal* incision may be considered for extensive tumours involving the gastric cardia or gastro-oesophageal junction. Goligher-type retractors or an Omnitract system improves access to the oesophageal hiatus and lower oesophagus.

A thorough abdominal examination is performed to determine the presence of metastatic disease, which may not have been identified with staging. Up to 20 per cent of gastric tumours are understaged in the preoperative assessment. Peritoneal deposits, liver metastases, or the presence of metastatic disease in para-aortic lymph nodes precludes curative resection. A frozen-section examination may help differentiate metastatic disease from inflammatory reaction when enlarged nodes are encountered. If a curative procedure is not possible, then the surgeon may still elect to proceed with a palliative resection for control of bleeding, or the relief of outlet obstruction, in which case retrieval of lymph nodes is of much less importance.

The first steps are to mobilize the splenic and hepatic colonic flexures, and to Kocherize the duodenum. The greater omentum is detached from the transverse colon along the avascular line about 1 cm from the bowel. The plane of dissection is continued deep to the anterior leaf of the transverse mesocolon (Fig. 16.21). This should be an

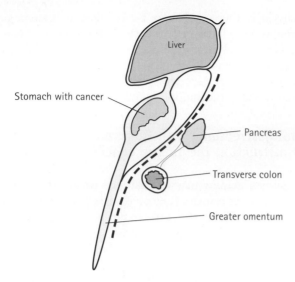

Figure 16.21 *Sagittal section showing the plane of dissection deep to the anterior layer of the transverse mesocolon, and deep to the peritoneum of the posterior wall of the lesser sac.*

avascular plane, but small vessels may be encountered. Avoid damaging the middle colic vessels or their branches. The omentum, and the anterior leaf of the transverse mesocolon, are removed en bloc with the stomach, thus keeping the lesser sac unopened at this stage. The dissection is continued on the right side until the right gastroepiploic vessels and subpyloric lymph nodes are identified. The right gastro-epiploic vessels are carefully ligated and divided at their origins, and the nodes swept up into the tissue to be excised. The dissection is carried onto the pancreas, taking the over-lying peritoneum/pancreatic capsule with the specimen. It is imperative to be in the correct plane. This plane on the sur-face of the pancreas is then followed laterally where it will allow access to the short gastric vessels which are divided.

The omentum is then returned to the abdomen and the liver elevated with a retractor to expose the gastrohepatic lig-ament. This is divided at its left extremity to provide access to the oesophageal hiatus. The division of the peritoneal reflec-tion onto the liver is then continued to the right, and the lesser sac is entered. In an antral carcinoma consideration should be given as to whether portal dissection, with retrieval of station 12 lymph nodes, is indicated (see Chapter 17). When these nodes are not to be dissected, the incision across the peritoneal reflection onto the liver stops to the left of the common bile duct and turns inferiorly towards the duode-num. When station 12 nodes are to be retrieved, the hepato-duodenal ligament is opened by the continuation of the peritoneal incision into Calot's triangle, providing exposure of the common bile duct, hepatic artery, and portal vein. The hepatic artery and its bifurcation are skeletonized, with retrieval of all lymph-bearing tissue. A tape around the hepatic artery with slight traction will provide exposure to the anterior portion of the portal vein. This dissection should

yield a significant number of lymph nodes, which are excised in continuity with the main specimen. Whether the portal nodes are retrieved or not, the line of dissection comes down onto the common hepatic artery. The right gastric artery, arising from it, is identified and ligated near its origin.

The duodenum must be fully Kocherized to allow access to the retropancreatic and hepatoduodenal regions. This exposes the inferior vena cava and abdominal aorta, and also allows retrieval of right para-aortic and retropancreatic lymph nodes. The duodenum is then divided and closed. This is most easily achieved with a linear cutting stapling device, but alternatively it can be divided between two non-crushing clamps and the distal limb closed using a continu-ous 3/0 absorbable suture. Duodenal division provides access to the infrapyloric group of lymph nodes. Elevation and cephalad traction on the stomach exposes the coeliac axis and the left gastric artery, and the lymph nodes associated with these vessels. The left gastric artery is divided near its origin with division of the left gastric vein along the superior border of the pancreas. Retrieval of tissue surrounding the left gastric artery, the hepatic artery and the coeliac trunk provides a high yield of lymph nodes. The ascending branch of the left gastric is divided just above the oesophagogastric junction so that the whole lesser curve arterial arcade and lymph nodes can be removed (see Fig. 16.2).

On the greater curvature the remaining short gastric ves-sels are divided as close to the splenic hilum as is safe, and the lymph nodes taken en bloc. As discussed in Chapter 17, it is sometimes justifiable to include the spleen, and even the pancreatic tail, en bloc in the resected specimen, in which case the dissection proceeds lateral to the spleen to mobilize it. The splenic vessels, rather than the short gastric arteries, must be ligated. With the stomach fully mobilized and any remaining adhesions divided, stay sutures are inserted into the lesser and greater curvatures. Stay sutures can also be inserted into the distal oesophagus to prevent its retraction after the stomach has been removed. It may be possible to apply a non-crushing clamp, proximal to the oesophageal stay sutures. The oesophagus is then divided using either a scalpel or straight scissors. When the gastrectomy is for a cancer close to the cardia, it is desirable to include at least a short segment of oesophagus in the resected specimen, along with a cuff of diaphragm. When a longer segment of oesoph-agus needs to be resected, a thoracoabdominal approach is preferable.

There are many options available for reconstruction. The present authors favour a Roux-en-Y loop and the formation of an end-to-side oesophagojejunal anastomosis. The first suitable loop of jejunum is divided using a linear stapler, and the distal end is brought up through the transverse meso-colon for an end-to-side anastomosis with the oesophagus. The anastomosis is formed using a single layer of absorbable monofilament sutures inserted in an interrupted fashion (Fig. 16.22a). The proximal end of the divided jejunum is then anastomosed 40–50 cm downstream to reduce subse-quent reflux. However, the anastomosis can also be per-

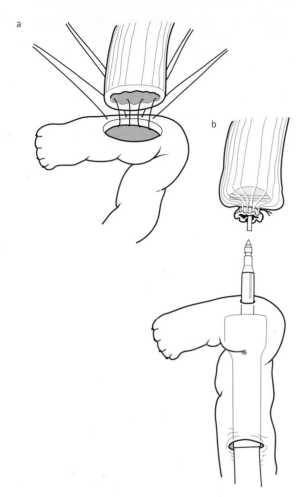

Figure 16.22 *Oesophagojejunal anastomoses after total gastrectomy. (a) Sutured. (b) Circular stapled through a separate enterotomy. Alternatively, the stapler can be inserted through the open end of the jejunal limb before it is closed. The stapled jejunal blind end should be oversewn.*

formed using a circular stapler. The head is carefully inserted into the oesophageal lumen where it is secured with a purse-string suture. The main portion of the stapler is then inserted, via an enterotomy, into the jejunum (Fig. 16.22b). The enterotomy is subsequently closed using a hand-sewn technique. There is also the option of using a longer segment of jejunum for the Roux loop, and making the end into a jejunal pouch using the linear stapler. This may improve the patient's postoperative capacity for food.[9]

Subtotal gastrectomy for gastric carcinoma

Subtotal gastrectomy with regional lymph node dissection (D2 or D3 lymphadenectomy) is particularly suitable for small gastric tumours involving the pylorus and distal third of the stomach. When macroscopic and microscopic clearance is obtained it provides equivalent survival rates compared to total gastrectomy, with a lower incidence of postoperative morbidity and mortality. The patient is left

with a gastric remnant, which in theory reduces the potential for post-gastrectomy syndromes. Additionally, an anastomosis onto a well-vascularized stomach remnant is more secure than an anastomosis onto oesophagus. Preoperative staging and general assessment are similar to that described for patients undergoing a total gastrectomy.

OPERATIVE PROCEDURE

This operation is very similar to that of the total gastrectomy described above, except that the final step of dividing all the short gastric vessels is omitted. The stomach is transected leaving a small gastric remnant with a blood supply from these remaining vessels. Once resection and lymphadenectomy are complete, reconstruction is usually performed with a Roux loop although, after the extensive mobilization needed for a radical lymphadenectomy, a Billroth I reconstruction may be an option.

OESOPHAGECTOMY

Oesophagectomy is performed almost exclusively for malignant disease. Benign conditions which occasionally warrant an oesophagectomy include long corrosive strictures and very late presentation of achalasia. When considering operative intervention for oesophageal carcinoma, the choice of incision and procedure are determined by tumour type, location, operability, and the patient's cardiorespiratory status. This is discussed in more depth in Chapter 17. The oesophagectomy may have to be combined with a partial, or even a total, gastrectomy to obtain adequate resection margins of a distal tumour. Similarly, a proximal oesophageal tumour may require the addition of a pharyngectomy to obtain local clearance (see Chapter 9). Three approaches to oesophagectomy are described below: the transhiatal; the left thoraco-abdominal; and the three-stage operation. Many other techniques have been described, but most are modifications of the above.

Transhiatal oesophagectomy

This involves abdominal and cervical incisions only, thus avoiding a thoracotomy. The stomach, gastro-oesophageal junction and distal oesophagus are mobilized via the abdominal incision. The intrathoracic component of the oesophagus is freed distally through the diaphragmatic hiatus and proximally via the cervical incision. The resected oesophagus is then reconstructed using the gastric remnant, or an intestinal loop as an oesophageal conduit. This is passed through the chest via the posterior mediastinum, allowing it to be anastomosed to the cervical oesophagus without tension.

Operative procedure

The patient is placed in a supine position with the neck elevated, supported in a head ring and turned to the right. Some surgeons favour turning the head to the left for a right cervical approach, and cite a lower incidence of recurrent laryngeal nerve injuries.

An upper midline laparotomy incision is made. A full laparotomy is performed to check for evidence of advanced disease, which might not have been apparent on imaging. This is particularly important in lower-third oesophageal cancers which have a greater propensity to spread intra-abdominally. The presence of liver metastases, retroperitoneal lymph nodes or disseminated disease means that no benefit is likely to be obtained by proceeding with oesophagectomy, and treatment should be palliative, aimed at symptomatic relief.

The greater omentum is mobilized outside the right gastroepiploic vessels, which must be preserved as an arterial supply to the stomach remnant. The left gastroepiploic and short gastric vessels are then divided along the greater curvature, taking care not to damage the gastric wall or spleen. The stomach is placed on stretch, allowing the gastrohepatic ligament to be incised. The right gastric artery is preserved which, with the right gastroepiploic artery, is the blood supply to the gastric remnant that will be used as the conduit. The left gastric vein and artery are identified and ligated near their origin.

When the stomach remnant is suitable to be used for the oesophageal conduit, the duodenum is Kocherized. The vagi will be divided during the oesophagectomy, and therefore a pyloroplasty is performed to reduce delay in gastric emptying. An alternative favoured by some is a pyloromyotomy, which is thought to be associated with a lower incidence of bile reflux and alkaline gastritis.

The oesophageal hiatus is then mobilized allowing a Penrose drain to be passed around the gastro-oesophageal junction. If the tumour involves the hiatus, a cuff of diaphragm surrounding the tumour may be removed en bloc, to ensure adequate margins of resection. Traction on the Penrose drain aids mobilization of the distal oesophagus under direct vision and, with good retraction, dissection under direct vision can be performed up to the level of the carina. The surgeon's hand is then inserted through the diaphragmatic hiatus and, using blunt dissection and staying close to the oesophageal wall, the posterior oesophagus is separated from the prevertebral fascia. Anterior blunt dissection is then performed, again staying close to the oesophageal wall, and avoiding cardiac displacement that may give rise to arrhythmias and hypotension. Communication with the anaesthetist is crucial at this point. If any haemodynamic instability ensues it will usually revert to normal if the hand is removed from the thorax, and all dissection must be halted until the patient has stabilized. The lateral oesophageal attachments must also be divided.

Attention is now turned to the neck. The cervical oesophagus is accessed by making an incision along the anterior border of the sternocleidomastoid (see Chapter 9). A low transverse cervical incision is a suitable alternative. The skin, subcutaneous tissue and platysma are incised. The carotid sheath is identified and retracted laterally, and the trachea is retracted medially. The middle thyroid vein and inferior thyroid artery may need to be ligated and divided, to avoid avulsion during dissection. It is imperative to avoid damaging the recurrent laryngeal nerve as it runs in the tracheo-oesophageal groove and retractors should not be inserted blindly. Even minor damage has significant implications beyond a temporary hoarseness as it increases the potential for aspiration pneumonia.

Posterior finger dissection will identify the prevertebral fascia and allow it to be separated from the posterior oesophageal wall. The recurrent laryngeal nerve is then identified and protected. Staying close to the oesophageal wall during anterior and right lateral dissection will reduce the risk of damage to the nerve and to the membranous posterior wall of the trachea. If a nasogastric tube is *in situ* this will be helpful for this part of the dissection. A Penrose drain is inserted around the oesophagus. This aids further dissection and allows the cervical oesophagus to be elevated out of the incision. Usually, a combination of dissection from the abdominal and cervical incisions will free all attachments. Small oesophageal arteries which are avulsed during these manoeuvres usually retract and thrombose spontaneously. However, substantial mediastinal bleeding may signify damage to a larger artery or the azygos vein and warrants a thoracotomy for control of haemorrhage.

The level of the oesophageal transection is then identified, and stay sutures are inserted proximal to this point into the lateral and medial walls. A latex drain is sutured to the oesophagus, distal to the line of transection. This will serve as a guide to bring up the oesophageal conduit from the abdomen. The nasogastric tube is then retracted proximal to the line of transection and the cervical oesophagus is divided cleanly using straight scissors or scalpel. Some surgeons prefer a GIA stapler. The divided oesophagus, with the attached latex drain, is then removed from the mediastinum via the diaphragmatic hiatus. The drain is now lying in the posterior mediastinum with one end at the cervical opening and one end in the abdomen.

The stomach must now be prepared as a conduit to be drawn up into the chest. The highest point on the fundus is identified and will be used for the anastomosis. It is therefore possible to remove the oesophagogastric junction, and the greater part of the lesser curve, without reducing available length. This has the advantage of removing upper gastric drainage nodes to which a distal oesophageal cancer may spread (Fig. 16.23). Division is usually undertaken using GIA staplers, going from the lesser curvature to the fundus to create a rotation gastroplasty, and the staple line of the gastric tube is then oversewn using an inverting stitch. The latex drain is now attached to the apex of the gastric conduit and used to guide the stomach up into the neck. This is aided by gentle manipulation of the stomach through the posterior mediastinum by the surgeon's hand. It is important to avoid gastric torsion.

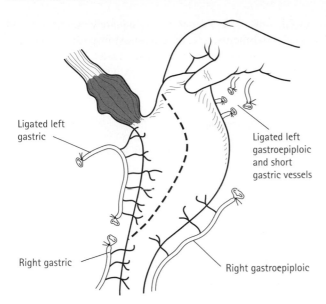

Figure 16.23 *Oesophagectomy: the preparation of a gastric conduit. The blood supply for the conduit is from the right gastric and gastroepiploic arteries. The left gastric, the short gastric and the left gastroepiploic arteries have all been ligated. Gastric transection along the dotted line enables the cardia, and the lesser curve and cardiac nodes to be removed en bloc with the tumour. The hand is holding the high point of the stomach which will be used for the anastomosis.*

The anastomosis can be created using a circular stapling device, introduced through a gastrotomy in a similar manner to that illustrated for a gastroduodenal stapled anastomosis in Figure 16.18d. However, the preference of the present authors is to make a small anterior opening near the highest point of the fundus and fashion the anastomosis with a single layer of interrupted sutures, using an absorbable suture. The posterior layer of sutures is inserted first. The nasogastric tube is then carefully advanced across the anastomotic line before closing the anterior layer. A small suction drain is placed close to the anastomosis prior to closing the neck incision.

Occasionally, the stomach cannot be used as a conduit. The tumour may have extended into the stomach such that a gastrectomy was necessary, or the mobilized stomach may have an inadequate blood supply. Alternative conduits in this situation include colon and jejunum (see below).

Finally, a feeding jejunostomy tube can be inserted (see Chapter 11), as this allows enteral nutrition to be started within 24 hours. Usually, the nasogastric tube remains *in situ* for approximately 6 days. A water-soluble contrast swallow should confirm oesophageal integrity prior to the commencement of oral fluids.

Intraoperative complications

The operating surgeon should be competent to convert to thoracotomy if, during the procedure, there is an unforeseen intrathoracic complication. These complications can in the main be avoided by correct selection of patients for a transhiatal approach (as discussed in Chapter 17). Bleeding from the azygos vein, or from oesophageal branches of the aorta, may not be manageable without a lateral thoracotomy. Other potential complications include damage to the membranous posterior wall of the trachea. A tracheal tear represents a life-threatening complication. This may be a small tear that is easily repaired at thoracotomy, or it may be extensive, where the tumour has abutted the trachea with the entire portion disrupted during the dissection. This latter variety is often fatal. When a tracheal tear occurs the endotracheal tube is deflated and advanced beyond the tear into the distal trachea, or left main bronchus. This provides ventilatory control while the oesophagectomy is completed. An upper sternal split will provide adequate access to the trachea to determine if repair is possible.

The management of late complications including gastric remnant necrosis, cervical anastomotic leaks, and chylothorax is discussed in Chapter 17.

Thoraco-abdominal oesophagectomy

This is a suitable approach for tumours involving the distal oesophagus, gastro-oesophageal junction and gastric cardia.

Operative procedure

The patient is placed in a right lateral decubitus position with the left arm flexed at 90 degrees to the body and placed in an arm-rest. It is a one-stage procedure that utilizes a single incision with the initial transverse, or oblique, abdominal incision extended over the left chest (see Fig. 12.15, page 207). The operating table is rotated as the surgical field moves from abdomen to chest, or vice versa. The choice of intercostal space is decided on exploring the abdomen, and may be through either the sixth, seventh or eighth space. The incision can extend to the edge of the erector spinae muscle, with the intercostals incised using diathermy to achieve good haemostasis. The cartilage of the costal margin is divided, while the rib above or below the chosen space may be divided to provide greater access. Once the pleural cavity is entered a rib retractor is inserted.

The diaphragm is incised to the oesophageal hiatus in a circumferential manner to reduce the potential for damage to the phrenic nerve or its branches. A radial incision carries a significant risk of diaphragmatic paralysis. The inferior phrenic artery is ligated. Adhesions to the lung base and the lower part of the pulmonary ligament are divided so that the lung can be retracted upwards. The stomach is then mobilized as described previously, and the lower oesophagus is freed through a longitudinal incision in the parietal pleura between the aorta and the pericardium. The vagi are identified and divided. Encircling the distal oesophagus with a Penrose drain aids its subsequent dissection. Vessels should only be divided if this is essential for oesophageal mobilization. The thoracic duct is ligated immediately above the diaphragm to prevent a chylothorax. Division of the diaphragm is now completed and a cuff is removed if this is required to ensure tumour clearance.

The thoracoabdominal approach is often chosen for more advanced oesophagogastric junction tumours where an oesophagectomy must be combined with a gastrectomy. However, the remaining stomach can often still be used as the oesophageal conduit, especially as it does not need so much length as it would for a cervical anastomosis. The division of the stomach and the formation of the gastric conduit are then undertaken in a similar manner to that described for the transhiatal operation. The anastomosis is performed beneath the aortic arch, and again this can be undertaken with a circular stapler, or by a hand-sewn technique. If a total gastrectomy is necessary, reconstruction is usually with a Roux loop and an oesophagojejunal anastomosis.

The diaphragm is closed with interrupted absorbable sutures. At the diaphragmatic hiatus the gastric tube, or other conduit, is sutured to the diaphragmatic edge to prevent herniation. Two drains are inserted into the chest, with a straight 28 French directed to the apex and a 32 French angled drain directed towards the base, prior to left lung re-inflation. Division of the costochondral cartilage may be a source of pain postoperatively. The divided edges must be closely approximated to prevent them rubbing together, with some surgeons favouring a miniplate attached by screws. Alternatively, 2 cm of costochondral cartilage is removed completely to prevent contact and friction.

Postoperative care is similar to that for the transhiatal oesophagectomy, but the thoracic incision makes these patients more prone to respiratory complications, including atelectasis and pneumonia. Pain relief and physiotherapy are therefore extremely important.

Ivor Lewis–McKeown (three-stage) oesophagectomy

The three-stage approach, as described by McKeown, consists of cervical, abdominal and right thoracotomy incisions.[10] Thus, it combines the excellent laparotomy and right thoracotomy exposure provided by the Ivor Lewis approach[11] with the safety of a cervical anastomosis.

ABDOMINAL COMPONENT

This is performed first, through a midline laparotomy incision and allows intra-abdominal spread which would preclude a curative resection to be excluded before proceeding further. If the tumour is still judged to be resectable, the stomach is mobilized with preservation of the right gastroepiploic and right gastric arteries. The duodenum is Kocherized, and a pyloroplasty or pyloromyotomy is performed, as described for the transhiatal oesophagectomy. The oesophageal hiatus is mobilized to provide access to the distal oesophagus, and the hiatal opening enlarged as required. Once the stomach is adequately mobilized and freed of attachments, a feeding jejunostomy tube is inserted and sutured to the anterior abdominal wall. The stomach is then partially delivered into the chest cavity. The abdomen is closed.

THORACIC COMPONENT

The patient is then placed in a left lateral position, which allows a right posterolateral thoracotomy to be performed through the fourth or fifth intercostal space (as described in Chapter 7). The double-lumen tube allows the right lung to be collapsed with ventilation maintained through one-lung anaesthesia.

The inferior pulmonary ligament is divided and the lung gently retracted by the assistant. The mediastinal pleura overlying the oesophagus is divided and the azygos vein is identified, and double-ligated before division. Dissection continues to free the oesophagus, and all para-oesophageal lymph nodes are included with the resected specimen. Oesophageal arterial branches are divided between clips. During superior dissection care must be taken to avoid damaging the recurrent laryngeal nerve. Many surgeons routinely identify and ligate the thoracic duct immediately above the diaphragm, on the right lateral aspect of the descending aorta, to reduce the subsequent incidence of chylothorax. Knowledge of the course of the duct and its potential anatomical variations is important if damage is to be avoided intraoperatively. The thoracic duct is the principal lymphatic drainage system. It commences as the cisterna chyli, in the midline, at the level of the twelfth thoracic vertebra to the right of the aorta. It passes through the diaphragmatic hiatus into the chest, and ascends on the right side of the thoracic spine until the level of the fourth or fifth thoracic vertebra where it crosses posterior to the aorta to ascend on the left side of the oesophagus. In the root of the neck, just above the level of the clavicle, it arches forwards and passes anterior to the left subclavian and common carotid arteries, eventually emptying into the left subclavian vein near its junction with the left internal jugular vein. The thoracic duct is thus particularly vulnerable to injury when the supra-aortic oesophagus is removed, or when there is dissection around the right side of the aorta as when the para-aortic mediastinal nodes are retrieved. Although some surgeons recommend routine ligation of the thoracic duct during oesophagectomy, others are selective. Those who are selective are most likely to ligate the duct when a right thoractotomy is employed for an oesophagectomy which is to be combined with a more extensive intrathoracic lymphadenectomy.

Once the intrathoracic oesophagus has been adequately mobilized, the stomach is fully delivered into the chest via the hiatus. The distal resection limit is identified. The resected specimen may involve a variable portion of the proximal stomach, as discussed above. The stomach is divided so that it can be closed to form a tubular conduit as described in the transhiatal oesophagectomy section.

CERVICAL COMPONENT

This is performed as described above for the transhiatal oesophagectomy. Once the oesophagus has been encircled by a Penrose drain, the distal dissection should not be too difficult, provided that adequate mobilization was performed at thoracotomy. The cervical oesophagus is divided and a latex drain attached to the distal portion. This is then pulled through from the thoracotomy opening. The latex drain is then attached to the gastric tube, or alternative conduit, and delivered into the neck avoiding torsion. The oesophagogastric anastomosis is then completed using a circular stapler, or hand-sewn anastomosis, as previously described.

OESOPHAGEAL CONDUITS

Resection and replacement of the oesophagus has been a source of great challenge to surgeons. The preferred conduit is usually the stomach, provided that this reaches the proximal oesophagus with a good blood supply and without undue tension. If the patient has undergone a total gastrectomy, then alternatives such as colonic interposition or jejunal grafts will have to be considered. The principles of the conduit are the restoration of gastrointestinal continuity with an adequate lumen and satisfactory function, while keeping the incidence of reflux, with the danger of aspiration, to a minimum. This is particularly pertinent when performing oesophageal surgery for benign disease in young people, whose quality of life is a major issue after surgery.

STOMACH

Stomach is the conduit of choice for oesophageal replacement in almost all situations. Following oesophageal surgery, most patients have a significant portion of a gastric remnant remaining, which will reach the proximal oesophagus. Kocherization of the duodenum, and division of the short gastric and left gastric vessels, adds to the length available for mobilization. One advantage of the stomach over other grafts is the need for only a single anastomosis. There is however, the risk of ischaemic necrosis at the apex of the gastric tube and, even in the absence of frank necrosis, a marginally adequate perfusion may contribute to anastomotic breakdown. A gastric conduit is associated in the long term with an increased risk of proximal oesophagitis and stricture.

COLON

The use of a colonic conduit involves three anastomoses, but the procedure is associated with a lower incidence of postoperative reflux symptoms, and patients may have an improved quality of life. Right, transverse, or left colon can be used as a colonic conduit (as discussed in Chapter 21). Preoperative colonoscopy and angiography are useful adjuncts to ensure that there is no underlying bowel disease, and to identify the

blood supply relevant to the conduit. The right colon is more satisfactory, and if the ileocolic segment is used there is little discrepancy between the lumen of the terminal ileum and the cervical anastomosis, ensuring a satisfactory end-to-end anastomosis. The right colon, the caecum and ascending colon are mobilized from their lateral peritoneal attachments. The hepatic flexure is freed, taking care not to damage the duodenum. The terminal ileum and the distal transverse colon are divided and an ileocolic anastomosis constructed (see Fig. 21.16, page 392). The ileocolic vessels are divided, and the conduit relies on its blood supply from the middle colic vessels, and variably also from the right colic vessels, although the latter may have to be divided to provide sufficient mobility.

JEJUNAL ROUX LOOP

This is a satisfactory alternative conduit when a lower-third oesophagectomy has been combined with a total gastrectomy for a tumour of the cardia. A left thoraco-abdominal incision has usually been employed and the anastomosis is below the aortic arch. This, however, is generally as high as it is possible to bring a Roux loop.

JEJUNAL INTERPOSITION

A segment of jejunum, with a suitable mesenteric vessel, is identified by mesenteric transillumination. The segment of jejunum, with its vascular supply still intact, is divided using GIA staplers, and the small bowel is anastomosed to restore intestinal continuity. The isolated segment of small bowel loop can then be used as an isoperistaltic interposition graft. However, its blood supply will seldom allow it to be brought up for an anastomosis above the aortic arch. When it is needed at a higher level it must be used as a free graft, but this requires considerable expertise and microvascular experience. It is therefore usually reserved for situations where other options are not possible, or have failed. Its routine use is restricted to pharyngo-oesophageal replacement (see Chapter 9). As the small intestine does not tolerate prolonged periods of ischaemia, it is usual to isolate the graft but to leave it *in situ* until all other dissection is completed, the recipient vessels have been identified, and everything is prepared for the microvascular reconstruction.

Route for the conduit

An oesophageal conduit can be brought up to the neck by the posterior mediastinal, the retrosternal or the subcutaneous route.

POSTERIOR MEDIASTINAL

This is the anatomical position of the native oesophagus, and the preferred route in most circumstances. It is slightly shorter than the alternatives, and the proximal oesophagus and the conduit are well-aligned for the anastomosis. When the native oesophagus is removed transhiatally a conduit can be tunnelled through the posterior mediastinum without a thoracotomy, as described above. However, this route may not be suitable when it is the site of dense adhesions. There may have been posterior mediastinal sepsis from a previous oesophageal perforation, or the failure of a previous conduit from ischaemic necrosis or anastomotic leakage. Corrosive damage, radiotherapy fibrosis and residual tumour can similarly exclude the posterior mediastinum.

RETROSTERNAL (ANTERIOR MEDIASTINAL)

This is usually the preferred non-anatomical route where the posterior mediastinum is unsuitable. A midline retrosternal tunnel can be created by blunt finger dissection through abdominal and cervical incisions. A narrow malleable intestinal retractor is then passed up the tunnel, keeping the tip immediately deep to the sternum. The conduit is then guided up to the cervical incision. The strap muscles are divided to allow the oesophageal substitute to pass to the oesophagus for an anastomosis. Unfortunately, the angulation of the conduit onto the cervical oesophagus, and its abnormal anterior relationship to the trachea, makes swallowing feel unnatural and unpleasant.

SUBCUTANEOUS (PRESTERNAL)

This route requires an even longer conduit than the retrosternal alternative, and is nowadays used only occasionally. It may however avoid any possible respiratory compromise in a patient with very poor lung function. It may also have to be considered in a patient whose anterior mediastinum is unsafe because of adhesions between the heart and a median sternotomy scar from previous cardiac surgery.

REFERENCES

1. *Surgical Laparoscopy*, 2nd edn. KA Zucher, L Blackbourne. Philadelphia: Lippincott Williams & Wilkins, 2000.
2. Johnson AJ, Baxter HK. Where is your vagotomy incomplete? Observations on operative technique. *Br J Surg* 1977; **64**: 583–6.
3. Pendower JE. A comparison of the Burge and Grassi intraoperative tests for completeness of nerve section in parietal cell vagotomy. *Br J Surg* 1981; **68**: 83–4.
4. Taylor TV, Gunn AA, Macleod DA, *et al.* Anterior lesser curve seromyotomy and posterior truncal vagotomy in the treatment of chronic duodenal ulcer. *Lancet* 1982; **2**: 846–9.
5. Orr IM, Johnson HD. Vagotomy for peptic ulcer. *Br Med J* 1949; ii: 1316–18.
6. McCulloch P. Description of the Japanese method of radical gastrectomy. *Ann R Coll Surg Engl* 1994; **76**: 110–14.
7. Lee HK, Yang HK, Kim WH, *et al.* Influence of the number of lymph nodes examined on staging of gastric cancer. *Br J Surg* 2001; **88**: 1408–12.
8. Qadir A, Trotter C, Park KGM. D2 gastrectomy for antral stomach cancer 'How I do it' series. *J R Coll Surg Edinb* 2000; **45**: 242–51.
9. Lehnert T, Buhl K. Techniques of reconstruction after total gastrectomy for cancer. Review. *Br J Surg* 2004; **91**: 528–39.
10. McKeown KC. The surgical treatment of carcinoma of the oesophagus. *J R Coll Surg Edinb* 1985; **30**: 1–14.
11. Crofts TJ. Ivor-Lewis oesophagectomy for middle and lower third oesophageal lesions – how we do it. *J R Coll Surg Edinb* 2000; **45**: 296–303.

17

OPERATIVE MANAGEMENT OF UPPER GASTROINTESTINAL DISEASE

OLIVER McANENA AND MYLES JOYCE

UPPER GASTROINTESTINAL TRAUMA

The stomach is seldom injured by blunt abdominal trauma, and the management of penetrating injuries to the stomach is usually straightforward. The stomach has good mobility, and an excellent blood supply, which makes primary closure almost always successful. Oesophageal and duodenal injuries are however more common, and they are much more difficult to treat. The management of blunt and penetrating duodenal trauma was covered in Chapter 14. The oesophagus is seldom injured by blunt trauma, but it is vulnerable to injury in penetrating trauma to the neck. This is discussed in Chapter 9. Similarly, the intrathoracic or abdominal oesophagus can also be injured by penetrating trauma. However, most oesophageal injuries are iatrogenic either at endoscopy, or during open or laparoscopic surgery.

Oesophageal perforation

Oesophageal perforation is a rare but life-threatening emergency. A high index of suspicion, coupled with prompt diagnosis and early surgical intervention, is the key to achieving a successful outcome. Patients undergoing oesophageal stenting and dilatation of strictures are at particular risk, especially if there is an underlying oesophageal malignancy. When a perforation occurs it may be a through-and-through injury or, alternatively, a mucosal tear that becomes infected with subse-

quent perforation, leading to a delay between the time of endoscopy and the onset of symptoms. Post-endoscopic perforations are more common at the three areas of oesophageal narrowing, namely the cricopharyngeus (upper oesophageal sphincter), at the level of the aortic arch/left main stem bronchus, and finally at the gastro-oesophageal junction.

Boerhaave's syndrome, named after Herman Boerhaave who first reported it in 1724, is a rupture of a normal oesophagus, following an episode of retching. The first successful repair of a post-emetic oesophageal rupture was performed by Barrett in 1946.

The optimal management of an oesophageal perforation is dependent on the site of the perforation, and the time interval between perforation and diagnosis.

CERVICAL OESOPHAGEAL PERFORATIONS

The initial symptoms may be mild, but include neck pain, dysphagia and regurgitation of a bloody discharge. Movement of the thyroid cartilage will often elicit significant pain. The patient may quickly become systemically unwell, with the development of subcutaneous emphysema, mediastinitis and respiratory compromise. When suspected, the diagnosis can be confirmed by water-soluble contrast studies or by direct visualization at endoscopy. Prompt exploration of the cervical oesophagus should be performed under general anaesthesia, but for very sick patients local anaesthesia may be an option.

An oblique incision is made along the anterior border of the sternocleidomastoid on the side of the perforation. The carotid bundle is then retracted posteriorly and the middle thyroid vein divided. The presence of oedema and inflammatory reaction will direct the surgeon to the site of perforation. Upper endoscopy is a useful guide, and also allows the performance of an insufflation test post-repair to confirm oesophageal integrity. In an early clean perforation it may be possible to close it, either with a single layer of absorbable sutures taking full-thickness bites or, alternatively, with a double layer consisting of an inner mucosal layer and an outer muscular layer. Copious washout is performed. Placement of an oesophageal suction drain to the neck and superior mediastinum is important. Often, the tissues are too friable to allow a safe primary repair; it may then be more prudent to allow the tissue to heal by secondary intention, with a drain left adjacent to the perforation.

Postoperatively a nasogastric tube is left *in situ* and the patient treated with broad-spectrum antibiotics and parenteral feeding. Oral intake is withheld until a contrast study, usually performed at around 7 days, confirms oesophageal integrity.

THORACIC OESOPHAGEAL PERFORATION

The contamination of the mediastinum results in a rapid onset of symptoms. Often, the first complaint is that of respiratory distress, with the development of a pleural effusion, usually on the left side. Cervical subcutaneous emphysema may be palpable. The chest X-ray may show mediastinal widening with pneumomediastinum, in addition to a pleural fluid collection or pneumothorax. Perforation can be confirmed by endoscopy, a water-soluble contrast study or a CT scan. A high index of suspicion is important if the diagnosis is to be established early, and this is important as prompt instigation of treatment is associated with a better outcome. The mortality rate is reported at 52 per cent for those explored after 24 hours, while it is 13 per cent for those who undergo surgery within 24 hours.

Surgical exploration as soon as the patient has been resuscitated is associated with the best outcome in most clinical situations. Lower oesophageal perforations are approached through the 6th or 7th intercostal space, on the side of the leak. If the perforation is recent, the contamination is minimal, and there is no underlying oesophageal disease then it may be closed primarily. The entire length of the mucosal defect must be exposed and closed. Thus, the muscle will have to be divided proximally and distally at the limits of the perforation. The type of suture material, and whether a one- or two-layer technique is used, are generally a matter of individual surgical preference. Closure is followed by extensive washout and the placement of chest drains for drainage of the mediastinum and pleura. If the perforation is less recent, or there is extensive contamination, attempts at repair are unwise. Treatment instead consists of the removal of all debris from the mediastinum, followed by lavage and drainage.

Occasionally, the thoracic oesophagus is extensively damaged, and this necessitates an emergency oesophagectomy. However, this carries a high mortality and if the patient is critically ill it may be prudent merely to drain the mediastinum and perform a cervical oesophagostomy. If the patient makes a satisfactory recovery, then oesophageal continuity may be restored at a later stage.

If the patient has a perforated carcinoma the overall prognosis is poor. Primary suture is not an option, and healing will not occur with lavage and drainage. A palliative emergency oesophagectomy can be considered if the patient is well enough but, rather than performing heroic surgery, it may be better to adopt a cautious approach and insert an endo-oesophageal prosthesis.

ABDOMINAL OESOPHAGEAL PERFORATIONS

These are almost exclusively iatrogenic, and in most cases there is a high index of suspicion at the time of injury. In addition to endoscopic instrumentation, perforation of the abdominal oesophagus may occur in association with upper gastrointestinal procedures such as a Nissen fundoplication, cardiomyotomy and, occasionally, splenectomy. When it is noted intraoperatively, it can be repaired immediately. This may sometimes require conversion from a laparoscopic to an open procedure. Abdominal perforations which present postoperatively usually require an upper midline laparotomy incision for peritoneal toilet and oesophageal repair. The repair can then be inspected with the endoscope and an insufflation test performed. As the oesophageal wall may be friable it is important, if possible, to buttress the repair with the fundus of the stomach, or with the omentum.

CONSERVATIVE MANAGEMENT

Prompt surgery generally carries a lower mortality than conservative management. However, there is occasionally a place for conservative treatment. It is only likely to be successful when leakage and contamination are minimal. Thus, it may be the appropriate management of a partial mucosal tear in the cervical oesophagus if it is identified early. Conservative management is also often the best course of action in patients who present late with radiological confirmation of a thoracic perforation, but with no clinical manifestations of severe sepsis. It may also be the better option in selected patients with an underlying malignancy who are critically ill. Conservative management consists of broad-spectrum antibiotics and parenteral nutrition. Such patients are closely monitored as they may require chest drain insertion for drainage of pleural effusions, or image-guided drainage of mediastinal collections.

Caustic oesophageal injury

Management depends on the severity of the caustic burn. Initially, treatment is supportive with analgesia, antibiotics and rehydration. Enteral feeding can be maintained if it is possible to establish a nasojejunal feeding tube; otherwise parenteral feeding should be started. A partial-thickness burn of the oesophagus will heal, but stricture formation may ultimately be so severe that an oesophagectomy, and reconstruction with an oesophageal conduit, becomes inevitable. In more severe full-thickness damage to the oesophagus the situation may be better managed by an early cervical oesophagostomy, and a feeding jejunostomy. The severely damaged oesophagus may be safer left *in situ* until a delayed reconstruction is performed, often by an extra-anatomical route. In the most severe cases there may be oesophageal and gastric necrosis, with oesophageal perforation and mediastinitis. This makes an emergency oesophagogastrectomy the only option. A late reconstruction with a colonic conduit can then be undertaken if the patient survives.

MOTILITY DISORDERS OF THE OESOPHAGUS

In recent years many advances have been made in the understanding of the pathophysiology of oesophageal motility disorders. This, in addition to minimally invasive laparoscopic and thorascopic techniques, has contributed to significant improvements in diagnosis and treatment. The more commonly encountered oesophageal motility disorders include achalasia, diffuse oesophageal spasm, and nutcracker oesophagus.[1] A variety of other non-specific oesophageal motility disorders are also recognized, but surgery is seldom helpful.

Achalasia

Achalasia is characterized by loss of peristalsis, typically affecting the distal two-thirds of the oesophagus in conjunction with failure of the lower oesophageal sphincter to relax in response to swallowing.

PRESENTATION AND DIAGNOSIS

Patients complain of progressive dysphagia, retrosternal chest discomfort and regurgitation of food. In many cases there is a delay in diagnosis, with symptoms being attributed to cardiac or respiratory pathologies. Often there is a response to nitroglycerine, which reduces the lower oesophageal sphincter pressure by its action as a smooth muscle relaxant, but unfortunately this symptomatic improvement is often attributed to anti-anginal effects leading to further delays in diagnosis. With time, patients may develop proximal oesophageal dilatation with retention of large amounts of food residue. Delays in diagnosis increase the risk of complications such as the development of oesophageal diverticulae, respiratory symptoms from aspiration, and squamous cell carcinoma secondary to chronic inflammation.

All patients in whom achalasia is suspected require extensive evaluation including chest X-ray, barium swallow, upper endoscopy and manometry studies. Endoscopy is an important investigation to exclude 'pseudoachalasia'. This term is used to describe an appearance on barium swallow typical of achalasia despite an underlying pathology such as an oesophageal malignancy or a benign peptic stricture. Manometry is the 'gold standard' in the diagnosis of achalasia. In the typical case it will identify a raised lower oesophageal sphincter pressure (>25 mmHg) with loss of peristalsis in the body of the oesophagus.

MANAGEMENT

Treatment options available include pharmacological measures, balloon dilatation and surgery. The mainstay of pharmacological therapy includes long-acting nitrates and calcium channel antagonists. Botulinum toxin injected under direct vision into the lower oesophageal sphincter will also decrease sphincter pressure, with over 90 per cent of patients obtaining symptomatic relief. Although the high pressures will return as the pharmacological effect of the injection wears off, this approach can be used as a diagnostic test in those patients for whom the diagnosis is uncertain.

Pneumatic dilatation

This is commonly used to disrupt the lower oesophageal sphincter, and in most centres has replaced the use of progressive dilators. A balloon is placed across the gastro-esophageal junction under fluoroscopic guidance and inflated to its maximum diameter. Given the risk of oesophageal perforation, all patients should have water-soluble contrast studies within 24 hours. Approximately 70 per cent of patients obtain symptomatic relief, but they may require a further procedure within three to five years. Pneumatic dilation is a viable option in the initial treatment of achalasia and is useful in elderly patients, and for those who are high-risk candidates for surgical intervention. As a myotomy is technically more difficult following pneumatic dilation, it is prudent to avoid a dilation as first-line treatment in younger patients who are suitable for surgery, particularly as surgery has better long-term results.

Heller's cardiomyotomy

The transient response to pneumatic dilation and pharmacological therapies gives surgery a prominent role in the long-term management of achalasia. This role has increased with the development of minimally invasive approaches to the surgery. Both the surgeon and the patient should be aware that the dissection may be more difficult when there have been previous dilatations causing fibrosis. The operation is described in Chapter 16. For a classical achalasia, surgery is usually performed using a laparoscopic approach. Due to the increased incidence of reflux symptoms, some surgeons routinely add an anti-reflux procedure to the initial myotomy.

The occasional patient with achalasia who fails to respond to myotomy, or who presents very late with a significantly dilated and tortuous oesophagus, may require an oesophagectomy.

Diffuse oesophageal spasm

This condition is characterized by uncoordinated oesophageal contractions, with several oesophageal segments contracting simultaneously and preventing the normal propagation of food. The diagnosis is established by manometry and the typical barium swallow finding of a corkscrew oesophagus secondary to segmental contractions. Mid-oesophageal diverticulae may be present.

Confirmation of the diagnosis, in conjunction with patient reassurance, may help to alleviate the symptoms, especially as there is often a coexistent psychological disorder. Pharmacological therapies again include the use of calcium channel antagonists and long-acting nitrates.

Operative intervention may be considered for patients with persistent dysphagia who have not obtained any symptomatic relief with pharmacological therapies, and whose quality of life is greatly impaired. Surgery consists of a long oesophageal myotomy extending to the level of the aortic arch, with manometry acting as a guide to the extent of myotomy required. This may be carried out via thoracotomy or thoracoscopy, and most surgeons also perform an anti-reflux procedure. It has been associated with a success rate of up to 80 per cent in the short term, but long-term results of surgery are more disappointing.

Nutcracker oesophagus

Nutcracker oesophagus is characterized by high-amplitude peristaltic contractions, which may be localized to the distal oesophagus or may affect the entire oesophagus. Pressures are found to exceed 180 mmHg, in contrast to pressures of approximately 90 mmHg for the general population. There may be associated gastro-oesophageal reflux disease. Only limited success has been observed with pharmacological therapies. Bougie and pneumatic dilatation have been reported to relieve the chest pain and dysphagia, but the benefits are often attributed to a placebo effect. Information on the benefits of oesophageal myotomy is limited.

GASTRO–OESOPHAGEAL REFLUX DISEASE

Patients whose symptoms have been confirmed to be secondary to reflux disease generally achieve a good outcome with anti-reflux surgery, thereby avoiding further need for acid-suppressing medication. Although anti-reflux surgery is undertaken mainly for the relief of the symptoms, it also prevents the long-term complications associated with reflux disease such as haemorrhage and strictures which can occur secondary to oesophagitis. Surgery may potentially reduce the progression of Barrett's oesophagus.

Patient selection

The ideal candidate for an anti-reflux procedure is a patient with reflux disease who has obtained symptomatic relief from proton-pump inhibitors or H_2-receptor antagonists, is not overweight, has no psychological disorders, and who wishes to avoid life-long medication. The operation is generally associated with a successful outcome, gives long-term symptomatic control and, as it can be carried out laparoscopically, it provides an attractive alternative to medical management. However, with the dramatic increase in referrals for anti-reflux surgery, it is important that indications for intervention are well-defined and that the operations are carried out by surgeons in institutions experienced in the procedure and who have the ability to deal with any operative complications.

Before embarking on operative intervention, patients should undergo a number of clinical and radiological tests to confirm the diagnosis of reflux disease and to identify any independent motility disorder. These tests allow the surgeon to decide on the appropriate intervention, and they also provide information on anatomical anomalies such as oesophageal diverticulae, shortened oesophagus and para-oesophageal hernia that will be deleterious to outcome if not discovered preoperatively and surgery planned appropriately. Investigations are particularly pertinent for patients with atypical symptoms and for those who continue to have significant symptoms despite the use of proton-pump inhibitors.

Typical investigations include:

- *Upper endoscopy*: this is critical as it identifies oesophagitis and other reflux complications such as stricture. Biopsies are taken if there is Barrett's metaplasia or suspected malignancy. It is important during endoscopy to note the presence of a hiatal hernia, as this may influence the choice of surgical approach.
- *24-hour pH monitoring* identifies oesophageal exposure to acid and its correlation with symptoms. It differentiates between supine and upright reflux disease. It is an objective test, and a good indicator of the potential response to surgery. It is particularly useful for confirming the presence of reflux disease in those patients in whom upper endoscopy was negative for oesophagitis. Disadvantages of the test include the need to discontinue proton-pump inhibitors prior to the test, and discomfort from insertion of the pH probe.
- *Manometry* will measure the lower oesophageal sphincter pressure, which in patients with reflux disease is usually reduced consistent with an incompetent lower oesophageal sphincter. It will help identify motility disorders such as achalasia, and may be useful in deciding the type of anti-reflux surgery that would best combat the individual patient's symptoms.
- *Barium swallow* is an important adjunct in the investigation of reflux disease. It provides specific

anatomical information on the presence of hiatal hernia, oesophageal stricture and shortened oesophagus. It will also help in the identification of motility disorders and delayed gastric emptying.

Open versus minimal-access surgery

Laparoscopic anti-reflux surgery is now the 'gold standard' for the surgical management of patients with gastro-oesophageal reflux disease. There is no difference in functional results between the open and laparoscopic approach, but the benefits of a minimal access approach include reduced postoperative pain, avoidance of a laparotomy or thoracotomy scar, early mobilization, and a shorter hospital stay. Patients undergoing a minimal access fundoplication may underestimate the operation, and should be aware of the risk of splenic injury, oesophageal perforation, pulmonary complications, and the occasional necessity to convert to an open procedure. Relative contraindications to the performance of laparoscopic anti-reflux surgery include a previous vagotomy or gastrectomy.

Abdominal versus thoracic approach

This debate has continued from the 'open' era. Most indications for one or other approach, whether by an open or a minimal access technique, are relative rather than absolute, and much depends on the surgeon's preference and experience. Some surgeons favour a transthoracic approach to anti-reflux surgery when reflux disease is complicated by a fixed hiatal hernia, or the patient has had a previously failed repair performed from below. It may also be a better approach in the morbidly obese.

Partial or complete wrap

Partial wraps have a lower incidence of dysphagia and gas bloat than the Nissen total wrap. However, partial wraps may be less effective in eliminating reflux. Trial outcomes have not been consistent and practice varies, but most surgeons favour a total wrap except in specific circumstances.

Elderly patients, and those with reduced oesophageal contraction amplitudes, may fare better with a partial wrap. For those patients in whom manometry identifies a specific coexisting oesophageal dysmotility disorder, a partial wrap, such as provided by the Toupet technique, may give a better outcome. A Dor partial wrap may be considered as an anti-reflux procedure in combination with a Heller's cardiomyotomy, and if it is sutured laterally to the edges of the myotomy it helps to keep the muscle fibres apart.

When a patient has had a complete wrap causing excessive dysphagia, then this may be taken down and converted to a partial fundoplication. Occasionally, a partial wrap is indicated by technical considerations, as when the patient has had previous gastric surgery limiting the fundus available for a wrap.

Surgery for Barrett's oesophagus

In gastrointestinal reflux disease the distal oesophagus may become lined with columnar epithelium as a consequence of the exposure to gastric juices. Intestinal metaplasia within this area is associated with an increased risk of adenocarcinoma of the oesophagus. Patients with the changes of Barrett's ocsophagus form a subgroup of patients with gastro-oesophageal reflux in whom symptom control is not the prime criterion of success. Management is mainly by gastroenterologists. Surveillance and biopsy of the area must be combined with intensive management to reduce the damage from reflux. Regression of these premalignant changes, by profound pharmacological acid suppression with proton-pump inhibitors, can be demonstrated but there is no clear evidence that the addition of anti-reflux surgery improves regression. Endoscopic ablation of dysplastic areas is practised. Unfortunately, high-grade dysplasia may still develop, and in a proportion of patients this finding predicts that early invasive cancer has already developed, though not within the biopsy specimen. Some 50 per cent of patients with Barrett's oesophagus who undergo oesophagectomy for an area of high-grade dysplasia have pathological evidence of invasive cancer in the resected specimen.[2] The risk of postponing intervention until there is unequivocal, but possibly incurable, cancer must be carefully weighed against the risks of major surgery in each patient, but many gastroenterolgists and surgeons believe that the finding of high-grade dysplasia is an indication to abandon surveillance and recommend oesophagectomy in fit patients.

HIATAL AND DIAPHRAGMATIC HERNIAE

Hiatal herniae

A hiatal hernia occurs when the stomach or other intra-abdominal organ herniates through the diaphragmatic oesophageal opening into the chest. They can be divided into sliding and rolling (para-oesophageal) herniae.

SLIDING HIATUS HERNIA (TYPE I)

This is the commonest type, accounting for over 90 per cent of cases (Fig. 17.1a). The cardia and gastro-oesophageal junction undergo cephalad migration through the diaphragm into the posterior mediastinum, but maintain their anatomical relationship. Patients commonly complain of reflux symptoms, which are attributed to functional disruption of the lower oesophageal sphincter. There is no true peritoneal sac, and in the initial stages the oesophageal length is normal. These hernias do not need to be considered for

a

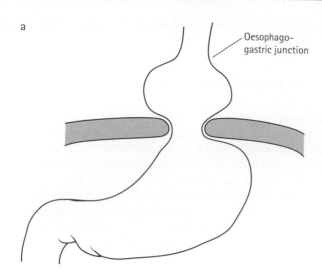

Oesophago-
gastric junction

b

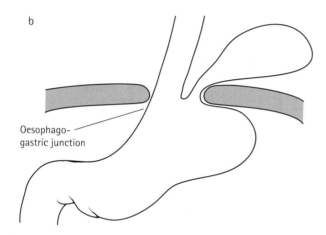

Oesophago-
gastric junction

Figure 17.1   *(a) Sliding hiatus hernia; (b) Rolling hiatus hernia.*

repair unless they are associated with pathological reflux that significantly interferes with the patient's quality of life.

When surgery is indicated, reduction of the hernia is combined with closure of the crural defect and an anti-reflux procedure. This is usually performed laparoscopically. If the hiatal defect is very large, then a synthetic mesh may be inserted giving a tension-free repair (Fig. 17.2). Prior to insertion a hole is cut in the mesh to accommodate the oesophagus. The mesh is then stapled to the diaphragm, taking care to avoid damaging the oesophagus and to avoid piercing the pericardium. Some surgeons strongly recommend an open approach to management of these large defects.

PARA–OESOPHAGEAL (ROLLING) HIATUS HERNIA

These are subdivided into three types.

Simple rolling hiatus hernia (type II)

Here, the gastro-oesophageal junction remains below the diaphragm, despite the gastric fundus rolling along the oesophagus (Fig. 17.1b). The gastro-oesophageal junction

remains tethered to the diaphragm by an intact phreno-oesophageal ligament and, again, oesophageal length is maintained. This type is found predominantly in the elderly. Iatrogenic para-oesophageal herniation is seen with increased frequency as a complication following anti-reflux surgery.

Mixed para–oesophageal hernia (type III)

This consists of a combination of type I and type II, in which both the fundus and the cardia migrate above the diaphragm.

Large para–oesophageal hernia (type IV)

In this case the spleen, colon, small bowel, stomach or other intra-abdominal organ herniate into the mediastinum through the hiatal defect. This type carries a significant risk of strangulation.

Most para-oesophageal herniae are asymptomatic and the diagnosis is often as a result of an upright chest X-ray which demonstrates an air–fluid level. However, they may present with gastrointestinal symptoms including dysphagia, regurgitation or chest pain. Bleeding from ulcerated gastric mucosa may result in a haematemesis or an iron-deficiency anaemia. Fatalities, secondary to gastric strangulation and perforation, have been well-described. Most surgeons would advocate repair in healthy patients, given the inherent risk of strangulation and gastric volvulus. Prior to the advent of minimally invasive techniques there was reluctance to advise surgery, especially in asymptomatic elderly patients. However, the long-term benefits of repair would now appear to outweigh the operative risks in most patients.

Preoperative investigations should include endoscopy to identify any underlying sinister pathology. It is also important to discover prior to intervention if there is a shortened oesophagus or motility disorder that will influence the type of repair. For example, patients with a shortened oesophagus may require the addition of a Collis gastroplasty to provide an adequate segment of intra-abdominal oesophagus. CT scans and barium studies are particularly valuable in type IV hernias to determine the type of hernia, and to show which abdominal organs have migrated into the hernial sac.

Traditionally, surgeons reduced the herniated contents and then performed a primary closure of the crural defect. However, a significant number of patients went on to develop reflux symptoms that greatly interfered with their quality of life. This may be related to the excessive dissection required to reduce the herniated contents with disturbance of the functional effect of the lower oesophageal sphincter. Thus, an anti-reflux procedure has since been added to the repair of most para-oesophageal herniae. The hiatal defect may be very large, and the crural fibres thinned, such that adequate closure of the defect will require a mesh to provide a tension-free repair.

Laparoscopic repair is now the preferred option in many centres. If the patient presents as an emergency, a minimal access approach can sometimes still be considered, depending on surgical experience and facilities, but there must be a low threshold for converting to an open technique.

LAPAROSCOPIC REPAIR OF A PARA-OESOPHAGEAL HERNIA

The position of the patient, and the placement of the ports, is similar to that described for a laparoscopic Heller's myotomy (see Chapter 16). The stomach, and any other herniated contents of the sac, are gently reduced using Babcock forceps inserted through the left lateral ports. Long-standing adhesions may have to be divided before this can be achieved. The gastrohepatic ligament is then divided, allowing visualization of the right crural fibres.

The hernia sac is dissected with care off the right crus and the mediastinal structures. This carries the risk of pleural damage with the formation of a tension pneumothorax. If this occurs, then the anaesthetist will develop difficulties ventilating the patient, who may become hypotensive. The pneumoperitoneum is released immediately, which should provide instant resolution. If not, then needle decompression of the affected pleural space followed by chest drain insertion will be required. Finally, the sac is dissected off the left crus and this is often difficult. Once the sac is freed and returned intra-abdominally, it is excised.

The next step is closure of the widened hiatus. The edges of the hiatal defect and posterior oesophageal window are identified. The right and left crural fibres must be adequately visualized, and this is greatly helped by elevation of the oesophagus anteriorly, using a Penrose drain if necessary. The posterior vagus nerve is elevated with the oesophagus. The upper short gastric vessels are divided to create sufficient mobility of the fundus to perform a Nissen fundoplication. The crura are approximated behind the oesophagus using 2/0 non-absorbable sutures (see Fig. 16.8b, page 265). Starting inferiorly, generous bites are taken and care must be exercised to avoid the underlying aorta. Very rarely, some sutures have to be inserted anterior to the oesophagus. Many surgeons favour the use of endo-suturing devices for crural approximation.

For very large defects (>10 cm in diameter), the cruroplasty is often inadequate and a mesh may have to be inserted (Fig. 17.2a). Once the mesh has been cut to size, a 3-cm circular defect with a radial slit is created to accommodate the oesophagus. The mesh is attached to the under-surface of the diaphragm using a stapling device, and care must be taken not to perforate the pericardium. As with any mesh insertion, the patient should receive prophylactic antibiotic cover. A Nissen fundoplication is then created (Fig. 17.2b). This is described in more detail in Chapter 16. When completed, the subdiaphragmatic surfaces are irrigated using 10 mL of 0.5 per cent bupivacaine in 500 mL of 0.9 per cent normal saline. This reduces the incidence of postoperative shoulder tip pain secondary to diaphragmatic irritation. The pneumoperitoneum is then released and port sites closed. If there is any question of damage to the pleura, then the patient should have a chest X-ray on the operating table to rule out a pneumothorax.

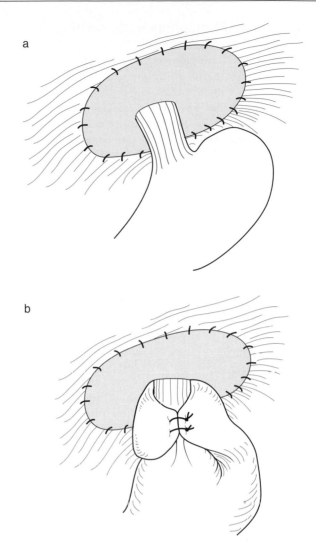

Figure 17.2 *Repair of a large para-oesophageal hernia. (a) A mesh can be used to close a large defect. (b) After the hiatal patch is in place, the repair is completed with a wrap to prevent gastro-oesophageal reflux.*

Patients are normally allowed oral fluids that evening, and a light diet on the next day. It is a procedure that is generally well-tolerated, even in elderly patients with a degree of co-morbidity.

The short-term results for the laparoscopic management of para-oesophageal hernias are encouraging. However, the open approach, using similar principles of dissection to those described above, enables a larger 'bite' to be taken of the diaphragm using stronger non-absorbable material. If necessary, a relaxing incision on the lateral diaphragm may be made to facilitate closure of the crura. Long-term results from open surgery for large para-oesophageal herniae still appear superior to the minimally invasive approach, but the increased morbidity of open surgery must be considered.

Congenital adult diaphragmatic hernia

The diaphragm is a musculotendinous structure which separates the thoracic cavity from the abdominal cavity. The pleuroperitoneal membranes close the communication between the pleural and peritoneal cavities at approximately the eighth embryonic week. Incomplete closure of the pleuroperitoneal canal, a phenomenon more common on the left side, gives rise to a posterolateral defect first described by Bochdalek in 1848. Usually, there is no hernial sac and the defect may be as small as 1 cm, but it may involve the entire hemidiaphragm (agenesis). Babies born with large defects usually present neonatally, and their management is discussed in Chapter 12. In contrast, a hernia of Morgagni is more common on the right side. It possesses a hernia sac and occurs through a parasternal defect at the site where the superior epigastric artery leaves the chest and enters the abdomen.

Presentation of Bochdalek and Morgagni hernias in adulthood is quite rare. Most are asymptomatic and only diagnosed when a routine chest X-ray demonstrates bowel within the chest. Some patients have non-specific symptoms, while others present as an emergency with obstruction, or strangulation, of the intrathoracic bowel or stomach. A CT scan is the investigation of choice to confirm the diagnosis, and it provides anatomical information on both the herniated organs and the site of the defect. Barium studies are also useful. Most surgeons would advocate repair, even in asymptomatic individuals, because of the danger of strangulation.

Traditionally, congenital diaphragmatic herniae have been repaired via a laparotomy or thoracotomy. The advent of minimally invasive surgery has facilitated the laparoscopic repair of diaphragmatic defects, but there should be a low threshold for conversion to an open procedure. The major danger associated with the laparoscopic repair of chronic diaphragmatic defects is damage to the lung, mediastinum or the herniated abdominal organs, which may include stomach, large bowel, greater omentum, spleen or liver. Dense adhesions are common and have to be divided prior to the reduction of the herniated tissue. Ultrasonic dissection, with coagulation shears, is useful for this. A small diaphragmatic defect can be closed by laparoscopic suturing, but a polypropylene mesh may be required to bridge a larger defect. The mesh is secured with staples. Thereafter, the greater omentum is placed over the mesh, preventing contact with intra-abdominal organs. It is advisable to insert a chest drain into the pleural cavity above the diaphragmatic defect until the lung has fully re-expanded.

Traumatic diaphragmatic hernia

The surgical management of this condition is discussed in the trauma section of Chapter 7.

GASTRIC VOLVULUS

Gastric volvulus is an abnormal rotation of the stomach that can cause a closed loop obstruction. It is usually associated with underlying pathology such as a para-oesophageal or diaphragmatic hernia. Patients may present with chronic non-specific symptoms including vomiting and postprandial epigastric pain. Once diagnosed, most surgeons would recommend repair, given the potential for catastrophe. A proportion of patients will present with severe pain and retching, without the ability to vomit. The inability to pass a nasogastric tube beyond the distal oesophagus completes *Borchardt's triad*. This is a closed loop obstruction which causes progressive gastric distension, and represents a surgical emergency as the blood supply to the stomach may be rapidly compromised. There are two types of gastric volvulus defined by their axis of rotation: organo-axial and mesentero-axial.

- An *organo-axial* volvulus occurs around a line between the pylorus and the gastro-oesophageal junction and is more common in elderly people (Fig. 17.3a). Occasionally, there is a gastric tumour at the apex of the rotation.
- A *mesentero-axial* rotation occurs in a plane running from the porta hepatis to the greater curvature of the stomach, and has a higher incidence in children (Fig. 17.3b). Very rarely, a combined form is encountered.

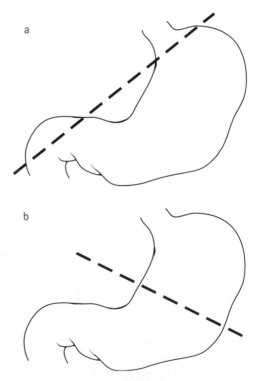

Figure 17.3 *Gastric volvulus. (a) Organo-axial rotation on an axis between the pylorus and the gastro-oesophageal junction. (b) Mesentero-axial rotation occurring on an axis from the porta hepatis to the greater curvature of the stomach.*

When a patient presents acutely with suspected gastric volvulus, an attempt should be made to pass a nasogastric tube. This may decompress the stomach and allow a subsequent elective procedure. If nasogastric deflation fails, endoscopic decompression may be successful but carries a risk of gastric perforation. If decompression is not achieved, an emergency laparotomy is essential to reduce the volvulus. If the stomach is viable, and there is no evidence of coexisting pathology, a simple gastropexy in which the anterior stomach wall is sutured to the anterior abdominal wall should suffice. If there are adhesive bands these are divided, and any associated diaphragmatic defect is repaired. In the presence of gastric necrosis or perforation, a subtotal or total gastrectomy may be unavoidable.

There are several other methods of fixing the stomach to prevent recurrent volvulus. It can be fixed to the anterior abdominal wall by a gastrostomy, or its mobility restricted by a gastrojejunostomy. In the elective setting a percutaneous endoscopic gastrostomy (PEG) tube is another method of fixation which may be the most suitable for high-risk patients.

PEPTIC ULCER DISEASE AND ASSOCIATED COMPLICATIONS

Historical perspective

Elective operations for peptic ulcer were among the commonest procedures performed by the general surgeon in the middle decades of the last century. The original operations of Billroth I gastrectomy, and gastroenterostomy alone, were replaced by the Polya gastrectomy, and later, to a greater extent, by vagotomy and drainage procedures. Gastroenterostomy and the Polya gastrectomy diverted gastric acid from the ulcer, but in general the main surgical objective was to reduce acid secretion. A partial gastrectomy reduced acid both by the removal of a portion of the parietal cell mass and by the excision of the gastrin-producing antrum, thus reducing stimulation of the remaining parietal cells. Vagotomy abolished vagal stimulation of the parietal cell mass. A vagotomy with antrectomy was probably the most effective operation, but it was associated with the side effects of both a truncal vagotomy and a partial, albeit limited, gastrectomy. Debate regarding the best operation for peptic ulceration focused on the balance between the incidence of recurrent ulceration, and the incidence and severity of side effects.

The whole situation changed with pharmacological advances. As the operations were designed to reduce the acid secretion of the stomach, their role became increasingly unimportant as more potent antisecretory drugs became available. Initially, there was concern regarding any long-term side effects of the new drugs, and for some years surgery was still advised for younger, fitter patients to avoid a lifetime of medication. The identification of *Helicobacter pylori* as a causative agent, combined with effective regimes for its eradication, further changed surgical practice. The majority of patients could be cured and did not require long-term acid suppression. The elective management of peptic ulcer disease is now almost exclusively medical. H_2 receptor antagonists, or proton-pump inhibitors, are used to block acid secretion, and *Helicobacter* is eradicated with antibiotics.

Surgery is now mainly confined to the management of the complications of peptic ulcer disease including perforation, haemorrhage and gastric outlet obstruction. Despite decreasing incidence, peptic ulcer perforation and haemorrhage are still major causes of morbidity and mortality. Surgery is also occasionally indicated for ulceration refractory to medical treatment, and for the complications of previous peptic ulcer surgery. The latter are discussed in the section on late complications of upper gastrointestinal surgery at the end of this chapter.

Refractory ulcers

With modern drugs, patients with refractory ulcers form a very small subgroup of those with peptic ulceration. This subgroup have ulcers that are also less likely to be cured by many of the standard operations that were effective for the majority of an unselected group of patients. This was first recognized in the 1980s, but with advances in pharmacology this must be an even more important consideration today.[3] An underlying pathology must be sought, and malignancy must always be considered, especially in gastric ulcers.

It is likely that if surgery has to be considered in patients with resistant duodenal ulcers, resection of the gastrin-producing mucosa of the antrum should be combined with either denervation of the parietal cell mass, or the excision of a major part of it. A subtotal gastrectomy is one possibility, but is associated with significant long-term morbidity. A truncal or selective vagotomy, combined with antrectomy, is probably the preferred option. Reconstruction can be either with a gastroduodenal (Billroth I) anastomosis, or with a gastrojejunostomy, either as a Billroth II anastomosis or as a Roux loop. A refractory gastric ulcer usually warrants a gastrectomy which will also excise the ulcer.

Zollinger–Ellison syndrome, in which a gastrin-secreting tumour is stimulating gastric hypersecretion, should be remembered. When these tumours are solitary, are located within the pancreas and have not metastasized, resection of the tumour can be curative. In many patients this is not the case, and management is by controlling acid hypersecretion. Before effective acid-suppressing drugs were available, a total gastrectomy was often necessary. However, with the emergence of H_2 receptor antagonists, a combination of these drugs with a parietal cell vagotomy was preferred. Nowadays, proton-pump inhibitors may be sufficient to control hypersecretion, without the necessity for surgery at all.

Gastric outlet obstruction

Chronic peptic ulcer disease can give rise to gastric outlet obstruction. The persistent inflammation causes intense fibrosis and scarring with subsequent channel narrowing. This presentation of chronic peptic ulcer disease is now less common in the Western world. In contrast, in the acute setting the obstruction may be secondary to oedema and inflammation associated with the ulcer, in which case symptoms tend to settle within a few days of conservative management.

The initial management of gastric outlet obstruction consists of the insertion of a wide-bore nasogastric tube, and the correction of fluid and electrolyte imbalance. Intravenous proton-pump inhibitor therapy is commenced. The diagnosis is established by barium meal or upper gastrointestinal endoscopy. A barium meal may identify a dilated, atonic stomach with an absent or narrowed pyloric channel, and it may take several hours for the stomach to empty of barium. Occasionally, an hourglass deformity of the stomach, secondary to a fibrous stricture from gastric ulcer disease, is demonstrated. On endoscopy the stomach may be dilated and visualization limited by undigested food. However, endoscopy has the advantage of enabling the mucosa at the site of the stricture to be inspected, and biopsies to be taken if there is a suspected malignancy. Malignant gastric outlet obstruction is considered later.

If the patient with active peptic ulcer disease fails to respond to conservative management, most surgeons would perform definitive surgery on the primary admission. Surgical options depend on intraoperative findings. The pylorus is usually too oedematous, or scarred, for a pyloroplasty to be an option. A gastroenterostomy is the simplest drainage option but, when carried out for active peptic ulcer disease, should be combined with a vagotomy. The avoidance of a full truncal vagotomy may reduce the incidence of post-vagotomy diarrhoea. If a resection is chosen, an antrectomy with vagotomy may be possible if the duodenal bulb is not too severely deformed. If the duodenum is considered unsafe for an anastomosis, then a Polya reconstruction or a Roux-en-Y loop may be indicated (see Chapter 16).

The decision is slightly different in the unfit elderly patient, with a fibrous stricture from previous ulceration but no active ulcer disease. It was for this latter group, who are decreasingly encountered in Western practice, that Eric Farquharson defended the old operation of gastroenterostomy alone.

Penetrating and giant ulcers

Giant peptic ulcers of the stomach, or duodenum, which penetrate the pancreas or liver, or fistulate into the transverse colon or other adjacent viscera, are now fortunately rare in the UK. They may however be encountered more frequently in other parts of the world. The surgery for these ulcers must usually involve a gastrectomy with a Polya, or Roux loop, reconstruction. As there will be no residual mucosa in the base of a gastric ulcer which has penetrated the liver or pancreas, it is simply circumcised and left *in situ* as the stomach is mobilized for the gastrectomy. A giant posterior penetrating duodenal ulcer usually precludes closure of the duodenal stump, and over-enthusiastic attempts may result in injury to the common bile duct. If closure involves any excess tension on the stump, or the tissue is unable to hold sutures adequately, then it may be better to create a controlled duodenal fistula. This is done by inserting a Foley catheter into the stump, and anchoring it with a purse-string suture (Fig. 17.4a). The area is then buttressed using greater omentum. Alternatively, a lateral duodenostomy tube can be inserted (Fig. 17.4b), or even a large-bore tube simply secured in the vicinity of the open duodenal stump. Once the catheter or T-tube has been removed the duodenal fistula should close spontaneously if there is no afferent limb obstruction.

When there is a fistula into the transverse colon, the colonic wall defect is often small and may be amenable to primary closure. Occasionally, a more extensive resection or a defunctioning stoma may be required (see Chapters 21 and 22).

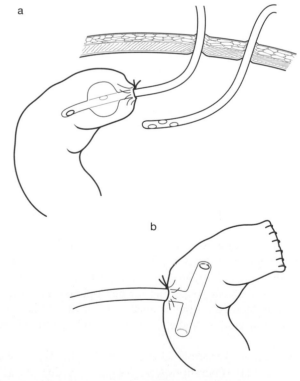

Figure 17.4 *Solutions for the difficult duodenal stump. A controlled fistula onto the skin surface can be created with: (a) a Foley catheter inserted into the duodenum or even with a drain left adjacent to an open duodenal stump; (b) a lateral duodenotomy using a T-tube.*

Emergency peptic ulcer surgery

Most operations nowadays for peptic ulcer are performed for acute complications. The surgeon must decide at the time of the emergency surgery whether any definitive acid-reducing procedure should be carried out at the same time. The debate regarding the correct policy in an emergency scenario has continued for over half a century. Even before medical treatment was so effective, it was recognized that many patients who presented with a perforation, or haemorrhage, did not require further medical or surgical treatment for chronic peptic ulcer disease. In these patients acid-reducing surgery was unnecessary; it exposed the patients to the long-term complications of the surgery, and it also prolonged an otherwise simple operation at a time when the patient might be septic, or haemodynamically unstable.

However, in other patients a definitive procedure simplified their subsequent management and avoided a later elective operation. With improvements in medical management, such that very few patients come to elective surgery for peptic ulcer disease, the argument for definitive surgery at the time of an emergency intervention has been weakened, but there may still be a case for it if the patient has developed a complication while receiving treatment, or has had a previous perforation or bleed. However, it should certainly only be considered if a patient's general condition is stable and the surgeon undertaking the procedure is experienced.

Sometimes a surgeon is forced into a more major procedure by the conditions encountered at the emergency laparotomy. For example, a large ulcer in a grossly scarred or stenosed pylorus may be causing an outflow obstruction in addition to a perforation. A gastroenterostomy becomes necessary for gastric drainage, and should not be performed in active peptic ulcer disease without a vagotomy, otherwise there is a significant risk of stomal ulceration. Giant duodenal ulcers which have perforated, are actively bleeding, or both, can sometimes only be managed by gastrectomy.

PERFORATED PEPTIC ULCER

The classical presentation of a perforated peptic ulcer involves sudden onset of epigastric pain. An erect chest X-ray will reveal free air in approximately 65 per cent of cases. Often, although a perforated ulcer is suspected, only a preoperative diagnosis of a perforated viscus, or generalized peritonitis, is possible. After resuscitation and elimination of non-surgical pathology, an emergency laparotomy is planned as discussed in Chapter 14. Turbid, bile-stained fluid confirms an upper, rather than a lower, gastrointestinal perforation.

In most cases the perforation is easily recognized. The anterior aspect of the first part of the duodenum and distal stomach are inspected first. A retractor is carefully inserted under the liver, and the stomach is drawn down, grasping it with a moist pack (Fig. 17.5a). Overlying omentum is peeled away. If no perforation becomes apparent, the remainder of the anterior aspect of the stomach and duodenum are inspected. On rare occasions a posterior ulcer has perforated into the lesser sac.

Duodenal perforation

Simple closure is usually the quickest and most appropriate method of dealing with a perforated duodenal ulcer. Closure is achieved by the insertion of three or four interrupted, absorbable, gauge 0 sutures. Generous bites, which pass through the entire thickness of the gut wall, should be taken. Care must be taken to ensure that they do not catch the posterior wall. Sutures should be inserted in the long axis of the gut to avoid narrowing (Fig. 17.5b). The closure may then be reinforced with an omental on-lay patch, a 'modified Graham patch' (Fig. 17.5c). If the ulcer is large and inflamed, the sutures tend to 'cheese-wire' through the tissues, and it is better not to attempt to draw the edges together. Instead, the defect is closed using an omental patch alone – a 'true Graham patch'.

In haemodynamically stable patients with a perforated

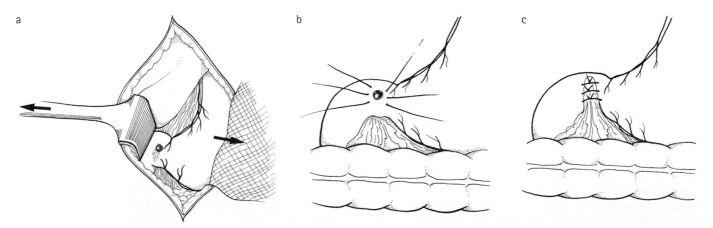

Figure 17.5 *Perforated duodenal ulcer. (a) Good retraction facilitates access to the duodenum and the identification of the perforation site. (b) Sutures in place for a primary closure of the perforation. (c) This can be reinforced with an omental patch using the same sutures.*

duodenal, pyloric or pre-pyloric ulcer the surgeon may decide on the criteria discussed above to proceed to a definitive acid-reducing procedure to lower the subsequent incidence of peptic ulcer complications. A truncal vagotomy and drainage procedure is usually the most appropriate. The choice between pyloroplasty and gastroenterostomy is dictated by the conditions prevailing in the pyloroduodenal area. Where possible, a perforation is incorporated in a pyloroplasty, but significant stenosis may mean that simple closure of the perforation and a gastroenterostomy is preferable.

Occasionally, the entire duodenal wall is eroded and it may be necessary to proceed to a Billroth II gastrectomy. In these circumstances closure of the duodenal stump is unlikely to be possible but a controlled duodenal fistula can be created by tube drainage (see Fig. 17.4).

Gastric perforation

Perforated gastric ulcers may be malignant and thus the ulcer is excised, or sufficient biopsies are taken prior to primary closure of the perforation. The closure is again reinforced using an omental patch. Occasionally, if the ulcer is very large, a gastrectomy may be required. A perforated, overtly malignant, gastric ulcer can pose difficult intraoperative decisions, especially if a gastrectomy cannot be performed through tumour-free planes. Any surgery, even for a small malignant ulcer which has perforated, is almost certainly palliative because of the contamination of the peritoneal cavity with malignant cells.

It is important to ensure thorough peritoneal toilet after the closure of any gastrointestinal perforation in order to reduce wound infections and intra-abdominal abscess formation. However, in recent years the concept of copious irrigation has been challenged. The concern is the noxious effect of irrigation fluid on neutrophils and peritoneal mesothelial cells which play a central role in the immune response to peritoneal infection.

Laparoscopic repair of a perforated peptic ulcer

This is becoming more popular in the patient who is haemodynamically stable and has no overt evidence of sepsis. The surgeon must be proficient with intracorporeal knot tying, although the development of fibrin glue and laparoscopic staplers may reduce the need for laparoscopic suturing. The camera is inserted through the umbilical port to establish the diagnosis. Three additional working ports are then inserted. The fibrin seal between the under-surface of the liver, gallbladder and the perforated ulcer is gently divided to expose the ulcer, with care being taken not to enlarge the existing perforation. The principles are similar to that for an open technique. The falciform ligament can be sutured over the ulcer as an alternative to the Graham patch. This repair is simpler to perform than a laparoscopic omental patch repair.[4] If there is a naturally occurring omental plug, peritoneal toilet alone may be sufficient. The laparoscopic approach allows better access and vision for peritoneal lavage, particularly in the subphrenic and pelvic spaces.

A definitive acid-reducing procedure is also possible when a perforation is treated laparoscopically, but feasibility is not the paramount consideration: there must be a sound indication for proceeding. It should only be considered by an experienced surgeon on a stable patient.

Postoperatively, as soon as it is possible patients should be commenced on triple therapy for *Helicobacter pylori* eradication. If the patient fails to settle postoperatively, the possibility of an intra-abdominal abscess must be considered. In most cases, when identified on ultrasound or CT scan, an abscess may be drained percutaneously under radiological guidance. The possibility that the patient has a persistent duodenal leak should be considered. This can be confirmed, or excluded, with water-soluble contrast studies.

Conservative management of perforated peptic ulcer

This may be considered for patients with a delayed presentation (i.e. greater than 24 hours) and extensive co-morbid factors. In patients who are haemodynamically stable with minimal abdominal symptoms, the ulcer may already be sealed by the greater omentum or adjacent organs. A non-operative approach involving adequate rehydration, nasogastric tube aspiration, broad-spectrum antibiotics, thromboembolic prophylaxis and acid suppression, has been shown to be effective in a selected group of patients. Patients are monitored closely, and any deterioration in clinical status will be an indication for operative intervention. The patient is susceptible to the development of subhepatic or subphrenic abscesses but, in the absence of generalized peritonitis, these can be managed by image-guided percutaneous drainage. Conservative management is unlikely to be successful for perforated gastric ulcers.

Peptic ulcer haemorrhage

Peptic ulcer disease, presenting as haematemesis and melaena, is a common cause of upper gastrointestinal tract bleeding. The three cardinal principles in the management are:

1. Vigorous resuscitation of the initial bleed to restore haemodynamic stability, followed by monitoring for re-bleeding and appropriate resuscitation if this should occur.
2. Prompt investigation to establish the cause.
3. Institution of appropriate measures to arrest bleeding and prevent further haemorrhage.

Gastroscopy has long been the diagnostic procedure of choice but now, increasingly, this has also become a therapeutic option. Depending on expertise and available resources, endoscopic treatment options include injection of the bleeding ulcer with adrenaline or sclerosant, laser photocoagulation or coagulation with bipolar diathermy. Surgery must always be considered when bleeding persists, or recurs despite endoscopic intervention. Although repeat endoscopic intervention may be successful, the mortality from salvage surgery, if it becomes necessary, increases with delay. The old lessons on the dangers of procrastination must not be forgotten. A large vessel, visible in the ulcer base, a major initial bleed, a re-bleed in hospital and advanced age are all factors which should encourage surgical intervention.

Operative procedure

Upper gastrointestinal endoscopy, except in hospitals where it is unavailable, is imperative prior to operative intervention to identify the site of haemorrhage, as this will direct surgical access towards the bleeding site. Very occasionally, the bleeding is so torrential that the patient must be taken directly to the operating theatre. In this situation, endoscopy can be performed in theatre after induction, but may be unhelpful if major haemorrhage is obscuring the view. A midline laparotomy, with division of the falciform ligament to allow upward retraction of the liver, should give good access.

Duodenal ulcer: If the bleeding is from a duodenal ulcer, two stay sutures are inserted either side of the pylorus using the prepyloric vein of Mayo as a guide. A longitudinal pyloroduodenotomy is made, and direct finger pressure on the bleeding site will control the haemorrhage, allowing the anaesthetist to resuscitate and stabilize the patient. If the bleeding site is not obvious, then careful inspection and palpation may identify an area of induration, which represents a thrombosed vessel. Careful lavage and gentle suction will help to dislodge clots which overlie the bleeding vessel. With a bleeding gastroduodenal artery, non-absorbable sutures should be inserted to gain control. A suture is placed proximally and distally on the gastroduodenal artery, and a third suture is inserted to control the transverse pancreatic branch of the gastroduodenal artery, which may be a cause of secondary haemorrhage if not identified and ligated (Fig. 17.6). The placement of sutures too deeply should be avoided due

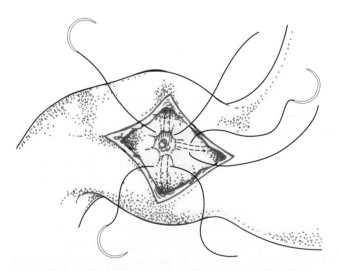

Figure 17.6 *Suture ligation of a bleeding gastroduodenal artery. The sutures must incorporate the artery proximal and distal to the site of the bleeding ulcer, and must also control its transverse pancreatic branch.*

to the risk of incorporating the pancreatic or common bile duct. Interrupted sutures are then used to close the pyloroduodenotomy incision transversely, to prevent narrowing of the pyloric channel. Thereafter, a definitive anti-secretory procedure to reduce the potential for re-bleeding and further peptic ulcer complications can be considered. The decision depends on a number of factors, and was discussed above. The options available include truncal, selective, or highly selective vagotomy (see Chapter 16).

Postoperatively, patients must be monitored closely due to the risk of re-bleeding, which tends to occur within the first 72 hours and carries a significant mortality. Some surgeons believe that a Polya gastrectomy is the better procedure for a bleeding duodenal ulcer as it carries a lower incidence of re-bleeding.

Gastric ulcer: Ideally, the precise site of the bleeding has been identified by preoperative gastroscopy, and an ulcer can be located by palpation of the relevant area of the stomach. When a posterior ulcer is suspected the lesser sac will have to be entered to examine the posterior aspect of the stomach. An antral or pyloric ulcer may be detected by digital palpation of the mucosa through a pyloroduodenotomy, if this has already been performed. If no bleeding site can be identified, it may be necessary to make a second gastrotomy. Intraoperative endoscopy can also be helpful in identifying the bleeding point and directing the placement of gastric incisions.

Once the bleeding point has been identified, the surgeon must decide on the most appropriate strategy. Under-sewing of the bleeding vessel from within should secure haemostasis, and this is often recommended for the small Diculafoy lesion. In contrast, a very large ulcer eroding into a major branch of the left gastric artery may necessitate a subtotal gastrectomy incorporating the ulcer. Some surgeons prefer a gastrectomy in all cases, because of the risk of re-bleeding and the concern that an ulcer might be malignant. The pylorus is divided between non-crushing clamps. The distal stomach is then elevated in a cephalad direction, which exposes the left gastric artery and facilitates the application of a vascular clamp. This should control bleeding from ulcers involving the lesser curvature and this can be confirmed by releasing the distal stomach clamp. Thereafter, the branches of the left gastric artery along the lesser curvature may be divided in a controlled fashion from the pylorus to a point proximal to the ulcer. The vascular clamp on the left gastric artery is then released. If haemostasis is achieved, the stomach may then be divided using staplers. If feasible, a Billroth I type anastomosis can be performed but if there is any risk of undue tension on the suture lines then a Billroth II anastomosis is safer.

An ulcer high on the lesser curve, which is eroding the left gastric artery, may not be included in a standard partial gastrectomy. It can be incorporated into the resection by a Pauchet manoeuvre, in which the ulcer is excised with a tongue of gastric wall. A new 'lesser curve' is created by apposing the cut anterior and posterior gastric walls with a continuous absorbable suture (Fig. 17.7).

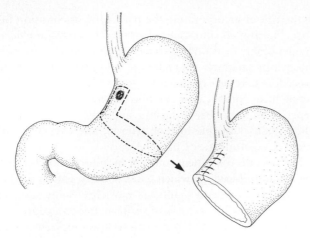

Figure 17.7   *Pauchet's manoeuvre.*

SURGICAL MANAGEMENT OF BLEEDING OESOPHAGEAL VARICES

Bleeding oesophageal varices, secondary to portal hypertension, can be a challenging emergency. The bleeding may be torrential, and many patients have severely compromised liver function.

Endoscopic treatment
Endoscopy is essential to rule out other causes for bleeding, as many patients with known oesophageal varices are bleeding from a duodenal ulcer or gastritis. Treatment options at endoscopy include sclerosant injection, clip placement or banding of the varices. In those patients in whom endoscopic treatment is either not possible, or is unsuccessful, and bleeding continues, a Sengstaken BlakeMore tube can be inserted. Such patients are usually intubated and ventilated, and this will provide airway protection as the tube is inserted. The tube must be well-lubricated, and can then be inserted either nasally or orally. The volumes to which the gastric and oesophageal balloons are inflated vary, and it is important to read the manufacturer's instructions and to inflate accordingly. In general, the gastric balloon is inflated with 250 mL of air and brought back onto the gastro-oesophageal junction. The oesophageal balloon is then inflated to approximately 120 mL of air, but this can be increased to 150 mL if the haemorrhage is not controlled. It should be remembered that in addition to bleeding oesophageal varices the patient may have bleeding secondary from gastric varices, which will not be controlled by the tube. After insertion, the position of the tube and balloons should be checked by chest X-ray.

Pharmacological management
Pharmacological management of an acute variceal haemorrhage consists of intravenous vasopressin, which constricts mesenteric arterioles reducing portal blood flow. An alternative drug with fewer side effects is octreotide, which inhibits the release of vasodilatory hormones and thus reduces splanchnic circulation. Oral neomycin and lactulose reduce

the incidence of encephalopathy by reducing nitrogen absorption from the gut.

Transjugular intrahepatic portosystemic shunt (TIPSS)
This may be used in patients who fail to respond to pharmacological and endoscopic therapy. It consists of an angiographically created shunt between the hepatic and portal veins which decompresses the portal system. A surgical total, or selective, portocaval shunt is a possibility if TIPSS is unavailable, but this carries a high mortality in the emergency setting (see Chapter 20).

Oesophageal transection
When a surgeon is faced with an exsanguinating patient, an oesophageal transection with end-to-end anastomosis using an EEA stapling device (as discussed in Chapter 20) is often the best emergency surgical option (see Fig. 13.16, page 229).

MORBID OBESITY

Morbid obesity is defined as a body mass index (BMI) greater than 40 kg/m^2, although many patients are well in excess of this. Morbid obesity is increasingly recognized as a medical condition, with serious implications for both health and longevity. As medical management of obesity frequently fails, surgical intervention has an important role. However, the increased morbidity associated with obesity places these patients in a high-risk group for surgery.

A minimal access approach has been particularly successful in the morbidly obese, and much of the recent expansion in bariatric, or obesity, surgery has been laparoscopic. It is imperative that any underlying medical conditions, or psychological disturbances, that may be contributing to the patient's weight gain are identified and addressed. Correct patient selection in conjunction with a multidisciplinary approach is the key to achieving a successful sustained weight reduction.

Surgical procedures for morbid obesity

These operations are based either on the concept of reducing the intake of food, or inducing malabsorption of the excessive intake. Most of the measures to reduce intake rely on reducing the storage capacity of the stomach, but less subtle measures – such as wiring teeth – and more sophisticated approaches – such as creating a situation where early dumping after the ingestion of a high refined carbohydrate load acts as aversion therapy – have also been tried.

In recent years bariatric surgery has become increasingly specialized. The most commonly performed operations include the vertical banded gastroplasty, the adjustable gastric band, and the Roux-en-Y gastric bypass. Laparoscopic approaches have significantly increased the demand for this type of treatment for morbid obesity. The options however are numerous, and patients should be referred to those surgeons with a special interest if good results are to be obtained.

JEJUNO–ILEAL BYPASS

This was one of the first operations for morbid obesity, and relied on malabsorption as its principle. The jejunum was divided, usually 25 cm from the duodenojejunal flexure. The distal end was closed, and the proximal end anastomosed end-to-side to the ileum, approximately 50 cm from the ileo-caecal valve (Fig. 17.8). The patient had a functional 'short bowel syndrome', combined with a blind loop of small bowel which was exposed to neither bile nor food. While the weight loss was dramatic, long-term complications were unacceptable. Many patients developed liver cirrhosis secondary to the increased endotoxin load from the bacterial colonization of the bypassed segment.

Later modifications, including pancreatobiliary diversion techniques, were an attempt to overcome these metabolic disturbances. A functional short bowel syndrome is still created, but a blind loop is avoided as bile and pancreatic juice traverse the segment of small bowel that the food bypasses (Fig. 17.9). These procedures are commonly combined with some form of gastric resection, and the weight loss induced is then dependent on a combination of restrictive and malab-sorptive factors.[5]

VERTICAL BANDED GASTROPLASTY

This is a 'restrictive' operation. The principle of restrictive operations stemmed from the clinical observation that

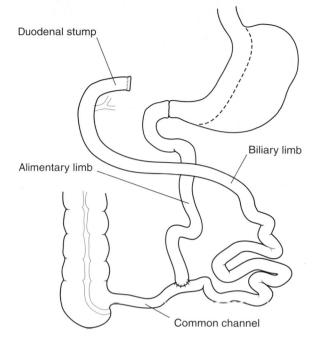

Figure 17.9   *Biliopancreatic bypass with a duodenal switch. The first part of the duodenum is transected and the distal end closed. The duodenum and jejunum form the biliary loop. A second division in the mid small bowel enables the distal divided end to be brought up and anastomosed to the proximal duodenum. The proximal divided end is then anastomosed end-to-side approximately 100 cm from the ileocaecal valve. The dotted line marks one type of gastric resection which can be combined with this procedure.*

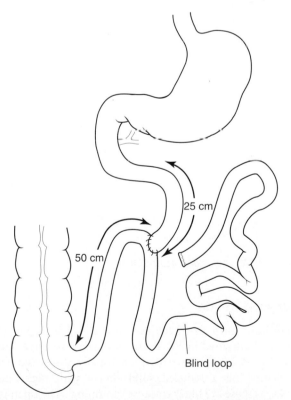

Figure 17.8   *Jejuno-ileal bypass. The jejunum is divided 25 cm from the duodenojejunal flexure, and the proximal end is anastomosed to the ileum 50 cm from the ileocaecal valve, creating a functional short bowel and a long blind loop.*

patients who had undergone a total, or subtotal, gastrectomy lost significant amounts of weight. The advantage of this procedure is that it works by limiting food intake rather than malabsorption, but the overall weight loss is less than after other procedures. The gastric pouch fills quickly and empties slowly, giving a feeling of satiety. The disadvantage is poorly motivated patients may opt for high-calorie drinks. In addition, with excessive food intake, it is possible to enlarge the proximal gastric pouch. The operation can be performed using either an open or a laparoscopic technique, although the latter can be technically challenging.

The gastrophrenic ligament is divided to open the angle of His, and an opening is made in the gastrohepatic ligament, close to the lesser curve, to enter the lesser sac. A stapled opening is then formed through both the anterior and posterior walls of the stomach, with a circular stapling device (Fig. 17.10a). This opening should be accurately positioned to lie 5 cm below the gastro-oesophageal junction, and 3 cm from the lesser curve. A vertical staple line is then created, using a 90-mm linear stapler, with three superimposed applications, extending from the circular stapled opening to the angle of His. Alternatively, the specially designed bariatric stapler which fires four parallel rows of staples can be used. A polypropylene mesh is passed through the opening,

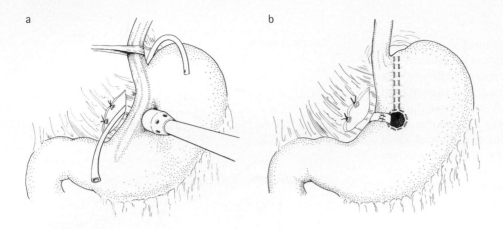

Figure 17.10 *Vertical banded gastroplasty. (a) A Penrose drain has been passed through the retrogastric tunnel. The circular stapler has been positioned accurately to make the opening through the stomach. (b) The upper gastric pouch is now defined by the vertical stapled closure and the restricting horizontal band.*

wrapped around the lesser curve, and then sutured to itself thus leaving only a small channel between the gastric pouch and the remainder of the stomach (Fig. 17.10b). The size of this channel can be gauged by the length of mesh used to encircle the lesser curve, and a 5 cm circumference is usually recommended.

Technical complications associated with the procedure include suture line dehiscence and mesh migration. Over time weight tends to return and this operation is going out of favour.

ADJUSTABLE GASTRIC BAND

This technique was developed from the vertical banded gastroplasty, over which it has several advantages. It is a more suitable operation for a laparoscopic approach, and the band is adjustable; this allows the outlet diameter from the gastric pouch to be varied according to patient needs. The band can also be easily removed, and no anatomical changes have been made that might interfere with future bariatric procedures. The high cost of the prosthesis is the main disadvantage.

Laparoscopic gastric banding is more technically challenging for patients with a BMI >60 kg/m², predominantly due to difficulty with upper abdominal access. This patient group may require a medically supervised diet during the weeks preceding surgery in order to achieve a temporary weight loss and make the surgery safer.

Laparoscopic access is established in a similar manner to that described in Chapter 16 for other gastro-oesophageal junction procedures. Prior to dissection, a calibration tube with an inflatable balloon is inserted into the stomach, filled with 15 mL of saline, and retracted until it lies just below the gastro-oesophageal junction. The gastrohepatic ligament is opened alongside the proximal lesser curve, the palpable balloon forming a useful landmark. The dissection continues behind the stomach towards the angle of His, creating a retrogastric tunnel. The gastric band is then introduced from the angle of His, brought through the perigastric opening and around the stomach. It is then locked in place around the distal end of the calibration tube beyond the balloon (Fig. 17.11). The band can then be secured to the anterior wall of the stomach with interrupted sutures. The tubing between the band and the reservoir is brought out through a port site. The reservoir, or access port, is placed at a site that allows easy access for percutaneous volume adjustments. A small incision is made, and the reservoir is placed directly on the rectus sheath to which it is sutured. The tightness of the band is adjusted according to the patient's weight loss, with larger volumes of saline resulting in a smaller stoma and more restriction of intake.

Long-term complications associated with the procedure include infection, band slippage, and erosion of the band into the stomach.[6]

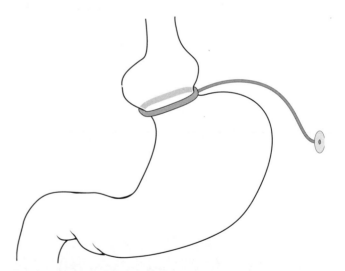

Figure 17.11 *Adjustable gastric band.*

ROUX-EN-Y BYPASS

In the Roux-en-Y gastric bypass (Fig. 17.12) the upper gastric pouch, drained by the Roux loop, is a restrictive operation. In addition, the patient is usually dissuaded from supplementing a reduced solid intake with high-calorie drinks, as these are likely to cause 'dumping'. The open procedure is performed through an upper midline laparotomy, but many surgeons have developed the skills to perform this operation laparoscopically. The gastro-oesophageal junction is mobilized. A retrogastric tunnel is created, starting from

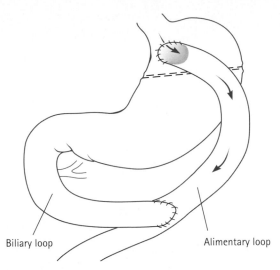

Biliary loop   Alimentary loop

Figure 17.12   *A Roux-en-Y gastric bypass for morbid obesity. Modifications to the Roux loop, which shorten the common channel, introduce an additional malabsorptive component.*

the gastrohepatic omentum, close to the lesser curvature and emerging lateral to the angle of His. A Penrose drain is passed through the tunnel to encircle the stomach, and is used as a landmark for the creation of an upper gastric pouch using linear staplers. The jejunum is transected approximately 40 cm beyond the ligament of Treitz, with the distal divided end anastomosed to the proximal gastric pouch with a restricted stoma outlet of 1 cm. The Roux loop is completed by forming a jejunojejunostomy approximately 50 cm downstream.

In patients with a BMI >50 kg/m², a greater weight loss can be achieved if a more distal loop of jejunum is used for the Roux loop, or if the jejunojejunostomy is performed further downstream. These manoeuvres decrease the length of small bowel through which food must pass, and also decrease the common channel where bile, pancreatic juice and food can mix. This is a similar principle to that employed in the biliopancreatic diversion techniques mentioned above. The increased weight loss is therefore attributable to an additional malabsorptive component. Many variations of this procedure have been described.

GASTRIC CANCER

Gastric cancer, despite a falling incidence in the Western world, is still a major cause of morbidity and mortality. In recent years the anatomical location of gastric cancer appears to have shifted from the antral portion to a more proximal part of the stomach, including involvement of the gastro-oesophageal junction. In Japan, gastric cancer is the commonest malignancy in both men and women, and this has led to the introduction of mass screening programmes to facilitate early detection. This approach appears to have successfully reduced mortality from the disease.

Outcomes for patients with gastric cancer who present with T1 and T2 disease, and no evidence of metastatic spread, are good. Unfortunately, many patients present with advanced disease. When a patient is diagnosed with gastric cancer, it must first be determined whether a curative resection is possible. It is important to identify those patients who will not benefit from any surgical intervention, prior to a laparotomy. A CT scan is pivotal in preoperative staging as it may show liver or omental deposits, or the involvement of pre-aortic nodes. Endoscopic ultrasonography is used in some centres to measure the depth of invasion and the involvement of adjacent nodes.

DIAGNOSTIC LAPAROSCOPY

Diagnostic laparoscopy is particularly valuable in the identification of peritoneal seedlings, and peripheral liver metastases, that are too small to identify by CT scanning. This should be performed several days prior to the intended surgery to allow time for pathological examination of suspicious lesions, and cytological examination of ascitic fluid. At laparoscopy, the surface of the liver and the peritoneum over the falciform ligament and under the diaphragm should be examined carefully for peritoneal deposits. Any suspicious lesions should be biopsied, and ascitic fluid sent for cytological examination to determine if malignant cells are present. While this places a further percentage of patients into a palliative category, it avoids unnecessary laparotomies, and also helps to identify those with the greatest potential for surgical cure. Despite preoperative investigations, gastric cancer is under-staged in approximately 20 per cent of patients.

Radicality of surgery

The reasons why apparently curative resections fail must be explored whenever the radicality of a surgical excision is considered. For example, changes in surgical technique are most unlikely to reduce failure from haematogenous spread, but may reduce failure if recurrence occurs solely at the anastomosis, in the tumour bed, or within the regional lymph nodes. Failure in gastric cancer occurs loco-regionally, but failures also result from dissemination throughout the peritoneal cavity, and from blood-borne metastases.

EXTENT OF THE GASTRIC RESECTION

For most patients, a potentially curative gastric cancer resection will involve either a subtotal or a total gastrectomy. Occasionally, a more conservative resection may be appropriate.

Subtotal or total gastrectomy

Gastric cancer spreads in the submucosal plane. At presentation, this infiltration may involve the whole of the stomach (linitus plastica), and in these cases the tumour infiltration may even extend into the duodenum or oesophagus. In most patients, however, there is a palpable edge to the tumour, and transection 5 cm clear of this edge will usually be free of tumour infiltration. In tumours which have breached the serosa, a 6-cm margin is recommended. Thus, in distal gastric cancer, a partial gastrectomy can offer a R0 resection. The proximal gastric pouch should include at least 2 cm of the lesser curve, and the palpable edge of the tumour must therefore be 7–8 cm from the oesophagogastric junction. A total gastrectomy thus becomes necessary for any tumour which encroaches to within 7–8 cm of the oesophagogastric junction if positive resection margins are to be avoided. In theory, a proximal gastric cancer can be resected with adequate margins, and the antrum and pylorus preserved. However, functional results after a proximal subtotal gastrectomy, and anastomosis of the distal stomach to the oesophagus, are poor, mainly due to alkaline oesophageal reflux. Most surgeons recommend a total gastrectomy in these circumstances.

Limited excision

Most of the research on gastric cancer confined to the mucosa and submucosa (T1) has come from Japan where, as a result of extensive surveillance programmes, around one-third of the gastric cancers are diagnosed at this stage. Limited resections, but still with curative intent, have been pioneered for small superficial cancers. Endoscopic resection, or laser ablation, has been used for those tumours which are judged on endoscopic appearance to be very superficial. Limited full-thickness gastric resections, either with or without the removal of the adjacent perigastric lymph nodes, is a slightly more radical option.[7] There are problems with these approaches, however. A superficial cancer can be more extensive locally than initially appreciated and, although superficial, may have spread in the submucosa beyond the resection margins. Accurate preoperative assessment of the depth of invasion is difficult, but it is crucially important as less than 5 per cent of mucosal cancers have nodal metastases, whereas in cancers which invade the submucosa up to 25 per cent may have nodal metastases, and around 5 per cent may have metastases in 2nd tier nodes.

Limited surgery for early gastric cancer has not generally been practised in the West. In the absence of screening programmes, suitable cases are only rarely encountered. It would seem, however, that it should be considered in those in whom a more radical operation would carry a significant risk.

THE EXTENT OF THE LYMPHADENECTOMY

It is known that lymphatic spread can occur early in gastric cancer, and that lymphatic recurrence in the gastric bed is a major area of failure. In some patients this occurs without simultaneous haematogenous or peritoneal spread, which raises the possibility that a more radical lymphadenectomy could have been curative. The Japanese have extensively mapped the patterns of lymph node metastases.[8] Gastric lymph nodes have been subdivided into numbered anatomical groups or 'stations' (Fig. 17.13), and then considered as

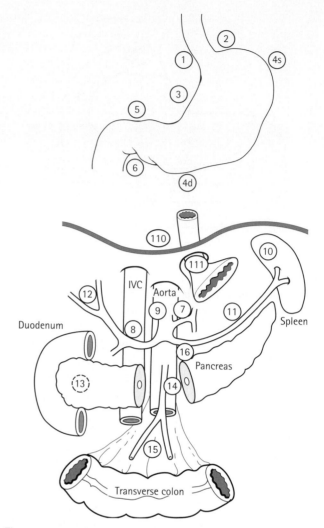

Figure 17.13   *Gastric lymph node stations. 1 = right cardiac; 2 = left cardiac; 3 = lesser curve; 4s = proximal greater curve; 4d = distal greater curve; 5 = suprapyloric; 6 = subpyloric; 7 = left gastric artery; 8 = common hepatic artery; 9 = coeliac axis; 10 = splenic hilar; 11 = splenic artery; 12 = hepatoduodenal; 13 = retropancreatic; 14 = root of mesentery; 15 = middle colic artery; 16 = para-aortic; 110 = para-oesophageal; 111 = diaphragmatic.*

'tiers' of nodes. The concept of a D1, D2 and a D2/D3 gastrectomy developed from this. The approach to lymphadenectomy in Japan became far more radical than in the West, and the Japanese were able to produce very impressive survival figures. A D1 gastrectomy implies the excision of all 1st tier nodes, a D2 gastrectomy the excision of all 1st and 2nd tier nodes, and a D2/D3 gastrectomy implies the additional removal of some 3rd tier nodes. The significantly better survival figures following these more radical lymphadenectomies in Japan has influenced Western practice. However, the true benefit from the more major surgery is less than it immediately appears. When a more radical lymphadenectomy is undertaken, metastases may be found in nodes which would not have been available for analysis after a standard, less radical operation. This places the cancer in a more advanced stage, and the apparent benefit from excision of more nodal tissue is then fallacious and merely a *stage migration phenomenon*. This can affect comparisons between the West and Japan, and also any comparison in clinical trials between D1 and D2 resections.

Other factors are also important. Patients in the West have generally less favourable disease as they not only present with more advanced disease, but there are more proximal cancers and more diffuse cancers – both of which carry a worse prognosis. A D2 gastrectomy for these cancers, involving the proximal stomach, is also a more major undertaking. Western patients are generally older, fatter, and have a higher risk of thromboembolism. These factors at least partly explain the higher inpatient mortality from the more radical lymphadenectomies in the West. Any gain in long-term survival must be balanced against a higher perioperative mortality.

The stomach is subdivided into an upper section (C), a middle section (M), and a lower section (A). The tumour is then classified according to the section of stomach in which it arose, and also any sections into which it has spread. For example, a localized antral tumour is designated 'A', and a middle-section tumour which has spread to the cardia 'MC'. The tiers of lymph nodes differ according to the position of the tumour. Standard surgical textbooks contain more detail on this.[9] However, as a simplification, the 1st tier nodes are perigastric nodes close to the tumour, and the 2nd tier nodes include both nodes along the proximal section of the arteries supplying the section of stomach involved in the malignancy and other more distant perigastric nodes. For example, stations 3, 4d, 5 and 6 are the 1st tier nodes for an antral cancer, and station 7, 8, 9 and 1 are the 2nd tier nodes. The standard subtotal D2 gastrectomy for antral cancer which excises all these nodes was described in Chapter 16. It is an operation which has been adopted in many specialist centres outside Japan. However, in upper third gastric cancer, the 1st tier nodes are 1, 2, 3 and 4s, and the 2nd tier nodes are 4d, 7, 8, 9, 10, 11, 5 and 6. Station 10 nodes are in the hilum of the spleen, and station 11 are along the splenic artery, behind the pancreas. A full D2 gastrectomy for proximal cancer is therefore a very major procedure. It involves the addition of a splenectomy and distal pancreatectomy, or a high-risk dissection if these nodes are to be retrieved but the organs retained.

The risk/gain balance for the individual node stations has been calculated, and this may be more important than a rigid classification into node tiers. This calculation is based on the likelihood of metastases within the nodes of a particular station, the possible survival benefit from removing them, and the additional mortality and morbidity from doing so. This has resulted in many surgeons performing the standard D2 subtotal gastrectomy for distal cancers with the additional removal of station 12 nodes (D2/D3 gastrectomy). Although these are 3rd tier (N3) nodes, they contain metastases in 9 per cent of distal tumours and 5-year survivals as high as 25 per cent have been reported from Japan in patients who have had positive station 12 nodes resected.

In proximal gastric cancers, most surgeons in the West have adopted a compromise between a D1 and a D2 operation. A full D2 gastrectomy for proximal cancers includes a splenectomy and distal pancreatectomy. This is associated with a higher in-hospital mortality, which approximately balances any improvement in long-term survival. However, in proximal cancers arising on the greater curve, a more major resection to include the retrieval of station 10, and possibly even station 11, nodes should be considered in younger fitter patients as there should be a survival benefit if the Japanese results can be matched.

Extended lymphadenectomies, in which the 3rd and 4th tier nodes (stations 13–16) are removed,[7] have only shown benefit in series from Japan. These radical lymphadenectomies can be combined with a more extensive clearance of the tumour. A left upper quadrant evisceration, in which the transverse colon is removed en bloc with the stomach, spleen, left adrenal and body and tail of pancreas, can be combined with Appleby's operation, in which the coeliac trunk and proximal segment of the common hepatic artery are excised to facilitate para-aortic lymphatic clearance. Liver perfusion is maintained from the superior mesenteric artery through the pancreaticoduodenal anastomotic arcade. These very radical procedures are very rarely undertaken in the West, and are probably also losing favour in Japan.[10]

SEROSAL SPREAD

This is a common area of failure in gastric cancer, and the reason that laparoscopy should be considered as part of the staging procedure in order to save patients with macroscopic peritoneal deposits from non-curative major surgery. Most patients in the West present with gastric cancer which has invaded the serosa. The peritoneal cavity is already contaminated with malignant cells, even if there are no visible metastatic deposits, and this is reflected in a significantly worse prognosis. Most of the lesser sac peritoneum is excised in a D2 gastrectomy, and this may be of some value in posterior tumours which have only contaminated this area. Intraoperative and postoperative intraperitoneal chemotherapy may have a place when there is serosal invasion. In some units in Japan this is used routinely if peritoneal malignant contamination is confirmed by the identification of free malignant cells on peritoneal cytology. This approach is still considered experimental in the UK.

Adjacent organs can adhere to the involved serosa overlying a gastric cancer. This may be followed by direct tumour invasion. General peritoneal contamination will have been minimized by the malignant adhesions, but the prognosis is still poor. Extended excisions to include other organs invaded by the primary tumour are seldom justified.

Palliative surgery

The survival of patients in whom a curative resection is not possible is poor, and in general, palliative surgery has a limited role. Chemotherapy can achieve a remission, with a reasonable quality of life, for a minority of patients.

If during the laparotomy conditions are discovered which preclude a curative resection, the surgeon must decide whether a palliative resection, a bypass or no further surgical procedure will offer the patient the best quality of life. This was a decision which had to be made frequently before preoperative staging was developed, and it may still be a common problem for those surgeons working in parts of the world where there is no access to sophisticated imaging modalities. The surgeon must be careful not to be influenced by the understandable desire 'to do something', and the perception of failure if an 'open and close' laparotomy is chosen. The decision is not always straightforward.

PALLIATIVE RESECTION

This can offer the best palliation for a bleeding tumour, for gastric outflow obstruction, and also for the non-specific, but distressing and unpleasant, symptoms associated with a fungating intragastric mass. It should certainly be considered for a small mobile distal tumour in a fit patient with a small metastatic load, especially as a palliative partial gastrectomy for malignancy does not need to include a radical lymphadenectomy. It should be remembered that if there is a heavy metastatic load the mortality and morbidity of any major resection will be significantly increased. No anastomosis should be attempted through macroscopically malignant tissue and, if the tumour cannot be cleared with a partial gastrectomy, a total gastrectomy is seldom justified as the quality of life with a total gastrectomy and metastatic malignancy is extremely poor.

BYPASS

A gastroenterostomy should be considered in any irresectable distal growth which is causing a gastric outflow obstruction. This is often undertaken electively in patients whose cancers are known to be too advanced for curative surgery, but who have developed obstructive symptoms, and in this situation it is often carried out laparoscopically. When the abdomen has already been opened and an irresectable tumour confined to the distal stomach is encountered, a gastroenterostomy is usually justified. Even in the absence of established outlet obstruction, there is a high risk of this developing as the cancer advances, unless the patient's life expectancy is severely limited by extensive metastatic disease. It is important to fashion the gastroenterostomy to a dependant part of the stomach, but as far from the tumour as possible to avoid later tumour obstruction of the anastomosis (see Chapter 16). A thorough abdominal examination should also be undertaken to determine the presence of peritoneal seedlings which might cause a future small bowel obstruction. This complication may sometimes be avoided if a stenosing serosal secondary is removed as a wedge excision (see Chapter 21).

Proximal tumours can cause dysphagia, and frequently present when they are locally irresectable, or the patient already has metastatic spread. Palliative surgical bypass is seldom a practical option, but fortunately these growths can usually be stented endoscopically with relief of distressing symptoms.

Prophylactic surgery in hereditary diffuse gastric cancer

The presence of familial clusters of gastric cancer following an autosomal dominant pattern has been observed for many years. Surveillance has been unsuccessful, mainly due to the diffuse, submucosal nature of the cancer, which makes it undetectable despite repeated endoscopies. Most patients, even when under surveillance, present at an advanced stage with unresectable disease. The penetrance rate of the gene is reported at 70–80 per cent and, in the absence to date of a successful surveillance mechanism, a prophylactic total gastrectomy with Roux-en-Y reconstruction is a viable therapeutic option. However, the mortality and morbidity risk is not insignificant, and genetic counselling in high-risk families is essential before offering any genetic testing.

When performing a total prophylactic gastrectomy for hereditary diffuse gastric cancer, it is imperative that all gastric mucosa is removed and that the transection is above the gastro-oesophageal junction and incorporates oesophageal squamous mucosa. This is confirmed intraoperatively by the pathologist with frozen-section examination. Any gastric mucosa left behind places the patient at a significant risk of cancer in the remnant tissue. The radical lymphadenectomy, which is usually associated with a total gastrectomy, is not required.

OTHER GASTRIC MALIGNANCIES

Gastrointestinal stromal tumours (GIST)

These mesenchymal tumours of variable malignant potential are most commonly encountered in the stomach. They were previously considered to be gastric leiomyomas or leiomyosarcomas (see Chapter 15). Although the tumour behaviour can be partially predicted histologically, this information is seldom available to the surgeon preoperatively. In general, a small tumour discovered as an incidental finding behaves in a benign fashion, and the larger tumours which present symptomatically are usually more aggressive. Many patients present at an advanced stage with extensive disease, and there may also be peritoneal and liver metastases.

Despite investigations it is often not possible to establish the diagnosis preoperatively, especially as, if a curative resection is planned, it is important to avoid biopsy with the risk of spillage of tumour cells. A common presentation is as an emergency with haemorrhage, and the bleeding is seen at endoscopy to be from an ulcer on the summit of a submucosal gastric mass. Complete surgical clearance is the main treatment objective, and this may require the removal of adjacent organs. Many patients who develop loco-regional recurrence have successfully undergone further clearance, and follow-up is therefore essential. Imatinib shows promise in the treatment of unresectable or metastatic GIST (see Chapter 15).

Gastric lymphoma

Primary gastric lymphoma accounts for approximately 2 per cent of gastric malignancies. It most commonly affects the distal stomach, and presentation is with epigastric pain or gastric outlet obstruction. Endoscopic biopsy confirms the diagnosis. Surgical resection of the involved gastric segment was traditionally the principal treatment, but chemotherapy has become increasingly effective in gastric lymphoma. Indeed, in patients with advanced disease chemotherapy is the mainstay of treatment, with surgery reserved for the control of symptoms such as bleeding or gastric outlet obstruction. Patients with a diagnosis of early gastric lymphoma should probably undergo surgical resection with adjuvant chemotherapy, although patients are sometimes treated with chemotherapy alone.[11] With chemotherapy as an additional treatment modality the surgery can be less radical, and a gastrectomy with en-bloc resection of the spleen is now seldom indicated.

Gastric carcinoids

Small tumours may be removed by endoscopic resection, whereas larger tumours (>2 cm) require formal resection with regular endoscopic follow-up.

MALIGNANT OESOPHAGEAL TUMOURS

Despite advances in care, oesophageal carcinoma still carries a poor prognosis which is attributed to its aggressive biological nature and late presentation. The world-wide incidence of oesophageal adenocarcinoma is increasing, and is now greater than that of squamous cell carcinoma. Adenocarcinoma predominantly affects the lower third of the oesophagus and the gastro-oesophageal junction. These tumours at the gastro-oesophageal junction should probably be considered as a separate group from either gastric or oesophageal tumours. Otherwise they are somewhat artificially divided into two separate entities when only a centimetre or two separates the one from the other.[12]

The surgery of oesophageal cancer is extremely challenging. It has now generally been centralized within the UK to regional centres in an attempt to improve results, and this surgery is certainly no longer within the remit of the general surgeon without a subspecialty upper gastrointestinal interest. Good results are only partly surgeon-dependent, and a multidisciplinary team approach to oesophageal cancer is essential – first to identify those patients who will benefit from neoadjuvant chemoradiotherapy, those suitable for surgery, and those requiring palliative care. Successful oesophageal surgery is dependent not only on skilled anaesthesia and intensive care, but also on physiotherapy and nutritional support.

PREOPERATIVE INVESTIGATIONS

In the absence of a screening programme, many patients in the Western world present with dysphagia. Diagnostic tests required for staging include barium swallow and endoscopy. These identify the tumour site and size, and allow biopsy for pathological determination of histological type. No surgery or intervention should be considered in the absence of a histological diagnosis. CT screening of the thorax, abdomen and neck will provide critical information on associated lymphadenopathy, or the involvement of adjacent organs. Bronchoscopy is useful in ruling out tracheal or bronchial extension. This was once considered essential for all tumours in the upper two-thirds of the oesophagus, but is now practised less frequently, due mainly to the increased accuracy of imaging modalities. Endoscopic ultrasonography, when performed by an experienced clinician, is accurate in determining extramural extension and the degree of associated lymphadenopathy. Positron emission tomography (PET) may be helpful in selecting a curative subgroup.

PRINCIPLES UNDERLYING OESOPHAGEAL CANCER SURGERY

Oesophageal lymphatic drainage is into a submucosal and peri-oesophageal plexus, in which lymph mixes from all levels of the oesophagus, before draining to regional nodes. This has two important implications for the surgeon:

1. The possibility of submucosal extension within the lymphatic plexus must be considered as this affects the margins of resection required. Even with a 10-cm macroscopic clearance, 10–20 per cent of specimens will have involved margins. For this reason a total or subtotal oesophagectomy is recommended even for lower-third tumours. Lower-third adenocarcinomas may invade extensively into the stomach, and oesophagectomy may have to be combined with proximal partial, or even a total gastrectomy, with or without splenectomy, to achieve an R0 resection. Similarly, oesophagectomy for a proximal oesophageal squamous cell carcinoma may have to be combined with a pharyngectomy to obtain complete local tumour clearance (see Chapter 9).
2. This mixing of lymph before drainage to nodes makes any form of very limited lymphadenectomy of little value. Debate continues over the survival advantages of a formal, more extensive lymphadenectomy. The lymphatic drainage from the oesophagus is divided into three fields: the abdominal; the intrathoracic; and the cervical:

- A *one-field lymphadenectomy* involves resection of the intra-abdominal nodes draining the proximal stomach and distal oesophagus. This follows similar principles to the D2 lymphadenectomy described for proximal gastric cancer.
- A *two-field lymphadenectomy* describes the additional clearance of the intrathoracic nodes. These include the nodes in the tracheal bifurcation, the right paratracheal nodes and pulmonary hilar nodes, in addition to the para-oesophageal and the para-aortic mediastinal nodes.
- A *three-field lymphadenectomy* includes, in addition, a neck dissection to clear the brachiocephalic, deep lateral and external cervical nodes.

Whilst some surgeons recommend a two-field lymphadenectomy, others believe that positive nodes are merely an indicator of incurable disease.

Surgery should be tailored to offer a patient the procedure that achieves minimal morbidity and mortality, but allows macroscopic and microscopic clearance. The choice of operative intervention depends on a number of factors including tumour type, location, extent of lymph node involvement, fitness for surgery, and surgeon preference. Resections are usually carried out with curative intent, as the role for palliative resections has diminished with advances in palliative management. However some patients who have involved margins (R1 resection) have good local disease control, and die of distant disease before the tumour recurs locally. The three main surgical approaches to oesophagectomy were described in Chapter 16. Each approach has both advantages and disadvantages.

Transhiatal approach

The transhiatal approach involves only abdominal and cervical incisions.[13] The patient does not have to be repositioned during surgery, the operative time is reduced, a thoracotomy is avoided, and it is thus associated with less cardiorespiratory dysfunction. This is the ideal approach for those patients with respiratory co-morbidity. Additionally, a cervical anastomotic leak is preferable to an intrathoracic leak.

However, patient selection is critical to outcome. The transhiatal approach is most suitable for cancers involving the distal oesophagus, and is unsuitable for tumours that are large and those that may have extensive extramural spread, involving adjacent organs such as the aorta or tracheobronchial tree. Particular care should be taken in selecting any middle-third tumour for this technique, where it is only suitable for those tumours that are confined to the oesophageal wall. Additionally, surgeons should be aware that fibrosis secondary to adjuvant therapies may make blunt dissection difficult, and more hazardous. Damage can occur during blunt dissection to intrathoracic vessels, the trachea and the recurrent laryngeal nerve. Another objection to transhiatal oesophagectomy is the quality of oncological clearance, given that much of the dissection is blunt and performed blindly, with a lower yield of lymph nodes compared to the thoracic approach. Despite the theoretical advantages of a formal lymphadenectomy, trials to date have shown no outcome differences in terms of long-term survival between the transhiatal and transthoracic approaches when patients are compared according to stage.[14]

Thoraco-abdominal oesophagectomy

Excellent access is obtained both to the infra-aortic oesophagus, and to the stomach, without the necessity of moving the patient during the operation. The standard technique however necessitates an anastomosis below the aortic arch, thus restricting the radicality of the oesophageal resection. Lymph node dissection may not be so radical as when the oesophagus is approached from a right thoracotomy. The incision, which crosses the costal margin, is associated with significant postoperative respiratory morbidity.

Several adaptations to the old thoraco-abdominal technique have been developed. It can be combined with a cervical incision to increase both the length of oesophagus removed and to carry the anastomosis into the neck. A left thoracotomy combined with a transhiatal approach to the stomach is a variant of the left thoraco-abdominal approach, and may be associated with a lower morbidity. This was the standard approach for a large series from China.[15]

McKeown and Ivor–Lewis oesophagectomy

These two- and three-stage oesophagectomies allow direct visualization of the whole length of the intrathoracic oesophagus. Proponents of the techniques quote a superior oncological clearance, with a greater yield of lymph nodes. These approaches are particularly suitable for large mid-oesophageal tumours that have breached the oesophageal wall and may lie in close proximity to adjacent structures. They may also be the safest option for patients who have had preoperative chemoradiotherapy that potentially limits oesophageal mobilization. In the Ivor–Lewis operation an intrathoracic anastomosis is performed[16]; this is less likely to leak than a cervical anastomosis, but the consequence of a leak is much more serious. In the three-stage McKeown oesophagectomy a third incision is made in the neck. The anastomosis in the neck is not only safer than in the thorax but also allows a greater length of oesophagus to be removed. However, the risk of recurrent nerve damage is increased when there is an additional cervical incision.

The main disadvantages of these operations is the morbidity associated with a thoracotomy. In addition, the patient must be turned during the operation as there is no access to the gastric cardia from the right thorax. A more modern variation on the McKeown technique involves performing the right thoracotomy first. Once intrathoracic oesophageal mobilization is complete, the thoracotomy is closed and the remainder of the operation is performed in a similar fashion to that described for transhiatal oesophagectomy through upper abdominal and left cervical incisions. This is thought to reduce the respiratory insult, but the benefit of the initial laparotomy to check for disseminated tumour is lost. A preoperative laparoscopy may therefore have an important place, particularly when this modification is planned for a distal oesophageal tumour.

Neoadjuvant therapy for oesophageal cancer

The poor long-term outcome of patients with oesophageal cancer has led to the search for neoadjuvant therapies. The more recent chemoradiation trials have reported complete pathological response in greater than 20 per cent of patients, with significant improvements in long-term survival. Thus, the combination of chemoradiotherapy followed by surgical resection appears to offer the best potential for cure.

Palliative management of oesophageal and gastro-oesophageal tumours

In the absence of any screening programmes, a high proportion of patients with gastric and oesophageal carcinomas present with advanced unresectable disease. Their management is principally palliative, aimed at symptom control. Some patients, despite having early cancer, may be unsuitable for radical surgery due to coexisting morbidity, and this subgroup also have to be managed using a minimalist approach.

In patients with unresectable and metastatic disease the addition of chemotherapy will prolong survival, but this must be weighed against the patient's fitness for such treatment and the quality of life obtained. Radiotherapy may also be used to ameliorate pain from metastatic bone disease. However, the predominant and most distressing symptom for patients with advanced oesophageal and proximal gastric cancer is dysphagia. Fortunately, there are several effective palliative options.

Oesophageal stents
A wide range of oesophageal stents is available, which will allow the restoration of oesophageal integrity. These have a success rate of over 90 per cent, and enable the patient to resume a liquid or semi-solid diet. In principle, a soft guidewire is placed through the lumen of the tumour under endoscopic visualization. The stent is then placed over the guide-wire, which directs it through the tumour so that a component of the stent lies both proximally and distally. The stent is then opened and gradually expands against the tumour. Oesophageal stent insertion may not be possible if the patient has a proximal oesophageal tumour near the cricopharyngeal sphincter.

Laser therapy
This consists of the application of thermal energy using a neodymium:yttrium-aluminium garnet (Nd:YAG) laser to the tumour. It is suitable for exophytic lesions in the middle or distal oesophagus. It provides relief of dysphagia in over 90 per cent of patients, requiring on average two treatment sessions. In more recent years, since the development of expandable stents, the use of laser therapy has diminished, although it is still used to control tumour overgrowth of the stents.

Palliative radiotherapy
Palliative radiotherapy is used to alleviate dysphagia, and is particularly useful for proximal oesophageal tumours, which are unsuitable for stenting. External beam radiotherapy is given at a dose of between 40 to 70 Gy in 20 to 30 fractions. However, inherent risks include the development of a tracheo-oesophageal fistula, and stricture formation. Patients should be aware that the dysphagia may be exacerbated in the initial treatment period, due to oedema, and no benefit may be seen for up to 2 months.

Brachytherapy
This involves the placement of a radioisotope within the lumen of the tumour.

Photodynamic therapy
This treatment also uses laser energy to restore oesophageal integrity. The principle involves the intravenous administration of photosensitizers that are taken up by malignant cells. The agent is then activated using light with a wavelength of 630 nm, generating oxygen free radicals that induce tumour necrosis. Sunburn is a common complication of this procedure because the photosensitive agent is retained in tissues for several weeks, making them hypersensitive to sunlight.

Surgical bypass
Although this carries a significant risk, it is a very effective method for alleviating dysphagia. It is also a useful procedure in the management of tracheo-oesophageal fistulae associated with oesophageal cancer, or its treatment. Either a gastric or a colonic conduit is suitable, and this must often be brought up by an extra-anatomical route (see below).

Tracheo-oesophageal fistulae in oesophageal cancer

An acquired tracheo-oesophageal fistula is almost always secondary to direct invasion by a primary or secondary tumour, or occurs as a complication of the treatment of a malignancy. The malignancy is most often an oesophageal tumour. The fistula may arise spontaneously with tumour advancement, or it may occur following oesophageal surgery or radiotherapy. The patient presents with extreme respiratory compromise and recurrent pulmonary infections, and despite aggressive intervention the condition is often fatal. The diagnosis can be confirmed by instillation of water-soluble contrast media into the oesophagus. The fistula may also be visualized using upper endoscopy or bronchoscopy, which helps to determine if there is a malignant cause for the communication. Acquired tracheo-oesophageal fistulae will not close spontaneously and require operative intervention if the patient is stable. In critically ill patients oesophageal ligation, with the creation of a high oesophagostomy and a gastrostomy, may offer the best outcome. If the fistulation is due to a primary or secondary malignancy, then management is principally palliative aimed at symptomatic relief.

Aggressive operative intervention should be considered in patients who have a fistula as a complication of oesophagectomy performed for an early cancer, and also in those who have had a complete pathological response following radiotherapy. High fistulae may be approached via a low collar incision. Fistulae at the level of the carina require a lateral thoracotomy for access. If the fistula is small, it may be divided and the oesophagus and trachea closed primarily. The strap muscles are mobilized and placed between the oesophagus and trachea to buttress the closure, thus reducing the potential for breakdown and recurrence. In the thorax the closure can be protected with a pleural and intercostal muscle flap. Large fistulae may require tracheal resection and reconstruction. When a tracheo-oesophageal fistula occurs as a complication of oesophagectomy the gastric tube may have to be removed and an interposition graft, using colon or jejunum, fashioned.

OPERATIVE MANAGEMENT OF COMPLICATIONS OF UPPER GASTROINTESTINAL SURGERY

Haemorrhage

EARLY POSTOPERATIVE HAEMORRHAGE

Intraluminal haemorrhage after a gastric resection or anastomosis is usually due to bleeding from a suture line. The patient may have melaena, or fresh blood in the nasogastric tube. Most bleeding is self-limiting and settles spontaneously, but if the bleeding is excessive or persists, then an endoscopy should be performed. Minimal insufflation is used, and diathermy should be avoided if the primary anastomosis was formed using staples. If endoscopic control of significant bleeding is unsuccessful, then re-laparotomy is mandatory.

In patients who have had a subtotal gastrectomy, a transverse incision is made in the stomach remnant just above the anastomosis. Alternatively, existing suture lines such as a gastrojejunal anastomosis, or a pyloroplasty, are reopened. Following gastric aspiration, and washout, a bleeding point can usually be identified, which can then be controlled by under-sewing the vessel. Occasionally, the bleeding point is from a duodenal ulcer, which will require an anterior duodenotomy to provide adequate access. There should be no hesitation in deciding to convert a Billroth I to a Billroth II anastomosis if there is difficulty in controlling a duodenal bleed.

A major intraperitoneal bleed most commonly results from an unrecognized splenic injury, or a ligature that has slipped from a gastric vessel. Laparotomy for control of haemorrhage is indicated. Mediastinal bleeding may be from the azygos vein or from oesophageal branches of the aorta. Even when the original oesophageal dissection has been performed transhiatally, access to deal with this emergency will require a thoracotomy.

SECONDARY HAEMORRHAGE

This usually occurs around 2 weeks after surgery, and is associated with intra-abdominal sepsis. The tissue is friable and any bleeding vessel is difficult to secure. As discussed in Chapter 14, interventional radiology and embolization may be a better solution than surgery. However, the haemorrhage may be sudden and torrential, and immediate laparotomy may then be the only option. A supra-coeliac aortic clamp will sometimes provide temporary control in this situation (see Chapter 6).

Anastomotic failure

Anastomotic failure presents as a wide range of clinical scenarios. At one end of the spectrum is a patient who is clinically well but has a subclinical leak, in which there is radiological evidence of extravasation of contrast. Generally, these settle by limiting oral intake for a few days. At the other end of the spectrum is a patient who is profoundly unwell, in whom the gastric remnant, or the oesophageal conduit which has been used for the anastomosis, has necrosed.

ISCHAEMIC NECROSIS OF THE GASTRIC REMNANT OR CONDUIT

Proximal gastric remnant

This serious complication of a distal gastric resection is fortunately uncommon. Predisposing factors include ligation of the left gastric artery, combined with excessive mobilization of the greater curvature with compromise of the blood supply from the short gastric vessels, particularly in association with a splenectomy. If the entire remnant has necrosed, then a completion gastrectomy with Roux-en-Y reconstruction will be required. If the ischaemia extends to the distal oesophagus then a primary anastomosis is problematic. A cervical oesophagostomy is performed, with colonic or jejunal interposition reconstruction at a later stage.

Gastric, colonic or jejunal conduit

The blood supply of the stomach, which has been mobilized to bring it up for an anastomosis to the proximal oesophagus, is vulnerable. Alternative oesophageal conduits are similarly vulnerable. Postoperative ischaemic necrosis of a conduit is associated with a high mortality, not least as surgical intervention in the form of a thoracotomy is usually necessary. The necrotic part of the conduit is resected and the viable portion returned intra-abdominally. A cervical oesophagostomy is then performed with future reconstruction possible if the patient survives.

ANASTOMOTIC DEHISCENCE

The presentation of anastomotic dehiscence is varied. Patients may have systemic sepsis from thoracic or peritoneal soiling, or a minor leak may only be demonstrated on contrast imaging. An anastomotic leak in the neck will usually present with localized sepsis, or the development of a fistula. Subclinical leaks will usually settle if commencement of oral intake is postponed. Generalized peritonitis or mediastinitis will require reoperation, but with the advancement of radiological techniques the vast majority of localized abdominal and thoracic abscesses secondary to minor anastomotic leaks can be successfully managed with antibiotics and percutaneous drainage. Failure to improve despite percutaneous drainage is an indication for an open procedure. When it is necessary to re-explore the abdomen or chest, great caution must be exercised, as often the tissues are oedematous, friable, and prone to bleeding. Abscesses are drained and any anastomotic breakdown defunctioned by fashioning an appropriate stoma. Re-suturing a leaking anastomosis in the presence of contamination is not recommended.

Oesophageal anastomotic leakage

This is a challenging complication, and the lethal consequences of an intrathoracic anastomotic dehiscence has led to an upsurge in popularity for transhiatal oesophagectomy with a cervical anastomosis. While the leak rate for cervical anastomosis is higher, it is associated with a better outcome. If leakage arises from a cervical anastomosis then the wound is opened, irrigated, and left on free drainage. The patient is commenced on jejunostomy feeding and is usually allowed oral fluids within a few days. Occasionally, the cervical anastomotic breakdown is associated with major ischaemia requiring reoperation.

Duodenal stump blow out

This is a life-threatening complication that may occur following any procedure that involves division and closure of the duodenum, as in a Billroth II or a total gastrectomy. An ultrasound scan may identify a fluid collection in the region of the duodenal stump, and aspiration of the collection confirms bile. Small collections may be managed by percutaneous radiological drainage, in combination with broad-spectrum antibiotics and parenteral nutrition. If radiological drainage is unavailable, or is unsuccessful, then a laparotomy is necessary. Unfortunately, on re-entering the abdomen there is often considerable inflammation and sepsis with anatomical distortion. Primary closure is not safe in this hostile environment. Instead, a controlled fistula should be created. A distal feeding tube to enable enteral nutrition is important for postoperative recovery. Octreotide may reduce the fistulous output. An adequately drained controlled duodenal fistula will usually heal unless there is local infection, mechanical obstruction of the afferent limb, associated pancreatitis, or a persistent duodenal ulcer.

Acute gastroparesis

Most patients, following upper gastrointestinal tract surgery, have a degree of gastric atony which generally recovers within 10–12 days. The condition is exacerbated in patients with underlying diabetes, hypothyroidism, preoperative gastric outlet obstruction, and in those who have undergone a truncal vagotomy. Delayed gastric emptying may also occur secondary to stomal oedema. Conservative management consists of nasogastric tube insertion to decompress the stomach, correction of electrolyte imbalances, maintenance of nutrition and the use of prokinetics, such as erythromycin. If symptoms do not respond to conservative management, which should be instigated for a minimum of 4 weeks, then surgical intervention may be required to rule out any underlying mechanical problem.

Chylous leak

Chylothorax is a collection of chyle within the mediastinum or pleural cavity. It occurs following damage to the thoracic duct or right bronchomediastinal trunk. Often there may be a delay of up to 10 days between the time of injury and onset of symptoms. Persistent output from the chest drain following an oesophagectomy or the development of a pleural effusion, usually on the right, should arouse suspicion. Biochemical analysis of the pleural aspirate will confirm a large triglyceride and chylomicron content. Chylothorax carries a mortality rate of 30 per cent and must be actively managed.[17]

- *Conservative management*, which includes total parenteral nutrition in addition to *somatostatin* to reduce chylous output, has a success rate of approximately 50 per cent. High-volume iatrogenic chylothorax – defined as over 1 L of chyle produced each day for 4–6 days – is most unlikely to respond to conservative management, and the patient becomes progressively metabolically and nutritionally compromised. Early surgery is therefore recommended for these high-volume leaks. A smaller volume leak which has persisted for over 2 weeks is another indication for surgical intervention.
- *Surgical intervention*: at re-exploration there are two main choices. The thoracic duct can be ligated just above the diaphragm or, alternatively, the laceration can be localized and repaired. Preoperative administration of cream via the nasogastric or feeding jejunostomy tube will increase the production of chyle and may help in the identification of the injured duct. The use of methylene blue dye is not recommended due to tissue staining that interferes with visualization.

Late complications of gastric surgery

Both resectional and non-resectional gastric surgery create permanent changes in gastrointestinal function. Some of the adverse consequences of these changes can be modified by further surgical intervention.

ALKALINE REFLUX GASTRITIS

Reflux of alkaline intestinal contents, particularly bile, into the stomach causes mucosal damage. Enterogastric reflux is most common after a Billroth II gastrectomy or a gastroenterostomy. Further reflux into the oesophagus can then cause an alkaline oesophagitis. Conservative management, including the use of bile-sequestering agents, provides little symptomatic relief, but further surgery can be very effective.

In those patients who have had a truncal vagotomy with gastroenterostomy, the simplest solution is to take down the gastroenterostomy. Gastric stasis is seldom a problem if more than a year has elapsed since the initial surgery, as poor post-vagotomy gastric tone improves with time. However, there is a risk of recurrent duodenal ulceration if the original vagotomy was incomplete. Reversal of the gastroenterostomy is contraindicated if there is any stenosis of the pylorus. Instead, an antrectomy with a Roux loop reconstruction should be considered.

After a Billroth II gastrectomy, the best method of controlling the patient's symptoms is to convert the gastric drainage to a Roux-en-Y gastrojejunostomy. The function of the Roux limb is to direct the alkaline contents 45–60 cm beyond the gastric remnant, thereby reducing the potential for bile reflux. A Billroth II anastomosis can easily be converted to a Roux loop (Fig. 17.14). However, this is an ulcerogenic manoeuvre as it diverts the buffering effect of the alkaline gastrointestinal secretions from the gastroenteric anastomosis. This is an important consideration if no vagotomy was performed, and the gastrectomy was relatively conservative with retention of much of the parietal cell mass. The addition of a vagotomy should therefore be considered, especially if the original operation was for peptic ulceration.

Enterogastric reflux can also occur in a retrograde fashion when the pyloric sphincter has been destroyed by a pyloroplasty, or has been excised and continuity restored by a Billroth I anastomosis. The reversal of a pyloroplasty is relatively straightforward and may be successful. The time that has elapsed since the surgery must again be considered. If the pylorus is too scarred to be reconstructed, an antrectomy with a Roux loop reconstruction is again the favoured option if the original operation was a vagotomy and pyloroplasty. When the previous surgery was a Billroth I gastrectomy this can be revised to a Roux loop anastomosis. The loss of buffering alkali to this anastomosis must again be considered. One manoeuvre for achieving Roux loop drainage without taking down the original anastomosis is with the De Meester duodenal switch procedure, which is illustrated in Figure 17.15. This can also be a useful operation for the alkaline reflux gastritis and oesophagitis, which can be particularly troublesome after an oesophagectomy that was combined with a proximal partial gastrectomy.

Interposition of an isolated isoperistaltic jejunal loop as a spacer between the gastric remnant and duodenal stump can also reduce bile reflux after a Billroth I gastrectomy (Fig. 17.16).

DUMPING SYNDROME

This is one of the commonest complications of gastric surgery, and is the result of the lack of an effective pyloric sphincter to control delivery of a glucose-rich meal into the small intestine.

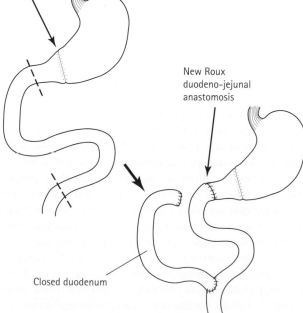

Original Billroth I anastomosis

New Roux duodeno-jejunal anastomosis

Closed duodenum

Figure 17.15 *De Meester duodenal switch operation after a previous Billroth I gastrectomy.*

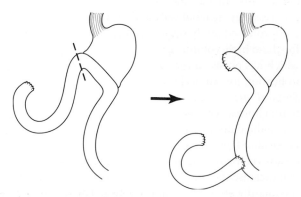

Figure 17.14 *A Billroth II anastomosis can be easily converted to a Roux loop.*

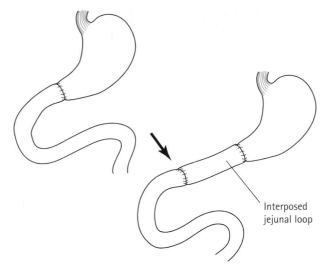

Figure 17.16 *An interposed isolated jejunal loop can reduce bile reflux into the stomach by acting as a spacer. If it is reversed it will slow gastric emptying.*

- *Early dumping* occurs within a few minutes of the meal, as the hyperosmolar intestinal contents cause significant fluid shifts into the intestinal lumen. This results in epigastric pain and explosive diarrhoea in association with systemic vasomotor symptoms secondary to the hypovolaemia.
- *Late dumping* occurs several hours after a meal. The large glucose load presented to the small intestine causes hyperglycaemia, followed by a compensatory hyperinsulinaemia which then results in a later hypoglycaemia and associated systemic symptoms.

The majority of these patients respond to dietary manipulation that consists of small-volume, frequent meals which are low in refined carbohydrate. Octreotide, when taken preprandially, is associated with a significant improvement in vasomotor and gastrointestinal symptoms. If symptoms persist, then surgical intervention should be considered to slow the delivery of gastric contents into the bowel. The reconstruction of a pylorus after a pyloroplasty, or the dismemberment of a gastroenterostomy as described above, can be successful. The conversion from a Billroth I or Billroth II reconstruction to a Roux-en-Y loop may be effective as it slows the delivery of gastric contents into the small bowel. The interposition of ante-peristaltic loops of jejunum has also been attempted (see Fig. 17.16).

AFFERENT AND EFFERENT LOOP SYNDROME

Afferent and efferent loop syndromes occur secondary to partial, or complete, loop obstruction.

- *Afferent loop syndrome* may present acutely early in the postoperative period following a Billroth II gastrectomy,

and is a surgical emergency. The closed loop is at imminent risk of perforation, usually as a duodenal stump blow-out. There may be an associated rise in serum amylase levels, giving rise to a misdiagnosis of acute pancreatitis. A sub-acute or chronic presentation, with non-specific symptoms, is more common. Endoscopy or water-soluble contrast studies will identify a dilated afferent limb. Surgical options include the conversion of a Billroth II to a Billroth I reconstruction, or to a Roux-en-Y reconstruction with a long afferent limb.
- *Efferent loop syndrome* is much less common, and usually occurs secondary to adhesions, internal herniation or jejunogastric intussusception. Patients present with symptoms of a proximal small bowel obstruction. Surgical intervention is indicated.

STOMAL ULCERATION

Stomal ulceration is most frequently seen after surgery for peptic ulcer disease. The ulcer occurs where the jejunum has been anastomosed to the stomach, and exposed to gastric acid. A gastroenterostomy is thus prone to stomal ulceration if a vagotomy has not been performed, and a Roux loop drainage is even more vulnerable as the buffering effects of alkaline intestinal secretions at the anastomosis are absent. A Roux loop should therefore ideally be used either to a small gastric remnant with less acid-producing potential, or in combination with a vagotomy. Management of recurrent and stomal ulceration is initially conservative and consists of proton-pump inhibition, eradication of *Helicobacter pylori* and avoidance of aggravating factors. If ulcers are refractory to medical management, the surgical options depend on the previous surgery. Completion vagotomy, combined with antrectomy is often the best option.

In both stomal and recurrent ulceration, an underlying malignancy, and also underlying pathologies such as Zollinger–Ellison syndrome, must be excluded. Ulceration associated with gastrinomas was discussed above in the section relating to peptic ulcer.

Gastrojejunocolic fistula

This is a fistula between a gastroenterostomy and the transverse colon (Fig. 17.17). It was once a well-recognized complication of a long-standing stomal ulcer, but is now very rare in the developed world. Patients present with intractable diarrhoea from the bacterial contamination of the small bowel, giving rise to severe nutritional deficiencies and weight loss. The situation is best managed by antrectomy, removal of the involved colonic segment followed by a gastroduodenal or gastrojejunal anastomosis and primary colonic anastomosis. In severely ill patients this may have to be a staged procedure.

A gastrocolic fistula can also occur secondary to a gastric or colonic neoplasm, or as a complication of gastric surgery.

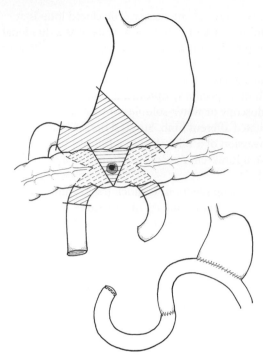

Figure 17.17 *Resection for a gastrojejunocolic fistula.*

UPPER GASTROINTESTINAL SURGERY IN INFANCY

Oesophageal atresia and tracheo-oesophageal fistula

This is a congenital failure of development of the mid-portion of the oesophagus, and in most instances the upper oesophagus ends blindly. Failure of intra-uterine swallowing by the foetus results in hydramnios and, as a result affected infants are often born prematurely. The accumulation of unswallowed saliva should further arouse suspicion of the diagnosis, which is confirmed by the failure to pass a naso-gastric tube into the stomach. Delay in diagnosis, until aspiration occurs with the first attempted feed, increases the mortality and morbidity of the subsequent surgery. In around 85 per cent of cases the atresia is associated with a tracheo-oesophageal fistula, and the two variants of the malformation are considered separately.

OESOPHAGEAL ATRESIA WITH A FISTULA

This is the commonest abnormality. The atretic segment is normally short, with the upper oesophagus ending blindly and close to the fistula between the trachea and the distal segment of oesophagus (Fig. 17.18a). This distal fistula is confirmed by the presence of gas within the stomach on X-ray. Surgical management consists of emergency repair of the fistula, combined with mobilization of the proximal and distal oesophagus, to allow a primary oesophageal anastomosis. The approach is via a right posterolateral thoracotomy

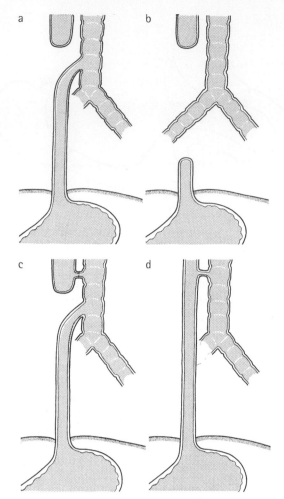

Figure 17.18 *Congenital tracheo-oesophageal anomalies. (a) Short segment atresia with a fistula to the distal oesophagus; (b) long segment atresia without fistula; (c) short atresia with double fistulae; (d) fistula without atresia.*

through the 4th intercostal space. The pleura is swept off the chest wall and the oesophagus approached extrapleurally. The azygos vein must be divided for adequate exposure. It is sometimes not possible to approximate the oesophageal ends even after mobilization, and any further management must be similar to the situation described below.

OESOPHAGEAL ATRESIA WITHOUT A FISTULA

This is confirmed by the absence of a gastric air shadow on X-ray. In many of these cases the atretic segment is of significant length, and a primary anastomotic repair is not possible (Fig. 17.18b). However, in the absence of a fistula the situation can be managed in the short term by gastrostomy feeding and drainage of the blind upper pouch, either by continuous suction or by the formation of a cervical oesophagostomy. The cervical approach to the oesophagus is described above and in Chapter 9. Later definitive reconstruction of the oesophagus may require the creation of a gastric tube, or the interposition of a jejunal or colonic conduit. A colonic conduit is associated with fewer problems with reflux.

OTHER VARIATIONS OF THE SYNDROME

These are all less common (Fig. 17.18c and d). The diagnosis may be more difficult, and delayed, but the surgical management follows similar principles.

The surgery and perioperative care of infants with this condition are complex, and the common associated gastrointestinal, cardiac or renal anomalies must be sought as they may alter management. Transfer to a specialist centre for assessment and surgery is mandatory. Before and during transfer a blind upper oesophageal pouch should be kept empty of secretions by repeated, or continuous, aspiration. Artificial ventilation may be necessary for coexistent respiratory distress, but unless the endotracheal tube can be placed sufficiently distal to occlude any fistula, increasing gaseous distension of the stomach via the fistula can compound the problems. Those surgeons unable to transfer such infants are unlikely to have anaesthetic and intensive care facilities to make a neonatal thoracotomy a viable undertaking.

Duodenal atresia

The infant presents with neonatal vomiting, which in two-thirds of cases will be bile-stained, reflecting the higher incidence of atresia distal, rather than proximal, to the ampulla of Vater. The diagnosis is confirmed by the 'double bubble' X-ray appearance of distension and gas restricted to the stomach and duodenum. There is a high incidence of other congenital abnormalities and a strong association with Down's syndrome. Surgery consists of restoring intestinal continuity with a duodenoduodenostomy (Fig. 17.19), or if this is impractical, with a retrocolic duodenojejunostomy. Gastrojejunostomy should be avoided because of stasis and ulceration in the proximal duodenum. A transanastomotic feeding tube should be considered. On occasion, a duodenal diaphragm, rather than an atresia, is the only cause of the obstruction, and a duodenotomy and excision of the diaphragm is then the more appropriate surgical manoeuvre. A malrotation (see Chapter 22) may present neonatally with duodenal obstruction and should be considered in the differential diagnosis.

Infantile hypertrophic pyloric stenosis

This is an acquired condition of unknown aetiology which classically presents at about 4 weeks after birth. The infant is hungry, but persistently vomits the whole of a feed in a characteristically projectile fashion. Visible gastric peristalsis may be observed during a feed, and the pyloric 'tumour' of hypertrophied muscle can be palpated after a vomit. Confirmatory diagnosis is now more often established by ultrasound examination. Treatment consists of correction of the dehydration,

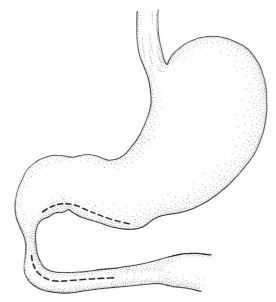

Figure 17.19   *Duodenal atresia. The incisions for a duodenoduodenotomy are marked.*

hypokalaemia and the metabolic alkalosis, followed by surgical relief of the obstruction with a Ramstedt's pyloromyotomy. The surgery is straightforward, but many general surgeons will have to transfer these infants to regional paediatric centres for optimum anaesthetic care. Before the advent of safe general anaesthesia for these babies, the operation was frequently performed under sedation, restraint and local infiltrative anaesthesia of the abdominal wall. This may still be the safest alternative for a surgeon practising in a hospital with very limited facilities, and no option of referral.

At operation, a 3- to 4-cm transverse incision is made in the right upper quadrant. This may be either a muscle-cutting or a muscle-splitting incision, but the former affords better access. The pyloric tumour is delivered into the wound, and the serosa and superficial muscle fibres of the tumour are incised in its long axis by scalpel or diathermy. The deeper fibres can be disrupted by distracting the edges of the incision, as great care must be taken to avoid breaching the mucosa, especially at the level of the duodenal fornix (Fig. 17.20). Blunt forceps can be used to push the mucosa gently down and out of danger as the last fibres are divided. On completion of the operation, the intact mucosa must be seen bulging into the depths of the whole length of the incision, as inadequate release will result in persistent pyloric obstruction postoperatively. Therefore, it is also important that the releasing incision extends over the whole length of the tumour, and it must be extended proximally for a few centimetres onto the gastric antrum, and distally onto the first part of the duodenum. A mucosal breach should be sought and, if one has occurred, it is closed with an absorbable suture. Wound dehiscence is not infrequent and abdominal closure must be meticulous, using an absorbable suture material which loses tensile strength slowly.

a

b

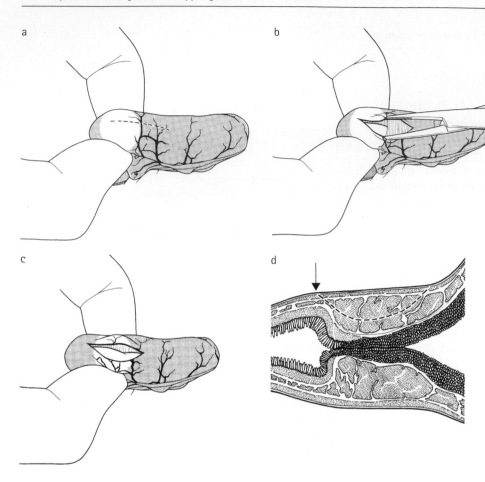

c

d

Figure 17.20 *Ramstedt's operation. (a) The posterior part of the tumour is held firmly pinched between finger and thumb. The dotted line indicates the incision. (b) Mosquito artery forceps introduced into the incision and spread will split the deepest hypertrophied muscle fibres. (c) The pyloromyotomy is complete when intact mucosa bulges into the base of the whole incision. (d) A cross-sectional view of the tumour shows the vulnerability of the mucosa of the duodenal fornix to inadvertent penetration.*

Gastro-oesophageal reflux

This condition is common in infancy and early childhood, and medical management of severe cases is not always successful. Presentation is most often with vomiting, but respiratory symptoms from aspiration, dental decay from increased intra-oral acidity and oesophagitis with stricture formation also occur. Severe gastro-oesophageal reflux is commonly encountered in infants with neurological impairment, where it can be a major cause of their failure to thrive. Many children who require long-term gastrostomy feeding also require anti-reflux surgery. The principles of surgery in infancy for this condition are similar to those in adults.

REFERENCES

1. Barham CP, Alderson D. Pathophysiology and investigations of GORD and motility disorders. In: MS Griffin, SA Raimes (eds), *Upper Gastrointestinal Surgery*, 2nd edn. London: Baillière Tindall, 2001.

2. Pera M, Trastek VF, Carpenter HA, *et al*. Barrett's esophagus with high-grade dysplasia: an indication for esophagectomy? *Ann Thorac Surg* 1992; **54**: 199–204.

3. Primrose JN, Axon AT, Johnston D. Highly selective vagotomy and duodenal ulcers that fail to respond to H2 antagonists. *Br Med J* 1988; **296**: 1031–5.

4. Munro WS, Bajwa F, Menzies D. Laparoscopic repair of perforated duodenal ulcers with a falciform ligament patch. *Ann R Coll Surg Engl* 1996; **78**: 390–1.

5. Scopinaro N, Adami GF, Marinari GM, *et al*. Biliopancreatic diversion. *World J Surg* 1998; **22**: 936–46.

6. Forsell P, Hallerback B, Glise H, *et al*. Complications following Swedish adjustable gastric banding: a long term follow-up. *Obes Surg* 2001; **9**: 11–16.

7. Sawai K, Takahashi T, Suzuki H. New trends in surgery for gastric cancer in Japan. *J Surg Oncol* 1994; **56**: 221–6.

8. Maruyama K, Gunven P, Okabayashi K, *et al*. Lymph node metastases of gastric cancer. General pattern in 1931 patients. *Ann Surg* 1989; **210**: 596–602.

9. (a) Ferguson JI, Paterson-Brown S. Staging of oesophageal and gastric cancer. In: MS Griffin, SA Raimes (eds), *Upper Gastrointestinal Surgery*, 2nd edn, pp. 57–91. London: Baillière Tindall, 2001. (b) Raimes SA. Surgery for cancer of the stomach. In: MS Griffin, SA Raimes (eds), *Upper Gastrointestinal Surgery*, 2nd edn. pp. 155–202. London: Baillière Tindall, 2001.

10. Yonemura Y, Kawamura T, Nojima M, *et al*. Postoperative results of left upper abdominal evisceration for advanced gastric cancer. *Hepatogastroenterology* 2000; **47**: 571–4.

11. Al-Akwaa AM, Siddiqui N, Al-Mofleh IA. Primary gastric lymphoma. *World J Gastroenterol* 2004; **10**: 5–11.

12. Wijnhoven BP, Siersema PD, Hop WC, *et al*. Adenocarcinomas of the distal oesophagus and gastric cardia are one clinical entity. Rotterdam Oesophageal Tumour Study Group. *Br J Surg* 1999; **86**: 529–35.

13. Gotley DC, Beard J, Cooper MJ, *et al*. Abdominocervical (transhiatal) oesophagectomy in the management of oesophageal carcinoma. *Br J Surg* 1990; **77**: 815–19.

14. Hulscher JB, Tijssen JG, Obertop H, *et al*. Transthoracic versus transhiatal resection for carcinoma of the esophagus: a meta-analysis. *Ann Thorac Surg* 2001; **72**: 306–13.

15. Liu JF, Wang QZ, Hou J. Surgical treatment of the oesophagus and gastric cardia in Hebei, China. *Br J Surg* 2004; **91**: 90–8.

16. Lewis I. The surgical treatment of carcinoma of the oesophagus with special reference to a new operation for growths of the middle third. *Br J Surg* 1946; **34**: 18–30.

17. Wemyss-Holden SA, Launois B, Maddern GJ. Management of thoracic duct injuries after oesophagectomy. Review. *Br J Surg* 2001; **88**: 1442–8.

18

GALLBLADDER AND BILIARY SURGERY

ROWAN PARKS AND FENELLA WELSH

ANATOMY

The gallbladder

The gallbladder is pear-shaped and about 10 cm in length. It is attached to the inferior surface of the right lobe of the liver and is enclosed within a peritoneal sheath. The extent of this attachment varies from a gallbladder that is embedded deeply within the liver, to one that presents on a mesentery, rendering it liable to volvulus. Commonly, the lower end or fundus of the gallbladder is completely covered with peritoneum and projects slightly beyond the free margin of the liver. The body and neck are usually covered only on three sides by peritoneum, the gallbladder being attached anteriorly to the liver by loose connective tissue and easily separated from it. The neck narrows down to form the cystic duct. If a gallstone becomes lodged in the neck of the gallbladder, it creates a dilatation at this point, known as Hartmann's pouch. The cystic duct, which is of variable length and width, runs backwards and medially and joins the common hepatic duct to form the bile duct. As the bile duct is still more often known to surgeons as the common bile duct, this name is used predominantly in the text. The mucosa of the cystic duct is arranged in spiral folds, the valve of Heister. The gallbladder is supplied by the cystic artery, which is usually a branch of the right hepatic artery, though this is very variable.

The bile ducts

The right and left hepatic ducts emerge from the liver through the porta hepatis and unite to form the common hepatic duct, which is in turn joined by the cystic duct to form the common bile duct (the bile duct). The common bile duct is about 10 cm long and up to 7 mm in diameter. It runs down behind the first part of the duodenum, then either lies in a groove on the back of the head of pancreas or tunnels the gland substance, and ends by passing obliquely through the posteromedial wall of the second part of the duodenum. The extreme lower end of the duct is accompanied by the main pancreatic duct (of Wirsung), running parallel to it and uniting with it to form the ampulla of Vater, which opens into the duodenum at the summit of a papilla. The ends of each duct and the ampulla are surrounded by circular muscle fibres, forming the sphincter of Oddi. Phasic contractions of the sphincter allow bile flow into the duodenum, and possibly prevent reflux of duodenal contents into the bile and pancreatic ducts.

Relations

The hepatic ducts and the supraduodenal part of the common bile duct lie in the right free border of the lesser omentum. The hepatic artery lies medial to the common bile duct, with the portal vein posteriorly. The right hepatic artery crosses behind the common hepatic duct, before it gives off its cystic branch (Fig. 18.1).

Anomalies

The above description of the anatomic relationship between the bile ducts and associated blood vessels is that given in standard textbooks of anatomy. It should be noted however, that considerable variation may exist, and those that occur most commonly are shown in Figure 18.2. A knowledge of such 'anomalies' is of great importance to the surgeon, as failure to recognize these at operation may lead to complications. Thus, the severance of an anomalous or accessory

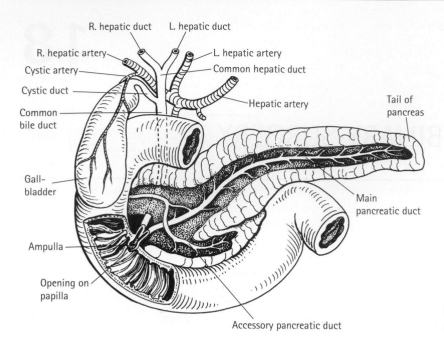

Figure 18.1   *The relationship of the gallbladder and bile ducts to the duodenum and head of the pancreas.*

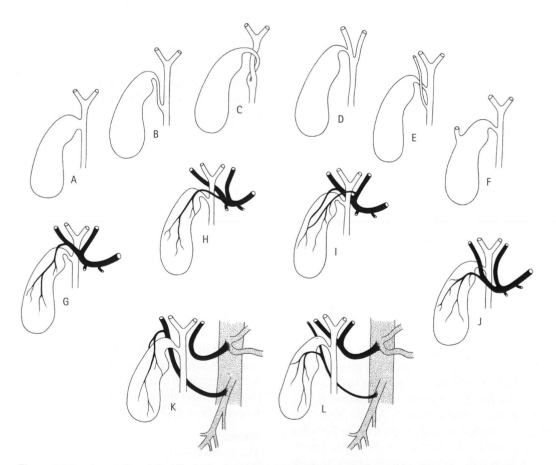

Figure 18.2   *Anomalies of the bile ducts. A = short wide cystic duct; B = long cystic duct; C = long cystic duct winding round the hepatic duct; D = cystic duct joining right hepatic duct; E = accessory hepatic duct joining common bile duct; F = accessory hepatic duct draining into gallbladder; G = right hepatic artery crossing in front of common hepatic duct; H = cystic artery arising low and crossing in front of common hepatic duct; I = accessory cystic artery from left hepatic artery; J = low division of hepatic artery; K = right hepatic artery arising from superior mesenteric artery (SMA); L = accessory right hepatic artery arising from SMA.*

hepatic duct would lead to a bile leak and consequent biliary peritonitis, while the ligation of an abnormally placed right hepatic artery might produce fatal hepatic infarction. Other anomalies render the right hepatic duct or common bile duct liable to injury.

GENERAL CONSIDERATIONS IN BILIARY SURGERY

Biliary physiology

Each day, between 0.5 and 1.5 L of bile are excreted from the ampulla of Vater, and most of the constituents are absorbed in the distal ileum. Hepatic bile is diverted into the gallbladder due to differential pressures within the biliary tree. Bile is concentrated within the gallbladder and intermittently expelled by spontaneous contractions, or in response to cholecystokinin release, which occurs after eating. Cholecystokinin and glucagon allow relaxation of the sphincter of Oddi to facilitate bile flow into the duodenum.

Investigation of biliary disease

Any operation on the biliary tract should be approached with the maximum possible information, and adequate time for investigation should be provided. Liver function tests include serum bilirubin (conjugated and unconjugated), serum enzymes (transaminases, alkaline phosphatase) and tests of synthetic function (albumin, prothrombin time, urea). Appropriate imaging of the biliary tract may include transabdominal ultrasonography (USS), endoscopic (EUS) or laparoscopic ultrasound (LapUS), endoscopic retrograde cholangiopancreatography (ERCP), percutaneous transhepatic cholangiography (PTC), radionucleotide scans (HIDA), computed tomography (CT) with vascular reconstruction, CTAP (CT angio-portography), magnetic resonance imaging (MRI) and magnetic resonance cholangiopancreatography (MRCP), angiography or portal venography and positron emission tomography (PET). The relative merits/ potential of each of these is summarized in Table 18.1.

Preparation for biliary surgery

The general preoperative preparation, and the intraoperative and postoperative management of patients is outlined in Appendices I–III. Broad-spectrum antibiotics are recommended in emergency biliary surgery, or if exploration of the common bile duct is anticipated. Subcutaneous heparin prophylaxis is indicated, except when coagulation is impaired.

ADDITIONAL PREPARATION IN THE JAUNDICED PATIENT

Both morbidity and mortality are higher following surgery in jaundiced patients, and patients must be meticulously opti-

mized for surgery.[1] The increased risks and appropriate therapeutic manoeuvres are as follows:

- *Haemorrhage.* In obstructive jaundice there is impaired absorption of the fat-soluble vitamin K due to failure of bile salts to reach the intestine. This results in failure to synthesize clotting factors II, VII, IX and X, and in turn to a coagulopathy which may manifest itself with a prolonged prothrombin time. This is corrected by administering intravenous vitamin K (10 mg per day), and there should be a low threshold for administering blood products such as fresh-frozen plasma during the perioperative period.

- *Infection.* The majority of patients with obstructive jaundice, and virtually all of those in whom the cause is gallstones, have infected bile. Parenteral antibiotics (ampicillin and gentamicin, a second- or third-generation cephalosporin, or piperacillin and tazobactam; Tazocin) should be given on induction of anaesthesia and continued or not, depending on the operation/operative findings.

- *Renal failure.* Renal tubular function is compromised in jaundiced patients due to: (i) direct action of bilirubin on the tubules; (ii) a degree of vascular shunting in the kidney leading to relative cortical ischaemia; (iii) preoperative hypovolaemia; and (iv) hypotension associated with biliary sepsis. Adequate preoperative hydration is essential to minimize the risk of acute renal failure. An intravenous infusion is set up to aim for a urine output of about 1 ml /kg per hour, which must be accurately recorded. All patients should be catheterized after induction of anaesthesia, in order to monitor urine output during the operation and hourly in the postoperative period.

  Hepatorenal syndrome. Patients with liver disease may also develop renal failure in the absence of clinical, laboratory or other known causes of renal failure – the hepatorenal syndrome. This unexplained renal failure in patients with liver disease is a clinical diagnosis of exclusion, and improvement of renal function appears to be dependent on recovery of liver function. Indeed, renal function in such patients who undergo liver transplantation returns to normal.

Biliary operations

POSITION OF THE PATIENT

The patient should be positioned supine on an operating table that allows radiographic screening for intraoperative cholangiography.

INCISIONS FOR OPEN PROCEDURES

The surgeon has a choice of several incisions, each of which allows good access to the biliary tree.

Table 18.1 *Imaging modalities in biliary disease.*

Imaging modality	Diagnostic potential	Therapeutic potential	Limitations
USS Trans-abdominal ultrasonography	Index investigation in the evaluation of biliary tree obstruction, gallbladder/bile duct stones, intrahepatic cysts/abscess/metastases, intra-abdominal collections/free fluid	Percutaneous drainage	Operator-dependent More difficult in the obese. Images can be obscured by bowel gas
EUS Endoscopic ultrasonography	Evaluation of (distal) biliary tree obstruction Bile duct stones. Biopsy (mass/lymph node)	None	Operator-dependent
LapUS Laparoscopic ultrasonography	Evaluation of malignant biliary strictures (size/relationship to portal vein/hepatic arteries/lymph node involvement/liver metastases/peritoneal disease) Biopsy (mass/lymph node)	None	Operator-dependent
ERCP Endoscopic retrograde cholangio-pancreatography	Evaluation of biliary tree obstruction Biliary brushings/biopsy Biliary manometry	Sphincterotomy. Stone extraction. Endobiliary stenting (plastic/metal).	Operator-dependent. Technically difficult if previous polya gastrectomy or duodenal diverticulum. Risk of bleeding/duodenal perforation/pancreatitis/cholangitis
PTC Percutaneous transhepatic cholangiography	Evaluation of biliary tree obstruction (particularly hilar cholangiocarcinoma) Bile for cytology	Percutaneous biliary drainage/stenting (plastic/metal).	Operator-dependent. Risk of bleeding/duodenal perforation/cholangitis
HIDA scan Radionucleotide scan	Demonstration of patent biliary tree or biliary–enteric anastomosis	None	No value in obstructive jaundice as isotope is not excreted into an obstructed system
Spiral CT Spiral computed tomography	Diagnosis and staging of disease – newer scanners provide biliary and vascular reconstruction Monitoring response to treatment	Percutaneous drainage	Quality of scanner
CTAP Computed tomographic angio-portography	Evaluation of hepatic metastases	None	Complications of arterial puncture. Flow artefacts
MRI Magnetic resonance imaging	Evaluation of liver lesions (HCC/haemangioma/intrahepatic cholangiocarcinoma), metastases	None	Claustrophobia Contraindicated with iron-containing implants
MRCP Magnetic resonance cholangio-panreatography	Biliary tree dilatation. Bile duct stones. Evaluation of malignant biliary strictures (particularly hilar cholangiocarcinoma) Avoids complications of ERCP	None	As for MRI. Small common bile duct stones may be missed Difficult to interpret if air in the biliary tree
Selective visceral angiography	Staging of cholangiocarcinoma (vascular involvement) Aetiology of haemobilia	Embolization	Complications of arterial puncture
PET Positron emission tomography	Recurrent malignancy, particularly detection of small volume disease. Monitoring response to treatment	None	Difficulty in distinguishing between inflammation/tumour, although this problem is becoming less with more selective tracers. Expensive/limited availability

- *Bilateral subcostal/roof-top*: this provides wide access to the upper abdomen and allows mobilization of the liver. The use of fixed subcostal retractors (e.g. Doyen's blades) and a fixed adaptable retractor system (e.g. the Omnitract) allows constant wide exposure. This is an incision which may be suitable for a major biliary procedure.
- *Kocher's subcostal*: this is the classic *oblique muscle-cutting* incision for an open cholecystectomy. It allows good access, especially in patients with a wide costal angle.
- *Right upper quadrant transverse*: this alternative to the Kocher incision provides a good cosmetic result.
- *Right paramedian*: this is either rectus-displacing or rectus-splitting, and is most suitable for patients with a narrow costal angle; it allows a full laparotomy.
- *Mayo-Robson (Hockey stick):* this is a combination of a paramedian and a medial subcostal incision.
- *Upper midline*: some surgeons prefer to operate on the biliary tree through a midline incision while standing to the left of the patient.

PRELIMINARY EXPLORATION

The stomach and duodenum are examined first. The duodenum is frequently adherent to the gallbladder or to an area of biliary stricture, and it is gently retracted down and the adhesions divided. The stomach and duodenum are then packed off, out of the operative field. The gallbladder is palpated for calculi, with particular attention being paid to the neck, in which a calculus may be overlooked, and the condition of the gallbladder wall is noted. In surgery for malignant disease, the entire abdomen must be carefully examined for evidence of tumour spread (nodal disease, liver metastases or peritoneal deposits).

In the presence of jaundice, special precautions must be observed. In view of the risk of haemorrhage, exploration is reduced to a minimum and gentleness is essential. Attention is directed to the common bile duct and to the pancreas, for it is here that the cause of the obstruction is most likely to be found.

INTRAOPERATIVE ULTRASOUND

Following preliminary exploration, intraoperative ultrasound, whilst being operator-dependent, can provide an invaluable aid to operative decision-making in the surgery for biliary disease. The examination starts by identifying the splenoportal junction behind the neck of the pancreas, with the superior mesenteric artery running posteriorly and the pancreatic duct anteriorly. The probe is passed over the head of pancreas, and any tumour mass within is noted, measured and its relationship with the portal vein determined. The portal vein, common bile duct and hepatic artery are traced upwards in the free edge of the lesser omentum, looking for the presence of aberrant arterial anatomy. The calibre of the common bile duct is noted, as are the presence of any stones or stent within. The probe is placed over the gallbladder and the thickness of the wall and presence of stones noted. Attention is then turned to the liver. The middle hepatic vein is identified and traced into the inferior vena cava (IVC). This marks the 'principle plane' of the liver – the true division between the right and left lobes. The liver is then examined in a systematic fashion, noting the presence and extent of biliary dilatation, liver cysts and tumours.

SPECIFIC BILIARY SURGICAL TECHNIQUES

Dissection
Even the simplest of biliary operations requires precise dissection in areas where there are important structures that must be preserved. Good access, illumination and assistance are all important. In the porta hepatis and in the lesser omentum, the bile ducts, the hepatic artery and its branches and the portal vein lie within the peritoneal fold. The isolation of these structures requires first the division of the overlying peritoneum with sharp dissection before the individual vessels and ducts can be cleared of fat, connective tissue and lymphatics. This clearance can be achieved by using a blunt dissection technique with, for example, a small 'peanut' swab, but this will not be possible until the peritoneum has been divided.

Suture material
Non-absorbable material should not be used in the biliary tree as it may form a nidus for stone formation. This is particularly important when suturing an opening into a large duct or when performing a biliary anastomosis, but it should also be avoided for bile duct closure or cystic duct ligation.

Anastomoses
The principles of biliary anastomoses are similar to those of other gastrointestinal anastomoses, which are discussed in more detail in Chapter 13. Interrupted absorbable sutures are suitable, but as the mucosa of the biliary tract is more adherent to the underlying muscle than that of the stomach and bowel, an extramucosal suture is not possible, and sutures have to be placed full thickness. The anastomoses are of small diameter structures, and early postoperative oedema can cause obstruction which may predispose to leakage. In the past, it was therefore standard practice to leave a stent or T-tube across an anastomosis, but many experienced biliary surgeons now believe that this is unnecessary, and may even cause further trauma.

SURGERY OF CHOLELITHIASIS

Although gallstones affect about 10 per cent of people in the Western world, more than 80 per cent of these people are asymptomatic. Cholecystectomy is not generally advocated in asymptomatic patients, but exceptions include those with sickle cell disease or hereditary spherocytosis, patients with a porcelain gallbladder (increased risk of malignancy) or those likely to be receiving long-term parenteral nutrition and who may rapidly develop sludge in their gallbladder. Diabetics respond particularly badly to emergency cholecystectomy, and whilst insufficient data are available to warrant prophylactic cholecystectomy, an aggressive surgical approach is advocated in diabetic patients with symptoms from gallstones. The commonest intervention for symptomatic cholelithiasis is removal of the gallbladder (cholecystectomy), as this is where almost all biliary calculi form. The indications and timing of cholecystectomy, or occasionally an emergency cholecystotomy, for symptomatic stones in the gallbladder varies with the presentation. Gallstones which have migrated into the common bile duct, but have failed to pass on into the duodenum, should be removed either surgically or endoscopically.

The complications of cholelithiasis are numerous, and include bilary colic, cholecystitis, obstructive jaundice, biliary strictures, cholangitis, pancreatitis and gallstone ileus.

BILIARY COLIC

The pain of biliary colic is due to gallbladder distension and contractions secondary to a gallstone occluding the cystic duct. The pain ceases when the gallstone drops back into the body of the gallbladder, or passes into the common bile duct. There may then be a transient episode of obstructive jaundice before the stone passes spontaneously into the duodenum. Following a single episode of biliary colic, the chances of further episodes of biliary pain or complications of gallstones are high (70 per cent), and these patients should be considered for elective cholecystectomy.

ACUTE CHOLECYSTITIS

The precipitating event is again a stone or sludge impacted in the neck of the gallbladder. If the stone does not become disimpacted (as in biliary colic), the resultant biliary stasis and gallbladder distension trigger the release of prostaglandins I_2 and E_2, which mediate an acute inflammatory response, even in the absence of superimposed bacterial infection. Cholecystectomy is indicated as recurrent attacks are likely, but recommendations regarding the timing of the surgery have undergone a change in recent years.[2] As more than 70 per cent of patients respond to conservative management, interval cholecystectomy can be undertaken after 6 weeks, when the acute inflammatory process has settled. Alternatively, the operation can be performed as a planned procedure during the first 48–72 hours of inflammation, when the associated oedema makes the tissue planes easier to dissect. Unfortunately, with a conservative approach, some patients will come to surgery in suboptimal circumstances. Those who develop gangrenous cholecystitis, an empyema of the gallbladder or peritonitis, will need emergency intervention which could have been avoided. In addition, those who fail to settle, and those who are readmitted to hospital with further complications of gallstones prior to their elective procedure, will have surgery beyond the 72-hour period, but before all inflammation has settled. Concerns that cholecystectomy, particularly laparoscopic, was more hazardous in the acute phase appear unfounded, and for both medical and economic reasons cholecystectomy within 72 hours of presentation is now generally advocated.

Acute acalculous cholecystitis

This occurs mainly in patients who are already critically ill. The condition tends to be more rapidly progressive, and frequently leads to gangrene of the gallbladder. Early intervention, by either cholecystostomy or cholecystectomy, is therefore indicated.

Mirizzi's syndrome

Type I Mirizzi's syndrome occurs when there is obstructive jaundice secondary to extrinsic compression of the common bile duct from a large gallstone impacted in the neck of an inflamed gallbladder or cystic duct. A type II Mirizzi's syndrome occurs when the disease progresses, and there is erosion of the stone into the bile duct, creating a fistula. If conservative treatment does not result in a rapid reduction in inflammation and resolution of the jaundice, early surgery may prove necessary, but a difficult cholecystectomy must be anticipated (see below).

Cholecystostomy

In cases of severe acute cholecystitis where the patient is unfit for general anaesthesia, percutaneous cholecystostomy may be performed by an experienced radiologist under ultrasound guidance and local anaesthesia either in the radiology department, or at the bedside. It is preferable if the drain is inserted transhepatically, in order to reduce the likelihood of spillage of bile into the peritoneal cavity.

Operative procedure

An open cholecystostomy may also be performed under local anaesthesia. However, it is more commonly undertaken as a salvage procedure in a sick patient with severe acute cholecystitis, where delineation of the biliary anatomy at a laparotomy for an intended cholecystectomy is difficult. The gallbladder is carefully surrounded by moist packs and a suction device inserted into the fundus of the gallbladder to aspirate the liquid contents. When no more bile can be aspirated, light tissue forceps are applied to the gallbladder wall on either side of the sucker, which is then withdrawn. The opening is enlarged with scissors to a length of 2–3 cm, and the remaining contents (usually gallstones and biliary sludge) are evacuated with a scoop or with fenestrated forceps, a receiver being held against the opening in order to catch any escaping bile or debris. Two fingers are then passed deeply along the outside of the gallbladder and its neck and the cystic duct carefully palpated. Any further calculi detected are milked upwards until they are within reach of the scoop or forceps (Fig. 18.3a). Care must be taken not to overlook a stone impacted in the cystic duct. The interior of the gallbladder is then explored with a finger and dried with

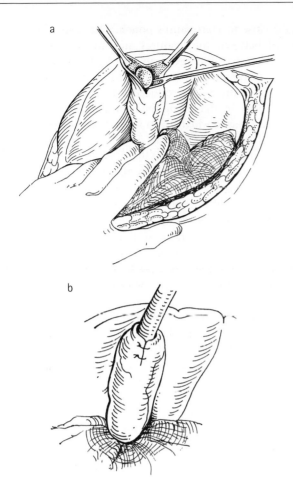

Figure 18.3 *Open cholecystostomy. (a) The fundus of the gallbladder is opened and all stones extracted. (b) The gallbladder is then repaired around a drainage catheter.*

a swab held on forceps; this is rotated in order to entangle and remove any small stones that remain.

A large Foley catheter, or other self-retaining catheter, is passed through a stab incision in the skin and muscle of the anterior abdominal wall, separate from the main wound. It is introduced into the gallbladder and the opening around the tube secured with a purse-string suture of 2/0 Vicryl or, if the gallbladder wall is thickened or friable, by insertion of one or two interrupted sutures (Fig. 18.3b). The area is lavaged with warmed saline solution and a tube drain placed in the right subhepatic space prior to closure of the wound.

Postoperatively, the cholecystostomy tube is attached to a closed-system bile drainage bag and allowed to drain freely for 7–10 days. A tubogram should then be performed to check for the presence of residual stones in the gallbladder or common bile duct. If the radiographs show no residual calculi and communication to a normal common bile duct, the tube drain may be spigoted and subsequently removed a few weeks later. Whether or not to perform an elective cholecystectomy will be determined by the patient's symptoms and clinical condition. More than 50 per cent of these patients will be asymptomatic during the next five years, so an expec-

tant policy is justified. If the tubogram demonstrates the presence of stones, or blockage of the cystic duct (most likely from a stone), the tube should be left *in situ* for a further 3–4 weeks and consideration is given to a planned cholecystectomy (likely to be a difficult procedure) or to instrumental removal of the stones via the tube track. Removal of the cholecystostomy tube in the presence of distal obstruction is likely to lead either to a persistent mucous fistula or to recurrent infection in the gallbladder. Should the tubogram reveal a gallbladder clear of stones or obstruction, but stones in the common bile duct, the ideal treatment is ERCP, sphincterotomy and endoscopic stone removal.

A fistula following cholecystostomy will usually close spontaneously within 7–10 days of tube removal. A persistent fistula is likely to be due to stricture of the cystic duct or to an impacted calculus, in which case the discharge will consist mainly of mucus. Cholecystectomy is usually curative.

Open cholecystectomy

The main indication for cholecystectomy is symptomatic gallstones. Cholecystectomy may be performed on its own, or combined with a common bile duct exploration to remove further stones. Removal of the gallbladder can be undertaken by either an open or a laparoscopic approach, and the latter approach is now the standard method used where facilities and skills are available. Cholecystectomy may also be undertaken as part of a major resection for hepatobiliary or pancreatic pathology, including hepatic, biliary and pancreatic malignancy. Surgery for tumours of the gallbladder and bile ducts is discussed later in the chapter.

All the steps of the operation must be carried out under direct vision. The patients are often obese and access is difficult, so good exposure of the gallbladder is essential. Suitable incisions have been described previously, and a Kocher incision is the one most frequently used, with the surgeon standing on the patient's right.

The first step consists of freeing any inflammatory intraperitoneal adhesions between the gallbladder and adjacent viscera or omentum. Careful packing and retraction can then achieve optimal exposure. A gauze roll or pack is placed over the duodenum, and this is retracted firmly downwards by the left hand of the assistant. A deep retractor is then placed under the right lobe of the liver and this is lifted gently upwards to expose the gallbladder.

There are two principal methods of removing the gallbladder, retrograde and fundus-first.

THE RETROGRADE METHOD

The generally advocated retrograde method involves early dissection and division of the cystic duct and artery, followed by retrograde dissection of the gallbladder off the liver towards the fundus. This early delineation of the key structures reduces the risk of injury to the common bile duct or right hepatic artery. When distension of the gallbladder prevents easy access to the ducts, or if there is risk of rupture, the contents should be aspirated and the puncture site closed with a stitch or clamp. Sponge-holding (Rampley's) forceps are then applied near the neck of the gallbladder and used to draw it gently forwards and to the right (Fig. 18.4a). Calot's triangle is dissected: this is a triangle bounded by the inferior surface of the right lobe of liver, the common hepatic duct, and the cystic duct and superior border of the gallbladder. The junction of the cystic duct and common duct is displayed by dividing the overlying peritoneum, and by gauze stripping. This dissection may take time, as the ducts are often obscured by fat or oedematous connective tissue. The cystic artery is found within Calot's triangle, and ligated and divided. An absorbable ligature is then passed loosely around the cystic duct close to its junction with the common bile duct. Any stones in the cystic duct should be milked towards the gallbladder and the cystic duct clamped or ligated (Fig.

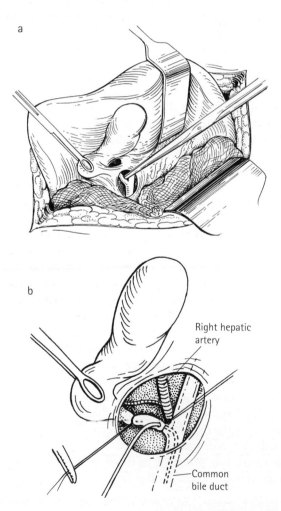

Figure 18.4   *Open cholecystectomy by the retrograde method. A longer incision in the peritoneum than illustrated here will allow better exposure of the anatomy. (a) Exposure of the cystic duct at its junction with the common hepatic duct, in the right free border of the lesser omentum. (b) The cystic duct has been ligated and a cannula has been inserted into the common bile duct for cholangiography. The cystic artery has been identified.*

18.4b) close to Hartmann's pouch. The cystic duct is then opened between the ligatures and any remaining stones removed. A bacteriology swab may be taken for culture. If intraoperative cholangiography is to be performed, a metal or plastic cannula is introduced through this opening and held in place by tightening the ligature with a single throw. The decision as to whether intraoperative cholangiography is indicated is discussed below in the section on choledochotomy. It is important that the cannula is flushed through with saline or contrast prior to placement, to eliminate air bubbles that may masquerade as stones on X-ray. Contrast is then injected whilst screening over the right upper quadrant. Points to note on the cholangiograms obtained are evidence of: (i) biliary tree dilatation; (ii) filling defects within the biliary tree; (iii) free flow of contrast into the duodenum; (iv) tapering of the distal common bile duct; and (v) normal filling of the intrahepatic ducts. After satisfactory images have been obtained, the cannula is removed, the ligature close to the common bile duct secured, and the cystic duct divided. If the cystic duct is particularly wide, it may be advisable to transfix the stump with a 2/0 Vicryl suture.

The gallbladder is now attached by little more than the peritoneal sheath that binds it to the inferior surface of the liver. The gallbladder neck is drawn forwards away from the liver and the plane between the two dissected. As the dissection continues, the peritoneum on each side is divided with scissors or diathermy. Some haemorrhage can occur from minute blood vessels that pass directly to the gallbladder from the substance of the liver, but if the separation is carried out in the correct plane (close to the gallbladder) the bleeding is minimal. If an accessory bile duct (of Lushka) is encountered entering the gallbladder directly from the liver bed, it should be secured and ligated. It is useful to delay the final separation of the gallbladder from the liver bed until adequate haemostasis has been achieved, as the partially separated gallbladder can provide useful retraction and aid visualization of bleeding points.

Drainage of the right subhepatic space with a closed-tube drainage system should be considered only in selected cases, if there is significant oozing after resection of a severely inflamed gallbladder, or if there is concern regarding a possible bile leak, either from the liver bed, or from a cystic duct which has been difficult to secure. Any drain should be removed after 24–48 hours, provided that there is no evidence of a bile leak.

THE 'FUNDUS–FIRST' METHOD

This method is advised only when difficulties (particularly severe inflammatory changes) prevent the ducts from being displayed in the first steps of the operation, thus exposing them to great danger if dissection near the cystic duct and common bile duct is continued. Paradoxically, the fundus-first method also carries risks of injury, particularly to the common bile duct and right hepatic artery. Excessive traction on the mobilized gallbladder may pull these structures out of their normal alignment, rendering them liable to be clamped or included in a ligature (Fig. 18.5).

Separation of the gallbladder from the liver bed is commenced at the fundus, the peritoneal sheath being divided (with scissors or diathermy) on both sides where it is reflected onto the liver. As the dissection proceeds, the gallbladder is finally attached only by the cystic artery and cystic duct. The cholangiogram is thus performed at a later stage in the dissection, when it cannot alert the surgeon to anatomical anomalies. More bleeding is encountered using this technique than using the retrograde method, where the cystic artery is controlled at an earlier stage. If, due to marked inflammation, isolation of the cystic duct and artery is thought to endanger the right hepatic artery or the common bile duct, it is better to leave part of the neck of the gallbladder *in situ* (a subtotal cholecystectomy) than to persevere with a hazardous dissection.

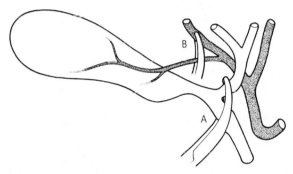

Figure 18.5 *The potential for injury to the common bile duct and right hepatic artery may be increased in the 'fundus-first' dissection, as traction on a fully mobilized gallbladder can distort the anatomy both at the termination of the cystic duct (A), and at the origin of the cystic artery (B).*

Difficulties and complications during cholecystectomy

CYSTIC DUCT

There is sometimes difficulty in isolating the cystic duct, or in following it to its confluence with the common hepatic duct. The difficulty may be caused by densely adherent planes in Calot's triangle making the anatomy impossible to elucidate. This may occur when a surgeon is forced to operate for complications of cholecystitis in a patient whose inflammation has been continuing for a week or more. The alternative strategy of cholecystostomy, as discussed above, should be considered as a safer alternative. Difficulty can also arise when the terminal portion of the cystic duct runs a long intramural course in the wall of the common hepatic duct before entering it, or when the cystic duct winds around the common hepatic duct (see Fig. 18.2c). It must be remembered that it is better to leave a portion of cystic duct *in situ*, or even to perform a subtotal cholecystectomy as described

above, than to persevere with a high risk of bile duct injury. Difficulty can also be due to a stone lodged in the neck of the gallbladder with intense inflammation around it. Combined pressure from the stone and the inflammation may also be obstructing the common hepatic duct and causing jaundice (Mirizzi type I). The stone must be released, by a lateral incision to minimize any risk to the common hepatic duct, but removal of the gallbladder neck will probably be unwise. A temporary bile leak should be anticipated with a drain placed to the area.

Simple ligation of a short wide cystic duct (see Fig. 18.2a) may be insecure, and it also has the potential to distort and narrow the common bile duct. A sutured closure with an absorbable suture may be a better alternative. It is sometimes impossible to pass a cholangiogram catheter through a very narrow cystic duct. It can be argued that any gallstone which was able to pass through such a duct would also have passed through into the duodenum without difficulty and that cholangiography can be abandoned. If, however, cholangiography is deemed essential it can be performed by direct needle puncture of the common bile duct.

HAEMORRHAGE

Haemorrhage from a torn cystic artery or from a slipped ligature is likely to be profuse, and injudicious attempts to stop it may result in damage to important adjacent structures. Instead, a large pack should be placed against the bleeding area and left *in situ* for several minutes. When the pack is removed, the bleeding vessel can usually be easily identified and secured. If necessary, the hepatic artery may be temporarily occluded by a soft bowel clamp placed on the free border of the lesser omentum (the Pringle manoeuvre). An injury to the right hepatic artery can also occur, and this should be considered when there is significant haemorrhage. Ligation of the right hepatic artery should be avoided and repair should be attempted. The right hepatic artery may be inadvertently ligated, being mistaken for the cystic artery, or may be included in the ligature applied to it (see Fig. 18.5). Although the patient may suffer no consequences, it may prove fatal due to massive hepatic necrosis.

IATROGENIC BILE DUCT INJURIES

Most injuries to the biliary tree are iatrogenic. They are usually due to inadequate demonstration of the anatomy of Calot's triangle at cholecystectomy, and they are the most feared complication of cholecystectomy. A segment of the common bile duct may be inadvertently clamped or included in a ligature (see Fig. 18.5), resulting in biliary obstruction, or a major bile leak. A partial circumference injury may heal, but cause a significant stricture of the duct. Common bile duct injuries can also occur during mobilization of the duodenum in a gastrectomy. When a surgeon suspects that a bile duct injury has occurred, it is very important not to compound the damage by making a hurried decision, or an inappropriate attempt at repair. If at all possible, the help and support of a colleague who was not involved in the initial injury should be sought. Such injuries are potentially serious and should be managed by a hepatobiliary surgeon, as there is good evidence that long-term results are significantly better if the initial repair/reconstruction is undertaken by a specialist.

Immediate repair

Primary repair and T-tube drainage may be an appropriate method of repair of a divided bile duct in selected circumstances. It is only practical when the injury is identified intraoperatively and if the trauma to the bile duct ends is minimal. Most authors would only advocate this type of repair for partial transection injuries. It is usually advised that the anastomosis should be performed over a T-tube, brought out through a separate opening in the lower segment of the bile duct, at least 1 cm below the suture line of the repair (Fig. 18.6). It must be emphasized that for such a primary repair to be successful, all the criteria for anastomotic healing must be met – that is a good blood supply, no tension, no surrounding infection, and no distal obstruction. In practice, the blood supply to the damaged common bile duct is frequently compromised, either because of diathermy injury, or because the periductal tissues containing the feeding arteries have been stripped away. This is often the reason for late stricturing of primary end-to-end repairs. A better solution is a biliary-enteric reconstruction.

Immediate reconstruction

The common hepatic duct is excised proximally until good bleeding tissue is obtained, after which an anastomosis is fashioned between this and a Roux loop of jejunum (see below: Late repair of bile duct injuries). Evidence suggests that long-term results from a primary hepaticojejunostomy are superior to those with a duct-to-duct anastomosis.

Choledochotomy

Choledochotomy describes the making of an opening into the common bile duct, in order to explore it and remove any

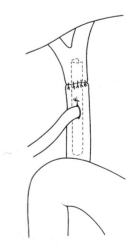

Figure 18.6 *Repair of a bile duct over a T-tube.*

stones within it. This procedure was initially performed when a stone could be palpated in the duct, or when the classical criteria were present which indicated a high probability of a common bile duct stone. These criteria included a dilated or thickened duct, recent jaundice, or multiple small stones in a gallbladder with a wide cystic duct. However, this policy resulted in a negative exploration rate of approximately 50 per cent, with increased mortality and morbidity. Intraoperative cholangiography in all patients then became routine, and exploration of the common bile duct was restricted to those in whom the cholangiogram revealed filling defects or strictures. Now the decisions are less clear, as calculi within the common bile duct can be removed using ERCP, as well as by choledochotomy. The management of patients with a high suspicion of, or proven, choledocholithiasis is dependent on local resources and expertise. One strategy is a pre-operative ERCP, which may be combined with endoscopic sphincterotomy and stone extraction if stones are confirmed, followed by a laparoscopic cholecystectomy. An alternative is to proceed directly to laparoscopic cholecystectomy with intraoperative cholangiography. If choledocholithiasis is confirmed, a laparoscopic or open exploration of the common bile duct can follow, or alternatively a postoperative ERCP and stone extraction can be planned.

SUPRADUODENAL CHOLEDOCHOTOMY

This approach is the method of choice, since the supraduodenal portion of the duct, lying in the free border of the lesser omentum, is relatively accessible. In the majority of cases exploration of the duct is for suspected calculi, and the gallbladder will have been removed earlier in the operation.

Operative procedure – open technique

The second part of the duodenum should be fully mobilized (Kocherized) after incision of the peritoneum lying lateral to it. This is usually avascular, though some vessels may require ligation close to the region where the common bile duct passes behind the duodenum. Mobilization of the duodenum and head of the pancreas should be carried out as far as the left side of the inferior vena cava, to allow the second part of the duodenum to be brought forward into the wound.

The peritoneum over the supraduodenal portion of the common bile duct is incised and the anterior surface cleared of peritoneum and fatty tissue over a distance of 1.5 cm. One or two small vessels in the immediate supraduodenal region may require to be controlled by fine sutures. If, due to gross inflammatory changes, there is some doubt as to the actual location of the common bile duct, it may be identified by aspiration of bile with a fine-calibre needle. Stay sutures of 4/0 polydioxanone (PDS) are inserted near the borders of the duct, and a 1.5–2.0 cm longitudinal incision is made between them (Fig. 18.7a). A bacteriology swab is taken of the bile escaping through the incision, and the bile is then aspirated. Some floating stones may emerge with the first rush of bile, and these should be retrieved. A gentle attempt should now be made to milk any palpable stones towards the chole-

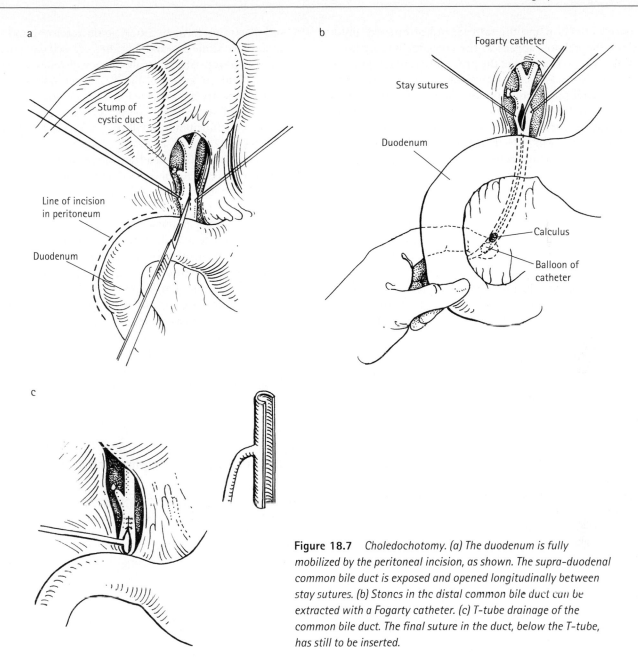

Figure 18.7 *Choledochotomy. (a) The duodenum is fully mobilized by the peritoneal incision, as shown. The supra-duodenal common bile duct is exposed and opened longitudinally between stay sutures. (b) Stones in the distal common bile duct can be extracted with a Fogarty catheter. (c) T-tube drainage of the common bile duct. The final suture in the duct, below the T-tube, has still to be inserted.*

dochotomy incision, where they may be removed using gallstone forceps.

The duct is now formally explored for residual stones, palpable or otherwise. A wide variety of instruments is available for this purpose. Rigid bougies or forceps (e.g. Desjardin's or Maingot's) are most frequently used, but unless great care is exercised damage to the duct, particularly at its lower end, may result, with subsequent stricture formation. It is therefore recommended that the initial exploration be made with a Fogarty balloon catheter (Fig. 18.7b). Retrograde exploration is performed first. The catheter is passed cephalad, guided into the right hepatic duct, and advanced as far as it will go. The balloon is then inflated until slight resistance to downward traction is felt and the catheter is pulled downwards, maintaining inflation to provide slight resistance. Any calculi appearing at the choledochotomy incision are removed by forceps. The procedure is repeated for the left hepatic duct and then repeated for both ducts in turn until the surgeon is satisfied that the proximal biliary tree is clear. Exploration of the distal common bile duct is now undertaken. The Fogarty catheter is passed into the duodenum (judged by the distance it has passed) and the balloon inflated. Confirmation of its position into the duodenum is made by palpation of the inflated balloon. The catheter is withdrawn until there is resistance signifying that the balloon is at the sphincter of Oddi. The balloon is partially deflated whilst maintaining upward traction until it is felt to come through the sphincter. It is then re-inflated to maintain slight resistance to traction and the catheter pulled upwards until calculi or the balloon appear at the choledochotomy incision. Calculi are removed and the procedure is repeated until the surgeon is satisfied that no calculi remain. Should the Fogarty catheter fail to enter the duodenum (usually due to an impacted and palpable stone), further gentle exploration with the biliary forceps, using the left hand to guide the instrument into position, will usually result in successful stone extraction. Management of the impacted and apparently unmovable stone will be considered later.

Given that at this stage in the operation the surgeon feels that the ducts have been cleared, the common bile duct and hepatic ducts are irrigated with saline to wash out any calculus debris or blood clots, and post-exploratory cholangiogram films are taken using a fine (8 Fr) Foley catheter. This is first inserted into the choledochotomy incision and directed upwards into the proximal biliary tree. The balloon is inflated and an occlusion cholangiogram obtained. The balloon is deflated, passed distally, and then re-inflated to occlude the distal bile duct and a further cholangiogram is performed. Provided that the ampulla is not occluded by a stone, the pressure obtained by using this technique will allow contrast to pass into the duodenum and fully display the lower portion of the bile duct. If a choledochoscope is available, cholangiography may be omitted and the surgeon can inspect the bile ducts under direct vision to ensure there are no residual calculi.

Following the demonstration of a satisfactory duct system, the common bile duct was traditionally closed over a T-tube. A relatively fine T-tube (10 or 12 Fr) should be used. The short limbs of the T-tube are inserted into the common bile duct via the choledochotomy incision (Fig. 18.7c), which is closed using interrupted 4/0 PDS sutures. The long limb of the T-tube is brought out to the surface through a stab incision, taking the most direct route. A small-calibre tube drain can also be placed in the subhepatic space. A T-tube cholangiogram is then taken on the 7th to 10th postoperative day to ensure there are no retained stones. If the cholangiogram is normal, the T-tube is clamped. Removal of the T-tube will depend on the material from which it is made, as this will determine the length of time for a track to form. If it is latex rubber, the T-tube can be removed at 10–14 days, but if it is silastic it should be left for 3–4 weeks before removal. Following removal of the T-tube, there may be a small bile leak that persists for 1–2 days. Many hepatobiliary surgeons no longer recommend the routine use of a T-tube if the duct has been seen to be clear on choledochoscopy.

THE IMPACTED STONE AT OPEN BILE DUCT EXPLORATION

If a stone remains impacted at the lower end of the common bile duct, despite routine measures to remove it, the surgeon has a numbers of approaches, depending on the fitness of the patient or availability of endoscopic skills:

- To leave the stone *in situ*, drain the common bile duct by T-tube for 2–3 weeks to allow inflammation to settle,

and then to perform an ERCP, sphincterotomy and endoscopic stone removal. For the very sick patient, this may be appropriate, but truly impacted stones can be very difficult to remove at ERCP, and certainly stones over 15 mm are not suitable for this technique.

- To leave the stone *in situ* and perform a hepaticodochojejunostomy Roux-en-Y (see below; Bile duct reconstruction).

- To remove the stone via a transduodenal sphincteroplasty. An oblique anterolateral incision is made in the second part of the duodenum. Stay sutures are then inserted in the medial wall of the duodenum on either side of the ampulla (Fig. 18.8). Using a blade, an incision is made directly over the stone, which is then extracted. The incision in the wall of the duodenum and lower end of the bile duct is then enlarged using Pott's scissors, to a minimum length of 15 mm and converted to a formal sphincteroplasty by approximating duodenal and bile duct mucosa using interrupted 4/0 PDS sutures. Care must be taken to ensure apposition of mucosa at the apex of the incision. The duodenotomy incision is then closed in a single layer. Supraduodenal T-tube drainage is not normally necessary following this procedure.

Laparoscopic cholecystectomy, on–table cholangiography and laparoscopic bile duct exploration

This procedure was first described in 1989, since when it has been adopted by the surgical community with enthusiasm. During the early years of its use, there was an unacceptably high incidence of bile duct injury, associated with the learn-

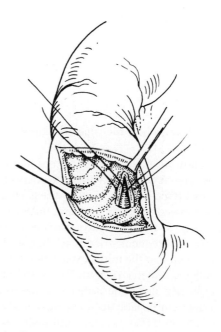

Figure 18.8 *Transduodenal sphincterotomy.*

ing curve of a group of self-taught surgeons. However, the clinical and economic benefits of laparoscopic cholecystectomy are now proven, with comparable or shorter operating times, shorter hospital stay (often a day case), more rapid return to full activity and less morbidity/mortality compared to open surgery.

The indications for laparoscopic cholecystectomy are the same as for the open approach. Relative contraindications include extensive previous upper abdominal surgery, portal hypertension and major cardiovascular or respiratory disease. Obesity is not a contraindication; indeed, laparoscopic surgery is more appropriate in the obese. Patients must be warned that there is a risk of conversion to the open procedure (approximately 2–5%), which is higher in those patients having an urgent cholecystectomy for acute cholecystitis (10–15%).

Operative procedure

The anaesthetized patient is placed supine on the operating table. The pneumoperitoneum may be achieved with an open (Hasson) or a closed (Verres needle) method, via an infra-umbilical longitudinal or transverse incision. The present authors advocate the open method described below. The central part of the umbilicus is elevated with a towel clip, and a 10-mm longitudinal infra-umbilical skin incision is made. The umbilical ligament is then identified, grasped, and a 0.5-cm incision made along its length. The abdominal cavity is then entered using artery forceps and the first port introduced over a graduated bougie. A gas leak is less common with this method. However, this procedure may not be appropriate if a patient has had multiple previous operations. Under such circumstances, the peritoneal cavity may be entered under direct vision by a cut-down in an area not associated with a previous incision.

Once the first port has been placed, the peritoneal cavity is carefully insufflated with warmed CO_2 to a pressure of 12 mmHg. A 30-degree laparoscope is introduced via the umbilical port and the peritoneal cavity is inspected. The second 10-mm port is inserted under direct vision in the midline in the epigastrium, passing just to the right of the falciform ligament, towards the gallbladder. Two 5-mm ports are introduced, one in the right mid-clavicular and one in the right mid-axillary line, angled towards the gallbladder (Fig. 18.9). Aids to vision and access include placing the

patient in a steep reverse Trendelenberg position with a left-down tilt and aspirating a distended stomach. Any adhesions between the gallbladder and omentum or duodenum are divided, and the gallbladder fundus grasped and retracted towards the patient's right shoulder. A 5-mm grasper is then placed on Hartmann's pouch and, using the operator's left hand, is retracted to the patient's right, opening up the porta hepatis. The anterior and posterior peritoneum over the neck of the gallbladder is then divided with a diathermy hook and Calot's triangle carefully dissected.

Once the cystic duct and cystic artery are clearly identified, a cholangiogram can be performed. Some surgeons perform cholangiography routinely, whilst others are selective, reserving cholangiography for patients with a high risk of common bile duct stones, or to define the biliary anatomy. A small cut is made in the cystic duct and a cholangiogram catheter introduced. A number of methods/catheter types have been described, but the present authors use an infant feeding tube introduced into the peritoneal cavity via an intravenous cannula and secured in the cystic duct with a clip. The cholangiogram is then performed as per the open method, after which the clip is removed and the catheter withdrawn. The cystic duct is clipped proximal and distal to the opening and then divided. If the cystic duct is wide, a ligature (e.g. Endoloop) may be used to secure the cystic duct stump. The cystic artery is then clipped and divided. The gallbladder is carefully dissected off the gallbladder bed. Prior to the final disconnection, and using the gallbladder as a retractor, haemostasis of the gallbladder bed is secured and the positions of the clips placed on the cystic duct and the cystic artery are checked. The dissection is then completed and the gallbladder is retrieved via the epigastric or umbilical ports. If the gallbladder has been punctured, it should be retrieved in a bag, with every effort being made to aspirate the bile and recover any spilt stones. The pneumoperitoneum is then released and the ports are removed. The wounds are infiltrated with local anaesthetic and closed with absorbable sutures.

LAPAROSCOPIC BILE DUCT EXPLORATION

If a filling defect is seen within the biliary tree on intraoperative cholangiography, the surgeon may: (i) explore the bile duct laparoscopically; (ii) convert to an open procedure; or (iii) perform an ERCP and stone extraction in the early postoperative period. Factors influencing this decision are the skills of the surgeon and the endoscopist, the size of the stone(s), and the diameter of the cystic duct and common bile duct. Approximately 60 per cent of patients may be explored via the transcystic route, and the stones either extracted or pushed into the duodenum using baskets or balloons. The cystic duct is then simply secured with clips or a ligature at the end of the procedure. The common bile duct may also be explored laparoscopically via a supraduodenal choledochotomy, followed by choledochoscopy and primary closure, or closure over a T-tube. Placement of a subhepatic

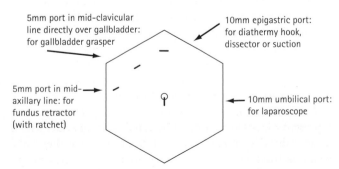

Figure 18.9 *Port-sites for laparoscopic cholecystectomy.*

5mm port in mid-clavicular line directly over gallbladder: for gallbladder grasper

10mm epigastric port: for diathermy hook, dissector or suction

5mm port in mid-axillary line: for fundus retractor (with ratchet)

10mm umbilical port: for laparoscope

drain is essential. Postoperatively, the T-tube is managed in a similar fashion to that after open surgery.

Any of the difficulties and complications described above for open cholecystectomy and common bile duct exploration can also occur at a laparoscopic operation. In most instances, if a significant difficulty or complication arises, then conversion to an open procedure is recommended, but this decision will be influenced by the experience of the surgeon in both the open and laparoscopic techniques.

POSTOPERATIVE COMPLICATIONS OF BILIARY SURGERY

The retained stone

Despite apparently satisfactory post-exploratory intraoperative cholangiography or choledochoscopy, the T-tube cholangiogram obtained 7–10 days later may demonstrate persistent choledocholithiasis (Fig. 18.10). Again, several management options are available:

- Leave the T-tube to drain for a further 7–10 days and repeat the cholangiogram. Up to 40 per cent of filling defects will have disappeared, either because they were not stones (air bubbles or blood clots) or if they were, they will have passed spontaneously.
- Institute irrigation of the common bile duct with saline via the T-tube. This is unlikely to be successful if the retained stone lies in the biliary tree above the level of the T-tube. It is also contraindicated if a stone is impacted at the lower end of the common bile duct and is preventing flow of contrast into the duodenum. Check cholangiograms are taken every few days to assess progress.
- ERCP and endoscopic sphincterotomy may be undertaken. The stone may be left to pass spontaneously, or extracted using a Dormia basket or balloon catheter. This technique may not be suitable for stones retained high in the biliary tree, and may be unsuccessful if the stone is firmly impacted at the lower end.
- Instrumental retrieval via the T-tube tract.[3] This technique, which should be delayed until 4 weeks after the operation to allow maturation of the T-tube tract, may be used for retained stones anywhere in the biliary tree, but it is particularly suitable for retained stones in the proximal ducts. Under fluoroscopic control, the T-tube tract is dilated using graduated dilators and a Dormia basket or balloon catheter is passed down the tract to extract the stone along the T-tube tract.
- Reoperation will be required in the event of failure or non-availability of the above techniques. This is technically demanding, particularly supraduodenal re-exploration, and thus a transduodenal approach with sphincteroplasty may be preferred for stones in the distal common bile duct (Fig. 18.8).

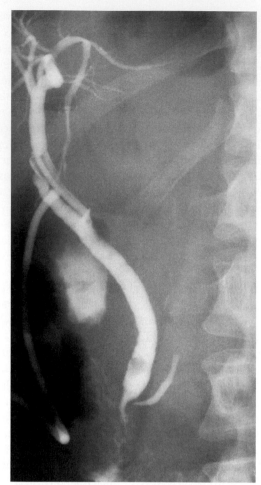

Figure 18.10 *A T-tube cholangiogram showing a retained stone.*

Postoperative bile leaks and biliary fistulae

A bile leak may occur into a subhepatic drain placed at the time of surgery, or the bile may collect intra-abdominally and present either as generalized biliary peritonitis or as a localized collection. The surgeon must have a high index of suspicion of a bile leak, or bile duct injury, in any patient who is not well after cholecystectomy. Upper abdominal or chest pain, associated with tachycardia and persistent hypotension (the Waltman Walters syndrome) are classical signs. Following resuscitation, an abdominal ultrasound should be performed and any free fluid or collection aspirated to determine if it is bile-stained. It may be appropriate to ask the radiologist to place a drain into a subhepatic/subphrenic collection. However, if the patient develops generalized biliary peritonitis, re-laparotomy should be performed once the patient's condition is optimized.

A minor discharge of bile from a subhepatic drain may represent a leak from a tiny undetected accessory duct which drained directly into the gallbladder. Alternatively, there may be a leak from an incompletely secured cystic duct, or from the closure of a choledochotomy. Many such leaks will cease spontaneously if there is no distal obstruction. Similarly, a fistula that follows cholecystostomy or choledochostomy usually closes spontaneously within 7–10 days of the removal of the tube, and a persistent fistula may close spontaneously even after a period of several months. However, before adopting a policy of conservative management, the anatomy should be defined by ERCP or PTC, and if large volumes of bile are being drained externally, then an early intervention is indicated. The nature of the intervention will depend on the underlying conditions present.

A biliary fistula following cholecystectomy is likely to be due to a bile duct injury. Often, the fact that such an injury has occurred is only apparent after a few days, with discharge of bile from the wound, or the development of a subhepatic collection. Management will depend on the type of injury (see below). If a fistula persists after choledochotomy, it is likely that the lower part of the common bile duct is obstructed, either by a retained stone or by fibrosis, and ERCP should be performed to aid further management.

A patient with a suspected bile duct injury during the early postoperative phase requires both stabilization and appropriate imaging, with ultrasound, ERCP or PTC, to define the nature and location of the injury. The principles of management are to control sepsis and achieve biliary drainage. Drainage of intra-abdominal collections must be achieved either percutaneously, or by laparoscopy or laparotomy. If a simple cystic duct leak is demonstrated on ERCP, the insertion of a plastic endobiliary stent should allow the leak to heal. Repair of a major bile duct injury should ideally be performed either within the first week before the development of sepsis, or after several months, when all sepsis has resolved and the patient is nutritionally replete.

Late repair or reconstruction of the bile ducts

Late repair of a severed or stenosed duct is one of the most challenging of operations. The duct is likely to be buried in dense scar tissue, and the ends may be widely retracted. The reconstruction performed depends on the level of injury, as classified by Bismuth and Majno.[4] The most successful method of reconstruction is to perform a hepaticojejunostomy, anastomosing the proximal biliary duct(s) to a Roux loop of jejunum.

HEPATICOJEJUNOSTOMY WITH A ROUX LOOP

This procedure is described here for the reconstruction of severed or stenosed ducts following iatrogenic injury, but the same technique is used for biliary reconstruction in a variety of other pathologies. It is the preferred method of surgical biliary drainage in most instances, and is the standard method of biliary reconstruction following bile duct resection.

The Roux loop is fashioned as described in Chapter 21. The jejunum is transected 25–30 cm distal to the duodenojejunal flexure, after which the closed distal end is brought up through a window in the transverse mesocolon to the right of the middle colic vessels, to be anastomosed to the proximal bile ducts as described by Voyles and Blumgart in 1982.[5] The biliary anastomosis is performed using a single layer of interrupted 4/0 PDS sutures. This is an end-to-side anastomosis of the common hepatic duct onto the jejunum. An incision into the side of the jejunum must be made of a size appropriate for the diameter of the transected bile duct (Fig. 18.11a). The anterior layer of sutures is passed from outside to inside through the bile duct. The needles are retained and they are held for completion of these anterior sutures after the back of the anastomosis has been finished (Fig. 18.11b). The anterior sutures are then elevated as retraction to expose the back wall of the duct, and the posterior sutures are all inserted, but not tied. These sutures are inserted from inside to out on the jejunum, and from outside to inside on the duct. After all are in place they are held taut and the jejunum is 'railroaded' down into place and the sutures tied (Fig. 18.11c). The knots of the posterior layer are thus on the inside. The first and last sutures of the back row are held to steady the anastomosis, and all the other sutures are cut short. The front of the anastomosis is then completed using the sutures which were placed in the front of the bile duct at the beginning of the procedure. The needles are passed from inside to outside through the jejunum (Fig. 18.11d). When all sutures are completed, the knots are tied (Fig. 18.11e). The enteroenterostomy is then fashioned approximately 70 cm distal to this anastomosis.

Sometimes, a hepaticojejunostomy cannot be performed because an injury, tumour or dense adhesions involves a considerable length of the common hepatic duct. In these circumstances adequate biliary drainage can only be obtained by a biliary-enteric anastomosis to the left or right hepatic ducts, or their intrahepatic branches. Occasionally, the confluence of the hepatic ducts is high and still intact, despite an absence of extrahepatic common hepatic duct suitable for a hepaticojejunostomy. The intrahepatic common hepatic duct and the confluence within the liver is approached by the same dissection as that employed to isolate the left hepatic duct.

The left hepatic duct is usually an extrahepatic structure, accessed at the base of segment 4 of the liver, by lowering the hilar plate. This involves dividing any liver tissue bridging the umbilical fissure between the base of the quadrate lobe (segment 4) and the left lobe of the liver (Fig. 18.12). The liver is then elevated and an incision made at the base of segment 4, at the point where Glisson's capsule reflects onto the lesser omentum. The dissection into the liver is then deepened in this plane from left to right, exposing the structures of the left portal triad. The position of the left duct is confirmed by needle aspiration. The duct is opened lengthwise with a scalpel, and the incision is extended using Pott's scissors. If the confluence is intact, both the left and right lobes of the liver can be drained by this approach.

If there is complete separation of the left and right ducts, the right lobe of the liver must be drained by a separate approach to the right duct through the base of the gall-

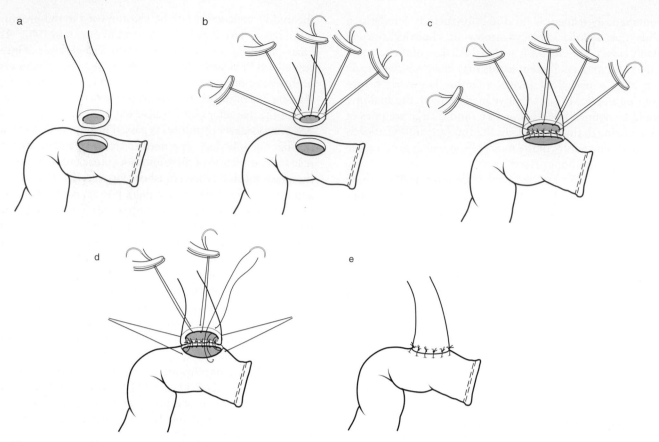

Figure 18.11 *Hepaticojejunostomy. (a) An incision is made in the Roux loop of jejunum. (b) The anterior sutures are only in the bile duct and are used to display the posterior wall of the duct while the posterior sutures are inserted. (c) The posterior sutures are tied. (d) The anterior sutures are completed. (e) The anastomosis is completed as the anterior sutures are tied.*

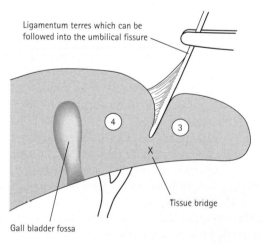

Figure 18.12 *Access to the right and left hepatic ducts may be necessary when there is no suitable extrahepatic common hepatic duct for a hepatojejunostomy. The tissue bridge between segments 3 and 4 is divided to expose the left portal triad. The right hepatic duct can be approached from the gallbladder fossa.*

bladder fossa. If the left duct is obliterated (e.g. by fibrosis or tumour), a biliary-enteric anastomosis can be performed onto the duct of segment 3, which runs in a relatively con-

stant position to the left of the umbilical fissure and is accessed by dividing the liver on its anterior surface just to the left of the base of the falciform ligament. Intraoperative ultrasound may be a useful adjunct to help identify the duct (see also Chapter 20).

SURGERY OF OBSTRUCTIVE JAUNDICE AND BILIARY STRICTURES

A complete obstruction of the biliary tree results in progressive obstructive jaundice. This obstruction can be due to a stone impacted in the lower end of the common bile duct. However, steadily deepening obstructive jaundice, without preceding biliary colic, suggests obstruction of the duct by malignant disease, a benign biliary stricture, or chronic pancreatitis. Malignant disease may be a primary tumour in the head of pancreas, bile ducts, gallbladder, or ampulla of Vater, or may be secondary to enlarged metastatic lymph nodes in the porta hepatis. Benign biliary strictures may be caused by primary or secondary sclerosing cholangitis, parasitic infections (*Ascaris, Clonorchis, Echinococcus*), traumatic injury (often post-cholecystectomy), or idiopathic inflammatory strictures. Non-malignant strictures often cause incomplete obstruction, and the morbidity is related to secondary biliary cirrhosis, sepsis and stone formation.

ACUTE CHOLANGITIS

Patients with complete, or partial, extra-hepatic biliary tract obstruction can become severely unwell with acute cholangitis, the classic symptoms and signs of which are right upper quadrant pain, jaundice and rigors (Charcot's triad). Acute (or ascending) cholangitis is due to secondary bacterial colonization of stagnant bile and subsequent bacteraemia. This is a surgical emergency, and patients must be resuscitated with fluids, oxygen, intravenous antibiotics and analgesia, followed by urgent decompression of the biliary tree by endoscopic, percutaneous, or surgical means.

Biliary strictures

The surgical management of a biliary stricture is dependent upon its aetiology and its anatomy.

Post-traumatic strictures

Most of these are secondary to iatrogenic bile duct injuries sustained during gallbladder surgery. Their management has been discussed above.

Inflammatory strictures of the biliary tree

These may result from injury or from fibrosis following inflammation (for example, secondary to an impacted common bile duct stone). When stenosis involves only the orifice of the duct, it may be dealt with either by transduodenal sphincteroplasty (see above) or by endoscopic sphincterotomy. When the stricture is thought to be too high or too long to be treated by simple incision of the duct orifice, a hepaticojejunostomy with a Roux loop of jejunum should be performed, as described above.

The extensive inflammatory biliary strictures associated with parasitic infestation of the biliary tree are often complicated by additional involvement of the intrahepatic bile ducts (see Chapter 20). Complications of intrahepatic strictures and calculi will continue even after excision of the extrahepatic ducts and reconstruction with a hepaticojejunostomy. In these patients, the addition of an access loop for radiological or endoscopic intervention is desirable.[6] Subsequent percutaneous access to a subparietal hepaticojejunal access loop can be facilitated by marking its position with ligaclips or wire for radiological identification (Fig. 18.13a). The gastric access loop allows easy endoscopic access,[7] and may be of particular value when endoscopic skills are available but interventional radiological facilities less well-developed (Fig. 18.13b).

Primary sclerosing cholangitis (PSC)

This is a chronic cholestatic syndrome of unknown aetiology which is characterized by diffuse fibrosing inflammation of the intra- and extrahepatic bile ducts. It is likely to have an autoimmune aetiology, and is associated with ulcerative colitis in about 70 per cent of cases. PSC is progressive, leading to biliary cirrhosis, portal hypertension and death from liver

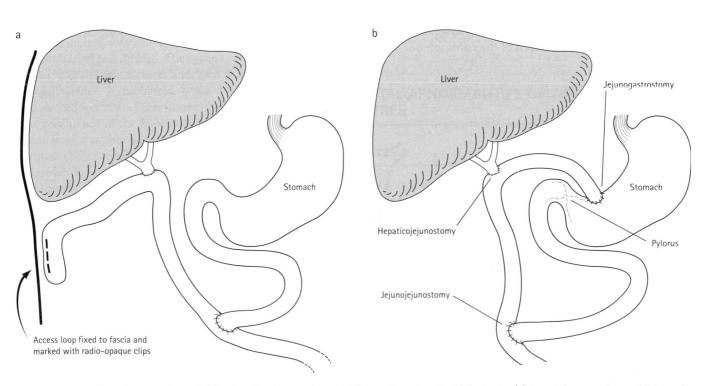

Figure 18.13   *Hepatic access loops. (a) A subparietal access loop which is easily entered radiologically. (b) A gastric access loop which can be entered at endoscopy.*

is urgent, as surgery before 8 weeks of age gives the best chance of good bile flow and long-term survival. Other causes of jaundice must be excluded, and confirmatory investigations include bile duct imaging and technetium-labelled hepatobiliary excretion scans. Currently, the most reliable test for diagnosing biliary atresia, aside from exploratory laparotomy, is percutaneous liver biopsy. A specimen containing five to seven portal tracts can be 93 per cent accurate for the diagnosis of this disease.

Treatment and outcome

The initial treatment is the surgical reconstruction of the biliary tree. At laparotomy, a shrunken fibrotic gallbladder suggests atresia and precludes operative cholangiography. If the gallbladder is patent, it is aspirated. If bile is obtained, this suggests either a type 1 atresia or a hepatitis syndrome, and a cholangiogram should be performed. If type 1 disease is confirmed, a hepaticojejunostomy is undertaken. Type 2 and 3 disease are treated by the portoenterostomy procedure described in 1959 by Kasai and Susuki,[9] who observed bile drainage from microscopic ductules in the porta hepatis after excision of the fibrosed hepatic ducts. Consequently, they developed a procedure whereby the atretic extrahepatic tissue is removed and a Roux-en-Y jejunal loop is anastomosed to the hepatic hilum.

Long-term outcome in these infants depends on the occurrence of ascending cholangitis, portal hypertension and the progress of intrahepatic inflammation. Age at operation and surgical experience are both critical prognostic factors. Short-term success, with restoration of bile flow and normalization of bilirubin, may result in a 10-year survival of up to 90 per cent with a native liver. If portoenterostomy fails, death before the age of 2 years is likely without liver transplantation.[10] Yet even with early surgery, most patients (70–80 per cent) eventually develop end-stage biliary cirrhosis and require liver transplantation. Biliary atresia is the most frequent cause of chronic end-stage liver disease in children, and is the leading indication for liver transplantation in the paediatric population, accounting for 40–50 per cent of all paediatric liver transplants. Advances in immunosuppression (tacrolimus), liver transplantation techniques (split-livers, reduced-size grafts) and living-related donors have resulted in a 5-year survival of more than 80 per cent in these children.[12]

Choledochal cysts

Choledochal cysts are not an isolated entity, but rather a spectrum of abnormalities in the pancreatohepatobiliary system. Choledochal cysts are more common in females, and have a high incidence in Japan and Asia. Their aetiology is unknown, but an abnormal pancreaticobiliary duct junction and the formation of a common channel is found in a high proportion of patients. It is speculated that this results in reflux of pancreatic enzymes into the biliary tree, causing inflammation, dilatation and fibrosis.

Classification

Choledochal cysts were classified in 1977 by Todani et al.[12] into five types (Fig. 18.15). The most common is the type I cyst, a solitary fusiform dilatation of the common bile duct into which the cystic duct enters; type II is a supraduodenal common bile duct diverticulum; type III is a choledochocele in the distal common bile duct; type IV is the second most common, with extra- and intrahepatic cysts; and type V is confined to the intrahepatic ducts and may merge into the syndrome of Caroli's disease, which in turn is associated with congenital hepatic fibrosis.

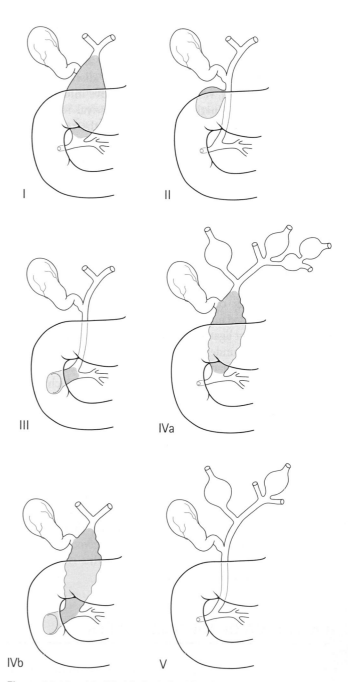

Figure 18.15   Modified Todani classification of choledochal cysts.

Presentation and treatment

Choledochal cysts may present in older infants and young children, or remain asymptomatic for many years. Clinical features include recurrent abdominal pain, jaundice, a right hypochondrial mass, recurrent cholangitis and pancreatitis. Emergency presentation with cyst rupture is a recognized complication in older infants. If choledochal cysts are left untreated, liver abscesses, cirrhosis, portal hypertension and malignant change can result.[13] The diagnosis is usually made by ultrasound, but definition of the anatomy of the biliary tree using ERCP, PTC or MRCP is essential. Treatment is surgical, based on cyst type and the associated hepatobiliary pathology. In principle, the extrahepatic biliary tree should be excised and bile flow re-established by a biliary-enteric anastomosis. For type IV intrahepatic cysts, liver resection may be necessary, and patients with Caroli's disease (type V) may require liver transplantation (see also Chapter 20).

Cystenterostomy is contraindicated. Long-term complications will still develop, and patients who have had a bypass still require definitive surgery. This will be more difficult and has a lower chance of success if a previous cystenterostomy has been performed. Occasionally, a temporary solution is required in an emergency for a patient who is unfit for a major procedure, or the necessary surgical skills are unavailable. Temporary T-tube drainage of the cyst is preferable in these circumstances to any anastomosis of the cyst onto the bowel.

FUNCTIONAL DISORDERS OF THE BILIARY TREE

Functional disorders causing pain of biliary origin in the absence of gallstones or other biliary organic disease, may be attributed to gallbladder dyskinesia or sphincter of Oddi dysfunction. Gallbladder dyskinesia may be diagnosed using radionucleotide scanning to demonstrate incomplete gallbladder emptying following a cholecystokinin stimulus. Cholecystectomy is usually curative. Patients with sphincter of Oddi dysfunction include those with spasm or dyskinesia. This dysfunction is diagnosed using biliary manometry, which may show a raised basal sphincter pressure, abnormalities in the direction and frequency of contractions, or a par-adoxical response to a cholecystokinin stimulus. Treatment involves division of the sphincter, either endoscopically, or by a transduodenal operation. The open, transduodenal approach may include sphincterotomy and sphincteroplasty (as previously described), or septectomy. This later, more radical, operation includes ablation of the high-pressure zone at outlets of both the pancreatic and bile ducts.

REFERENCES

1. Diamond T, Parks RW. Perioperative management of obstructive jaundice. Leading article. *Br J Surg* 1997; **84**: 147–9.
2. Indar AA, Beckingham IJ. Acute cholecystitis. Clinical review. *Br Med J* 2002; **325**: 639–43.
3. Burhenne HJ. Garland Lecture. Percutaneous extraction of retained biliary tract stones: 661 patients. *Am J Roentgenol* 1980; **134**: 889–98.
4. Bismuth H, Majno PE. Biliary strictures: classification on the principles of surgical treatment. *World J Surg* 2001; **25**: 1241–4.
5. Voyles CR, Blumgart LH. A technique for the construction of high biliary-enteric anastomoses. *Surg Gynecol Obstet* 1982; **154**: 885–7.
6. Beckingham IJ, Krige JEJ, Beningfield SJ, *et al.* Subparietal hepaticojejunal access loop for the long-term management of intrahepatic stones. *Br J Surg* 1998; **85**: 1360–3.
7. Sitaram V, Perakath B, Chacko A, *et al.* Gastric access loop in hepaticojejunostomy. *Br J Surg* 1998; **85**: 108–10.
8. Shoup M, Fong Y. Surgical indications and extent of resection in gallbladder cancer. *Surg Oncol Clin North Am* 2002; **11**: 985–94.
9. Kasai IM, Susuki S. A new operation for 'non-correctable' biliary atresia; hepatic porto-enterostomy. *Shujustsu* 1959; **13**: 733.
10. Ohi R. Biliary atresia: Long-term results of hepatic portoenterostomy In ER Howard *Surgery of Liver Disease in Children.* Oxford: Butterworth-Heinemann, 1991, pp. 60–71.
11. Diem HV, Evrard V, Vinh HT, *et al.* Pediatric transplantation for biliary atresia: results of primary grafts in 328 recipients. *Transplantation* 2003; **75**: 1692–7.
12. Todani T, Watanabe Y, Narusue M, *et al.* Congenital bile duct cysts; classification, operative procedures, and review of thirty-seven cases including cancer arising from choledochal cyst. *Am J Surg* 1977; **134**: 263–9.
13. Atkinson HDE, Fischer CP, de Jong CHC, *et al.* Choledochal cysts in adults and their complications. *Hepatopancreaticobil Surg* 2003; **5**: 105–10.

19

SURGERY OF THE PANCREAS, SPLEEN AND ADRENAL GLANDS

ROWAN PARKS AND JAMES POWELL

THE PANCREAS: ANATOMY, HISTOLOGY, EMBRYOLOGY AND PHYSIOLOGY

Anatomy

The pancreas is a solid organ which is located in the retroperitoneum. Its internal anatomy and relationship to the duodenum and bile ducts are illustrated in Chapter 18 (see Fig. 18.1, page 318). The pancreas consists of a head, uncinate process, neck, body and tail. The head and uncinate process are located within, and are intimately associated with, the concavity of the duodenum. The body and tail pass upwards and backwards covered with the peritoneum of the posterior wall of the lesser sac, with the tail terminating at the splenic hilum. The anterior surface of the pancreas is for the most part in contact, through the lesser sac, with the posterior aspect of the stomach. The posterior surface of the pancreas is associated with the inferior vena cava, aorta, portal vein, splenic vein, the left renal vessels and the left kidney. The portal vein is formed by the confluence of the superior mesenteric vein and splenic vein behind the neck of the pancreas. The splenic artery has a wavy course along the upper border, and the splenic vein lies behind the body and tail of the pancreas. The superior mesenteric artery and vein pass over the anterior aspect of the uncinate process and lie posterior to the neck of the pancreas. The neck of the pancreas lies in front of the vertebral bodies and is at risk of damage during compression-type injuries to the abdomen. An accessory or 'replaced' right hepatic artery arising from the superior mesenteric artery may run upwards behind the head of the pancreas.

Blood supply

Most of the blood supply to the pancreas is derived from the coeliac axis through the splenic artery and the superior pancreaticoduodenal artery. The inferior half of the head of the pancreas and the uncinate process are supplied by the superior mesenteric artery through the inferior pancreaticoduodenal artery. The superior and inferior pancreaticoduodenal arteries anastomose to form an arcade around the head of the pancreas. This anastomotic arcade forms an important collateral circulation between the superior mesenteric artery (SMA) and the gastroduodenal artery in occlusive disease of the common hepatic artery, and may be the sole arterial blood supply to the liver in this situation.

The venous drainage of the pancreas is via the portal system, and the lymphatic drainage follows the arterial supply.

Nerve supply

The pancreas receives innervation from the autonomic nervous system. Parasympathetic innervation is derived from the vagus nerve, and may stimulate pancreatic exocrine secretion. Sympathetic innervation is through the greater splanchnic nerves (T6–T10), and provides vasomotor function and pain sensation.

Histology

The pancreas is a composite gland with both exocrine and endocrine components. The exocrine component forms the bulk of the gland with the serous acinar cells comprising 80 per cent of the gland volume. In contrast, the endocrine component within the islets of Langerhans, comprises a mere 2 per cent of the gland structure. The remaining 18 per cent is comprised of ducts, nerves, vessels and connective tissue.

Embryology

The pancreas is formed from two outpouchings of the developing intestinal tract termed the dorsal and ventral pancreatic buds.[1] The superior part of the pancreatic head, the body and the tail of the pancreas, all develop from the dorsal pancreatic bud. The dorsal pancreatic duct forms the main pancreatic duct, and initially drains at the site of the minor duodenal papilla. The inferior half of the pancreatic head and the uncinate process develop from the ventral pancreatic bud. This arises in common with the bile duct at the site of the major duodenal papilla (which marks the junction between the fore and mid-gut). The ventral pancreatic bud rotates posteriorly to fuse with the dorsal pancreatic bud. Following fusion of the ventral and dorsal buds, there is reorganization of the two pancreatic ductal systems, with the result that the dorsal (main pancreatic duct) drains mainly through the major duodenal papilla. Fusion of the two pancreatic ductal systems fails to occur in 5–10 per cent of individuals, giving rise to pancreas divisum in which the main pancreatic duct drains through the minor duodenal papilla, situated 2–3 cm above the major duodenal papilla. Pancreas divisum is a relatively common anomaly of which the pancreatic surgeon must be aware (Fig. 19.1). The consequences of pancreas divisum remain contested, although it is believed that it may give rise to main pancreatic duct hypertension resulting in recurrent episodes of abdominal pain and acute pancreatitis.

Pancreatic physiology

Exocrine secretion of digestive enzymes (amylase, proteases, lipase, nuclease) from pancreatic acinar cells, along with bicarbonate rich fluid from centro-acinar and ductal cells, is important for digestion. The secretion of pancreatic enzymes is stimulated by a number of hormones, although the predominant influence is cholecystokinin, which is secreted in response to fat and amino acids within the duodenum following a meal. The bicarbonate-rich secretion of centro-acinar cells is controlled by the hormone secretin, which is secreted in response to acid within the duodenum.

Endocrine secretion from the islets of Langerhans is important in carbohydrate metabolism. The α cell secretes glucagon, the β cell secretes insulin, and the δ cell secretes somatostatin. Blood glucose concentration is the stimulus for β-cell secretion of insulin.

The surgeon must remember the dual exocrine and endocrine roles of the pancreas, especially when undertaking a pancreatectomy.

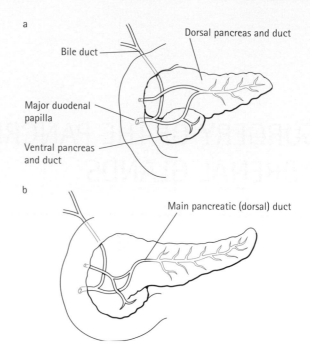

Figure 19.1 *Pancreatic ducts. (a) Developmentally, the pancreas consists of a separate dorsal and ventral organ, each with its own duct. The larger dorsal pancreatic duct opens into the duodenum above the opening of the bile duct. In pancreas divisum there is a failure of communication between the two ductal systems, and this anatomical arrangement persists. (b) Fusion of the two parts of the pancreas and reorganization of the ducts results in the normal adult anatomy. The main dorsal pancreatic duct now drains through the major duodenal papilla.*

GENERAL PANCREATIC SURGICAL TECHNIQUE

Pancreatic surgery is highly specialized and patients should, if at all possible, be transferred to a specialist pancreatic unit. This is even possible in many cases of pancreatic trauma, the management of which was discussed in Chapter 14, page 244. However, the general surgeon with a different subspecialty interest must still understand the challenges posed by the pancreas. Unwelcome encounters with the pancreas can arise in a number of operations, and all experienced surgeons have a healthy respect for a viscus which has a justifiable reputation as an organ which is extremely unforgiving of surgical encroachment. Injury to the pancreas can occur during any dissection in its vicinity, and care must be taken to avoid damage during gastric, colonic, aortic, splenic and adrenal surgery.

Identification

The edge of the pancreas is usually fairly easy to distinguish from the surrounding extraperitoneal fat in ideal operating conditions, as it is slightly pinker, and usually a little firmer. However, the surgeon must be aware of the proximity of the gland, and the dissection has to be meticulous with good haemostasis, for this to be an obvious tissue plane.

Haemorrhage

Small, thin-walled vessels are frequently encountered over the anterior surface of the pancreas. These can be particularly troublesome over the head of the gland during the final dissection for the mobilization of the right colon for a radical right hemicolectomy. Ideally, the vessels should be identified and ligated before division using a fine ligature. Unfortunately, they are often torn and subsequent diathermy coagulation is often unsuccessful with the vessel continuing to bleed. A fine Prolene suture is often a better solution.

Parenchymal tears

An inadvertent minor tear in the pancreas, or an area of trauma, which is not bleeding may be best left alone, as sutures in the pancreas can sometimes compound an otherwise minor injury. There is still a risk of a pancreatic fistula and the area should be drained (see below). Larger tears should be treated in a similar manner to a transection.

Transection

A small portion of the tail of the pancreas may be removed either unintentionally during a splenectomy, or as a planned excision when it is adherent to a colonic splenic flexure tumour. If a pancreatic duct is visible on the cut surface it should be secured and ligated. The remainder of the parenchyma can then be oversewn or sealed with a haemostatic endoGIA. Whichever method is employed, pancreatic leaks are common and the area should be drained.

Pancreatic drains

Any incision into the pancreas releases digestive enzymes with the potential for autodigestion. These enzymes inhibit healing, and late leakage of pancreatic juice is common even when at first the closure appeared sound. The enzymes cause intense inflammation, and it is essential that any collection is drained. It is therefore recommended that a drain is placed to any pancreatic resection, or area of injury, and that the drain is left *in situ* for at least a week, even if initially there is no drainage.

Pancreatic fistulae

A pancreatic leak may persist for many weeks as a pancreatic fistula. Eventually, most pancreatic fistulae will seal spontaneously, provided that there is no obstruction in the proximal pancreatic duct. The drain is left *in situ*, cut short and a stoma bag fixed over it so that the skin is protected and the volume of the fistula effluent can be measured.

PANCREATIC NEOPLASIA

Pancreatic neoplasms may arise from any of the cell types that constitute the pancreas. The biological behaviour of pancreatic neoplasms may range from benign indolent tumours to aggressive malignant cancers.

Benign pancreatic neoplasms

Benign tumours of the pancreas are rare. Cystic tumours are the most common benign neoplasms arising from cells of the exocrine pancreas. A serous cystadenoma may grow to such a size that it may cause local pressure effects, or present as a palpable mass. Resection of a serous cystadenoma is usually curative and malignant change is uncommon. In contrast, mucinous cystadenoma often have foci of invasive adenocarcinoma.

Malignant pancreatic neoplasms

Ductal adenocarcinoma is the commonest neoplasm, accounting for 90 per cent of all pancreatic neoplasms. It arises predominantly in the head of the gland, and is the most prevalent of the *peri-ampullary* tumours considered below. The commonest presenting features are jaundice, weight loss and pain. Progressive obstructive jaundice, frequently associated with marked and disabling pruritis, is due to compression or infiltration of the common bile duct as it passes through the head of the pancreas. Epigastric pain or discomfort is common and may radiate to the back, although the presence of back pain is a poor prognostic sign suggesting advanced local disease. Adenocarcinoma of the body or tail of the pancreas typically presents with pain and weight loss, and is almost invariably non-resectable because of either advanced local disease or the presence of metastases. The presence of an abdominal mass suggests non-resectable disease, although a malignant mass must be distinguished from a palpable enlarged gallbladder due to distal biliary obstruction (Courvoisier's sign).

Endocrine neoplasms

Tumours arising from cells of the endocrine pancreas are very rare. They are often small, and present with symptoms of endocrine hypersecretion rather than with symptoms from any mass effect of the growth itself. They may be benign or malignant, and solitary or multiple.

INSULINOMAS

Insulinomas are the most common pancreatic endocrine neoplasm, with an incidence in the United Kingdom of one case per million population per year. The majority (90 per cent) of insulinomas are small (<1 cm diameter) and do not demonstrate malignant features, whereas larger lesions may metastasize. Most insulinomas are solitary and occur anywhere in the pancreas. Multiple pancreatic insulinomas also occur and have an association with the multiple endocrine neoplasia type 1 syndrome (MEN I). The diagnosis of insulinoma may be difficult, and patients often undergo numerous investigations before a correct diagnosis is made. A history of neuroglycopaenic symptoms (e.g. altered consciousness, confusion, seizures) provoked by exercise and/or fasting, and relieved by eating, in the absence of other identifiable causes of hypoglycaemia (Whipple's triad) forms the clinical basis for the diagnosis of insulinoma. The biochemical demonstration of inappropriate secretion of insulin (raised serum insulin and C-peptide levels) in the setting of hypoglycaemia confirms the diagnosis. It is important to exclude factitious hypoglycaemia due to covert administration of insulin or oral hypoglycaemic agents. Although a large number of imaging modalities can be utilized in an attempt to localize suspected insulinomas before surgery, the most accurate method of localization remains a laparotomy and intraoperative ultrasound undertaken by an experienced pancreatic surgeon. Insulinomas identified at laparotomy may be successfully treated by enucleation of the tumour.

GASTRINOMAS

In contrast to insulinomas, 60 per cent of gastrinomas are malignant. Moreover, gastrinomas are not confined to the pancreas and commonly occur in the wall of the duodenum. Preoperative localization is of benefit, and somatostatin receptor scintigraphy has been demonstrated to be particularly useful. Resection of the tumour should be undertaken where possible as even palliative resection may provide useful control of symptoms.

Peri-ampullary neoplasms

At the time of presentation and during assessment it is often not possible to determine the exact nature, or tissue of origin, of tumours arising in the region of the head of the pancreas, and indeed the distinction may be difficult even following histological analysis (Table 19.1). Therefore, neoplastic lesions found in the region of the head of the pancreas are frequently considered together as peri-ampullary neoplasms.

Table 19.1 *Peri-ampullary neoplasms.*

Pancreatic adenocarcinoma
Cholangiocarcinoma
Adenocarcinoma of the ampulla of Vater
Duodenal adenocarcinoma

STAGING OF PERI-AMPULLARY NEOPLASMS

Preoperative staging investigations are undertaken in an attempt to reduce the number of patients subjected to a laparotomy at which a non-curative procedure is undertaken.[2] Furthermore, preoperative assessment identifies comorbidity which would contraindicate major resectional surgery.

Staging investigations aim to determine the presence of either advanced local disease (e.g. involvement of portal vein or superior mesenteric vein/artery) or metastases, both of which would be a contraindication to resectional pancreatic surgery. An advanced tumour may be obvious clinically in a patient who has a palpable mass and ascites at presentation, but sophisticated imaging is necessary to demonstrate more subtle signs of irresectability, such as a cuff of tumour surrounding the mesenteric vein or local infiltration of tumour into the mesenteric vessels and the aorta. Triple phase contrast-enhanced computed tomography (CT) is the most frequently used imaging modality, although it does have limitations. Although gross vascular involvement or occlusion by a pancreatic neoplasm may be easily determined by contrast-enhanced CT, the distinction between early vascular invasion and adherence of a neoplasm to the vessels may be difficult. In units where the philosophy is not to resect an involved portal vein this distinction is important; however, this differentiation is less of a concern if the surgeon is willing to consider portal vein resection. Furthermore, contrast-enhanced CT may not detect small hepatic metastases or low-volume peritoneal disease. For these reasons, a number of centres undertake laparoscopy and laparoscopic ultrasound in addition to contrast-enhanced CT.

PREOPERATIVE BILIARY DRAINAGE

The majority of patients with a peri-ampullary neoplasm present with jaundice. These patients frequently undergo endoscopic retrograde cholangiopancreatography (ERCP), and insertion of a biliary stent in order to relieve the biliary obstruction. The benefits of preoperative biliary drainage have been debated, however. Although obstructive jaundice is associated with a number of postoperative complications, several studies have demonstrated that preoperative biliary drainage is associated with an increase in septic complications. Therefore, if preoperative staging has shown a potentially resectable lesion and a delay to surgical intervention can be avoided, it is reasonable to proceed without preoperative biliary drainage in patients with uncomplicated obstructive jaundice. In those patients with acute cholangitis it is wise to achieve adequate biliary drainage and resolution of the acute cholangitis before contemplating resection. If preoperative biliary drainage is undertaken, then surgical intervention should be delayed for 3–4 weeks to allow resolution of the pathophysiological disturbances associated with obstructive jaundice (see also Chapter 18).

PREOPERATIVE TISSUE DIAGNOSIS

Preoperative histological confirmation of a peri-ampullary neoplasm is not mandatory before undertaking resectional surgery. The indication for surgery is based on a clinical picture and radiological imaging consistent with pancreatic neoplasia. Radiologically guided percutaneous core biopsy is not generally recommended because of concerns about tumour implantation along the biopsy track and false-negative results. Upper gastrointestinal endoscopy may allow confirmatory biopsies to be obtained in patients with duodenal and ampullary tumours. Furthermore, a cytological diagnosis may be achieved from biliary brushings or endoscopic ultrasound-guided fine-needle aspiration. Negative cytological and histological results should not in themselves contraindicate resection if significant concerns still exist regarding the possibility of an underlying malignancy. Indeed, up to 10 per cent of pancreaticoduodenectomies undertaken for presumed malignancy are found to have non-neoplastic pathologies (e.g. chronic pancreatitis, inflammatory bile duct stricture).

Pancreaticoduodenectomy

Pancreaticoduodenectomy is the procedure of choice for surgery with curative intent in patients with a peri-ampullary neoplasm. This technique was described by Whipple in 1946, and the resection bears his name.[3] The extent of the resection is shown diagrammatically in Figure 19.2. It is a major undertaking, and although current published series report mortality rates under 5 per cent, it should be remembered that during the 1960s mortality rates approached 25 per cent. Therefore, in an era of increasing sub-specialization within general surgery, pancreatic resectional surgery should be concentrated in specialist pancreatic units.

Indications
Indications for pancreaticoduodenectomy include:

1. Resectable peri-ampullary neoplasms.
2. Chronic pancreatitis with disease confined to the head of the gland.

Incision
Excellent access to the pancreas is afforded by a transverse upper abdominal or roof-top incision. To aid exposure, fixed

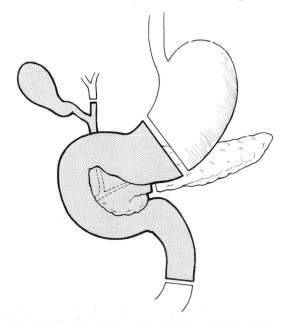

Figure 19.2 *The extent of the resection in a standard Whipple's pancreaticoduodenectomy. In a pylorus-preserving resection the proximal intestinal tract transection is through the proximal duodenum.*

costal margin retraction is employed, whilst the lower wound edge may be sutured to the lower portion of the anterior abdominal wall.

A midline incision may be useful in those patients with a high costal margin.

Assessment
A full laparotomy is undertaken. In malignant disease, special attention is directed towards the exclusion of peritoneal and hepatic metastases, the presence of which would be a contraindication to a major procedure. Invasion of tumour through to the infracolic aspect of the transverse mesocolon or invasion into the portal vein or superior mesenteric vein generally precludes resection, although some centres advocate portal vein resection when this is involved. Intraoperative ultrasound may be utilized in the assessment of vascular invasion and liver metastases.

Operative procedure
The ascending colon and hepatic flexure are mobilized towards the midline by division of the lateral peritoneal reflections. The duodenum is completely Kocherized with subsequent mobilization of the head of the pancreas from the inferior vena cava and anterior surface of the aorta. The lesser sac is entered through the mid portion of the gastrocolic omentum with serial ligation and division of epiploic vessels. Entry into the lesser sac may also be facilitated by dissection of the greater omentum from the transverse colon (see Chapter 13 and Fig. 13.4). The lesser sac dissection is continued to the right towards the head of the pancreas, allowing identification of the right gastro-epiploic vessels. Continuation of the dissection of the colon from the 2nd and 3rd parts of the duodenum across the anterior surface of the pancreas reveals the superior mesenteric vein (SMV) with the artery lying on its left lateral aspect. As the SMV passes over the uncinate process it receives a number of fragile veins on its anterior surface, including the right gastro-epiploic vein. These veins are easily torn, and should be ligated and divided at the earliest opportunity in order to prevent bothersome bleeding.

The gallbladder is dissected from the gallbladder bed in a fundus-first fashion, but the cystic duct is not divided. The cystic artery is ligated and divided. The anterior peritoneum of the hepatoduodenal ligament is divided with mobilization of tissues down towards the duodenum. The common hepatic duct is identified and transected. Any previously placed biliary stent is removed. Transection of the common hepatic duct exposes the portal vein lying behind it. The peritoneum overlying the lateral and posterior edge of the portal vein is divided. Care must be employed to avoid injury to an accessory or replaced right hepatic artery. The common hepatic artery and the gastroduodenal artery (GDA) are dissected free in a retrograde fashion. Tissue cleared from the vessels is removed en bloc with the resection specimen. The GDA is temporarily occluded in order to confirm that arterial inflow to the liver is maintained. If the pulse in the hepatic artery is lost on occlusion of the GDA, pancreaticoduodenectomy is not possible without vascular reconstruction. The GDA is then divided between ligatures and the stump is suture ligated.

The site of the proximal intestinal tract transection depends on whether a classical Whipple's procedure or a pylorus preserving pancreaticoduodenectomy (PPPD) is being undertaken. PPPD was initially introduced in an attempt to reduce postoperative complications due to dysfunctional gastric emptying following classical Whipple's resection.[4] However, randomized trials have not demonstrated superiority of one technique over the other, and therefore for the most part the choice is operator-dependent. However, for tumours abutting the pylorus, a classical Whipple's procedure must be performed in order to obtain adequate oncological clearance.

Antrectomy is performed in a classical Whipple's procedure. At the level of the incisura, the lesser omentum is divided onto the lesser curve of the stomach, ligating the vessels running parallel to the gastric wall. A suitable point is identified on the greater curve of the stomach and the gastroepiploic arcade is divided. The stomach is then transected. The use of a linear cutting stapling device simplifies the division.

The small bowel is divided in the proximal jejunum, with the use of a linear cutting stapling device again simplifying the division. The small bowel proximal to the transection line is devascularized with serial ligation and division of the vessels as they enter the wall of the small bowel. Two layers of vessels may be identified in the region of the distal duodenum and proximal jejunum. Peritoneum around the duodenojejunal flexure is divided allowing the small bowel, distal to where it has been transected, to be passed through the transverse mesocolon into the supracolic compartment.

The superior mesenteric vein is identified. Using careful blunt dissection, the plane between the SMV and the neck of the pancreas is developed. Continued dissection in this plane frees up the SMV and portal vein. Invasion of the SMV or portal vein most often denotes non-resectable disease, although portal vein resection may occasionally be appropriate. The tunnel behind the neck of the pancreas marks the pancreatic transection line. Stay sutures are placed on the superior and inferior borders of the pancreas on either side of the proposed transection line (Fig. 19.3). These sutures facilitate the control of bleeding following pancreatic transection. Transection of the pancreas is undertaken using a scalpel. Haemostasis is achieved by under-running bleeding pancreatic vessels.

Tissue between the pancreatic head and the right border of the SMV and portal vein is serially ligated and divided, allowing delivery of the resection specimen. During this stage care must be taken to ensure that the SMA is not rotated around to the right lateral aspect of the SMV placing it at risk of injury.

Following resection, intestinal continuity with the stomach, biliary tree and pancreas must be restored. Numerous methods of reconstruction have been described. The pancreaticoenteric anastomosis is at greatest risk of failure, and

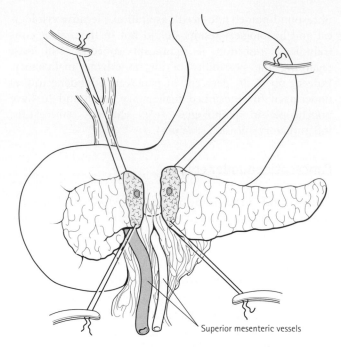

Figure 19.3 *The tunnel behind the neck of the pancreas, and in front of the superior mesenteric vessels, marks the line of the pancreatic transection. Stay sutures in the pancreas are useful at this stage.*

therefore a number of techniques for this have been tried in an attempt to reduce the risk of anastomotic leakage, though none has been proven to be clearly more effective than another. The present authors favour reconstruction to a single loop of small bowel; the pancreaticojejunostomy being fashioned just distal to the small-bowel transection line, followed by the hepaticojejunostomy and finally the gastrojejunostomy (Fig. 19.4). The proximal jejunum is brought up through a window in the transverse mesocolon (retrocolic) into the supracolic compartment. An end-to-side pancreaticojejunal anastomosis is fashioned using a single-layer interrupted parachute technique with an absorbable monofilament suture. Mucosa-to-mucosa apposition is straightforward in patients with a dilated pancreatic duct and a firm pancreas, but in those patients with a non-obstructed pancreatic duct and normal pancreatic parenchyma, formation of the pancreaticojejunal anastomosis requires meticulous technique. Biliocnteric continuity is restored by an end-to-side hepaticojejunostomy fashioned using a single-layer interrupted parachute technique with an absorbable monofilament suture (see Chapter 18 and Fig. 18.11). The gastrojejunostomy is fashioned using a single-layer, full-thickness technique with an absorbable monofilament suture. A nasogastric tube may be placed through the gastrojejunostomy into the afferent loop in order to decompress the proximal jejunum; however, stents are not placed across the pancreatic or biliary anastomoses. It is the present authors' practice to position two drains, anterior and posterior to the pancreaticojejunal anastomosis, but in such a

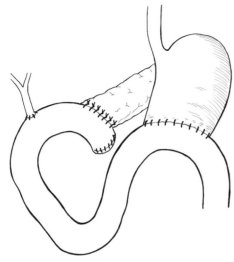

Figure 19.4 *A satisfactory arrangement for the anastomoses of stomach, bile duct and pancreas to the jejunum.*

fashion as to cover all three anastomoses. However, it should be noted that the routine use of drains has been questioned.

Despite meticulous surgery, there is a high incidence of failure of pancreaticoenteric anastomoses. *Octreotide* is a somatostatin analogue which reduces pancreatic secretion, and has been used prophylactically following pancreatic surgery in an attempt to reduce the risk of complications such as pancreaticojejunal anastomotic leak or pancreatic fistula. However, although randomized trials have been undertaken, the role of prophylactic octreotide in reducing the risk of pancreaticojejunal anastomotic failure is still not clear. Prophylactic octreotide may be beneficial in high-risk situations where the pancreas is soft and the pancreatic duct is not dilated. It is not present policy to use prophylactic octreotide routinely. Octreotide may also be prescribed with therapeutic intent in order to treat complications of pancreatic disease and surgery.

Palliative surgery

The majority of patients presenting with pancreatic cancer have non-resectable disease because of local vascular invasion, metastatic disease or significant medical co-morbidity. Current management aims to identify contraindications to resection prior to laparotomy, and to provide appropriate palliation in those patients. Although it has been suggested that surgical palliation should be undertaken in patients who are felt to have a good chance of prolonged survival, studies have failed to demonstrate any survival benefit from surgical palliation when compared to non-operative palliative procedures such as endoscopic or percutaneous biliary stenting (see Chapter 18). In patients presenting with evidence of non-resectable disease and gastric outlet obstruction, a palliative gastroenterostomy should be performed. This will usually be undertaken at open surgery, but where sufficient expertise exists, this may be performed laparoscopically. Endoscopic duodenal stenting is another alternative. Percutaneous biliary stenting may be undertaken at a later date if obstructive jaundice develops. In those patients undergoing open gastroenterostomy, a hepaticojejunostomy Roux-en-Y should also be performed. Cholecystojejunostomy is to be avoided because it is associated with a higher failure rate when compared to hepaticojejunostomy, as the cystic duct frequently becomes occluded with progression of the underlying malignancy.

For those patients in whom a radical resection was planned but non-resectable disease is discovered at laparotomy, a gastroenterostomy and hepaticojejunostomy Roux-en-Y double bypass should be undertaken (Fig. 19.5). Further descriptions of these procedures are provided in Chapters 16 and 18.

Distal pancreatectomy

Indications
Indications for distal pancreatectomy include:

- Neoplasia involving the body/tail of the pancreas.
- Chronic pancreatitis affecting the body/tail of the pancreas only.
- Pancreatic pseudocyst or pancreatic fistula arising from a pancreatic duct disruption in the body/tail of the pancreas.

Preoperative management
Because of the high probability of undertaking a splenectomy at the time of distal pancreatectomy, patients should have preoperative immunizations if time allows, as discussed later in the chapter (see Splenectomy).

Incision
An upper abdominal transverse incision extending more to the left provides excellent exposure. Alternatively, an upper midline incision may be employed.

Operative procedure
A distal pancreatectomy with splenectomy is represented diagrammatically in Figure 19.6. The lesser sac is entered through the gastrocolic omentum, allowing exposure of the pancreas. The whole length of the pancreas is exposed through the serial ligation and division of the epiploic vessels. Access to the lesser sac may also be obtained following dissection of the greater omentum from the transverse mesocolon, and the vascular arcade along the greater curve of the stomach preserved. The short gastric vessels are ligated and divided, allowing separation of the spleen from the stomach. The splenic flexure of the colon is mobilized, which allows full access to the tail of the pancreas.

When possible, the splenic artery at the level of the upper border of the pancreas is isolated and followed towards its origin. Ligation of the splenic artery at the level of planned transection may be undertaken prior to dissection of the spleen and tail of the pancreas in order to reduce blood loss.

On occasion, closure may only be achieved through the use of a prosthetic material. A planned second-look laparotomy and necrosectomy is performed at 24–48 hours. Further debridement may be undertaken if required.

- Open laparostomy: the abdominal wound is left open allowing free entry into the lesser sac. 'Marsupialization' of the lesser sac may also be undertaken, whereby the stomach is sutured to the upper part of the abdominal wound, whilst the transverse colon is sutured to the lower part of the wound. Following the initial procedure, further lesser sac debridement may be undertaken in the intensive care environment, and need not be performed in theatre. This management strategy can be complicated by secondary haemorrhage. Furthermore, because the wound is left to heal by secondary intention the development of an incisional hernia is almost inevitable.

Minimally invasive pancreatic necrosectomy[7]

Minimally invasive or percutaneous necrosectomy may be undertaken in some patients. Percutaneous necrosectomy involves the radiological placement of a percutaneous drain into the infected pancreatic necrosis, preferably using a retroperitoneal approach. In theatre and under general anaesthesia, the retroperitoneal drain is changed for a guide wire and the track is dilated, allowing insertion of an operating nephroscope through which the pancreatic necrosectomy is undertaken, taking great care to minimize the risk of haemorrhage. Once completed, a large drain is inserted along the track into the lesser sac cavity. It is possible to place two drains down the track, thereby allowing post-procedure lesser sac lavage. Further 'drain track' necrosectomies may be performed following the initial percutaneous necrosectomy.

SURGERY FOR CHRONIC PANCREATITIS

The majority of patients with chronic pancreatitis do not require intervention and may be managed conservatively. Conservative management consists of elimination of the aetiological agent where possible, and medical treatment of the complications, namely pain and pancreatic exocrine and endocrine insufficiency. Where alcohol excess is the cause, abstinence from alcohol must be encouraged. Analgesics appropriate to the level of pain should be prescribed, although this may result in both physical and psychological dependence on opiate analgesia. Exocrine insufficiency is treated by the prescription of pancreatic enzyme supplements (e.g. Creon). Endocrine insufficiency may require prescription of oral hypoglycaemic agents or insulin therapy. A multidisciplinary approach is frequently required.

Chronic pain is a common feature. Although pain may arise as a consequence of a specific complication of chronic pancreatitis such as a pseudocyst, for the majority of patients the cause of the pain is not clear, and management may be difficult. The proposed mechanisms of pain include increased pancreatic duct and/or pancreatic parenchymal pressure, pancreatic ischaemia, pancreatic fibrosis, alteration of pancreatic nerve function and, most recently, a neuroimmune interaction. For those patients with a specific complication giving rise to pain, the management is directed towards that complication. For the remainder of patients with pain, an appropriate approach to management is shown in Table 19.2. It should be noted however that the majority of patients with chronic pancreatitis and pain are managed conservatively. Procedure selection for pain is dependent on the presence or absence of pancreatic duct dilatation and pancreatic inflammation. A dilated duct demonstrated on CT scan, especially if there are also stones within the duct, suggests an obstructive component. Drainage procedures are undertaken in those patients with a dilated pancreatic duct, whilst resectional procedures are undertaken for inflammation. Drainage and resectional procedures may be combined. For those patients without pancreatic inflammation and a normal-sized pancreatic duct, the role for pancreatic surgery is uncertain. A period of abstinence from alcohol is mandatory for those in whom alcohol is the aetiological agent before surgical intervention for pain is considered. Significant improvement in both symptoms and radiological signs may be obtained following withdrawal of alcohol.

Table 19.2   *Surgical management of pain in chronic pancreatitis.*

		Involvement of the head of the pancreas?	
		Yes	**No**
Dilated main pancreatic duct?	**Yes**	Lateral pancreaticojejunostomy with partial excision of the pancreatic head (Frey)	Lateral pancreaticojejunostomy (Puestow, Partington-Rochelle)
	No	Duodenal-preserving pancreatic head resection (Beger) or Pancreaticoduodenectomy	Thoracoscopic splanchnicectomy or Medical management

IMAGING

Computed tomography is the mainstay of pancreatic imaging, and may demonstrate features such as pancreatic calcification, inflammation and pancreatic duct dilatation. It may also detect complications such as pseudocysts, false aneurysms and splenic vein thrombosis. ERCP may be undertaken to delineate pancreatic duct morphology and identify pancreatic duct strictures and sites of duct disruption. Magnetic resonance cholangio-pancreatography (MRCP) may also identify these features, and is being used with increasing frequency, although ERCP allows both dynamic interpretation of duct irregularities and endoscopic intervention where appropriate.

Surgical procedures in chronic pancreatitis

PARTINGTON-ROCHELLE OR PUESTOW PROCEDURE: LATERAL PANCREATICOJEJUNOSTOMY[8]

Lateral pancreaticojejunostomy aims to provide drainage of the main pancreatic duct. The operation may be undertaken in patients with intractable pain and radiological evidence of pancreatic duct dilatation with or without pancreatic duct calculi. In addition to treating the pain, there is some evidence that early pancreatic duct drainage may reduce the risk of the development of pancreatic endocrine insufficiency.

Operative procedure

The full length of the pancreas is approached via the lesser sac after division of the gastrocolic omentum. Although the bulging pancreatic duct may be seen through the anterior surface of the pancreas, aspiration with a syringe and needle ('seeker' needle) is frequently used to identify the dilated pancreatic duct. The duct is then incised using diathermy and opened along its length into the head of the gland. The insertion of a probe or Lahey forceps may facilitate the opening of the duct. A Roux loop is fashioned and brought up into the lesser sac through the transverse mesocolon to the right of the middle colic vessels. The blind end of the Roux loop is laid on the tail of the pancreas (Fig. 19.7). A side-to-side pancreas to small-bowel anastomosis is fashioned using a single-layer technique with absorbable sutures (e.g. polydiaxanone, PDS). If access is difficult, the blind end of the Roux loop may be parachuted into position. The original descriptions are of an anastomosis between the edges of the opened jejunum and the capsule of the pancreas on either side of the opened duct. If technically possible, a mucosa-to-mucosa apposition is now considered superior, but in a grossly thickened gland this may not be an option. Intestinal continuity is restored with an enteroenterostomy 40 cm below the transverse mesocolon.

In the original Puestow operation the drainage of the distal duct was combined with a splenectomy and distal pancreatectomy, but the later modification by Partington-Rochelle preserves both the pancreatic tail and the spleen.

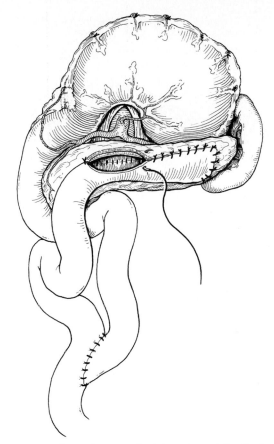

Figure 19.7 *Lateral pancreaticojejunostomy – 'Partington-Rochelle'. The pancreatic duct is opened along its length and unastomosed side-to-side to a Roux loop of jejunum.*

BEGER'S PROCEDURE: DUODENAL-PRESERVING PANCREATIC HEAD RESECTION[9]

This procedure is indicated for a symptomatic inflammatory mass in the head of the pancreas that has failed to respond to conservative treatment. This procedure is not appropriate where concern exists regarding the possibility of an underlying malignancy, in which case pancreaticoduodenectomy is the procedure of choice.

Operative procedure

The pancreatic head is resected leaving the duodenum *in situ*. The end of the Roux loop is anastomosed to the transected neck of the pancreas (Fig. 19.8). In cases with very severe inflammation, particularly in patients with cholestasis, the posterior limit of the resection in the region of the head of the pancreas may include the anterior wall of the common bile duct. The edges of the pancreatic defect left by the resection are then used for the anastomosis to the Roux loop.

FREY'S PROCEDURE

This operation is a lateral pancreaticojejunostomy with partial excision of the pancreatic head[10]. It combines a pancreatic duct drainage procedure with resectional surgery, and is

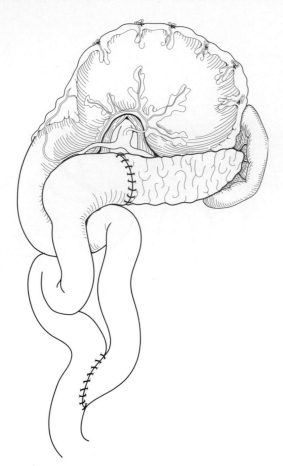

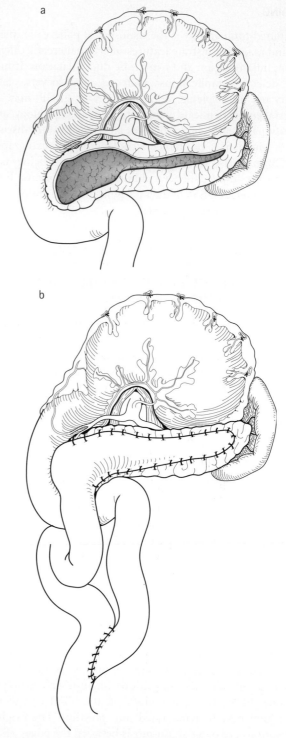

Figure 19.8   *Duodenal-preserving pancreatic head resection – Beger's procedure. A Roux loop of jejunum is anastomosed to the site of the pancreatic head resection.*

indicated in those patients with an inflammatory mass in the head of the pancreas with an associated dilated pancreatic duct. The Roux loop is anastomosed to the opened duct and to the edges of the pancreatic defect left by the resection of the inflammatory mass in the head (Fig. 19.9).

PANCREATICODUODENECTOMY

A pancreaticoduodenectomy is indicated for those patients in whom an isolated inflammatory mass in the head of the pancreas exists, especially if it is associated with either gastric outlet or biliary obstruction. In these patients, there is usually concern about the possibility of a pancreatic neoplasm. Indeed, focal chronic pancreatitis is part of the differential diagnosis for a peri-ampullary neoplasm. In those patients with chronic pancreatitis the dissection is made difficult because of the fibrous obliteration of the tissue planes following episodes of inflammation. However, the pancreatico-jejunal anastomosis is made easier because of pancreatic fibrosis. Some authors advocate pylorus-preserving pancreaticoduodenectomy over a Whipple's procedure in chronic pancreatitis, although there is no good evidence as to its superiority.

Figure 19.9   *Frey's procedure. (a) The pancreatic duct is opened along its length and the pancreatic head is cored out. (b) A Roux loop is used for a side-to-side pancreaticojejunostomy both to the opened duct and the edges of the defect in the head.*

TOTAL PANCREATECTOMY

There are few indications for total pancreatectomy in chronic pancreatitis. This is due in part to the significant metabolic and nutritional complications of total pancreatectomy. Diabetes mellitus is inevitable after total pancreatectomy and is often 'brittle', with poor glycaemic control. Total pancreatectomy has however been advocated for those patients with hereditary pancreatitis who are at high risk of the development of a pancreatic neoplasm.

THORACOSCOPIC SPLANCHNICECTOMY

Pancreatic pain is mediated through the greater splanchnic nerves which are formed by the postganglionic sympathetic nerves arising from segments T6–T10. Division of the greater splanchnic nerves may therefore provide relief from pain in chronic pancreatitis. The greater splanchnic nerves and the sympathetic chain may be divided in the chest at thoracoscopy. It is possible to undertake bilateral splanchnicectomy utilizing spontaneous ventilation with a single-lumen endotracheal tube whilst the patient is in the prone position.

COMPLICATIONS OF NON-NEOPLASTIC PANCREATIC DISEASE

Biliary obstruction

Biliary obstruction may arise as a consequence of a pseudocyst, or an inflammatory mass, in the head of the pancreas. It may also be due to fibrosis of the bile duct as a consequence of recurrent episodes of inflammation. Biliary obstruction from the pressure of a pseudocyst can be relieved by drainage of the pseudocyst. Resectional surgery of an inflammatory mass or bile duct stricture is indicated if there is concern about neoplasia. However, because of its lower associated morbidity and mortality rates, a bypass procedure in the form of a hepaticojejunostomy Roux-en-Y is indicated when there is no concern about malignancy (see Chapter 18). Although biliary stenting may provide temporary relief of jaundice and allow time for the resolution of any inflammatory element, it is not a long-term solution. Prolonged biliary stenting is associated with recurrent episodes of acute cholangitis and secondary biliary cirrhosis.

Gastric outlet obstruction

A pseudocyst or inflammatory mass in the head of the pancreas may give rise to gastric outlet obstruction. In some cases, gastric outlet obstruction may improve with conservative measures, including the withdrawal of alcohol where appropriate. In those patients requiring surgical intervention, an attempt should be made to treat the cause of the obstruction, although usually a gastroenterostomy is undertaken.

Splenic vein thrombosis

Pancreatic inflammation can cause splenic vein thrombosis that may lead to segmental portal hypertension. Haemorrhage from gastric fundal varices or hypersplenism are possible sequelae. Operative intervention should be considered in those with complications of splenic vein thrombosis, and splenectomy is curative. Portal vein thrombosis and its ensuing complications can also occur.

Pancreatic pseudocysts

A pancreatic pseudocyst is a non-epithelialized collection of pancreatic juice, which is surrounded by fibrous or granulation tissue. Pseudocysts may arise following acute pancreatitis, chronic pancreatitis or trauma. In patients with acute pancreatitis, a pancreatic pseudocyst must be differentiated from an acute fluid collection, which does not have a well-developed wall, and occurs within 6 weeks of the initial episode of acute pancreatitis. Although acute fluid collections may mature into pseudocysts, their initial management is conservative unless they become infected.

DIFFERENTIAL DIAGNOSIS

The differential diagnosis of a pancreatic pseudocyst includes a pancreatic cystic neoplasm. It is therefore important to be confident that a pancreatic cystic lesion is indeed a pseudocyst, before embarking on either conservative management or operative drainage. Although the presence of radiological features such as septation, cyst wall calcification, focal wall thickening and papillary projections should raise concern about a diagnosis of neoplasia, perhaps the most important guide to making the correct diagnosis of a pancreatic pseudocyst is a prior history of pancreatitis.

ASSESSMENT

The following factors influence decisions in the management of pancreatic pseudocysts.

Size

Traditional teaching was that pseudocysts >6 cm, or those present for more than 6 weeks, required operative intervention. However, recent observational studies have suggested that asymptomatic pseudocysts may be managed conservatively and followed with serial imaging. Intervention is warranted in symptomatic, complicated or enlarging pseudocysts.

Acute or chronic status

Pseudocysts arising in the context of acute pancreatitis may differ from those developing as a consequence of chronic pancreatitis. Because of the peripancreatic inflammation and necrosis that is associated with acute pancreatitis, pseudocysts which arise following an episode of acute pancreatitis frequently contain debris or necrotic material. In contrast, debris in a pseudocyst secondary to chronic pancreatitis is unusual, and should raise the possibility of previous haemorrhage into the pseudocyst. It should be noted that the amount of necrotic material is frequently underestimated on

CT scan, but can be readily appreciated by using ultrasonography. The presence of necrotic material within a pseudocyst may influence management decisions, as endoscopic drainage may not effect adequate access to allow successful drainage of necrotic material. This may therefore result in the development of infected pancreatic necrosis or a pancreatic abscess. Thus, for those with an appreciable volume of pancreatic necrosis and debris, open or laparoscopic pseudocyst drainage with debridement of necrotic material may be the procedures of choice.

Spontaneous resolution of pseudocysts in the setting of acute pancreatitis occurs more frequently than in those related to chronic pancreatitis.

Pancreatic duct morphology

Endoscopic pancreatic duct stenting may be utilized in the management of patients with either pseudocysts or pancreatic ascites, especially those arising in the context of chronic pancreatitis. Successful treatment is dependent upon the satisfactory determination of pancreatic duct morphology, and in particular the presence and location of pancreatic duct strictures and disruption. Pancreatic duct disruption distal to a pancreatic duct stricture that cannot be crossed with a stent will not respond to endoscopic management. However, if there is no pancreatic duct stricture, decompression of the pancreatic duct with a stent should permit healing of the duct disruption and resolution of the pseudocyst. The stent does not have to traverse the pancreatic duct defect; indeed, effective drainage may be achieved with a small transampullary stent. (The long-term placement of pancreatic duct stents may induce changes within the pancreatic duct.)

Extent of the cyst

Internal drainage of pancreatic pseudocysts should be between a dependent portion of the pancreatic pseudocyst and the intestinal tract, regardless of the methods used. For those pseudocysts confined to the lesser sac, adequate drainage may be achieved by internal drainage into the stomach. If the pseudocyst extends down behind the transverse mesocolon into the infracolic compartment, drainage should be by the formation of a pseudocyst-jejunostomy Roux-en-Y.

DRAINAGE OF PANCREATIC PSEUDOCYSTS

Prior to undertaking any intervention for a pancreatic pseudocyst, up-to-date abdominal imaging should be available in order to ascertain the morphology of the pseudocyst and to determine whether spontaneous resolution has occurred.

Pseudocyst-gastrostomy

This is suitable for pseudocysts lying behind the stomach. Adequate access is achieved through a roof-top incision. A longitudinal anterior gastrotomy is performed between stay sutures. Aspiration through the posterior wall of the stomach with a needle and syringe helps to localize the pseudocyst. Following this, deep stay sutures are placed in the posterior stomach wall and an incision is made through the wall (Fig. 19.10). As soon as entry into the pseudocyst is achieved,

absorbable sutures should be placed encompassing all layers of the stomach and the pseudocyst wall. The pseudocyst-gastrostomy is lengthened along with the sequential placement of sutures. When required, removal of necrotic material within the pseudocyst may be undertaken through the pseudocyst-gastrostomy. A nasogastric tube is placed within the stomach. The anterior gastrotomy is closed.

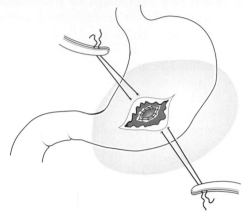

Figure 19.10 *Pseudocyst-gastrostomy.*

Pseudocyst-jejunostomy Roux-en-Y

This is suitable for pseudocysts that have a significant component which would not have adequate dependent drainage into the stomach. A side-to-side pseudocyst-jejunostomy is undertaken using a 60-cm Roux loop.

Laparoscopic internal drainage

Techniques for both laparoscopic pseudocyst-gastrostomy and pseudocyst-jejunostomy have been described. There have been no formal comparisons between open and laparoscopic techniques.

Endoscopic internal drainage

Internal drainage of pseudocysts may be achieved by using endoscopic methods. Transmural stents may be inserted into the pseudocyst to achieve either trans-gastric or trans-duodenal drainage. Endoscopic transmural drainage is suitable for pseudocysts occurring in either the pancreatic head or body, and with a distance of less than 1 cm between the enteric lumen and the pseudocyst. The presence of a significant amount of solid material in the pseudocyst is a relative contraindication for endoscopic drainage because of the risk of inadequate drainage and the development of infective complications. Endoscopic ultrasound is a useful adjunct for confirming wall thickness, the nature of the pseudocyst contents, and the presence of intervening vascular structures that may give rise to haemorrhagic complications during endoscopic drainage.

Pancreatic fistulae and pancreatic ascites

Pancreatic fistulae and ascites occur as a consequence of pancreatic duct disruption. As with pseudocysts, fistulae and ascites arise as a consequence of acute or chronic pancreatitis, surgery and pancreatic trauma. The basis for successful management of both conditions is the attainment of effective pancreatic duct drainage using an approach similar to that for the management of pancreatic pseudocysts. For the majority, endoscopic pancreatic duct stenting results in resolution of a pancreatic duct disruption, as long as a stricture does not exist between the site of disruption and the pancreatic stent. In cases where a stricture exists proximal to the site of duct disruption, surgical resection may be required. Effective pancreatic duct drainage may be supplemented by the use of parenteral nutrition, a nil-by-mouth regimen, and the prescription of octreotide to reduce pancreatic secretion.

SURGICAL ANATOMY OF THE SPLEEN

The spleen lies between the fundus of the stomach and the diaphragm, under cover of the 9th, 10th and 11th ribs, its long axis being in the line of the 10th rib. Normally, the organ lies entirely behind the mid-axillary line, and does not project below the costal margin. Its concave medial surface is related to the fundus of the stomach in front, and to the upper part of the left kidney behind. Its lower part is related to the splenic flexure of the colon, and the phrenicocolic ligament.

Peritoneal connections
The spleen is almost completely invested by the peritoneum. At its hilum, it is connected to the upper part of the greater curvature of the stomach by the *gastrosplenic omentum (ligament)*, and to the posterior abdominal wall in front of the left kidney by the *lienorenal ligament*. These ligaments each consist of two layers, one layer being formed by the peritoneum of the lesser sac (Fig. 19.11). The tail of the pancreas extends forwards to a variable extent into the lienorenal ligament, and may lie in direct contact with the spleen at the hilum.

Vessels
The splenic vessels are large in proportion to the size of the organ, and are very thin-walled. The splenic artery arises from the coeliac axis, and runs laterally at the upper border of the pancreas until it can turn forwards between the layers of the lienorenal ligament to the splenic hilum. The splenic artery commonly divides into five to eight branches before entering the splenic parenchyma. The *short gastric* and *left gastro-epiploic* branches of the splenic artery pass on between the layers of the gastrosplenic ligament to reach the stomach. The splenic vein runs parallel to the splenic artery, but lies below it, and behind the pancreas. The inferior mesenteric vein drains into it behind the body of the pancreas, and the splenic vein then joins the superior mesenteric vein behind the neck of the pancreas to form the portal vein.

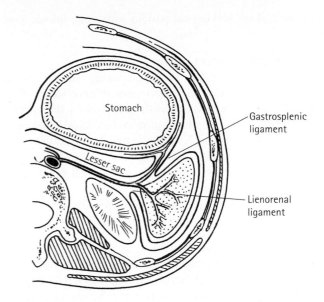

Figure 19.11 *The spleen is anchored at its hilum by two peritoneal folds (ligaments). Large vessels run within these ligaments.*

SPLENECTOMY

There are both short- and long-term effects of splenectomy, but the importance of the long-term effects was not initially appreciated. It was first recognized that young children who had had a splenectomy were at increased risk of overwhelming infections, but only later was it realized that adult patients were at similar risk.[11] This knowledge has led to the development of techniques to preserve an injured spleen, and also to the modification of standard resections to exclude the spleen from the resected specimen, unless its inclusion is necessary on oncological grounds.

INDICATIONS

Trauma
Splenectomy for trauma was discussed in Chapter 14, as well as a variety of splenorrhaphy techniques which can be used to preserve an injured spleen. These techniques can also be employed for a spleen injured during colonic, gastric or pancreatic surgery. However, the risks of splenic haemorrhage during the postoperative period must be weighed against the disadvantages of its loss, and many surgeons will opt for splenectomy whenever there has been any significant iatrogenic damage.

Spontaneous splenic rupture
This emergency may be associated with very minor trauma which ruptures an abnormally fragile spleen, or it may be completely spontaneous. Underlying pathology includes malaria, infectious mononucleosis and distal pancreatitis. Splenectomy is usually unavoidable but, as in trauma, functioning intraperitoneal splenunculi may develop from the

shattered spleen, leaving the patient with some splenic function.

Malignancy in adjacent organs

The spleen may have to be sacrificed during radical resection for cancers of the stomach, pancreas or splenic flexure of the colon due to direct invasion of the pancreas by the tumour. The spleen was also often included in the radical resection of a tumour of the stomach or distal pancreas because it was technically easier to do so, although it was of no oncological benefit. More recently, as the benefits of splenic preservation have become appreciated, some radical excisions have been modified to preserve the spleen as described in the section of this chapter relating to the pancreas, and also in Chapter 16.

Enlarged or overactive spleen

Splenectomy is undertaken for a spectrum of disorders, including infective, metabolic and malignant pathology, in which the spleen becomes enlarged. The decision that a splenectomy is advisable will normally be made by the physician or the haematologist who is managing the underlying condition. The indication for surgery may be either hypersplenism or, more commonly, the discomfort and pressure effects of an enlarged spleen. Repeated infarction within a grossly enlarged spleen can also produce recurrent episodes of severe pain. Hypersplenism can occur in a spleen which is only moderately enlarged from another pathology, but the increased rate of destruction of white and red blood cells, and of platelets, becomes the predominant clinical problem. A splenectomy is also sometimes indicated when a spleen is only undertaking its normal physiological role of removing damaged or malformed red blood cells or platelets. This can be counterproductive in conditions such as hereditary spherocytosis and immune thrombocytopenic purpura. However, with advances in medical treatment, and more awareness of the adverse effects of splenectomy, surgery is now seldom advised for hereditary spherocytosis, and in immune thrombocytopenia splenectomy is reserved for a subgroup of drug-resistant cases.

The aetiology of the giant spleen of tropical splenomegaly is probably multifactorial, with malaria and other infections all implicated. Other causes of giant spleen include myelofibrosis, chronic myeloid leukaemia, schistosomiasis and Kala-azar. Earlier treatment of the underlying pathology can prevent this complication, but once giant splenomegaly has developed splenectomy may have to be undertaken in addition to any medical treatment.

Miscellaneous

Splenectomy for primary splenic, or splenic artery, pathology is relatively rare, but may be necessary in the management of splenic cysts, pyogenic and tuberculous abscesses, splenic lymphoma, and splenic artery aneurysms. Other indications for splenectomy are declining. It is no longer part of the staging procedure for Hodgkin's lymphomas, and most malignant and non-malignant haematological pathologies can now be managed with other treatment modalities.[12]

Splenectomy combined with the formation of a lienorenal shunt for portal hypertension is also now a rare procedure (see Chapter 20).

PREOPERATIVE AND POSTOPERATIVE CONSIDERATIONS

When splenectomy is unavoidable, patients should be immunized against a number of organisms which are implicated in overwhelming post-splenectomy sepsis.[13] Where possible, this should be given at least 2 weeks before surgery. Current UK guidelines recommend immunization against *Streptococcus pneumoniae* (*Pneumococcus*), *Haemophilus influenza* type b (Hib) and *Neisseria meningitidis* (*Meningococcus*) group C conjugate. Appropriate influenza immunization should also be given. When an emergency or urgent splenectomy is required, immunization should be delayed until 2 weeks after surgical intervention in order to ensure the most effective immune response. In addition, life-long prophylactic antibiotics are recommended (oral phenoxymethylpenicillin or erythromycin). The reduced resistance to malaria is an additional consideration for those living in endemic areas.

Patients undergoing splenectomy for drug-resistant immune thrombocytopaenic purpura who are still significantly thrombocytopaenic preoperatively may require perioperative platelet transfusions (see Appendix II). Postoperatively, the short-term adverse effects of splenectomy must also be considered. Mortality and morbidity are increased after abdominal surgery in which a splenectomy becomes necessary as an additional procedure. This does not appear to be merely a reflection of a more difficult operation, or of more advanced pathology. Infective complications are increased, and in addition the early postoperative rise in platelets can increase thromboembolic complications. The platelet count must be carefully monitored after splenectomy so that appropriate action can be taken.

Open splenectomy

A left subcostal or a midline incision is suitable for the removal of a spleen of normal size, or one which is moderately enlarged. A hand is passed over the lateral surface of the spleen, between it and the diaphragm; the organ is lifted forwards and medially, and the posterior layer of the lienorenal ligament is divided (Fig. 19.12a). This allows the spleen to be delivered up into the wound.

Attention is then turned to the gastrosplenic ligament stretching between the splenic hilum and the upper part of the greater curve of the stomach. Within this ligament run the short gastric and the left gastro-epiploic vessels. They are divided between artery forceps, and the vessels are ligated as both layers of the gastrosplenic ligament are divided and the lesser sac is entered (Fig. 19.12b). The fundus of the stomach and the splenic flexure of the colon lie against the spleen. Any adhesions to a normal spleen are minimal, and they are easily separated from it and safeguarded. Occasionally, they are

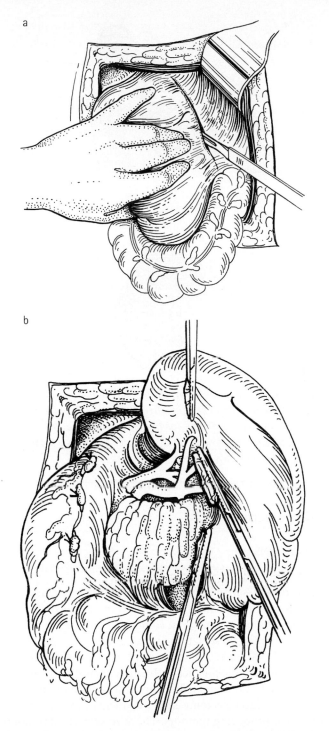

vein which must be isolated, clamped, divided and securely ligated. This dissection can be completed either from in front or from behind. The splenic vessels are very thin-walled and must be handled with care. They are often multiple in the splenic hilum, and it is then easier to ligate them a few centimetres more proximally. However, this increases the risk of pancreatic injury unless the tail of the pancreas has been accurately delineated and separated from the vessels. The hilar vessels may be clamped and ligated as a single pedicle, but it is recommended that the artery and vein are secured separately. This is probably more secure, but it also avoids the theoretical risk of an arteriovenous fistula. The artery should be clamped before the vein in order to prevent splenic engorgement.

MODIFICATIONS FOR GIANT SPLEENS

A bilateral subcostal incision or the oblique incision, as illustrated in Figure 19.13, may be necessary for access to a giant spleen. This incision was traditionally extended up as a thoraco-abdominal extension when additional access was needed, but this is seldom now considered necessary.

If there are no adhesions and the spleen is mobile, the splenectomy can be very straightforward as the splenic ligaments are already stretched. The spleen can be delivered out of the wound and the posterior layer of the lienorenal ligament brought into view. The splenectomy then proceeds in the standard manner.

Some giant spleens are associated with adhesions, particularly vascular adhesions between the anterior surface of the spleen and the diaphragm, preventing the standard initial mobilization. The first step in these circumstances is to divide the gastrocolic ligament and the short gastric vessels to enter the lesser sac. The splenic artery should then be sought at the upper border of the pancreas and ligated in continuity to reduce vascularity. The adhesions are then divided between the spleen and the stomach, colon and diaphragm so that the spleen can be delivered. If an oblique incision has been made there is the option of conversion to a thoraco-abdominal incision, but a bilateral subcostal incision will usually provide good access.

Figure 19.12 *Splenectomy. (a) The peritoneum is incised lateral to the spleen which can then be delivered up into the wound. (b) The tail of the pancreas is closely related to the splenic hilar vessels, and is easily injured by blind application of clamps.*

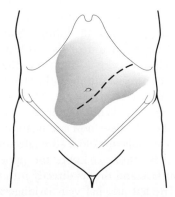

Figure 19.13 *Access for a splenectomy in giant splenomegaly can be difficult. A long oblique incision is recommended.*

more densely adherent to a pathological spleen and time must be taken to release them with care.

The spleen is still attached by the structures within the lienorenal ligament; the tail of the pancreas which must be carefully identified and preserved, and the splenic artery and

MODIFICATIONS FOR RUPTURED SPLEENS

Whether the laparotomy is undertaken as a emergency for splenic rupture, or for a spleen damaged unintentionally during intra-abdominal surgery, there is some urgency to control the blood loss, which may be profuse. Once the posterior leaf of the lienorenal ligament has been divided it is possible to limit splenic inflow and haemorrhage by finger compression of the hilar vessels until the dissection has reached a stage where it is possible to clamp the splenic vessels without damage to the tail of the pancreas. Emergency splenectomy and the techniques for preserving a damaged spleen are described further in Chapter 14.

Laparoscopic splenectomy

Laparoscopic surgery is an increasingly popular option for elective splenectomy, though it is only suitable for spleens which are of normal size or only slightly enlarged. The dissection commences with mobilization of the splenic flexure of the colon so that it can be moved out of the left hypochondrium, before the posterior leaf of the lienorenal ligament can be visualized and divided. The splenic vessels in the hilum are divided with a vascular stapling device, and similar caution to that needed in open splenectomy must be exercised to avoid inclusion of the pancreatic tail. Clips, ties or vascular staples can then be used to complete the division of the gastrocolic ligament. The spleen is too large to be delivered intact through a port site, and must first be macerated within a waterproof retrieval bag.

SURGERY OF THE ADRENAL GLANDS

Anatomy

The adrenal glands lie over the upper pole of each kidney, where they are embedded in fat and enclosed within the renal fascia. The glands lie superomedial to the kidneys, with the diaphragm posteriorly. The right gland – which is triangular in outline – is in contact anteromedially with the vena cava, and anterolaterally, with the liver. The left gland – which is more semilunar in outline – extends further down the medial border of the kidney towards the hilum. Its anterior surface is covered by the peritoneum of the posterior wall of the lesser sac, and below it is closely applied to the pancreas and splenic vessels. The arterial supply of the glands is from multiple variable small arteries which are of little concern during surgery. In contrast, the venous drainage is usually by one large vein, and the safe dissection and ligation of this can be the main technical challenge of an adrenalectomy. The right adrenal vein is very short; it leaves the upper part of the anteromedial surface and drains directly into the vena cava (Fig. 19.14a). The left adrenal vein is longer; it leaves the anterior surface of the gland and runs downwards and medially to drain into the left renal vein (Fig. 19.14b).

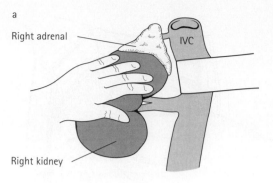
a

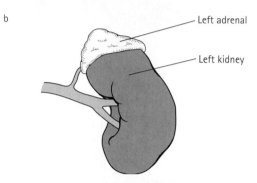
b

Figure 19.14 *Adrenalectomy. (a) The right adrenal gland lies against the cava. The short right adrenal vein is displayed by gentle lateral retraction of the kidney and medial retraction of the cava. (b) The left adrenal vein is more easily visualized as it runs a longer course, obliquely down to the left renal vein.*

Adrenalectomy

INDICATIONS

Hormone-producing tumours

These tumours may be either benign or malignant, and may arise from the adrenal cortex, or from the medulla. The tumours are often small, but sometimes they are multifocal and bilateral. Presentation with a hormone-producing tumour is with a recognizable clinical syndrome, which is then confirmed biochemically. Imaging then shows the position of the tumour and either confirms or excludes multifocal lesions. Adrenalectomy is the treatment of choice for these hormone-producing tumours. The adrenal cortical tumours include those that cause Cushing's syndrome and Conn's syndrome, and the rarer tumours which can cause virilization or feminization. The pharmacologically active tumour of the adrenal medulla is the *phaeochromocytoma*. Patients with some variants of familial endocrine neoplasia (MEN IIa and IIb) have such a high risk of developing phaeochromocytoma that they are screened regularly. It is this group of patients which is most likely to develop bilateral tumours.

Non-hormone-producing tumours

Tumours which do not produce hormones may grow to a large size and only present when they cause compression, or invasion, of adjacent structures. They can arise from either the cortex or the medulla. *Ganglioneuromas* arise in neural crest cells, and a small percentage of these tumours are from the adrenal medulla. The tumours are relatively benign and are often very large at presentation. The more aggressive *neuroblastoma* of infancy and early childhood more often arises from the adrenal medulla than from other neural crest cells. It also grows to a large size and an abdominal mass is the most common presentation. Unfortunately, 70 per cent of these lesions will already have metastasized before diagnosis. Adrenalectomy is indicated if these tumours are still technically resectable, and there are no metastases.

Non-hormone-producing 'incidentalomas'

A management dilemma was posed by the introduction of high-quality abdominal imaging. Computed tomography scans performed for unrelated abdominal pathology sometimes show a small adrenal tumour as an incidental finding. The malignant potential of these *incidentalomas* was unknown, and initially there was debate as to whether they should be ignored, or watched, or excised. A general policy now exists to advise an adrenalectomy for those lesions of over 3 cm, and to monitor smaller lesions with serial imaging.

Bilateral adrenal hyperplasia

Pituitary-dependent Cushing's disease is now seldom treated by bilateral adrenalectomy. Rather, the pituitary adenoma is treated by pituitary ablation or radiotherapy. Alternatively, its secretions are blocked pharmacologically. Bilateral adrenalectomy is reserved for those cases where these interventions have failed. Adrenalectomy is, however, occasionally undertaken for the rarer autonomous adrenal hyperplasia.

Adrenal hormone-dependent tumours

The most frequent indication for a bilateral adrenalectomy used to be the palliation of metastatic breast cancer. However, advances in pharmacological hormone manipulation have relegated this indication to history.

Adrenal metastases

Particularly in colorectal malignancy, isolated metastases may develop in the adrenal gland, or the right adrenal may be involved by a metastasis in the adjacent liver. Resection may still be a potentially curative option. Adrenal metastases are also common in other disseminated malignancies, but surgical resection is generally of no therapeutic benefit due to widespread disease.

MEDICAL AND ANAESTHETIC CONSIDERATIONS

Surgery on those patients with hormone-producing tumours is complicated by the biochemical effects of the excess circulating hormones. Haemodynamic instability from high levels of catecholamines can be particularly challenging in those patients with phaeochromocytoma. However, preoperative and perioperative pharmacological blockade of the excess circulating hormone can now make this surgery relatively uneventful. The patient is usually referred to the surgeon after full investigation and treatment by the endocrine physician, and the anaesthetist is fully prepared for any unexpected instability. Nowadays, the danger is with the patient who has no preoperative diagnosis and a surgeon unexpectedly discovers an adrenal lump at laparotomy. The anaesthetist should be warned before any dissection is undertaken, and any such lump should be handled extremely gently as manipulation can result in a sudden bolus release of pharmacologically active secretions into the circulation.

Those patients who have a bilateral adrenalectomy require lifetime cortisol and adrenocorticoid replacement therapy.

Surgical approaches to the adrenal glands

The adrenal glands can be approached either transabdominally or from the loin. A transabdominal approach is more appropriate when access to both glands is required. It was therefore the standard approach for bilateral adrenalectomy for metastatic breast cancer. In addition, before accurate preoperative imaging was available, bilateral surgical exploration was often necessary so that both glands could be inspected and palpated. The loin approach provides limited access for the excision of a large tumour, and some surgeons favoured a thoraco-abdominal incision. However, excellent access can be obtained with a long subcostal incision, and few surgeons would now choose a thoraco-abdominal incision, other than in exceptional circumstances, as the postoperative morbidity is greater.

The deep-seated position of these small glands has always required a disproportionately large incision for access and, as a consequence in recent years, an increasing proportion of adrenalectomies have been performed laparoscopically. A laparoscopic approach is, however, unsuitable for large tumours or for suspected adrenal cancer. The laparoscopic surgery can also be either transabdominal or through a retroperitoneal loin approach.

TRANSABDOMINAL APPROACH

When access is required to both adrenal glands, a transverse upper abdominal incision is satisfactory; alternatively, it can be a curved incision, convex upwards. A subcostal incision is suitable for the removal of one gland. The adrenal glands lie behind the posterior parietal peritoneum which must be divided for access. The transabdominal open and laparoscopic operation follow similar principles.

Right adrenal gland

The right adrenal gland is exposed by a peritoneal incision between the upper pole of the kidney and the lateral edge of the inferior vena cava (IVC). Usually, the right adrenal gland lies just cranial to the duodenum, but it can be overlain by both the duodenum and the hepatic flexure of the colon. When necessary, the duodenum and hepatic flexure are

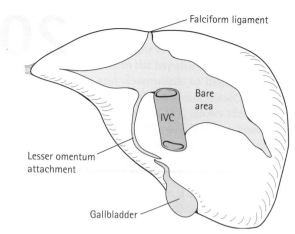

Figure 20.2   *The bare area of the liver viewed from behind. After full mobilization the liver is only fixed by the hepatic veins draining into the IVC and the attachment of the lesser omentum around the structures of the porta hepatis.*

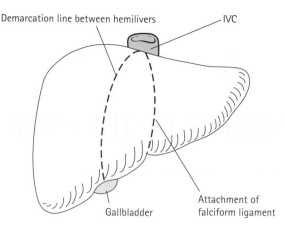

Figure 20.3   *The plane between the right and left halves of the liver lies at around 20–30 degrees from the vertical, and extends from the gallbladder fossa anteriorly to the insertion of the middle hepatic vein into the IVC posteriorly.*

rows to end as the right triangular ligament (Fig. 20.2). The surgical importance of these ligaments is simply the need to divide them in order to mobilize the liver, to improve access during resection.

The *porta hepatis* is a transverse cleft far back on the inferior surface of the right lobe. It transmits the portal vein, the hepatic artery and the hepatic ducts. The lesser omentum is a peritoneal fold which is attached to the liver around the porta hepatis. From there it stretches to the lesser curvature of the stomach and the first part of the duodenum, with the hepatic artery, the portal vein and the bile ducts lying in its right free border. The common bile duct lies anteriorly and to the right, and the hepatic artery lies anteriorly and to the left. The portal vein lies behind. This free border forms the anterior boundary of the epiploic foramen into the lesser sac. The only other obvious surface landmark on the liver is the gallbladder, which lies directly against the inferior surface of the right lobe, and is covered on its inferior surface, and also on a variable percentage of its circumference, by the peritoneum of the liver. The fundus of the gallbladder is the anterior landmark for the division between the two halves of the liver as defined by the internal anatomy. The posterior landmark between the two hemi-livers is the insertion of the middle hepatic vein into the inferior vena cava (IVC), and the line between lies at around 20–30 degrees from vertical (Fig. 20.3). The IVC is closely applied to the posterior surface of the liver. Frequently, it is partially covered by the peritoneum of the posterior wall of the lesser sac, and it is also partially in direct contact with, or even buried within, the bare area of the liver. The hepatic veins drain directly into the vena cava.

SEGMENTAL ANATOMY

The hepatic artery and the portal vein divide into left and right branches in the porta hepatis, just outside the liver sub stance. At the same level the right and left hepatic ducts converge to form the common hepatic duct. The right portal

structures run a near-vertical course in the hilum and enter the liver substance within a few millimetres. The left hilar structures run a longer and more horizontal course before entering the liver parenchyma, and then turn to follow a more vertical course. The three portal structures are surrounded by a fibrous sheath, and this sheath also splits to enclose the diverging right and left structures as they enter the right and left halves of the liver respectively. This extension of the vascular biliary fibrous sheaths continues to surround the second and third divisions of the portal triad, which finally terminate in the separate functional units, or segments. The second-order divisions divide the liver into four distinct parts or sections, a medial and lateral section on the left, and an anterior and posterior section on the right. The third-order division divides the liver into eight segments (Fig. 20.4). This anatomical arrangement allows the main bulk of the liver to be considered as either two halves, four sections or eight segments, each based on a portal pedicle, when a resection is planned. Further divisions of the portal triad allow some segments to be considered as separate sub-segments. For example, segment 4 can be divided into segment 4a and 4b and the caudate lobe (segment 1) may be considered as two further segments – a left half (segment 1L) and a right half (segment 1R). Segments 2 and 3 (lateral section) lie to the left of the falciform ligament. Segments 4a and 4b (medial section) are to the right of the ligament and up to the main plane of a line from the gallbladder fossa to the insertion of the middle hepatic vein. Segments 5 and 8 (anterior section) are lateral to the main plane and occupy roughly half of the right hemi-liver. Segment 5 lies immediately next to the gallbladder. The posterior section of the right half contains segments 6 and 7. The relative size of all segments varies between individuals.

Whereas the portal pedicles run within the segments, the hepatic veins run mainly between segments and converge posteriorly to drain into the inferior vena cava (Fig. 20.4). The right hepatic vein drains most of segments 6 and 7, and

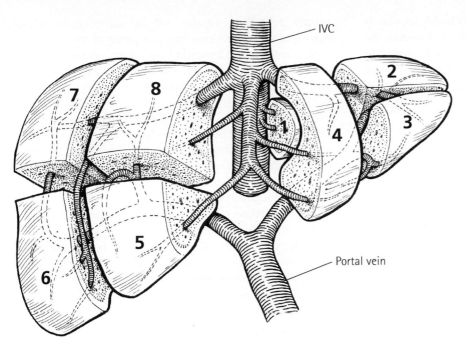

Figure 20.4 *Diagrammatic representation of the liver segments as viewed from the parietal surface (after Couinaud). The portal vein is the only structure in the portal triad that has been shown in the drawing.*

part of segments 5 and 8. A variable posteroinferior vein drains from segment 6 directly into the vena cava, and there are also multiple small veins draining the right liver adjacent to the IVC directly into it. The middle hepatic vein lies in the plane between the two halves of the liver and drains segments 4, 5 and 8, before usually joining the left hepatic vein just before it in turn drains into the vena cava. The left hepatic vein drains segments 2 and 3. There is usually a small umbilical vein, running in a plane deep to the umbilical ligament, which may be useful in maintaining venous drainage of segment 4b in cases where the middle hepatic vein is taken. The caudate lobe drains directly into the vena cava, via one or more separate veins. The details of the biliary, portal, hepatic arterial and venous anatomy, and the common variants which can produce challenges to the surgeon are discussed further in the sections on individual resections.

Physiology

The major role of the liver as a metabolic organ must not be forgotten, despite the challenges of its anatomy. Its blood supply is 25 per cent of the resting cardiac output, and its importance as a processor of the nutrients absorbed from the gastrointestinal tract is emphasized by the fact that 75 per cent of its blood supply is from the portal vein. Glycogen is stored in the liver, proteins and peptides are synthesized, and waste products are broken down to be eliminated in the bile, or excreted by the kidneys. The liver has great powers of regeneration. This was recognized in ancient Greek mythology in the Prometheus legend. Prometheus was tortured by a vulture that, each day, ate a proportion of his liver which then regenerated in time for the next attack. As much as 60–70 per cent of a healthy liver can be removed without precipitating liver failure. However, the situation is not so favourable if the liver is already permanently damaged by cirrhosis, or temporarily impaired by biliary obstruction or cytotoxic chemotherapy.

PREOPERATIVE INVESTIGATIONS

Imaging

Until the advent of computed tomography (CT) and ultrasound scans, contrast studies of the intrahepatic bile ducts were the only useful preoperative anatomical imaging available to the surgeon. No information could be obtained about lesions within the liver parenchyma, except where there was distortion of a main duct, and no information was available on the relationship of a mass to major intrahepatic vessels. An unenhanced CT scan provided only limited information, but the addition of contrast and the careful timing of images became increasingly sophisticated. In CT angioportography, images are taken of the same 'slice' of liver at two separate times after injection of contrast into the abdominal aorta. The first image is in the phase when contrast is perfusing the liver parenchyma from the hepatic artery. The second image is taken when contrast, which initially went to the gut, is returning to the liver via the portal vein. The increased sensitivity of these images is mainly dependent on the difference in blood supply between normal liver and malignant tumours. In contrast to normal liver, a tumour derives most of its blood supply from the hepatic artery.

In recent years, liver magnetic resonance imaging (MRI) scans have generally superseded CT angioportography. The technique is less invasive, and the images are better with fewer false positive findings arising from perfusion defects. Both the triple phase-contrast CT and the MRI with liver-specific contrast agents have the ability to identify accurately abnormal lesions in the liver, and also to delineate the relationship of such lesions to the intrahepatic anatomy. In addition, MRI has greater ability to differentiate lesions and thereby help to distinguish between those that are benign and those that are malignant.

Physiology

The preoperative preparation of a patient for surgery is discussed in Appendix I. When planning any liver surgery, it is important to know whether the essential metabolic functions of the liver are impaired by the underlying pathology. Particular care in assessment is important in patients with cirrhosis and those with obstructive jaundice (see also Chapter 18). When a major resection is planned, the reserve physiological capacity of the liver, and regeneration potential of the remnant, are important, or an apparently successful resection may be followed by fatal liver failure. Temporary liver decompensation frequently occurs after major liver resections, but improves as liver regeneration progresses. Biochemical measurements can provide some indication of both the physiological reserve of the liver, and of its regeneration capacity, but are not always an accurate prediction of the metabolic complications of the postoperative period.

Histological proof

There is frequently doubt over the pathology of lesions within the liver, especially when they are small and do not show classic features on imaging. However, biopsy should always be avoided if there is the potential for a curative resection. All techniques, whether open, laparoscopic or image-guided needle biopsies, spill malignant cells into the peritoneal cavity. A percutaneous needle biopsy has the additional capacity to implant malignant cells along the needle track with resultant abdominal wall or diaphragmatic secondary deposits.[2] Small lesions in the liver should be monitored by serial scans as an increase in size not only suggests malignancy, but slightly larger lesions are also easier to differentiate on imaging modalities. Occasionally, a surgeon must decide to proceed to a liver resection where doubt still remains. Both the surgeon and the patient must be prepared to accept that the surgery may, in retrospect, prove to have been unnecessary in that the resected abnormality is histologically benign (less than 1% in our series[2]).

GENERAL LIVER TECHNIQUES

Historical perspective on liver surgery

Until the closing decades of the twentieth century, liver surgery carried a daunting mortality and morbidity. This was mainly related to major intraoperative haemorrhage. Attempts to reduce blood loss concentrated more on speed than on precision. The need to work very quickly in an operative field where visibility was obscured by bleeding was probably at least in part responsible for some of the other complications which were more common in this era. Precision has proved more important than speed, but this precision has only become possible with advances in both knowledge and technology. The anaesthetist can now provide optimum intraoperative physiological conditions for the surgeon. In turn, the surgeon must be armed with knowledge of the segmental anatomy of the liver and discern additional information on any anatomical anomalies, using both preoperative and intraoperative imaging. With these two criteria met, combined with the improvements in surgical technique which have become possible with technological advances, it is now possible to operate on the liver with minimal blood loss and a low mortality and morbidity.[3]

Anaesthesia

The tendency for bleeding during transection of the liver is related to the level of the central venous pressure (CVP). When the CVP is below 6 mmHg, bleeding can be minimal, whereas if it is above 13 mmHg bleeding will almost certainly be troublesome, even with the most careful surgical technique.[4] The anaesthetist should therefore attempt to keep the CVP as low as possible during liver surgery by restricting fluids and with a glyceryl trinitrate infusion.[3]

Access

A long transverse, or oblique, subcostal incision with the patient placed supine, or partially lateral, is now the favoured approach. The thoraco-abdominal incisions advocated previously are seldom necessary, and are responsible for significant postoperative morbidity. Fixed retraction of the costal margin as illustrated in Fig. 13.1a (page 217) is helpful.

Mobilization of the liver is essential for adequate surgical access, especially when the pathology is in the posterosuperior portion of the right lobe. The falciform and triangular ligaments are divided. Small vessels in the free edge of the falciform ligament will need to be secured by ligation of the ligamentum teres. As the dissection to complete the division of the three ligaments converges posteriorly, the vena cava and hepatic veins can be damaged (see Fig. 20.2). Accidental division of smaller phrenic veins can also cause troublesome bleeding. The left half of the lesser omentum is divided and the lesser sac entered. After full mobilization, the liver is attached only by the hepatic veins to the vena cava, and by the structures in the porta hepatis. It can be rotated out from its normal anatomical position into the wound and packs placed behind it to maintain its position. These packs have the additional benefit of holding the liver in a position such that the anatomical plane between the two halves of the liver is vertical rather than oblique. A vertical plane is easier for the surgeon to identify and follow.

Intraoperative ultrasound

This is now a standard part of many liver resections. It can be used to identify intrahepatic lesions which have not been visualized on preoperative imaging, but with improvement in imaging this is becoming of lesser value. Of greater value is the ability to map the segmental anatomy by the identification of intrahepatic structures.

Liver dissection

A liver incision bleeds profusely from multiple small vessels in the liver parenchyma. Bleeding can be reduced by lowering the CVP, and by temporary occlusion of the inflow to the liver with a Pringle clamp, as outlined below. It can be reduced by following the planes between the two halves of the liver, or the planes between liver segments. This can be done more accurately if the inflow to the area to be removed has been previously ligated, and the surgeon is able to follow a line of demarcation. In addition, technological equipment advances allow more precise dissection.

THE PRINGLE MANOEUVRE

This procedure has stood the test of time since its first description in 1908.[5] It consists of the placement of a soft occlusion (non-crushing) clamp across the free edge of the lesser omentum, thus occluding the inflow to the liver from both the hepatic artery and the portal vein. The assessment of an injury, or the dissection for a liver resection, can then proceed with greatly reduced bleeding. The present author favours partial inflow occlusion using three light 'clicks' on the clamp, and which in his experience has prevented thrombosis of the hepatic artery or portal vein. If the occlusion does not arrest arterial inflow into the liver, an aberrant hepatic artery arising from the left gastric artery should be sought in the lesser omentum, and an additional soft clamp placed across it. The 'safe' time for such occlusion is difficult to quantify. During elective resection of a segment of otherwise healthy liver, total occlusion for as long as 90 minutes may be tolerated without detriment. The physiological reserve of the remnant, and the ability to regenerate, may however be compromised by as little as 20 minutes of occlusion when a more major resection is undertaken in a liver which is already compromised by cirrhosis, or other pathology. There is evidence that longer times can be tolerated if a short period of occlusion is undertaken initially, and a variety of occlusion regimes have been recommended. The present author favours transection of the liver with removal of the clamp and reperfusion of the liver for about 5 minutes after each 20-minute period of occlusion. The length of occlusion is reduced to 10 minutes if the liver is compromised or cirrhotic.

EARLY LIGATION OF INFLOW

This has long been practised in right and left hepatectomies where the hepatic artery and portal vein to the hemi-liver to be excised is ligated in the porta hepatis before division of the parenchyma is commenced. The advantage of this approach is that the line of demarcation becomes apparent between well-perfused and ischaemic liver. This underlines the fact that there is little collateral flow between the two halves of the liver, and that a surgical plane between the two halves should be relatively bloodless. The surgeon can then follow the plane accurately during dissection. The realization that the perfusion of each liver segment is equally discrete, in theory should allow a similar technique to be employed for segmentectomy, but it is often not possible to isolate the inflow vessels for occlusion until some parenchymal dissection has been undertaken.

CAVITRON ULTRASONIC SURGICAL ASPIRATOR (CUSA)

This has become the standard instrument for optimal division of liver parenchyma. Traditionally, the liver parenchyma was divided by 'finger fraction'; this disrupted the liver cells, and exposed larger vessels intact which could then be ligated and divided. However, this method is imprecise, smaller vessels are disrupted, and bleeding is still profuse. The CUSA divides the liver following a similar principle, but is much more delicate and precise. The liver cells are vaporized by the sound waves and aspirated, whilst all fine tubular structures, including small vessels and bile duct radicles, are skeletonized and can be seen straddling the most recent parenchymal division.

LIGATION OF VESSELS AND BILE DUCTS WITHIN THE LIVER

Structures of less than 1 mm in diameter, skeletonized by the CUSA, can be secured by diathermy. Any larger structures should be ligated with fine absorbable material (e.g. 3/0 Vicryl) and divided between the ligatures. Larger vessels and ducts to segments or sub-segments of the liver may also appear in the line of division. As a general rule, any structure of a size which merits a name should have two ligatures on the end which is to be left inside the patient.

HEPATIC VEIN DIVISION

Simple ligation is usually contraindicated as the veins are so short and wide that a ligature would be insecure. A transfixion ligation, although theoretically more secure, is also unsatisfactory as it inevitably bunches and distorts the wall of the vena cava. The only satisfactory method, other than a stapled closure, is a sutured closure. The vein is divided between clamps, and is oversewn with a fine Prolene vascular suture. A monofilament suture which slides through tissue without tearing is essential, as all of the continuous suture must be in place before the clamp is removed and the suture tightened (Fig. 20.5). If the clamp should slip during this

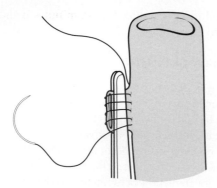

Figure 20.5 *Sutured closure of a short wide hepatic vein.*

manoeuvre, haemorrhage from the vena cava can be torrential. Air embolism is also a potential danger, especially in a patient with a low CVP. Techniques for controlling and suturing an inadvertent venotomy in the inferior vena cava are described on page 489, in relation to a similar complication that can arise during nephrectomy. A stay suture applied to both the superior and inferior border of any large vein prior to division between clamps is recommended.

Endo GIAs

These are small cutting linear stapling devices which have revolutionized the difficulties in the control and division of hepatic veins. These thin-walled veins draining directly into the vena cava have always been technically challenging, not least due to restricted access.

THE ARGON BEAMER

This is a spray diathermy which produces superficial coagulation to a depth of only a few millimetres. It has proved extremely valuable in arresting the surface ooze from a large raw area, and has found one of its main applications in liver surgery.

HAEMOSTATIC MATERIALS

Absorbable, pharmacologically active materials which enhance clotting are particularly helpful when there is persistent low-volume ooze from the large raw surface of a major resection. There is a wide range of proprietary products available, including sheets and teased-out fibres which can be laid against the surface, and 'tissue glue' or fibrin which can be spread or sprayed onto a bleeding area.

Drains

After a liver resection, drains are recommended as the best method of both detecting, and treating, an early bile leak. An early leak represents a technical failure in identifying or securing a bile duct radicle. If there is no leak, a drain should usually be removed within 72 hours as it can cause trauma to the tissues. Late bile leaks, which are associated with tissue

sloughing, occur at about 10–14 days and long after any drain has been removed. Excessive bleeding during the immediate postoperative period may also be detected earlier if there is a drain in place.

Specialization

By accurate preoperative assessment – and by using a knowledge of intrahepatic anatomy and employing all available operative strategies – the surgeon can reduce blood loss to a minimum. It should now be possible to perform liver surgery with a low mortality and morbidity. This is however only possible in centres specializing in liver surgery, and it is therefore important that patients are referred to these centres. In the developed world this should be possible for all elective cases, and for most patients with liver trauma who need a resection. There are, however, surgeons practising in remote hospitals in countries with restricted health budgets. If referral to a major centre is not possible, the general surgeon should be very wary of embarking on any but the most minor elective liver surgery. Despite good surgical technique and attention to detail, the morbidity and mortality from major liver surgery will remain unacceptably high in suboptimal surgical circumstances.

LIVER RESECTION

Anatomically based partial hepatectomies involve the removal of one or more segments of liver parenchyma by isolation and division of the relevant portal pedicle and hepatic veins. They are employed for most major resections, whereas non-anatomically based resections still have a place for some small tumours.

Small non-anatomical resections

These resections are not based on the intrahepatic anatomy, but they are suitable for the removal of small, peripherally situated tumours. Traditionally, these excisions were wedge-shaped, to allow a sutured closure for haemostasis (as illustrated in Fig. 14.3, page 242). They were therefore often described as 'wedge resections'. Today, they are more frequently cut as a circular defect which may be shallow and saucer-shaped, or deeply indented from the removal of half a sphere of tissue to include a lesion further from the surface. As the excision does not follow the anatomical boundaries of vascular inflow, no preliminary ligation of inflow vessels to reduce haemorrhage is possible. Instead, the surgeon must rely on CUSA dissection and the individual ligation of parenchymal vessels and bile radicles. The liver wound is left open. Care must be taken to avoid a non-radical excision with this technique. It is well-documented that the surgeon may underestimate the extent of resection required and hence get a 'positive' or involved margin.[6]

Right hepatectomy

This excision is along the anatomical plane between the two halves of the liver. The operation commences with division of the falciform, triangular and coronary ligaments. The assistant rotates the liver to the left and the retrohepatic IVC is cleared. Care must be taken to separate the right adrenal gland from the bare area of liver. At this stage it may be convenient to secure the small hepatic veins draining directly into the IVC from the back of the right liver, but the main right hepatic vein should be left until the end of the operation to prevent venous engorgement. However, a band of fibrous tissue – the hepatovenacaval ligament – can be divided. This structure is said to be bloodless, but occasionally harbours a significant venous tributary which must be secured. The liver is then returned to a more neutral position, but with packs behind the right liver to lift it forwards into the wound. In this way the packs rotate the right lobe of the liver so that the plane between the two halves is in the vertical plane. A cholecystectomy is then performed. The anterior leaf of peritoneum of the lesser omentum is then divided in the porta hepatis, thus exposing the right hepatic duct, the right branch of the portal vein and the right hepatic artery. The right hepatic artery is easily identified and then suture-ligated and divided. This exposes the right branch of the portal vein. It is safer to secure this vessel with either an endo GIA or by a sutured closure rather than with a simple ligature. A small caudate branch to the right must also usually be divided. Division of the right hepatic artery and the right portal vein produces a line of demarcation between the two halves of the liver. Whilst the right duct can be divided at this stage, it is the author's preference to take the duct later, during the parenchymal transection to avoid inadvertent damage to the left duct. An alternative strategy is only to occlude the right hilar vessels with a soft clamp, at the initial dissection in the porta hepatis. This will produce the same line of demarcation without the finality of a division, and all the structures of the portal triad can then be divided more distally at a later stage in the dissection as illustrated in Figure 20.6. This may prove a safer option, especially if there are anatomical anomalies.

Transection of the liver parenchyma is then commenced, as described above. This transection should be in the ischaemic half of the liver, approximately 5 mm from the line of demarcation. However, the line of transection will often have to encroach into the left hemi-liver to ensure radical excision of more centrally based tumours. If a Pringle clamp is to be used, the surgeon should mark the intended line for the transection on the capsule of the liver with diathermy before the Pringle clamp is applied, as demarcation will no longer be obvious once an occlusion clamp is across all structures at the porta hepatis. The middle hepatic vein lies in the plane of dissection (see Fig. 20.4) and is best preserved if possible as it can provide venous drainage of part of the left liver. However, several veins drain into it from the right liver, and cross the plane of the dissection.

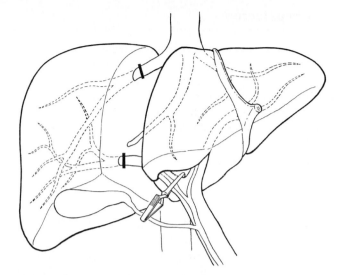

Figure 20.6 *A right hepatectomy. Temporary inflow occlusion to the right half of the liver has been secured with a clamp at the porta hepatis. Definitive ligation of the structures of the right portal triad can wait until they are encountered in the plane of the dissection.*

Each of these must be ligated and divided. The larger right hepatic vein which drains directly into the IVC requires meticulous division and suturing. Alternatively, the vein may be divided with a haemostatic stapling device. In addition, several small veins draining directly into the vena cava must be secured, if this has not been done at an earlier stage. In 25 per cent of people there is also a larger posteroinferior vein draining directly from segment 6 into the vena cava, which must also be divided.

The right hepatic vein may be divided and sutured by an extrahepatic approach, after the right hepatic artery and portal vein have been secured. Alternatively, the right hepatic vein may be dealt with from within the liver during the later stages of parenchymal transection. The present author preferred the latter approach for his first 100 right hepatectomies, but now favours the extrahepatic approach using the newer vascular stapling devices for dividing and stapling the vein.

After division of the portal structures to the right hemi-liver, together with all parenchyma between the two hemi-livers, and the division of all hepatic veins draining the right liver, the right hepatectomy has been completed. The cut surface must be checked for bile leaks from any unsecured biliary radicle. Typically, a white swab is used in order to identify any spot of green bile. Any leak thus identified is then sutured with fine Prolene sutures. Finally, haemostasis must be ensured after removal of any occlusion clamp. Time should be taken to allow the anaesthetist to administer fluids to raise the arterial and central venous pressures to normal levels. Any bleeding site is sutured and the cut surfaces are covered with haemostatic aids, the present author's preference being fibrin glue.

Left hepatectomy

This excision is along the anatomical plane between the two halves of the liver. Segments 1, 2, 3 and 4 are removed. Full mobilization of the right lobe enables it to be rotated forwards with packs behind it, thereby making the transection plane between the two halves of the liver easier. However, the retrohepatic IVC does not need to be cleared on the right side. The left half of the lesser omentum is divided, and it is important to check within it for an accessory left hepatic artery arising from the left gastric artery. The gallbladder is removed if necessary. The principles of the portal dissection to ligate or control the structures in the left portal triad is similar to that required for the right portal triad in a right hepatectomy. As before, the left hepatic artery and the left portal vein are suture-ligated first, and the duct divided during transection. The dissection along the plane between the two halves of the liver is similar to that described for a right hepatectomy, but on this occasion the dissection, which is made 5 mm inside the ischaemic half, is to the left of the middle hepatic vein. The vein is preserved, but tributaries to it from the left half of the liver are ligated and divided. The left hepatic vein must be secured with a sutured or stapled closure. There are additional hepatic veins draining directly into the vena cava from the caudate lobe (segment 1) which must be secured if the caudate lobe is to be removed. This is normally done at the outset by developing a plane between the left side of the IVC and the left caudate.

Segment 2/3/4 segmentectomy

This is a modification of a left hepatectomy in which the caudate lobe (segment 1) is retained. This is a more common procedure as most tumours do not encroach on to the caudate lobe. In the porta hepatis the left hepatic artery and portal vein are ligated, but preferably distal to the branches which run posteriorly into the caudate lobe. The anatomy of the caudate lobe is complicated.[7] However, this lobe receives arterial and portal inflow from both halves of the liver, and the biliary drainage is similarly split. The venous drainage is directly into the IVC. Part or all of the caudate lobe can therefore be retained in a left hepatectomy.

Left lobectomy (segment 2/3 segmentectomy)

This is the excision of the two segments lying to the left of the falciform ligament. The falciform ligament, the left triangular ligament and the left end of the lesser omentum are all divided to increase mobility, and the left liver is rotated forwards and packs placed behind it. The resection is immediately on the left side of the falciform ligament, and is a relatively easy plane to follow. CUSA dissection is ideal for the small bridge of liver parenchyma which crosses the fissure between the lobes. The umbilical ligament is first followed deep into the umbilical fissure. This brings the

dissection directly onto the left portal triad, and its main biliary and vascular branches to the segments of the left liver (Fig. 20.7). The segmental branches to the segments to be excised are ligated and divided. The branches of the portal triad which turn back to segment 4 are preserved (see Fig. 20.4). Superiorly, the left hepatic vein is in the plane of the dissection, lying near the upper end of the fissure between the lobes. It is more superficial than is sometimes anticipated, and care must be taken not to injure it before it can be safely isolated, ligated and divided.

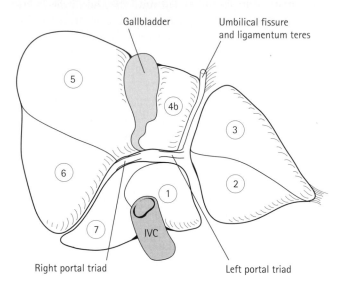

Figure 20.7 *The liver viewed from its inferior aspect. The ligamentum teres (umbilical ligament) can be followed to the left portal pedicle deep in the umbilical fissure. Gallbladder tumours can invade segments 4 and 5. Hilar cholangiocarcinoma can also invade segment 1, while adrenal tumours can invade the adjacent liver of segments 1 and 7.*

Extended right hepatectomy

In this resection, segments 5, 6, 7 and 8 of the right liver are excised with the addition of segment 4 from the left liver. Segment 1 may be included in the resection if segments 2 and 3 are of a size to leave a physiologically competent remnant. The first step is to mobilize the whole liver and rotate it to the left to secure the small tributaries draining into the vena cava, as described for a right hepatectomy. The gallbladder is removed and the dissection in the porta hepatis isolates the right branches of the portal triad in a similar manner to the dissection for a right hepatectomy. They are then usually ligated and divided at this stage rather than merely controlled. The dissection to divide the liver is then similar to that for a left lobectomy (segment 2/3) excision, but the plane of dissection is on the *right* side of the falciform ligament. The vascular and biliary structures supplying, or draining, the segments to be retained, should lie protected on the left of the falciform ligament during the initial dissection, but great care must still be exercised to avoid any damage. The branches turning back from the right portal triad to segment 4 are isolated. Once the segmental branches to segment 4 can be identified and ligated a line of demarcation will aid further dissection.

Extended left hepatectomy

This resection includes the removal of segments 5 and 8, in addition to the left hemi-liver. However, segment 1 is often retained. The operation commences with a dissection in the hilum, as for a left hepatectomy. The position of the ligatures on the structures of the left portal triad will depend on whether segment 1 is to be excised or preserved; a ligature can be placed more distally to preserve a vessel or duct to this segment. The line of the parenchymal dissection is at the anterior border of segments 6 and 7. There are no reliable surface markings to identify this nearly horizontal plane between the anterior and posterior portions of the right liver. It is usually not possible to obtain early control of vascular inflow to create a line of demarcation. However, intraoperative ultrasound can show the position of the right hepatic vein, which drains from all four segments of the right liver and lies in the horizontal intersectional plane between segments 5 and 8 anteriorly and segments 6 and 7 posteriorly. In practice packs are placed behind the right lobe of the liver to shift the liver as far forward as possible. As a consequence the anatomical plane between 5/8 and 6/7 moves from horizontal to as near vertical as possible, similar to the orientation shown in Fig. 20.4. Please note the position of the right hepatic vein is also shifted forwards putting it at risk during dissection. The vein is thus a useful landmark also for right-sided segmentectomies. When early inflow occlusion is not possible, a Pringle clamp is of particular value. An extended left hepatectomy is extremely challenging, and an accurate map of the right-sided portal structures is crucial.

Segment 6 and 7 segmentectomies

These segments may be excised together, or one segment may be excised on its own. The planes between segments are difficult to identify by external landmarks, and the anatomy does not always lend itself to vascular control to show lines of demarcation before parenchymal dissection. Ultrasound identification of the right hepatic vein is often the only landmark. Alternatively, the intersectional plane (between segments 5 and 8 anteriorly and segments 6 and 7 posteriorly) runs in a horizontal plane between the gallbladder and the right extreme edge of the liver.

Segment 1, 4, 5 and 8 resections

These resections may be performed in isolation as single segmentectomies, or as part of a major resection of the central liver. Both the caudate and the quadrate lobe can be divided

into segments, which can be preserved or removed independently. Segment 4a is superior or cranial and may be removed in isolation or in combination with a right hepatectomy. This preserves segment 4b as an extra 5–10 per cent of functioning liver. This usually entails excision of the middle hepatic vein, but great care must be taken to preserve the umbilical vein. Segment 4b is caudal and inferior. It may be removed in isolation, as for a small secondary colorectal deposit, or combined with the adjacent segment 5 if this is also involved in the pathology (see Fig. 20.7). A radical resection for cancer of the gallbladder may necessitate either a segment 4b/5 segmentectomy or a 4b/5/6 segmentectomy. Resections in the central portion of the liver may be confounded by the proximity of the lesion to be excised to the structures of the porta hepatis and the IVC. Intact vascular inflow and outflow – as well as biliary drainage – must be preserved, or reconstructed, to any remaining liver, and an understanding of the anatomy is essential both in the planning and in the execution of these resections. Vascular anomalies can sometimes make a resection impossible, but on other occasions they may make a resection unexpectedly feasible. For example, a large postero-inferior accessory right hepatic vein draining directly into the IVC allows the sacrifice of both the middle hepatic and right hepatic veins if they are involved in tumour.

The dissection for these central segmentectomies follows the planes already described but, as selective inflow occlusion to the individual segments before parenchymal division is not possible, there is no line of demarcation to follow. Portal control of vascular inflow with a Pringle clamp will be essential to reduce blood loss. Further details of these resections is beyond the scope of this book, but further reading on this subject is recommended.[8]

LIVER TRANSPLANTATION

This specialized subdivision of liver surgery must only be attempted within the discipline of a transplant unit. Many specialist liver surgeons will practise outside such a unit and will have no involvement in this field. However, an understanding of the issues involved is important for all surgeons specializing in the liver, as liver transplantation is sometimes one of the treatment options. In addition, if the possibility of a future transplant has not been considered, surgery which is undertaken in the interim may make a transplant more difficult.

The commonest indication for liver transplantation in the adult is deteriorating liver function from progressive chronic liver disease, including primary biliary cirrhosis and primary sclerosing cholangitis, in addition to cirrhosis secondary to viral infection or alcohol. In children, the commonest indication is biliary atresia, and the progressive cirrhosis which ensues when a porto-enterostomy performed for this condition fails to establish adequate biliary drainage (see Chapter 18). A transplant can sometimes make the excision of an

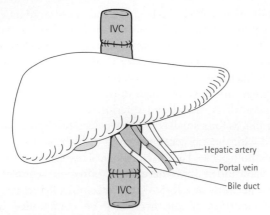

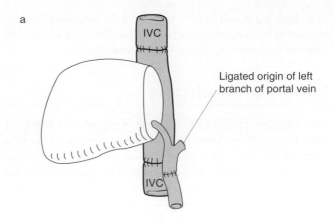

Figure 20.8   *A liver transplant. The donor IVC is anastomosed end-to-end to the recipient IVC above and below the excised diseased liver. Anastomoses are constructed between donor and recipient hepatic artery, portal vein and bile duct.*

intrahepatic malignancy possible, and is also occasionally an option in fulminant liver failure as, for example, after a paracetamol overdose.

Surgical options
The standard cadaveric liver transplant includes the donor liver with the retrohepatic IVC. It also includes the donor common bile duct, portal vein and hepatic artery. The recipient liver is excised with the retrohepatic IVC. The recipient common bile duct, portal vein and hepatic artery are divided close to the porta hepatis. The anastomoses as shown in Figure 20.8 are then performed. Alternatively, a piggy-back technique is used wherein the recipient IVC is retained, to which the donor supra-hepatic IVC is anastomosed end-to-side.

The need for paediatric donor livers always outstrips the availability, and a variety of techniques have been developed to implant a portion of an adult liver.[9] A left hemi-liver or a segment 2/3 graft are suitable. From this developed the expertise to split a donor liver and use the larger part for an adult recipient and the smaller for a child (Fig. 20.9). More recently, the practice of using live, related donors for children has become increasingly popular, though the not insignificant risk to the donor has deterred other surgeons from utilizing this approach.

POSTOPERATIVE AND POST-TRAUMATIC COMPLICATIONS

Emergency surgery for liver trauma was discussed in Chapter 14. The emphasis of management has shifted in favour of a more conservative approach. Often, no action is required other than careful monitoring, with the occasional addition of radiological endovascular intervention. Any surgery is frequently restricted to packing of the liver to control bleeding, but the occasional patient will require either an emergency resection for uncontrollable haemorrhage or a later interven-

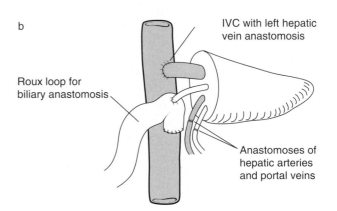

Figure 20.9   *Split liver transplant techniques enable an adult to receive the right liver and a child to receive segments 2/3. (a) The right liver is transplanted with the donor vena cava. The donor portal vein and hepatic artery, with the origins of their left branches ligated, are anastomosed to the recipient portal vein and hepatic artery. The donor common bile duct, with its left hepatic duct confluence ligated, is anastomosed to the recipient common bile duct. For clarity, only the portal vein reconstruction is shown and the donor and recipient hepatic arteries and bile ducts have been omitted from the drawing. (b) Segments 2/3 of the liver are harvested with the left hepatic vein, the left hepatic duct and artery, and the left branches of the portal vein: ducts or vessels to segments 1 and 4 are ligated. The left hepatic vein is anastomosed end-to-side onto the recipient IVC, and the left hepatic artery and the left branch of the portal vein are anastomosed to the recipient hepatic artery and portal vein. The left hepatic duct is frequently anastomosed onto a Roux loop.*

tion for a post-traumatic complication. The range of complications following trauma are similar to those that may be encountered after liver surgery, and they will therefore be considered together.

Haemorrhage

Early post-traumatic and postoperative haemorrhage can often be managed expectantly with blood replacement.

However, a coagulopathy must first be excluded or corrected. If time allows and there is radiological expertise available, significant haemorrhage is best managed by angiography and embolization of a bleeding artery. If the patient decompensates and interventional radiology is not available, then a laparotomy is mandatory. In the trauma situation packing of the liver is advised. In contrast, after surgical resection oversewing of bleeding points is necessary. Secondary postoperative or post-traumatic haemorrhage is often associated with infection. The tissues are extremely friable and the only surgical intervention possible is usually packing of the bleeding area. Angiography and embolization of the bleeding vessel is a much better alternative if the radiological skills are available.

Haemobilia

Haemobilia – haemorrhage into the biliary tree – may follow trauma or surgery, and can also be a complication of almost any hepatobiliary pathology. It implies the existence of a fistula between a vessel and a bile duct. Subsequent bleeding is into the gastrointestinal tract through the duodenal ampulla. A bleed may be major with haematemesis and melaena, or persistent and of low volume, resulting in anaemia. Diagnosis is initially one of exclusion of other sources of gastrointestinal blood loss. Haemobilia is sometimes confirmed if blood is seen at endoscopy to be coming from the duodenal ampulla. Angiography can be confirmatory in showing the anatomical site of the fistula. However, if there is no active bleeding at the time of the examination the angiogram may be normal, although an area of abnormal vascular anatomy may still be demonstrated. Unless an underlying pathology which requires surgical intervention is identified as the cause of the haemobilia, the treatment is by embolization at angiography.

Liver failure

Liver decompensation after a major resection requires expert supportive management until the liver can recover. If anticipated at the time of surgery, the effects may be ameliorated by intravenous acetylcysteine (Parvolex; as used for paracetamol overdosage). This may improve oxygen delivery to the hepatocytes. Liver function must be carefully monitored, and any metabolic abnormalities or coagulopathy treated. The prothrombin time is the most sensitive measure of liver function during this period. A gradual rise in serum bilirubin of 20–40 μmol/L per day is usually indicative of liver failure as a consequence of a small liver remnant. When the bilirubin level reaches a plateau it indicates a favourable prognosis. During this period the initial rise in liver transaminase activity, seen as a consequence of the Pringle clamp injury, should fall if there is no concomitant injury to vascular structures. By a week after surgery the serum alkaline phosphatase level should start to rise, indicating liver hypertrophy that continues for two to three months. During this period oral administration of the choleretic, ursodeoxycholic acid (250 mg, three times daily), may help.

An unexpected decompensation should alert the surgeon to the possibility of a surgical complication. An area of liver may be ischaemic or have necrosed. A portal vein thrombosis may have developed. If the liver remnant was not secured at the time of surgery, it may have rotated and kinked its vascular inflow or drainage. There may be a bile leak or an infection. These complications are best identified by ultrasound and CT examination. Any collection must be drained. Likewise, a bile duct obstruction which presents as a sudden rise in both serum bilirubin and alkaline phosphatase must be drained percutaneously.

Liver necrosis, cysts and abscesses

A small area of liver necrosis may absorb spontaneously, and progress can be monitored on serial imaging. If a cyst forms, or if infection supervenes and a liver abscess develops, these are treated as outlined below. A large area of necrotic liver may be better excised early, or better still identified and dealt with at the time of the original resection.

Bile leaks

Bile that is leaking from the biliary tree must be drained. In practice, the majority of leaks occur immediately after liver resection, and are managed expectantly by leaving the drain placed at operation *in situ*. Bile in the peritoneal cavity must be drained by percutaneous image-guided placement of a drain or, if this service is unavailable, by laparotomy. If bile is draining through a drain left at the time of surgery it must be established by imaging that it is draining all the leaking bile, and that there is no additional collection. Many bile leaks will seal spontaneously, and a steady reduction in the volume that drains is reassuring while spontaneous closure is awaited. The management of larger volume leaks which fail to close depend on the underlying problem. Biliary imaging is necessary to define the anatomy of the leak and exclude biliary obstruction distal to the leak which is preventing spontaneous closure. Surgery to repair a large duct or secure a small duct is seldom indicated in the acute situation. Persistent or high-volume leakage may imply injuries to larger ducts. This may require endoscopic retrograde cholangiopancreatographic (ERCP) stenting, or a sphincterotomy to reduce biliary pressure. Bilary reconstruction at a later date may have to be considered. Peripheral leaks will usually eventually close, but a persistent biliary fistula should be re-explored. If the duct cannot be satisfactorily closed a Roux loop can be brought up to the area to secure internal drainage of the fistula back into the gastrointestinal tract. This is fortunately rare as most bile leaks after trauma or resection settle by good conservative management.

SURGERY FOR LIVER INFECTIONS

Pyogenic liver abscesses

These may develop as a result of bacteria in the systemic circulation, portal vein or within the bile ducts. A systemic bacteraemia can occur from a variety of underlying pathologies, including bacterial endocarditis and intravenous drug abuse. A portal pyaemia can occur with any infective pathology in the gastrointestinal tract including appendicitis, and a liver abscess is occasionally the presenting feature of a colonic cancer or intestinal Crohn's disease. Ascending cholangitis may also be complicated by the formation of liver abscesses. The patient has symptoms and signs suggesting sepsis, but often none that localize the source of the sepsis to the liver. To make the diagnosis, a liver abscess must first be suspected and then excluded or confirmed.

Treatment is with image-guided drainage and antibiotics, adjusted by sensitivity testing of any bacteria grown from the pus drained. A drain should be secured into the abscess cavity and left on free drainage until all drainage has ceased, and the cavity has been shown to have collapsed on repeat imaging. Occasionally, the drain becomes blocked and may require unblocking by saline injection under sterile conditions. The antibiotic regime should also be intensive and prolonged as otherwise recurrence of infection can occur. Initially, intravenous therapy is instituted to ensure high blood levels. Oral antibiotics should then be continued for up to 6 weeks; the choice of antibiotic regime will depend on culture of the pus drained.

The management of pyogenic liver abscesses is more difficult for surgeons who are practising in areas with no access to sophisticated imaging. The diagnosis is often delayed and, even with a high incidence of clinical suspicion, a liver abscess is still difficult to confirm. At laparotomy, pus can be confirmed and the abscess localized by needle aspiration. Open drainage of pus can then be instituted with the introduction of a soft drain into the abscess cavity. The drain is brought to the abdominal wall by the shortest intraperitoneal route, and out to the skin through a separate stab wound. Thereafter, the management is similar. If more sophisticated modalities to check shrinkage of the cavity are unavailable, a slow removal or 'shortening' of the drain over a period of a week or more is recommended. A sinogram can also be of value.

Amoebic liver abscesses

Although the treatment of amoebic liver infection is primarily medical with metronidazole, large collections of amoebic pus still require drainage. Ideally, the accumulation of pus should be confirmed by imaging, and the aspiration performed with the guidance of ultrasound, or other imaging modality. In areas of the world where amoebiasis is common, the drainage of an amoebic liver abscess is often a routine ward procedure carried out without imaging. A point is chosen over the grossly enlarged liver where there is maximum tenderness. This is usually laterally just above or below the right costal margin. A local anaesthetic agent is infiltrated into the skin. A wide-bore needle, attached to a large syringe with an intervening three-way tap, is then advanced into the liver. The abscess is aspirated of pus until it is empty, and frequently quantities of over 1 L are removed. The 'pus' consists of necrotic liver cells mixed with blood, and is traditionally described as resembling 'anchovy sauce'. The needle is then withdrawn, and medical treatment continued. A repeat aspiration may be indicated a few days later, but it is not recommended that a drain is left *in situ* as tracking of the infection into the skin can be problematic. Although aspiration is often undertaken as a ward procedure – similar to the aspiration of a pleural infusion – it is extremely important that full sterility is maintained to prevent a superimposed iatrogenic pyogenic infection.

Ascaris

These intestinal worms can enter the biliary tract through the duodenal ampulla.[10] In the biliary tract they cause intermittent partial obstruction, irritation and infection. This in turn leads to a combination of calculi and fibrous strictures which may involve both the extrahepatic and the intrahepatic ducts. Some patients with severe disease eventually require replacement of their extrahepatic ducts with a Roux loop hepaticojejunostomy. Occasionally, bypass may have to be on to a dilated intrahepatic duct above a stricture (see Chapter 18). Repeated endoscopic or radiological access may still be necessary for the dilatation of recurrent intrahepatic biliary strictures and the retrieval of further biliary stones. Useful access loops are illustrated in Figure 18.13, page 333.

Hydatid disease

Hydatid disease is caused by *Echinococcus*, a parasite which has a life cycle that passes through dogs and sheep alternately as the two hosts. The parasite is in a different form in each host. In the sheep, it is within visceral cysts, whilst in the dog it is a small worm in the gut. The human infection is contracted from an infected dog, and occurs only where there is a close association between dogs, sheep and man. The incidence of the disease thus shows great occupational and geographical variation. Additionally there are two varieties, *E. granulosus* and *E. multilocularis*, which have a different distribution and different behaviour. The latter is more aggressive and requires a more active approach to management. A cyst containing viable parasites develops in the liver, and there may be one or more smaller adjacent 'daughter cysts'. The cysts grow slowly and may be asymptomatic for many years. Larger cysts may cause pain or jaundice from pressure. The cysts may become secondarily infected, and rupture occasionally occurs.

Treatment requires excision of the cyst in addition to medical eradication of the parasitic infection.[11] Most liver surgeons will now advocate a formal liver resection for the removal of the affected area. The older technique of excising only the cyst may however be a safer option for a surgeon unable to transfer a patient to a specialist unit. With a Pringle clamp in place, an incision is made through the liver parenchyma overlying the cyst until the ectocyst is exposed. This appears as a discrete capsule, but consists only of condensed liver tissue around the cyst. The ectocyst is incised to expose the rubbery endocyst, which is only lightly adherent to the ectocyst, and is separated gently from it so that the endocyst with the parasites inside can be delivered intact. Initial aspiration of the cyst from within a controlling purse-string suture may make the removal easier. It is very important not to rupture the endocyst with subsequent spillage of viable parasites. To reduce the consequences of such a mishap the liver is surrounded by packs, which may be soaked in a scolicidal solution such as hypertonic saline. Traditionally, scolicidal agents were also injected into the cyst, but this practice is now condemned as there is almost always a connection from the cyst into the biliary tree, and a risk of such an agent causing secondary sclerosing cholangitis. This communication with the biliary tree is also the cause of the bile leaks which are common after this procedure. Bile leaks may be avoided by a formal liver resection and ligation of the segmental bile ducts draining the cyst. After the cyst has been excised, mobilized omentum is frequently packed into the liver cavity, but alternatively the area can be left open to the peritoneal cavity.

SURGERY FOR NON-INFECTED LIVER CYSTS

Simple cysts

Single or multiple liver cysts are often visible, or palpable, at laparotomy or laparoscopy. There is sometimes initial diagnostic uncertainty and concern about malignancy. They are also a common incidental finding on imaging. Small asymptomatic cysts require no treatment. The occasional cyst may grow to a large size, compress the surrounding liver, and distort the vascular or biliary anatomy. Pain, and less commonly jaundice, precipitate intervention. Percutaneous aspiration should not be attempted as the cyst invariably re-accumulates, and may bleed or become infected. Total excision is the treatment of choice, whether by dissection on the surface of the cyst or, more satisfactorily, by a formal liver resection. Conservative surgery, whether fenestration or marsupialization, is often disappointing as recurrence is likely if a significant portion of the cyst wall is left *in situ*. However, as these cysts are large, and have caused compression and distortion of the intrahepatic anatomy, a segmentectomy or hemi-hepatectomy required for their removal may be technically challenging. Cysts that hang off the infe-rior aspect of the liver may be managed by laparoscopic deroofing as long as the majority of the cyst wall can be easily removed. Occasionally cysts are malignant. Whilst imaging characteristics may highlight the possibility of malignancy, it can be extremely difficult to distinguish with certainty between a benign and a malignant cyst. It is the author's preference therefore to excise symptomatic cysts intact if at all possible.

Biliary cysts

Occasionally, a cyst in the liver is found on preoperative imaging to communicate with the biliary system. These rare cysts, which are most often a complication of biliary surgery or trauma, can be drained internally with a cystoenterostomy onto a Roux loop.

SURGERY FOR LIVER TUMOURS

Haemangiomas and benign neoplasms

The advent of scanning the liver by ultrasound, CT and MRI has led to the coining of the term 'incidentaloma'. In other words, innocent abnormalities are discovered as a by-product of scans performed for non-related symptoms, or for the monitoring of unrelated pathologies. The culprits include haemangiomas, adenomas, focal nodular hyperplasia and cysts. Characterization of these lesions may be straightforward, but can be extremely difficult even for specialist hepatobiliary radiologists. If doubt remains then a trial of time with repeat scanning at three- to four-month intervals will identify enlarging lesions that may be malignant. Surface bile duct adenomas, haemangiomas and cysts may also be encountered as incidental findings when the liver is inspected or palpated during laparotomy. Larger lesions may have a characteristic appearance enabling a reasonably confident diagnosis to be made, but small benign lesions can be difficult to differentiate from secondary deposits. A 'trial of time' and repeat scans are again appropriate. As explained further below, the temptation to biopsy such a lesion for histology should be resisted.

Small capillary haemangiomas and bile duct adenomas can be safely left *in situ*. Larger cavernous haemangiomas may present with pain or obstructive jaundice and require excision, by either segmentectomy or hemi-hepatectomy. Liver cell adenomas are associated with the contraceptive pill; they may grow to a large size, and major haemorrhage, both into the tumour or into the peritoneal cavity, is sufficiently common that their removal is usually advised. They are excised as a hemi-hepatectomy or segmentectomy, depending on their location. A patient with a haemangioma or a liver cell adenoma may present as an emergency with a major intraperitoneal bleed. If at laparotomy a general surgeon encounters this situation the treatment is packing to control haemorrhage, followed by transfer to a specialized hepatobiliary unit for a resection.

Very large cavernous haemangiomas in infancy can present with high-output cardiac failure. Spontaneous regression of an infantile haemangioma will often occur, and hepatic artery embolization may be used to reduce the arteriovenous shunt and avoid the need for a resection. If this is unsuccessful and resection is not possible, then a liver transplant is a further option.

Hepatocellular carcinoma (HCC)

These tumours mostly arise within a liver that is already damaged by viral hepatitis or alcohol. There is great geographical variation in incidence, and this tumour is much more common in Asia than in the West. This is partly related to the increased incidence of chronic viral hepatitis, but food carcinogens are a probable additional factor. Many patients are already under medical management for impaired liver function associated with cirrhosis, and the diagnosis is frequently made following investigations for a deterioration in liver function. Smaller, presymptomatic tumours detected on liver imaging are often initially difficult to differentiate from the regenerative nodules within a cirrhotic liver. Although there may be multifocal hepatic cell carcinomas at presentation, they often metastasize late and a potentially curative liver resection, which can offer around a 35 per cent five-year survival, is the first option to be considered. Unfortunately, many of these lesions are irresectable at presentation, either because of their proximity to vital structures or, more frequently, because the physiological and regenerative reserve of the cirrhotic liver will not permit any major resection.

Excision and liver transplantation has become an increasingly attractive option in the surgical management of small tumours in severely cirrhotic livers with significant impairment of function and portal hypertension. Liver transplantation has been less successful when the indication is a large tumour which cannot be resected without the removal of most of the liver. Transplantation is now considered to be contraindicated if the patient has a hepatocellular carcinoma greater than 4 cm. Palliative non-surgical tumour destruction can be a very effective therapy but, as it cannot match the prognosis possible with resection, it should not be considered unless resection is contraindicated. There are many methods of tumour destruction but those most frequently used in HCC are either percutaneous injection of alcohol into the tumour, or tumour embolization via the hepatic artery with lipiodol, either on its own or in combination with cytotoxic agents. Percutaneous ablation by radiofrequency-generated heat is being increasingly used and is under ongoing evaluation.

HCC can present as an emergency with rupture and major intraperitoneal bleeding, and this complication is usually fatal. Liver packing to control haemorrhage, followed by transfer of the patient to a specialist liver unit for an emergency resection, may occasionally be successful.

Cholangiocarcinoma

Cholangiocarcinoma may arise from the extrahepatic ducts, from major intrahepatic ducts, or from peripherally placed small bile ducts. Peripheral tumours, for reasons as yet unidentified, are increasingly common, and are resected as a hemi-hepatectomy or segmentectomy. The more centrally placed tumours within the liver may be amenable to resection by a central segmental approach. The surgery of hilar tumours was discussed in Chapter 18.

Secondary liver tumours

The pattern of metastatic spread of a malignancy can to a great extent be predicted by the origin of the primary tumour. For example, if a breast cancer spreads to the liver it is commonly in the form of many hundreds of tiny deposits, and it usually occurs at the same time as secondary deposits also develop in the lungs, the bony skeleton and the bone marrow. In contrast, a metastatic colorectal cancer may result in only one or two secondary deposits in the liver, with no metastases to other organs. Whilst the deposits from the former tumour are obviously unsuitable for surgical excision, excellent results have been obtained from excision of the latter. Cures are undoubtedly achieved, and the five-year survival figures after resection are of the order of 30 per cent. Most liver resections for secondary malignant deposits are for colorectal cancer, but other tumours, especially secondary sarcomas and carcinoid tumours, should also be considered.

DETECTION

If a colorectal surgeon waits for a liver secondary to become palpable or symptomatic, it is usually too late to offer a resection. Therefore, it is now routine to screen the liver at the time of the initial bowel resection, and to include regular liver imaging during follow-up. The frequency and the modality of such imaging varies in different units, but a yearly ultrasound scan for five years is a reasonable compromise between what is desirable and what is affordable. The limitation of ultrasound has prompted increased use of 6-monthly CT scans if available and affordable. When an abnormality is detected, further, more sophisticated imaging with MRI will usually clarify whether the abnormality represents a secondary deposit. In cases of doubt the situation is watched and scans repeated in 3 to 4 months time. There is however no justification for watching a solitary secondary growing over a number of years before considering surgery. A large solitary secondary, even when fully excised, carries a worse prognosis than an R_0 resection of multiple smaller deposits.[12] This is because of metastases from the metastasis. Secondary deposits in the liver may invade intra-hepatic veins with resultant tumour emboli and systemic spread. The invasion of portal vein branches results in metastases within the liver itself, both locally in the same segment and also in adjacent segments.

SELECTION

Most patients who were fit enough for the original bowel resection should be considered for surgery for resectable liver secondaries. Age in itself is not a contraindication. A liver resection in the presence of extrahepatic metastases is seldom justified. It should however occasionally be considered, as when an adrenal deposit can be excised en bloc, or where there is an abdominal wall needle track deposit which can be excised. A coexistent lung secondary may also be potentially resectable, and patients with up to four discrete pulmonary deposits should be considered. However, multiple pulmonary metastases are a contraindication to a liver resection, and should be excluded by preoperative chest CT scanning. Para-aortic nodal disease, local pelvic recurrence or peritoneal seedlings are also contraindications to a liver resection. The two former metastatic situations can be diagnosed on pre-operative abdominal and pelvic CT or MRI scans, but peritoneal seedlings are best excluded by a laparoscopy before an abdominal laparotomy incision is made. The present author would recommend a laparoscopy in patients whose primary tumours were originally unfavourable, such as those that had perforated or invaded through the peritoneum, and in those which had extensive nodal involvement. The availability and cost of positron emission tomography (PET) scanning still limits its place in the detection of extrahepatic disease. False-positive and false-negative results are also still a problem, but PET scans may become an increasingly valuable investigation in the future.

It was originally believed that only solitary secondaries should be considered. This was then extended to include multiple secondaries, provided that they were in only one half of the liver. It is now accepted that resection may be a curative option even when there are secondaries in both the right and left liver, provided that all the secondaries can be removed whilst preserving sufficient liver. Resections may take the form of hemi-hepatectomies, segmentectomies or localized excisions. Local excisions are most often used for an additional small secondary not included in the major resection. There is however seldom any place for a resection which does not remove all the intrahepatic disease. Preoperative imaging can be used to predict operability and to plan the surgery with accuracy. However, at the time of laparotomy, 5–15 per cent of patients may still be found to be inoperable.

It must be remembered that patients who have liver secondaries at the time of presentation of the primary do not necessarily have incurable disease. The liver resection can be carried out at the same time as the bowel resection, except when both require a major procedure. For example, a right hemicolectomy can be combined with a right hepatectomy and an anterior resection with a segment 2/3 left lobectomy, but if a patient requires an anterior resection and a right hepatectomy the liver resection should be deferred for a second operation. A temporary defunctioning stoma in the right hypochondrium, and the timing of its closure, can be an additional surgical challenge.

Repeat resections when a patient develops further secondary deposits in the liver following a previous liver resection should be considered on the same criteria as those used for a first liver resection. The prognosis is at least as good as on first presentation with liver secondaries. A repeat resection is made more difficult by the distortion of anatomy following regeneration of the remnant, in addition to adhesions and fibrosis.

Surgery is not the only effective treatment for liver secondaries. The lesions can be reduced in size, or even occasionally obliterated, by chemotherapy. There are also a large variety of techniques available for thermal or chemical ablation. However, for those metastases which can be completely removed by surgical excision, no other modality can offer as good a prognosis as a liver resection.

EXTENDING THE POSSIBILITIES

The percentage of patients with colorectal liver metastases who are considered suitable for a liver resection is steadily rising. Some patients who are initially unsuitable may still have a potentially curative resection by using some of the following strategies.

- *Preoperative chemotherapy*, especially with the newer more potent agents including Oxaliplatin and Irinotecan, can shrink the periphery of a tumour away from vital intrahepatic structures which must be preserved and thus make a resection feasible. The liver is more difficult to handle at operation after chemotherapy, and it must be remembered that a liver after chemotherapy will have its functional and regenerative capacity at least temporarily impaired. These patients are also more vulnerable to postoperative septic complications if the preoperative course of chemotherapy is prolonged.
- *Staged resection* can be useful when there are metastases in both halves of the liver. For example, an initial right hepatectomy can be followed by a delay while the left liver hypertrophies to allow one or more segmentectomies to be undertaken on the left hemi-liver, without embarrassing liver function. The accelerated growth of the remaining deposits in the regenerating liver during this delay must be taken into account.
- *Portal vein embolization* will induce a 40–60 per cent increase in the size of that part of the liver that has not been embolized. This is an image-guided procedure carried out by an interventional radiologist, and may be of value when, for example, an extended right

hepatectomy is planned but the remnant to the left of the falciform ligament is small. A disadvantage is that the portion to be removed has only hepatic artery inflow, which will favour the metastases that may grow preferentially during the delay before surgery.

Extrahepatic malignancies invading the liver

An extrahepatic malignancy may invade the liver by direct extension. When this occurs in a renal, gastric, oesophageal or colonic cancer it almost always represents an irresectable situation. However occasionally, including when an adrenal, gallbladder or hilar cholangiocarcinoma is invading the liver, a resection is still sometimes appropriate, including resection of the affected segment of liver.

CYSTIC DILATATION OF THE INTRAHEPATIC BILE DUCTS

There is a wide range of aetiologies, including Caroli's disease, which probably represents an intrahepatic variant of choledochal cyst (see Chapter 18, page 336). In addition, any condition which causes fibrous strictures can be associated with proximal dilatation. Presentation is with obstructive jaundice and recurrent biliary sepsis. There are often intrahepatic calculi. Drainage can sometimes be secured onto grossly dilated sections of the intrahepatic biliary system, but when the pathology affects only a localized area of liver a resection is the treatment of choice. More often, the liver is more extensively involved. Repeated radiological or endoscopic access to the intrahepatic biliary tree will often be necessary. Therefore, consideration should be given to the provision of an access loop as described in Chapter 18 (Fig. 18.13, page 333). In some patients the only effective solution is liver transplantation.

PORTAL HYPERTENSION

Surgical management of portal hypertension is now mainly historical. Portal hypertension is caused by obstruction to venous drainage. This may be post-hepatic from hepatic venous thrombosis in the Budd–Chiari syndrome, intrahepatic from cirrhosis, or pre-hepatic from obstruction of the portal vein. Whatever the aetiology, the pressure within the portal venous system rises and collateral channels open up between the portal and systemic venous beds. Many of these channels, such as those in the retroperitoneum, are harmless, but those at the gastric cardia produce oesophageal varices which can present with torrential intraluminal haemorrhage. Historically, the surgery of portal hypertension was focused either on interrupting the portosystemic venous anastomosis at the cardia and direct ligation of the varices in an emergency, or on the reduction of portal pressure as an elective procedure.

Interruption of the portosystemic anastomosis at the cardia, and direct ligation of the varices from within the opened oesophagus, was a formidable undertaking in an emergency. Even before the oesophagus has been isolated there is often major bleeding from the upper abdominal wound from anastomotic venous channels around the attachment of the falciform ligament, and the surface of the stomach has dilated subserosal veins coursing up toward the oesophagus. If a laparotomy has to be performed nowadays for uncontrolled variceal bleeding, the alternative transection and re-anastomosis of the distal oesophagus with a circular stapling device introduced through a separate gastrotomy (as illustrated in Fig. 13.16, page 229), is an easier solution. However, for those surgeons still forced to tackle this emergency due to a lack of facilities for endoscopic sclerotherapy, a circular stapling device may not be an available option either.

The creation of a shunt between the portal and systemic veins reduces portal venous pressure and is effective in reducing the incidence of variceal bleeding. However, any shunt which reduces portal pressure also reduces portal venous perfusion of the liver, and this proves critical in some patients with significant hepatic impairment from cirrhosis. In an attempt to reduce the proportion of blood which was shunted, there was a move away from the original end-to-side portocaval shunt to a variety of other shunts (Fig. 20.10). These included a splenectomy followed by the formation of an end-to-side anastomosis of the splenic vein onto the left renal vein (a proximal lieno-renal shunt), the fashioning a side-to-side shunt between the superior mesenteric vein and the IVC with a prosthetic graft (a mesocaval H-graft shunt) or the formation of an end-to-side anastomosis of the distal splenic vein onto the renal vein (distal lieno-renal shunt) as popularized by Warren. These more limited shunts were less effective in the prevention of variceal bleeding, but were associated with a lower incidence of liver failure precipitated by the surgery.

In recent years the focus of management has returned to that of the varices themselves. They can be effectively sclerosed by endoscopic injection, both as an emergency measure to arrest haemorrhage, and as an interval procedure to obliterate the varices and prevent a subsequent bleed. Very occasionally, a portosystemic shunt is still indicated, most commonly in patients with normal liver function and severe post-hepatic venous obstruction. A transjugular intrahepatic portosystemic shunt (TIPSS) is performed as an interventional radiological procedure, and is created within the liver substance. This has the additional advantage that there is no distortion of the extrahepatic vascular anatomy, which is an important consideration if a liver transplant might be an option at a later stage. The place for an open surgical shunt is limited to situations where the facilities or skills to undertake a TIPSS are unavailable.

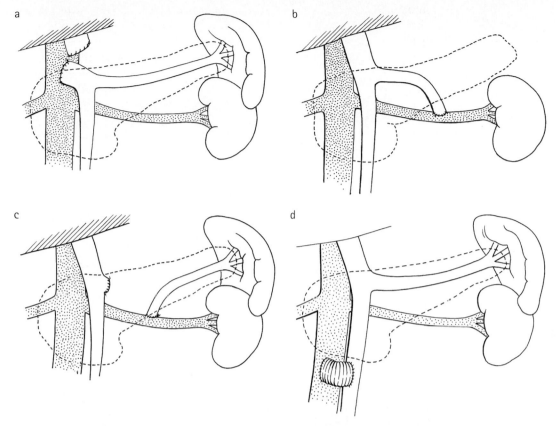

Figure 20.10   *Portacaval shunts. (a) An end-to-side portocaval anastomosis. (b) A proximal lienorenal shunt with splenectomy. (c) A Warren distal lienorenal shunt in which only the splenic component of the portal venous blood is diverted from the liver. (d) A mesocaval shunt with a Dacron 'H' graft. The diameter of the graft can be selected so that there is only partial portal-systemic diversion.*

REFERENCES

1. Bismuth H, Houssin D, Castaing D. Major and minor segmentectomies – Réglées in liver surgery. *World J Surg* 1982; **6**: 10–24.
2. Jones OM, Rees M, John TG *et al.* Biopsy of resectable colorectal metastases causes tumour dissemination and adversely affects survival following liver resection. *Br J Surg* 2005 (in press).
3. Rees M, Plant G, Wells J, Bygrave S. One hundred and fifty hepatic resections: evolution of technique towards bloodless surgery. *Br J Surg* 1996; **83**: 1526–9.
4. Johnson M, Mannar R, Wu AVO. Correlation between blood loss and inferior vena caval pressure during liver resection. *Br J Surg* 1998; **85**: 188–90.
5. Pringle JH. Notes on the arrest of hepatic hemorrhage due to trauma. *Ann Surg* 1908; **48**: 541–9.
6. Scheele J, Strangl R, Altendorf-Hofmann A. Hepatic metastases from colorectal carcinoma: impact of surgical resection on the natural history. *Br J Surg* 1990; **77**: 1241–6.
7. Murakami G, Hata F. Human liver caudate lobe and liver segment. *Anat Sci Inst* 2002; **77**: 211–24.
8. *Surgery of the Liver and Biliary Tract*, 3rd edn. Y Fong, LH Blumgart. Philadelphia: Elsevier, 2000.
9. Strong RW. Liver transplantation: current status and future prospects. Clinical review. *J R Coll Surg Edinb* 2001; **46**: 1–8.
10. Khuroo MS, Zargar SA, Mahajan R. Hepatobiliary and pancreatic ascariasis in India. *Lancet* 1990; **335**: 1503–7.
11. Buttenschoen K, Carli Buttenschoen D. *Echinococcus granulosus* infection: the challenge of surgical treatment. *Arch Surg* 2003; **388**: 218–30.
12. Rees M, Plant G, Bygrave S. Late results justify resection for multiple hepatic metastases from colorectal cancer. *Br J Surg* 1997; **84**: 1136–40.

21

CLASSIC OPERATIONS ON THE SMALL AND LARGE BOWEL

ANATOMY

The small intestine

The *jejunum* begins as a direct continuation of the predominantly retroperitoneal duodenum at the duodenojejunal flexure. Distally, it is continuous with the *ileum*, with no line of demarcation. The ileum joins the medial wall of the caecum at the ileocaecal valve. The jejunum and ileum have a complete peritoneal covering and lie as free loops in the peritoneal cavity suspended on their mesentery. The *mesentery* contains, between its two layers, the arteries, veins, lymphatics and nerves of the small intestine. Its root, or line of attachment to the posterior wall, extends obliquely from the duodenojejunal flexure to the caecum.

The large intestine

An understanding of the surgical anatomy of the colon is dependent on an appreciation of intrauterine folding and rotation of the gastrointestinal tract, which is outlined in the embryology section in Chapter 13, page 218.

The *caecum* normally occupies the right iliac fossa; it is completely enveloped in peritoneum, but has no mesentery so that it is relatively fixed in position. The *appendix* is attached to the posteromedial aspect of the caecum just below the ileocaecal junction, and the three taeniae coli of the caecum converge to end at the base of the appendix. The appendix is variable in position, but most commonly lies retrocaecally, or less frequently lies with the tip free in the pelvis. A retrocaecal appendix may lie retroperitoneally, but in most cases the appendix has a complete peritoneal cover-

ing and its own mesentery in which runs the appendicular artery (Fig. 21.1). An additional avascular fold of peritoneum extending from the front of the terminal ileum to the proximal appendix may be present.

The *ascending colon* is bound down to the posterior abdominal wall, and is covered with peritoneum only on its anterior surface and sides. The *hepatic flexure* lies on the right kidney and the second part of the duodenum. The *transverse colon* is again freely mobile since it has a complete peritoneal investment and a mesentery. A long transverse colon may hang down into the pelvis, but is easily distinguishable from the sigmoid colon by the attachment of the greater omentum to its lower border. The complex peritoneal folds around the transverse colon are easier to understand from an embryological viewpoint. At the *splenic flexure* the colon is again

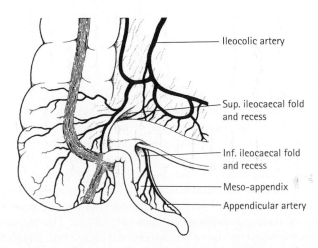

Figure 21.1 *Anatomy of the appendix and ileocaecal region (after Grant).*

Ileocolic artery

Sup. ileocaecal fold and recess

Inf. ileocaecal fold and recess

Meso-appendix

Appendicular artery

bound to the posterior wall and overlies the left kidney and is closely related to the spleen which lies superolateral to it. The *descending colon* is related to the posterior abdominal wall in a similar fashion to the ascending colon. The colon again becomes mobile on a mesentery as the *sigmoid* (or *pelvic*) *colon.* The sigmoid colon is of variable length and mobility and, as its extremities lie fairly close together, it is liable to volvulus. The large intestine again becomes fixed and finally totally retroperitoneal as the rectum.

The *recto-sigmoid junction* has been defined as opposite the third segment of the sacrum, as the point where the taeniae spread out to form a continuous longitudinal muscle layer and as a measured distance from the anal verge. The distance used for the definition of this rather artificial junction has varied from between 12 and 15 cm. Standardization is important for communication between surgeons with regard to the treatment of rectal and sigmoid cancer, and the junction between sigmoid colon and rectum has now been accepted as 15 cm from the anal verge when measured with a rigid sigmoidoscope.

The *rectum* lies in the concavity of the sacrum, and ends by making an acute posterior angulation to become the anal canal. The upper third of the rectum is covered with peritoneum anteriorly and on each side; the middle third is covered only in front, while the lower third is entirely devoid of peritoneum, because it lies below the pelvic peritoneum. Below the peritoneal reflection, the rectum is related anteriorly in the male to the base of the bladder, the seminal vesicles and the prostate, and is separated from them by Denonvillier's fascia. This fascial layer may represent the fused anterior and posterior peritoneum of the deeper rectovesical pouch which was present during embryological development. In the female, the rectum is related anteriorly to the posterior vaginal wall with a thin rectovaginal septum between them. The rectum has its own discrete 'mesentery' or *mesorectum* which encircles the rectum, but the bulk of the mesorectum lies posteriorly in the concavity of the pelvis. There is an areolar plane between the mesorectum and the structures of the pelvic side wall. This was not initially appreciated, but is of great importance in the surgery of rectal cancer.

BLOOD SUPPLY

The small and large bowel are supplied almost exclusively from branches of the *superior* and *inferior mesenteric arteries.* The jejunal and ileal branches of the superior mesenteric artery run in the small bowel mesentery. Three main branches from the superior mesenteric artery supply the large bowel proximal to the splenic flexure. The middle colic artery runs in the transverse mesocolon, and the right colic and ileocolic arteries are retroperitoneal as they run towards the ascending colon and caecum (Fig. 21.2). The inferior mesenteric artery runs a retroperitoneal course but, after full mobilization of the sigmoid colon, it can be appreciated that in reality it is lying posteriorly within the pelvic mesocolon.

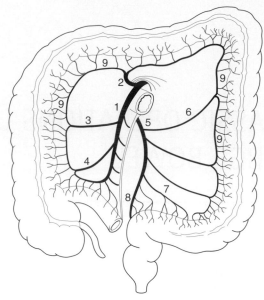

Figure 21.2   *The arterial supply of the large bowel. (1) superior mesenteric; (2) middle colic; (3) right colic; (4) ileo-colic; (5) inferior mesenteric; (6) ascending left colic; (7) sigmoid arteries; (8) superior rectal; (9) the 'marginal' artery which consists of anastomotic arterial loops between individual arteries. It may form an inadequate anastomotic channel at the watershed between the supply from the superior and the inferior mesenteric arteries around the splenic flexure.*

It supplies the large bowel distal to the splenic flexure via the ascending left colic artery, the sigmoid arteries and its own continuation as the superior rectal artery into the mesorectum. The rectum also has a blood supply from the inferior rectal (haemorrhoidal) arteries, but the middle rectal arteries, which are described in older anatomy texts, are small and often absent. The arterial vasculature within the large bowel mesentery is arranged in a series of loops with interconnecting anastomoses. The large anastomotic channel close to the bowel is the *marginal artery.* It is this arterial anatomy which makes many large bowel resections possible and enables the surgeon to sacrifice the inferior mesenteric artery in infrarenal aortic prosthetic replacement surgery with only infrequent compromise to left colonic perfusion.

The venous drainage of the intestines initially follows the arteries. The *superior mesenteric vein* lies on the right side of the superior mesenteric artery until it unites with the splenic vein to form the portal vein behind the neck of the pancreas. The *inferior mesenteric vein* lies lateral to the inferior mesenteric artery, and as it ascends above the level of origin of the artery it lies progressively more lateral. It disappears behind the pancreas in the vicinity of the duodenojejunal flexure to join the splenic vein (Fig. 21.3).

LYMPHATIC DRAINAGE

The lymphatic drainage of the intestines follows the arterial supply. The only exception is the rectum which, although it

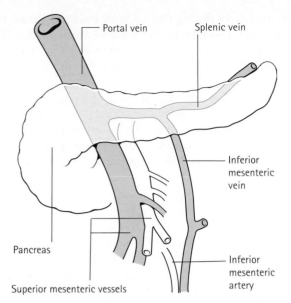

Figure 21.3 *Venous drainage of the bowel. The veins are lateral to the arteries.*

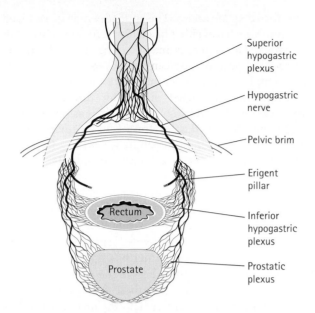

Figure 21.4 *The superior hypogastric plexus on the front of the aorta and the common iliac vein, the two hypogastric nerves at the pelvic brim, the inferior hypogastric plexus on the pelvic side walls and the prostatic plexus lying on the anterior surface of Denonvillier's fascia are all at risk in rectal surgery.*

has an arterial contribution from the inferior rectal arteries, its lymphatic drainage is almost exclusively upwards alongside the superior rectal artery. Lymph nodes are along the lymphatic channels throughout the mesentery and drainage is finally into the pre-aortic lymph nodes.

PELVIC AUTONOMIC NERVES

The multiple sympathetic fibres of the *superior hypogastric plexus* lie over the anterior surface of the bifurcation of the aorta and the left common iliac vein. They condense to form the two hypogastric nerves which diverge as they cross the brim of the pelvis to the pelvic side wall where each merges with the parasympathetic outflow from S2, 3 and 4 to form the *inferior hypogastric plexus* (Fig. 21.4). This combined autonomic plexus lies as a fenestrated plaque on the pelvic side wall. The largest parasympathetic contribution to the inferior hypogastric plexus is from S3, and this erigent nerve can be demonstrated during pelvic surgery as a sidewall pillar running up to the plexus. Anteriorly, the inferior hypogastric plexi turn medially and finally coalesce anteromedially on the anterior surface of Denonvillier's fascia as the *prostatic plexus*.

The parasympathetic and sympathetic innervation of the pelvic organs is from small nerves from these pelvic autonomic plexi. Autonomic innervation of the bladder and sexual organs is from the prostatic plexus anterior to the rectum. Sympathetic innervation is essential for ejaculation, and parasympathetic innervation for erection. Rectal autonomic innervation is from both inferior hypogastric plexi. The small rectal branches cross the areolar plane, between the parietal structures in the pelvis and the visceral contents, to enter the mesorectum. These nerves are the only autonomic nerve fibres which are intentionally sacrificed when

the rectum is mobilized by dissection on the surface of the mesorectum. All other autonomic nerves, although vulnerable to injury, are just outside this anatomical plane.[1]

APPENDICECTOMY

An appendicectomy is most commonly performed during an attack of acute appendicitis. If the preoperative diagnosis is fairly certain, the surgeon will probably choose a small right iliac fossa incision (see Chapter 12). Pus may be encountered on opening the peritoneum, and is removed by suction. The first step is to deliver the caecum into the wound, and this can be difficult through the small incision. Small bowel loops, lying anterior to the caecum, are often repeatedly delivered to the surface. They can be differentiated from the caecum by their absence of taeniae. Occasionally, a long transverse colon is delivered in error, but can be recognized by the attached greater omentum. The simplest method of isolating the caecum is to introduce an index finger lateral to all bowel loops, and down into the paracolic gutter lateral to the caecum. It is then usually possible to hook the finger under a caecal taenia and to draw a portion of the caecum gently out of the wound. The taenia is then followed to its termination and the appendix delivered. If the appendix does not immediately deliver into the wound at this stage, a finger is re-inserted into the wound along the taenia towards the caecal pole, where it is usually possible to feel the appendix as a tense cord, hook the finger around it, and gently deliver it. If there is still difficulty, the wound must be enlarged for adequate access. The appendix may be wrapped in omentum which can either be gently freed, or excised with the appendix. The appendix may be lying retroperitoneally in a retrocaecal position and can be delivered only after lateral caecal mobilization allows the caecum to be turned over and the appendix dissected out under direct vision. A superolateral muscle-cutting wound extension will be required to give sufficient access for this manoeuvre.

Once safely delivered, the appendix is held in a Babcock's forceps while the mesentery is viewed against the light to identify the anatomy of the appendicular vessels. A window in the mesentery near the base of the appendix allows application of an artery forceps and division of the mesentery (Fig. 21.5a). It is often advisable to divide the mesentery in separate bites if the artery has divided early into individual branches, and this may also be safer in a fat-laden, or oedematous, mesentery. The arteries held in the artery forceps are then ligated. It is important that these forceps do not slip during ligation, or the mesentery with the unsecured vessels may retract inside the abdomen and be difficult to re-secure. Back-bleeding from the cut distal end is usually minimal but, if troublesome, can be controlled temporarily with artery forceps. Care must be taken not to injure the terminal ileum or its mesentery during dissection of inflamed tissue. It is also important to remove the *whole* of the appendix. If an over-generous appendix stump is left *in situ*, a further attack of appendicitis, with a dangerous delay in diagnosis, is possible.

The appendix is now attached only by its base. This is ligated with an absorbable suture (Fig. 21.5b). Traditionally, the appendix base was crushed with an artery forceps prior to ligation. This was to reduce the swelling in the tissue to be ligated over a wider area than that compressed by the subsequent ligature, and thus reduce the likelihood of the ligature cutting through the oedematous tissue. Many surgeons no longer recommend this preliminary crushing manoeuvre. An artery forceps is placed 5 mm distal to the ligature. The appendix is then divided with a knife cutting against the artery forceps (Fig. 21.5c). The traditional purse-string suture has also lost popularity. It is a seromuscular suture encircling the appendix stump. It can be inserted after ligation of the meso-appendix, and either before or after the appendix is removed. Care must be taken when inserting a purse-string suture not to catch the vessels in the base of the divided meso-appendix. As the purse-string suture is tightened and ligated, the stump is inverted by pressure with

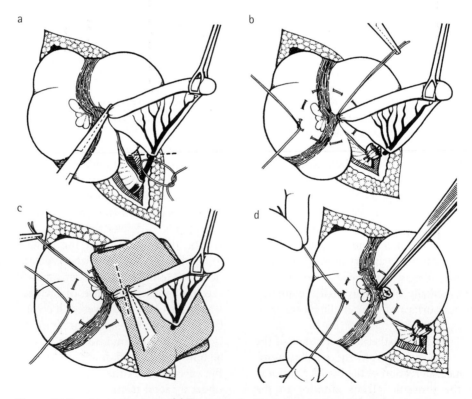

Figure 21.5 *Appendicectomy. (a) The appendicular vessels are ligated and the mesoappendix divided (the artery forceps on the appendicular vessels has been omitted for clarity). (b) The base of the appendix is ligated. If a seromuscular purse-string suture is used, it must be placed so that injury to vessels in the transected mesoappendix is avoided. (c) Artery forceps have been applied to the appendix distal to the basal ligature and the appendix is divided. Any spillage will be on to the underlying swab. (d) Pressure with the artery forceps invaginates the appendix stump as the purse-string suture is tightened.*

artery forceps (Fig. 21.5d). The argument for an invaginating purse-string is the possible deleterious effect of infected stump mucosa left exposed to the peritoneal cavity. It is also an extra closure should the ligature on the base of the appendix fail. Those who do not favour a purse-string suture argue that there is no evidence that the infected mucosa is harmful if left exposed, and that a purse-string suture merely traps any infection to form an intramural caecal abscess. All, however, agree that any attempt to place a purse-string suture in thickened oedematous tissue is contraindicated as it will fail to invert the stump and will only cause damage to the friable caecal wall.

Frequently, the base of the appendix is more accessible than the tip. If an inflamed retroperitoneal tip cannot be delivered into the wound, a retrograde appendicectomy is a useful manoeuvre (Fig. 21.6). Two pairs of artery forceps are insinuated through the meso-appendix and applied to the base of the appendix, 5–6 mm apart. The proximal forceps is then removed and the appendix ligated in the groove that has been crushed. The appendix is then divided close to the distal forceps which are left on for retraction as the appendix is freed by dissection, and by successive clamping and cutting of its mesentery.

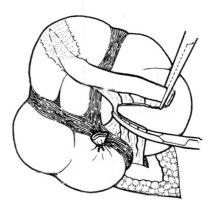

Figure 21.6 *A retrograde appendicectomy is a useful technique when the base of the appendix can be drawn into the wound but the inflamed tip is difficult to deliver.*

Special considerations in appendicectomy

GENERALIZED PERITONITIS

An acutely inflamed appendix which has burst free into the peritoneal cavity causes a generalized peritonitis. This is common in children as the ability to localize and wall off an intra-abdominal infection is less well-developed, at least in part explained by the shorter omentum. In addition, in the pre-school child, presentation of appendicitis is often atypical and the diagnosis delayed. Surgery is urgent but relevant preoperative resuscitation should not be overlooked. The appendix is commonly easily accessible and is removed in the standard manner. All pus should be sucked from the peritoneal cavity, which is then further irrigated with saline or a bactericidal solution. A general peritoneal drain is of little value but a wound drain is recommended. A course of broad-spectrum antibiotics greatly reduces postoperative septic complications (see Appendices II and III).

LOCALIZED APPENDIX MASS OR ABSCESS ENCOUNTERED AT APPENDICECTOMY

An acute appendicitis may be walled off from the general peritoneal cavity by adherent omentum or small bowel. Alternatively, if the appendix is lying retrocaecally, the inflammation is localized by the overlying caecum. Pus may form within the mass and the resultant appendix abscess may thus be either intraperitoneal, or retrocaecal and mainly retroperitoneal, dependent on the position of the appendix. An inflammatory appendix mass is frequently palpable in the right iliac fossa preoperatively, but often only after the patient is anaesthetized and the abdominal wall relaxed. The presence of a mass is an indication that the operation may be more difficult, and that more extensive access than usual may be necessary. Loops of small bowel involved in an appendicular inflammatory mass must be freed very gently as the bowel will be friable. Omentum can either be separated from, or excised with, the appendix. When localized pus is encountered within the inflammatory mass, a drain is placed into the depths of the abscess cavity after the appendix has been removed. This drain should be brought out through a separate incision.

DELAYED PRESENTATION

If a patient presents with a history of several days' duration, and a large appendix mass without any signs of generalized peritonitis, conservative management with antibiotic therapy is often safer. As a future attack of appendicitis is likely, an elective appendicectomy is usually planned for 3 months later, when all inflammation has settled. In an older patient it is advisable during this delay to take the opportunity of excluding an inflammatory episode associated with a caecal carcinoma by a barium enema or colonoscopy.

If a patient, with a delayed presentation and an appendix mass fails to improve on antibiotics, a significant collection of pus within the inflammatory mass should be suspected. This pus requires drainage. Where the equipment and skills are available, ultrasound or computed tomography (CT) imaging can confirm a collection and, if confirmed, radiological image-controlled drainage is now an alternative for many surgeons. After drainage, the acute episode should resolve on conservative management, and an interval appendicectomy can be planned. When this radiological service is not available, the diagnosis must be made on clinical criteria and open operative drainage becomes indicated. This may be safely combined with an appendicectomy in most situations. However, the surgeon may encounter an inflamed appendix densely adherent to loops of friable small bowel which are also forming the wall of the abscess. Simple drainage of the localized abscess, antibiotic therapy and an elective appendicectomy 3 months later is safer than attempting an appendicectomy in these circumstances. Injudicious attempts to mobilize the appendix at the initial operation may result in haemorrhage, or small bowel injury with resultant fistulae.

APPENDICITIS IN PREGNANCY

Surgery is often delayed in pregnancy for fear of an unnecessary laparotomy inducing a miscarriage or premature labour. However, it is the intra-abdominal inflammatory process itself, rather than the surgery, which will most frequently precipitate uterine contractions. Early surgical intervention is therefore indicated. In late pregnancy the caecum and appendix will be displaced upwards by the gravid uterus, and this can cause diagnostic confusion. It should also be remembered that in late pregnancy the incision for appendicectomy will need to be made higher on the abdominal wall.

AVOIDANCE OF POSTOPERATIVE SEPTIC COMPLICATIONS

Before the advent of antibiotics, wound infections and pelvic abscesses were common after appendicectomies. Great care was taken to change instruments and gloves after contact with mucosa, which was itself then inverted with a purse-string suture. However, contamination of the pelvic peritoneum had already occurred preoperatively, and the wound was inevitably contaminated as the appendix was delivered. It is now standard practice to administer prophylactic, peroperative antibiotics for all appendicular and colonic surgery, even in the absence of an infective pathology, and when a grossly inflamed or perforated appendix is found, a postoperative treatment regime of antibiotics is instigated (see Appendix II). As a result of this change in practice the infective complications following appendicectomy are now comparatively rare.

Peroperative diagnostic dilemmas

Pelvic peritonitis from another pathology, such as diverticulitis or salpingitis, will often have an appendix lying within the pus, and such an appendix will show serosal inflammation. Awareness of this possibility is usually sufficient to prevent a mis-diagnosis. If there is some anxiety after the removal of a relatively mildly inflamed appendix associated with pelvic pus, a useful test is to open the appendix. A pale, non-inflamed mucosa confirms the suspicion that the appendix is inflamed from without by another pathology which must then be sought. Extension of the wound, or a separate midline laparotomy incision, is often necessary.

An entirely normal appendix may be encountered and should be removed to prevent future diagnostic difficulties in a patient with an 'appendicectomy' scar. In the absence of peritonitis, the original incision is adequate for a limited laparotomy. Distal ileal loops should be delivered and

mesenteric adenitis, a Meckel's diverticulum or terminal ileal Crohn's (see Chapter 22) may be apparent. The right ovary and Fallopian tube are also accessible for examination. Occasionally, an unexpected finding of a caecal carcinoma is made, and a radical right hemi-colectomy should be undertaken. An inflammatory mass in the right iliac fossa, from an inflamed or perforated caecal diverticulum, also requires a right hemi-colectomy, which should be a radical dissection if a carcinoma cannot be excluded.

An *appendicular tumour* is occasionally encountered, and may coexist with an acute appendicitis, distal to where the tumour has obstructed the lumen. The commonest of these is a carcinoid, and if a tumour is less than 2 cm in diameter and well clear of the base a simple appendicectomy is still appropriate. Larger, or more proximal, tumours require a formal right hemi-colectomy, as malignant carcinoids and adenocarcinoma can both occur.[2] A true mucocoele of the appendix is occasionally encountered and represents a non-inflamed, obstructed appendix filled with mucus. A mucinous cystadenoma of the appendix is a separate entity. It must not be ruptured during the appendicectomy as it is the primary tumour of pseudomyxoma peritonei (see Chapter 15). If the tumour has already ruptured, or ruptures during surgery, follow-up should be arranged at a specialized centre, as early surgical treatment of the disseminated intraperitoneal pseudomyxoma will be more successful than treatment delayed until there is clinical evidence of the established syndrome.

Laparoscopic appendicectomy

This is an increasingly popular option.[3] The advantages of a laparoscopic approach include a faster postoperative recovery in most studies. This encourages the surgeon who wishes to increase his or her laparoscopic experience, especially as patients generally prefer the cosmetic result of the small laparoscopic scars. The difference in cosmesis can, however, be a more important consideration in an obese patient who would otherwise require a substantial incision for adequate access. Laparoscopy also has the advantage of allowing better inspection of the pelvic organs for other pathology. For this reason, some surgeons recommend an initial laparoscopic examination of young women with suspected appendicitis, even if appendicectomy, if indicated, is to be undertaken by the open method. Interestingly, many laparoscopic surgeons will then leave a non-inflamed appendix *in situ*. It must be remembered however, that a laparoscopic scar and a history of a suspected attack of appendicitis may also cause diagnostic problems and the patient must understand that the appendix is still *in situ*.

The disadvantages of a laparoscopic appendicectomy are mainly those of cost. It is also possible that in the long term the incidence of umbilical port site herniae could compare unfavourably with the low incidence of incisional herniae from Lanz incisions.

Operative procedure

A three-port technique is favoured by most surgeons. The first port is a 10-mm port for the camera, and is established at the umbilicus. Additional 5-mm ports are positioned to give access to the right iliac fossa for dissection. A suprapubic port, and a port close to the left anterior superior iliac spine, will achieve this. The patient is placed in a Trendelenberg position so that the small bowel falls into the upper abdomen. When the appendix is lying retrocaecally, the first step in the dissection is release of the peritoneum lateral to the caecum so that the appendix can be delivered. The caecum is grasped and retracted upwards to expose the base of the appendix, which is then encircled with a laparoscopic Johan's forceps. These forceps have the advantage over a laparoscopic Babcock's forceps in that they can be passed through a 5-mm port; this avoids the necessity of establishing a second 10-mm port.

A window is then developed through the appendix mesentery, close to the base of the appendix. These two structures are secured separately. The appendix mesentery can be secured with clips but, as this was not possible through a 5-mm port, other options were explored. Diathermy coagulation of the appendix mesentery has proved to be secure, and is now generally preferred. A tissue grasper is then passed through the noose of a pre-tied suture to hold the appendix. The appendix is delivered through the noose which is then guided down to the base of the appendix and tightened. This manoeuvre is repeated and the appendix cut between the ligatures.

Port site contamination, as the inflamed appendix is withdrawn, should be minimized and a specimen bag should be employed. This is particularly important when there is a distended, severely inflamed or gangrenous specimen. An alternative manoeuvre is to substitute the 10-mm camera at the umbilicus for a 5-mm one placed through a port in the left iliac fossa. The appendix can then be grasped through the 10-mm port and usually withdrawn through it, without any risk of contaminating the wound.

SMALL BOWEL RESECTIONS

A small bowel resection may be indicated for a non-viable segment which has been damaged by trauma or ischaemia. Alternatively, the bowel wall may be involved in an inflammatory or malignant process. The radicality of a resection must be tailored to the pathology. For example, if only the anti-mesenteric border of small bowel is involved in a benign pathology, a limited 'V' resection will suffice (Fig. 21.7a). The advantages of this include an intact strip of bowel at the mesenteric border with no ligation of mesenteric vessels required, and the angulation after closure of the defect protects the suture line from forming adhesions with other peritoneal surfaces. This form of resection may be suitable for a strangulated Richter's hernia or the excision of a Meckel's

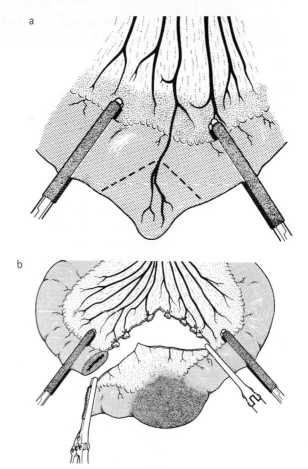

Figure 21.7   *(a) A limited V resection which leaves the mesenteric border intact is sometimes appropriate. (b) More often, a full circumferential resection is required associated with the excision of a V of mesentery.*

diverticulum, although a chance finding of the latter is now considered better ignored. It may also be suitable for the palliative excision of a malignant peritoneal deposit on the small bowel which is narrowing the lumen.

More frequently, the whole circumference of the small bowel must be excised and, even when this is only a few centimetres in length, a V of mesentery must also be removed (Fig. 21.7b). Division of the mesentery is most simply carried out by clamping it with a succession of artery forceps, and cutting with scissors. The vascular pattern of the mesentery can be displayed by means of trans-illumination with a bright light. Windows can then be made through the avascular areas between the vessels, and the artery forceps applied to the tissue between the windows. The tissue held in the forceps is then ligated. The temptation to include a large bulk of mesentery in each clip should be resisted, as this nearly always results in tearing and bleeding as the ligature is tightened. When a curable malignancy of the small bowel is suspected, the V of mesentery removed should give the maximum lymphadenectomy without damage to the main superior mesenteric vessels.

The technical details of a bowel resection and an end-to-end anastomosis are described in more detail in Chapter 13.

FORMATION OF STOMAS

An enterocutaneous stoma is a controlled iatrogenic fistula.[4] A stoma may be fashioned as an alternative outlet to the gastrointestinal tract after the excision of all distal bowel, or when restoration of continuity after a resection is contraindicated. Stomas are also used as a temporary or permanent diversion of the faecal stream from distal pathology or a healing anastomosis. A temporary stoma is commonly a loop stoma which can be closed without a major laparotomy when it is no longer required. An end stoma is preferable when permanence is anticipated. A loop stoma may be left as a permanent stoma, but is more prone to complications. An *end stoma* has a single opening into the proximal bowel, and the epithelial continuity is between the skin and the whole circumference of the bowel mucosa (see Figs 21.9 and 21.11). A *loop stoma* is formed by an enterotomy on the anti-mesenteric border of a loop of bowel which has its continuity maintained by an intact mesenteric border. There are two openings, one into the proximal bowel and one into the defunctioned distal bowel. The epithelial continuity is between the skin and the mucosa around the edge of the enterotomy (see Figs 21.10 and 21.12).

Colostomies and ileostomies are both in routine use. Colostomy effluent is 'faecal' and intermittent. A sigmoid colostomy may only empty once daily with formed stool and is the easiest to manage, whereas an ileostomy may empty continually. Ileostomy effluent is thickened small bowel contents, and patients often prefer it as it is 'non-faeculent' and usually less malodorous. However, dehydration may be a problem, especially in elderly patients, in the early weeks when effluent volumes are highest. A transverse colostomy is the least popular stoma as it produces a large volume of soft offensive faecal effluent. It does, however, have a useful role as a temporary defunctioning loop stoma. The importance of good stoma management is essential if the patient's preoperative quality of life is to be regained. The expertise of stoma nurse specialists, together with advances in appliances, have greatly reduced the problems of leakage and skin excoriation. The first essential, however, is for the surgeon to site the stoma optimally and to fashion it correctly. If at all possible, the preferred site for a stoma should be marked preoperatively by the stoma therapist in conjunction with the patient. An apparently ideal site in a patient on the operating table may be buried in a skin crease when he or she sits, or be out of sight and dependent on the under-surface of a protuberant abdomen when standing. The stoma should be through an area of smooth flat skin in order that a good seal with an appliance can be achieved. The vicinity of the umbilicus and abdominal scars should therefore be avoided.

A stoma is usually brought through the rectus sheath a few centimetres either above or below the umbilicus. More lateral stomas were thought to be associated with a higher incidence of incisional herniae, but this is uncertain. A disc of skin and subcutaneous fat is excised. It is inadvisable to bring a stoma out through a wound as the incidence of wound infection, parastomal herniation and problems with appliance fixation to irregular scarred skin are all increased.

Left iliac fossa end colostomy

This stoma is formed after a resection which leaves no distal bowel to which an anastomosis can be made, or when a restorative procedure is contraindicated. It is therefore the final step in an abdominoperineal resection, or a Hartmann's operation. An end left iliac fossa colostomy may also be used as a permanent diversion of a rectum irretrievably damaged by tumour, inflammation or trauma, and as a final solution for faecal incontinence or a rectovaginal fistula. The rectum is closed and left *in situ* (Fig. 21.8). However, this is an unsuitable operation if there is distal obstruction as the rectal stump may distend with mucus, and the closure disrupt with resultant peritonitis. Instead, either a loop stoma should be used or, in addition to the end colostomy, the distal defunctioned end should be brought out as an additional stoma described as a *mucous fistula*.

At the end of an abdominoperineal resection, or a Hartmann's procedure, the surgeon has only to bring the divided proximal bowel out through the abdominal wall as a stoma. Adequate length is essential or stoma retraction will

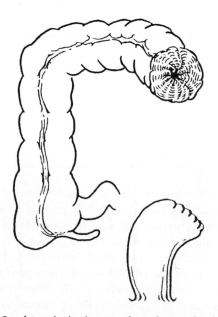

Figure 21.8   *A terminal colostomy. An end stoma has been formed and the rectum has been closed and left* in situ. *This is a satisfactory solution when there is no distal obstruction. When there is a distal obstruction, either a loop stoma should be formed or the distal end brought out as a separate mucous fistula.*

occur, and allowance must be made, particularly in fat patients, for the anterior abdominal wall protuberance which will occur when standing. Postoperative distension from ileus will also increase any tension. If the bowel division has been high in the descending colon, mobilization of the colon by incision of the peritoneum lateral to the bowel will increase the length of colon available, and can be extended to a full mobilization of the splenic flexure if necessary.

The optimal site on the colon for the stoma is chosen and the bowel divided with a mechanical linear stapling device. This has the advantage of closing the distal end definitively, and producing a temporarily sealed proximal end for delivery through the abdominal wall without the extra bulk of a clamp. (If such a device is not available the distal end is closed with sutures and a small clamp used to seal the proximal bowel.)

The disc of skin and subcutaneous fat is excised at the chosen stoma site, and a horizontal or vertical incision is made through the anterior layer of the rectus sheath. The rectus muscle is split and the incision extended through the posterior sheath and the parietal peritoneum. The size of the opening is difficult to judge; it should be snug, but not tight, around the bowel. Too small an abdominal fascia incision produces a dusky oedematous stoma, whilst too large an incision predisposes to a parastomal hernia. It is easy to damage the inferior epigastric artery within the rectus muscle, and the pulsations should be palpated from within in an attempt to avoid incising the vessel. If cut, the ends retract and are difficult to locate. When injury occurs and there is a separate laparotomy incision, deep suture ligations placed from within, a few centimetres above and below the stoma incision, will include the severed vessel, and is the easiest method of control.

A Babcock forceps is introduced through the stoma incision to hold the proximal bowel end and to guide it gently through the abdominal wall to the skin. The main incision is then closed before the stoma is opened. The few millimetres of colon which is crushed in the clamp, or held with staples, is excised. Bleeding points may have to be coagulated, and the free edge of bowel is then sutured to the skin around the defect. Catgut was an ideal suture material as it is absorbed quickly, but it has now been replaced by synthetic absorbable material with similar properties. Interrupted sutures are used, and each bite should include the full thickness of bowel wall and a bite of skin, although it is important to deliver the needle close to the skin edge (Fig. 21.9).

If no resection is planned, the surgeon will wish to avoid a major laparotomy. It may be possible to perform a *trephine stoma*, in which a loop of mobile sigmoid colon is delivered through the definitive incision for the stoma. This is not always possible however, and it may be dangerous if there is tension due to inadequate mobilization. The colon is delivered outside the wound, divided, and the sealed distal end replaced. It is imperative that at this stage the surgeon is sure which end is the proximal, and which the distal bowel. When access is too limited for certainty, insufflation of the rectum

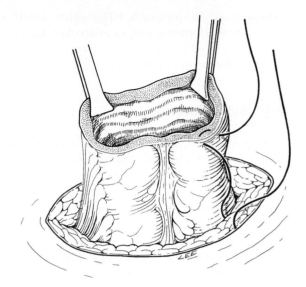

Figure 21.9 *An end colostomy. The closed end of colon has been brought through the abdominal wall and trimmed. Skin mucosal apposition is then achieved with interrupted absorbable sutures. This is illustrated here with a suture passed extramucosally in the bowel and subcuticularly in the skin; this may be a superior refinement to the simpler suture described in the text.*

with air from below will confirm the distal limb. The limited division of the sigmoid mesentery, to allow sufficient separation of the ends without devascularization, is also more difficult with a trephine technique. Injury to the inferior epigastric vessels is both more difficult to avoid, and more difficult to treat, when there is no separate abdominal incision.

A small laparotomy to mobilize the sigmoid is therefore often safer. A lower abdominal midline incision is the approach usually recommended, but a low left iliac fossa oblique muscle-cutting incision has the advantage of giving better access to the peritoneum lateral to the sigmoid colon. This incision can be placed so that it will lie outside the fixation of the appliance. It must be below, lateral, and at a sufficient distance from the skin mark of the proposed site of the stoma.

An increasingly popular alternative is to combine a laparoscopic mobilization with a trephine stoma technique. The mobilization is completed and the pneumoperitoneum is released, whilst the sigmoid loop, or sealed end, is held just under the site of the stoma by an instrument retained within a port site. Identification and delivery of the colon through the small trephine incision is thus much easier.

Left iliac fossa loop colostomy

This is the appropriate stoma when there is a rectosigmoid obstruction and no resection is planned as it can also decompress the distal colon immediately above the obstruction. If, however, a later resection is planned a more proximal colonic stoma may be preferable. The pelvic colon is mobilized, as for the formation of an end colostomy. The bowel is not divided but brought out as a loop in a similar manner to the fashioning of a transverse loop colostomy.

Transverse loop colostomy

This is a temporary stoma, and was traditionally the standard emergency treatment of a left colon obstruction. It may still have a place in this situation (as discussed in Chapter 22), but a primary resection is now the preferred option. The defunctioning loop colostomy is most often indicated as a temporary diversion to protect a left colon anastomosis. Coloanal anastomoses are particularly vulnerable to anastomotic leakage, and some surgeons routinely defunction with

a loop stoma. Surgeons are divided in their preference for either a loop transverse colostomy or a loop ileostomy as a temporary measure. The colostomy is less pleasant for the patient to manage, and is probably associated with more wound infections and incisional herniae after closure. These disadvantages may be offset by a reduced likelihood of early fluid and electrolyte loss and a lower long-term risk of late adhesion obstruction. In addition, if there should be a leak the more distal stoma may provide a better defunction of the anastomosis and reduce contamination from the leak.

A suitable site in the proximal transverse colon is selected which will reach the abdominal skin without tension. The greater omentum is separated from this portion of the colon, and a pericolic window is made close to the bowel wall. An artery forceps is passed through the window to grip a soft catheter which is guided through (Fig. 21.10a). A stoma inci-

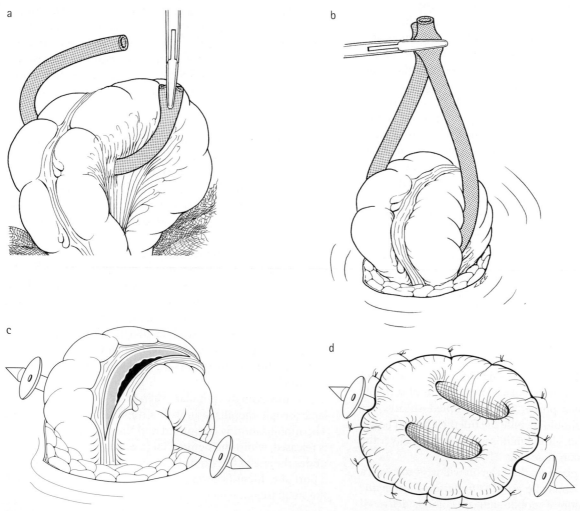

Figure 21.10 *A loop colostomy. This is illustrated with a colostomy bar, which many surgeons now reject on the grounds that if there is no tension it is of no value, and argue that it merely causes difficulty with early appliance fixation, and may cause additional scarring which could make subsequent closure more difficult. (a) An artery forceps has been passed through a mesenteric window close to the bowel and is now drawing a catheter through. (b) An artery forceps has been passed into the abdomen through the prepared stoma site and the ends of the catheter grasped. The bowel is gently delivered to the exterior. (c) The colostomy bar has been guided through the mesenteric window by its insertion into the open catheter end. A longitudinal incision is made in the colon. (d) The bowel edges are folded back to the skin edges and skin-mucosal apposition is achieved with interrupted sutures, except where the stoma bar emerges.*

sion is then made in the same fashion as for a left iliac fossa colostomy, but in the right hypochondrium. A forceps passed through the stoma incision can grip the catheter and guide the loop of colon through the abdominal wall while it is eased through from inside (Fig. 21.10b). The main incision is then closed. A colostomy bar is then guided through the mesenteric window by inserting one end, which has been swivelled to lie in line with the bar, into the open end of the catheter. The catheter is removed and the end of the bar swung back to right-angles (Fig. 21.10c). The bar is removed at about 10 days postoperatively and until then provides support to the colonic loop, preventing retraction. Severe tension will, however, result in the bar ulcerating through the bridge of intact bowel wall and will not prevent retraction in this situation. The main abdominal wound is now closed. Earlier concerns regarding immediate opening of a colostomy are unfounded, and it should be opened and sutured to ensure skin-mucosal apposition and healing without stenosis. A longitudinal incision along a taenia can be made with scalpel and scissors, or with diathermy, with care being taken to avoid injury to the opposite wall of the bowel (Fig. 21.10c). The bowel is then opened and the cut edge of bowel apposed to the skin edges of the colostomy incision with interrupted absorbable sutures in the same fashion as when suturing an end colostomy. Skin mucosal apposition is only deficient where the stoma bar emerges (Fig. 21.10d).

End ileostomy

This is the stoma created at the completion of a total colectomy. The optimal stoma site, high in the right iliac fossa, should have been marked preoperatively.

At surgery, a disc of skin is excised, and an incision made through the abdominal wall as described for an end colostomy. The terminal ileal stump is then drawn through the abdominal wall in a similar manner, with care being taken to avoid rotation. There will inevitably be some mesentery drawn through with the ileum, as complete division of this from the bowel will result in an ischaemic stoma. Skin mucosal apposition is again achieved with interrupted absorbable sutures, but a 'spout' to the stoma should be created so that the more liquid stoma effluent drops into the bag, beyond the flange of the appliance. A flush ileostomy can result in excoriated skin due to leaks as the flange separates from the skin. A spout of 2–3 cm is sufficient, and is fashioned from the terminal 6 cm of the bowel, which has been drawn out through the abdominal wall. The spout is created by an eversion manoeuvre, in which the first four skin-mucosal apposition sutures include a seromuscular bite of more proximal bowel wall (Fig. 21.11a). Care must be taken not to include mucosa in this seromuscular bite as it may create a fistula at the stomal edge. When placing these sutures, care must also be taken to avoid injury to the mesentery of the bowel. The mesentery often distorts the stoma initially, but after eversion it is normally no longer a problem. These four

sutures are left untied until all are in place, and then as they are tied the stoma everts. The stoma must sometimes be gently eased into position, as complete reliance on the sutures to achieve eversion may cause them to tear through the bowel. The stoma should ideally face downwards, and this can be achieved by placing the superior everting suture with its seromuscular bite 6 cm from the free edge, an inferior suture with a bite at 4 cm, and two lateral sutures with bites at 5 cm. Precise measurements of the distance of these bites from the open bowel end make the creation of an optimal stoma easier. After eversion, a further skin mucosal apposition suture is placed between each of the everting sutures (Fig. 21.11b).

Loop ileostomy

This stoma is most frequently used to defunction an empty colon to protect a vulnerable distal anastomosis. The abdomen is already open, and the terminal loop of ileum is drawn through the prepared stoma site. Few surgeons use a stoma rod for a loop ileostomy, and it is therefore preferable not to use a catheter through a mesenteric window as

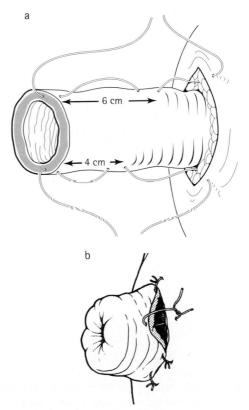

Figure 21.11 *An end ileostomy. (a) Lateral view of the stoma as the everting sutures are inserted. These sutures include a seromuscular bite of the ileal wall between the bites of skin and bowel edge. To produce a 2.5-cm spout, facing slightly downwards, these seromuscular bites should be 6 cm from the end of the ileum superiorly and 4 cm inferiorly. Laterally, they should be at 5 cm. (b) The everting sutures are tied, the spout is formed, and skin mucosal apposition is completed with additional sutures.*

described for the delivery of a loop of colon. A Babcock forceps passed through the stoma incision is usually sufficient to guide the loop through. Before closure of the main wound, the loop is orientated so that the distal limb is inferior and three sutures are placed apposing the unopened wall of the distal loop to the skin edge (Fig. 21.12a). After the main wound is closed, the stoma is opened by an incision 2–3 mm above the three sutures. The incision is extended to just over half the diameter of the distal limb. Eversion sutures are then

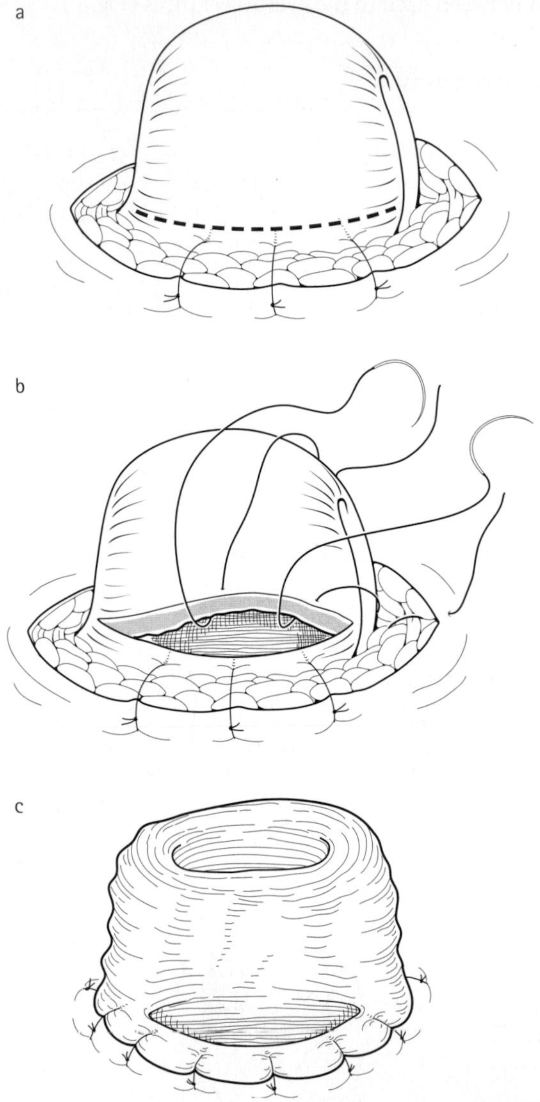

Figure 21.12 *A loop ileostomy. (a) Three sutures are placed between the skin edge and the seromuscular coat of the distal limb prior to closure of the main wound. This manoeuvre prevents any rotation of the loop and confusion as to which is the proximal and which the distal limb. (b) An incision has been made a few millimetres above the three seromuscular skin apposition sutures. The superior and the first lateral eversion sutures are in place but untied. (c) As the sutures are tied, the stoma everts as a spout. Viewed from below, the distal bowel opening is visible, flush with the skin.*

placed superiorly and laterally, exactly as for a terminal ileostomy (Fig. 21.12b), and the proximal limb of the stoma drawn out as a spout (Fig. 21.12c).

STOMA COMPLICATIONS

Some patients have a trouble-free stoma, while others have recurrent problems for which they may need further surgery.

Retraction and stricture

Retraction of a stoma in the first 2 weeks is often in conjunction with separation of the skin to mucosa suture line. It is most commonly caused by excessive tension on the afferent bowel, and therefore no local operation on the stoma will be helpful. Re-laparotomy is indicated if there is cellulitis around the stoma indicating escape of bowel contents into the abdominal wall, or if signs of peritonitis indicate escape into the peritoneal cavity. Reoperation will be difficult as a new stoma will have to be fashioned with bowel which will be more friable to handle, and problems of tension will be increased by postoperative oedema. Fortunately, more minor degrees of early retraction can usually be managed conservatively, although a stricture may develop as healing occurs by secondary intent.

A late retraction of a colostomy, often with an associated stricture, or an ileostomy which has lost its spout, can usually be corrected by a local refashioning operation. The skin immediately adjacent to the stoma is incised circumferentially and the stoma mobilized as for a stoma closure (see below), and refashioned. A re-laparotomy can be avoided unless adequate length can not be obtained without deeper mobilization. An intermittently retracting ileostomy can be fixed in position by linear stapling at two or three positions around the circumference. One blade of the stapler is introduced into the ileostomy and the other blade is on the outside. It is important that the linear cutting stapler is not used in error!

Conservative management of a stricture with dilation is sometimes successful, but more often, revision surgery is required. A stricture at the mucocutaneous junction, without stoma retraction, can be solved very simply by a minor operation under local anaesthesia as minimal dissection is required. The skin is circumcised just outside the stenosed orifice, and the stoma is then mobilized down to the abdominal fascia. The stenosed mucocutaneous junction is trimmed from the end of the stoma, and a fresh apposition of skin and bowel secured with interrupted sutures. At this stage, the surgeon often realizes that the incision around the stenosed stoma has removed too large a disc of skin.

Prolapse

Prolapse of an end colostomy can be dealt with locally by a circumferential skin incision. After minimal dissection the redundant bowel is drawn out and amputated. The new end is sewn to the skin edges. Unfortunately, recurrence is common. A prolapse is sometimes associated with an incisional hernia, and is then best managed by re-siting of the stoma (see below). Colostomy prolapse is more common in loop stomas, and can usually be managed conservatively until closure can be safely undertaken. If closure is not an option, full mobilization of the stoma will allow division of the loop. The distal end, which is often the end that is prolapsing, is then closed and dropped back into the abdomen. Proximal redundant bowel can be excised before re-suturing the bowel to the skin edges. This is, of course, only an option when there is no distal obstruction.

Prolapsing end ileostomies are uncommon, and any local excision procedure is likely only to offer a temporary solution due to the mobility of the small bowel. To prevent prolapse, the bowel adjacent to the stoma must be fixed to the parietal peritoneum over a distance of about 10 cm with non-absorbable sutures. The old technique of extraperitoneal routing of an ileostomy to obliterate the lateral space produced a similar fixation of the terminal ileum.

Parastomal herniae

Parastomal herniae are difficult to treat, but strangulation, although possible, is fortunately uncommon. Surgeons are therefore often reluctant to advise any action, especially if the hernia is easily reducible. Patients, however, are often troubled with both the difficulty in securing the appliance, and the prominence of the device showing through their clothes when it is secured to the summit of a protruding hernia. Patients may also complain of abdominal wall discomfort on exertion, or colic from small bowel loops within the sac. Occasionally, a specially fitted corset will be of value.

Local mobilization of the stoma and excision of the hernial sac, followed by one or more sutures placed to narrow the abdominal wall opening, and finally resuturing of the bowel end to the skin is simple, but usually fails. The addition of encircling mesh after this dissection is generally contraindicated as a mesh infection is likely. The most satisfactory alternative is often to re-open the abdomen, and re-site the stoma through a separate area of abdominal wall. The stoma and the associated hernia can be dissected from both within and without, the hernial sac excised and the old stretched stoma defect closed completely. If necessary, a mesh may be used for this closure but, even with the stoma moved to another site, there will still be some concern over a mesh infection.

Re-siting may be impractical if the abdomen is extensively scarred, or if there will be insufficient length of bowel to reach another abdominal site. A third alternative is to approach the parastomal hernia from without, but through an incision placed well lateral to the stoma itself.[5] Incisions on both sides of the stoma may improve access to the sac for dissection, reduction and closure. The stoma is excluded from the operative field with a skin adhesive covering, and the skin-mucosal apposition of the stoma is left undisturbed. Contamination of the abdominal wall defect can thus be avoided and a mesh may be used to encircle the bowel of the stoma at the level of the fascia.

CLOSURE OF LOOP STOMAS

A temporary stoma, which has protected an anastomosis, may be closed as soon as the anastomosis is soundly healed. Early closure, at around 2 weeks, is practised by some surgeons but is technically more difficult at this stage. A delay of 6–8 weeks allows the stoma to mature and the planes around the stoma to become better defined. The additional wait will also allow the patient to regain nutritional and immunological status after a major operation, and will also reduce the risk of thromboembolic complications. However, the patient has to learn to manage the stoma in order to return home.

Bowel preparation is normally only necessary before closure of a sigmoid loop colostomy, which has formed stool. An elliptical incision allows linear closure of the skin (Fig. 21.13a), but some surgeons prefer a circular skin incision which cicatrices to a circular scar. The skin incision is deepened into subcutaneous fat and the bowel wall identified. Two artery forceps, placed on the skin to be excised, provide useful counter-retraction while the assistant retracts the skin and subcutaneous fat. The plane is followed between the bowel and the subcutaneous fat, and then between the bowel and the abdominal wall until the peritoneal cavity is reached. The assistant retracts progressively deeper as the dissection continues. It is easier to identify the correct plane adjacent to the bowel than to its mesentery, and the plane will be particularly difficult around the scarring from a colostomy bar, if one was used. If the surgeon dissects in one area until the plane becomes difficult, and then moves to another again until difficulty is encountered, it will be found that on returning to the previous area the dissection is now easier as mobility has increased. Some difficulty is sometimes encountered deep in the abdominal wall dissection, as dissection may enter an extraperitoneal plane rather than entering the peritoneum. After the peritoneal cavity is entered, a finger, introduced and swept around the fascial defect, can identify further bands to be divided. Adhesions can be broken down with the finger, but great care must be taken not to tear a loop of adherent small bowel. The stoma can now be lifted further out into the wound, and the dissection to free the stoma has also prepared the abdominal wall for a satisfactory closure of the fascia. If extreme difficulty is encountered, or damage has occurred to adjacent bowel, the surgeon must extend the wound to convert to a mini-laparotomy. Alternatively, a separate midline incision is made.

A *colostomy stoma* is prepared for closure by excision of the mucocutaneous junction (Fig. 21.13b). Difficulties are more often encountered if too little rather than too much is racic oesophagus, and can seldom provide adequate length. The stomach is most commonly used following resections for cancer, but an alternative is the ascending colon mobilized as an isoperistaltic loop, based on the middle colic vessels (Fig. 21.16). The isolated colon on its vascular pedicle may be brought up to the cervical oesophagus by the anatomical posterior route, or alternatively, either retrosternally or subcutaneously, as discussed in Chapter 16. Other colonic segments may be used, but a left colon conduit will only reach if it lies in an anti-peristaltic direction and function will be poor.

ISOLATED ILEOCOLIC SEGMENT

This segment, which includes a few centimetres of terminal ileum, the caecum and the ileocaecal valve, has a good blood

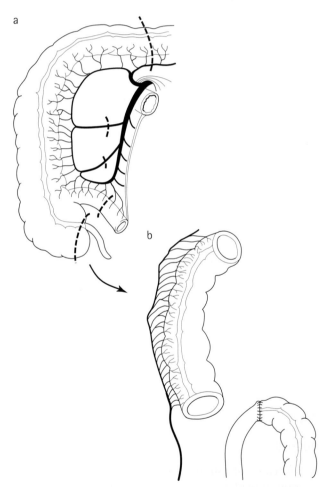

Figure 21.16 *(a) The anastomotic arcades close to the bowel wall allow isolation of the ascending colon and the hepatic flexure perfused by the middle colic artery. The right colic and ileocolic vessels are divided. The terminal ileum is divided and the appendix removed (alternatively the caecum is transected to remove both the appendix and the ileocaecal valve). (b) The caecum is swung up and an iso-peristaltic conduit which will reach the neck has been created. The caecum or terminal ileum can then be anastomosed to the cervical oesophagus and the divided transverse colon to the stomach. Intestinal continuity is restored with an ileocolic anastomosis.*

supply from the ileocolic vessels. Intestinal continuity is restored by an ileocolic anastomosis. The isolated segment has good mobility, and can be rotated over into the left iliac fossa and pelvis as a caecal interposition when, after a distal large bowel resection, the divided left colon will not reach the pelvic floor. The ileal end of the segment is anastomosed to the descending colon, and the caecum to the rectal stump. The place for this technique is, however, limited.

UROTHELIAL SUBSTITUTION

The colon has proved generally unsuitable as a urothelial substitute as the long-term risk of neoplasia in colonic mucosa exposed to urine is substantial.

RADICAL COLONIC RESECTIONS

Small bowel resections are almost exclusively for benign pathology, whereas resections of the large bowel are more frequently undertaken for malignancy. Adenocarcinoma of the colon (as discussed in Chapter 15) is a malignancy which at presentation often has lymph node involvement in the absence of distant metastases. It is, therefore, still potentially curable if the primary tumour is excised en bloc with its lymphatic drainage. As the lymphatic drainage follows the arterial supply, radical lymphadenectomy is planned on the arterial anatomy of the colonic mesentery (see Fig. 21.2). The ascending and descending colon, and the rectum, have retroperitoneal mesenteries, and large bowel resections are therefore predominantly concerned with accurate dissection to isolate these mesenteries.

The length of bowel to be excised is determined by considerations of reconstruction. The ends must reach for a tension-free anastomosis, and the blood supply of the ends must be adequate for healing. The radical lymphadenectomy inevitably compromises the vascularity of a longer segment of bowel than that which would have to be excised to clear a tumour which has minimal ability to spread intramurally. The extent of the lymphadenectomy is thus the important determinant of the length of colon that has to be excised.

The anastomosis after a large bowel resection may be more technically challenging than a small bowel anastomosis due to poor access, but the same general anastomotic principles apply. The blood supply is more critical in the colon than the small bowel, and is one reason why the anastomoses are more vulnerable. Solid intraluminal material with a high bacterial content is an additional adverse factor. An ileocolic anastomosis is safer than an anastomosis of colon to colon, and a coloanal anastomosis is the most vulnerable of all. Preoperative mechanical emptying of the colon (except in obstruction) is recommended for all left-sided resections, and perioperative antibiotics should be given to reduce septic complications in all colonic resections (see Appendix II). A midline incision is favoured by most surgeons, and the operations commence with a general laparotomy to check for previously undetected tumour spread, or other pathology. Good intraperitoneal access is then obtained by retraction, and small bowel exclusion from the operative field (see Chapter 13).

Every operation must be tailored to the vascular anatomy, and the length and mobility of the colon in the individual patient. The exact position of the tumour may dictate adaptations of a standard resection. A more radical excision may be justified for a locally advanced, but still potentially curable tumour, and loops of adherent small bowel or other organs may have to be excised en bloc. Conversely, a less radical lymphadenectomy may be a justifiable alternative in the presence of inoperable liver secondaries, or in a frail elderly patient. In these instances the primary lesion can be excised with only a limited wedge of mesentery, thus minimizing the dissection for mobilization. All modified resections are, however, based on the standard resections described below.

Right hemi-colectomy

A radical right hemi-colectomy is performed for malignant tumours of the caecum, ascending colon and hepatic flexure, and also for the less common malignant tumours of the appendix or terminal ileum. Radical lymphadenectomy involves the excision of the lymphatic drainage from the tumour to the proximal mesenteric nodes which are around the origin of the ileocolic and right colic arteries from the superior mesenteric artery. The ligation of these arteries at their origin determines the length of colon to be excised (Fig. 21.17). The right colon must be mobilized with its retroperi-

toneal 'mesentery' from the right paracolic gutter, as described in Chapter 13. The white line on the peritoneum lateral to the right colon is a guide for entering the plane between this mesentery and the truly retroperitoneal structures.

The incision is extended around the right colon (Fig. 21.18), and the areolar plane identified by retraction of the ascending colon forwards and medially. This avascular plane is followed medially by sharp dissection, allowing the gonadal vessels and ureter to fall back into place. An injured gonadal vessel may have to be ligated, and no adverse effects on the testis need be anticipated after ligation within the abdomen. The ureter must be identified and protected from injury. Inadvertent ureteric injury or the need to sacrifice a ureter on oncological grounds is discussed in Chapter 25. As the dissection is continued medially, the second part of the duodenum and the anterior surface of the head of the pancreas are exposed, and care must be taken to prevent tears to small delicate vessels in this area. If bleeding does occur, it is best treated initially by the application of an adrenaline-soaked swab which is left undisturbed for 5 minutes. Continuing bleeding should be controlled by a fine suture, as the application of artery forceps or diathermy may cause further pancreatic trauma. The superior mesenteric artery and vein are identifiable just below the pancreas, as they enter the root of the mesentery.

The line of the mesenteric transection is lateral to the main trunks of the superior mesenteric vessels, which must be pre-

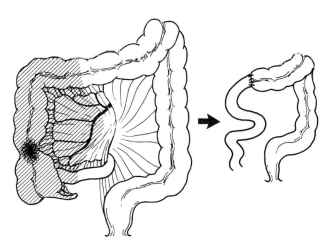

Figure 21.17 *A right hemi-colectomy. The right colic and ileocolic vessels are divided, and the tumour excised en bloc with the lymphatic drainage alongside these arteries. The bowel supplied by these arteries is excised, and continuity restored by an ileocolic anastomosis to the proximal transverse colon. A right hemi-colectomy for a caecal pole tumour should include in the resection specimen the lymphatic channels alongside the terminal arcade of the mesenteric root, and a longer segment of terminal ileum may have to be sacrificed.*

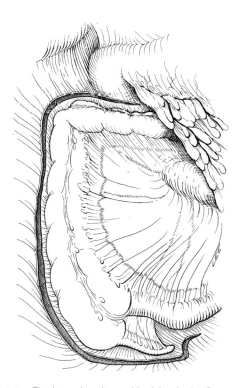

Figure 21.18 *The lateral peritoneal incision is the first step in mobilizing the right colon with its retroperitoneal mesentery. Note the relationship to the second part of the duodenum.*

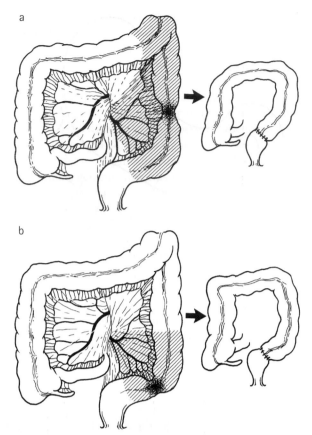

Figure 21.23 *A left hemi-colectomy is based on the lymphatic drainage around the inferior mesenteric artery. (a) The whole left colon with the exception of the rectum has been excised. (b) Even after a high ligation of the inferior mesenteric artery a good marginal artery may be sufficient to allow retention of the whole descending and proximal sigmoid colon.*

access when releasing the splenic flexure. In addition, retraction from this position is useful if pelvic dissection is required. Also, if the anastomosis has to be lower than anticipated, and access is difficult for a hand-sewn anastomosis, a circular mechanical stapler can be inserted per anum.

The principles of mobilization of the left colon are similar to that of the right. Before the lateral peritoneum is divided it may be necessary to divide adhesions between the sigmoid colon and the anterolateral abdominal wall, or pelvic organs. These peritoneal adhesions may be congenital, but more often they are inflammatory or post-operative adhesions, for example following previous gynaecological surgery. If, however, the tumour is in the sigmoid colon, and these adhesions are dense, they may represent local malignant infiltration. The resection must therefore be more radical in order to prevent rupturing the tumour. An ovary, a disc of abdominal wall muscle, or dome of the bladder may have to be excised en bloc with the tumour. A sigmoid tumour may be folded down into the pelvis with malignant adhesions to the anterior rectal wall. In this situation an anterior resection will be necessary for a tumour which was seen even as high as 30 or 40 cm at endoscopy.

The left colon mobilization is then continued by incision of the peritoneum lateral to the distal descending colon (Fig. 21.24) and the plane entered behind the retroperitoneal 'mesentery'. The lateral mobilization of the descending colon is continued up towards, and finally round, the splenic flexure. It is easy at this stage to damage the spleen. Damage is most commonly caused through tearing an omental adhesion off the lower pole of the spleen by excessive retraction on the colon, or more frequently on the omentum. Good access is essential for a difficult mobilization of a high splenic flexure, and any reluctance to extend the wound should be overcome. A high splenic flexure is best approached from both sides. The plane between transverse colon and greater omentum is opened, and followed laterally towards the flexure. This manoeuvre allows the omentum to be retracted anteriorly, releasing any tension on adhesions between the omentum and the spleen, and guides the dissection into the correct plane. With gentle traction on the colon, the peritoneum is divided around the flexure. If visualization is still poor, a finger inserted under the peritoneum to draw down and protect the colon is also helpful in displaying the final strands to be divided (Fig. 21.24). A splenic flexure tumour

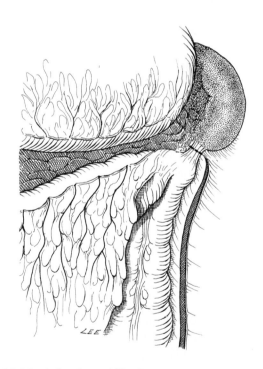

Figure 21.24 *Left colon mobilization commences with an incision of the peritoneum lateral to the distal descending colon. Above the transverse colon the greater omentum has been separated from the stomach by division of epiploic vessels. (Except for splenic flexure tumours, the alternative plane between the transverse colon and the omentum is preferable.) A finger introduced along the distal transverse colon and round the flexure, deep to the remaining peritoneum which is tethering it, will define the remaining tissue to be divided and protect the colon from injury. Excessive traction on the colon may tear adhesions off the spleen and damage it.*

will require the left side of the omentum to be excised en bloc with the specimen. The greater omentum is not separated from the colon, but instead it is separated from the stomach by division of the epiploic vessels, as shown in Figure 21.22. The spleen may have to be excised with the specimen in a locally advanced splenic flexure tumour. In addition it can be damaged inadvertently during splenic flexure mobilization. A damaged spleen can sometimes be saved, but unfortunately a splenectomy is often required (see Chapters 14 and 19). Once the splenic flexure has been fully released it can be lifted forwards and medially, and its 'mesentery' released from the underlying pancreas and duodenojejunal flexure.

Mobilization of the descending and sigmoid colon is continued medially by following the areolar plane between mesenteric structures anteriorly, and gonadal vessels and ureter posteriorly. A damaged gonadal vessel can be sacrificed with impunity, but the ureter should be identified early in this dissection and carefully preserved (Fig. 21.25a). The ureter is occasionally involved in tumour and has to be sacrificed (see Chapter 25). When the dissection has reached the midline, it is helpful to insert a swab into the extremity of the dissection before turning the colon back to the left, and making a peritoneal incision, posteriorly on the right of the sigmoid mesentery (Fig. 21.25b). The swab is visible immediately on dividing the peritoneum, and aids identification of the window behind the inferior mesenteric artery, but in front of the hypogastric nerve plexus on the surface of the aorta. This plane is then followed up until the origin of the inferior mesenteric artery can be felt between finger and thumb. The artery and the vein are clamped, ligated and

divided separately; many surgeons prefer a transfixion ligation for the artery. Care should be taken to preserve the sympathetic nerve fibres on the anterior surface of the aorta and for this reason ligation of the inferior mesenteric artery 1–2 cm from its origin is preferable to a flush tie on the aorta. As the artery is skeletalized prior to clamping, the fat and lymphatic tissue of the proximal centimetre of mesentery can be drawn into the specimen.

At this stage a 'division of convenience' of the colon improves access for the final dissection. Division with a mechanical stapler, or between small crushing clamps, is suitable. It is important not to divide the colon too proximally, remembering that excessive length can be trimmed but colon which will not reach the rectum may pose a major challenge to a restorative anastomosis. The mesentery is then divided between the inferior mesenteric root and the colonic division. The sigmoid colon can now be retracted anteriorly to display the continuation of the posterior areolar plane over the pelvic brim and into the pelvis behind the mesorectum. The autonomic nerves lying on the aorta and the posterior pelvic brim should be carefully preserved. Only minimal dissection is required in the pelvis, and is employed simply to gain rectal mobility for the anastomosis. Division of the peritoneum, lateral and anterior to the rectum, will also allow further upward mobilization of the rectum (Fig. 21.25b). The level of the distal resection site is finalized. This should be below the pelvic brim and not more than a few centimetres above the peritoneal reflection. A higher division carries a risk of inadequate perfusion of the distal end of the anastomosis. The mesentery behind is divided between forceps and

a
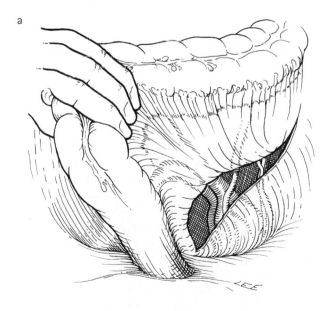

b
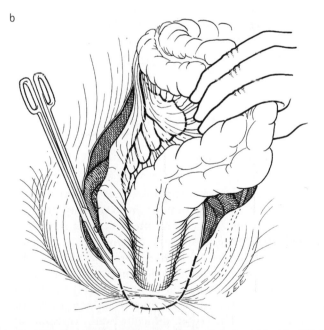

Figure 21.25   *A left hemi-colectomy. (a) The descending and sigmoid colon mobilization starts on the left, and the ureter must be identified early. (b) When the dissection from the left has reached the midline, the colon is swung to the left. The right leaf of the peritoneum is incised to form a window in front of the aorta and behind the mesenteric package which contains the inferior mesenteric artery, its branches and the lymphatic drainage of the hind gut. The inferior mesenteric artery is then ligated and divided close to its origin. The anterior and lateral peritoneal incisions around the rectum allow it to be drawn up to make an anastomosis easier.*

ligated. A right-angled clamp is placed across the bowel to prevent contamination from above, and the bowel is divided. The rectum is emptied by suction and liberally washed with a tumouricidal solution.

Attention is now turned to the proximal end, and its viability is checked. If there is any doubt, it must be resected back to well-vascularized bowel. It should reach without tension to the anastomotic site and, if difficulty is encountered, a second higher division of the inferior mesenteric vein below the body of the pancreas, as routinely performed in an anterior resection, provides extra length. The anastomosis may be performed using either a hand-sewn technique or a circular stapling device (see Chapter 13). The surgeon will find a difficult hand-sewn anastomosis easier if the first suture is placed on the posterior wall furthest away, taking the initial bite from the rectal side of the anastomosis. If this suture is accurately placed, then each subsequent suture, when working along the back wall, becomes easier. The anterior wall poses no difficulty unless mobilization has been inadequate and there is unacceptable tension. No drain is recommended unless there has been more extensive pelvic dissection.

VARIATIONS

A radical lymphadenectomy, with ligation of the inferior mesenteric artery close to its origin, will often still allow preservation of the entire descending and sigmoid colon on the marginal artery. It is sometimes therefore possible in a distal sigmoid tumour to perform a radical resection and still have sufficient length to anastomose without the need to mobilize the splenic flexure (see Fig. 21.23b).

A locally advanced left colonic neoplasm may be unresectable. Obstruction can be relieved by an intraluminal stent or a proximal loop colostomy. A splenic flexure tumour can sometimes be bypassed (Fig. 21.26).

RADICAL RECTAL RESECTIONS

Historical perspective

A radical resection for a carcinoma of the rectum requires excision of the primary tumour in continuity with its lymphatic drainage. The earliest attempts at excision were performed from the perineum, or through a *posterior* approach (see Chapter 23). These approaches do not offer sufficient access for a radical lymphadenectomy. In addition, it is not possible to mobilize the colon sufficiently to undertake a restorative procedure, or even to fashion a left iliac fossa colostomy. This latter difficulty was overcome by performing a prior, or synchronous, laparotomy merely to establish the colostomy.[6] In contrast to the later abdominoperineal excision, none of the dissections to mobilize the rectum was undertaken from above.

Abdominoperineal excisions of the rectum later became

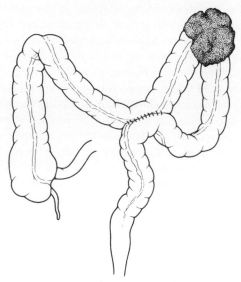

Figure 21.26 *An irresectable splenic flexure tumour with invasion of spleen, pancreas and kidney can be bypassed with a side-to-side anastomosis between the transverse and sigmoid colon.*

the standard radical excision for rectal cancer, with the opportunity to include a radical lymphadenectomy. However, an increasing understanding of the mode of spread of rectal cancers has demonstrated that a purely abdominal, or *anterior resection* of the rectum is oncologically sound. There is no significant submucosal spread of rectal or colonic tumours, and it is therefore safe to resect a rectal cancer with a distal bowel wall margin of around 1 cm. The lymphatic drainage of the rectum is almost exclusively in a proximal direction along the inferior mesenteric artery. Lymphatic drainage in association with the inferior or middle rectal arteries appears only to occur late in the disease process, and is associated with advanced and incurable tumours. However, the initial lymphatic drainage of the tumour fans out into the mesorectum, and at least 5 cm of mesorectum distal to the tumour must be excised (Fig. 21.27). Therefore, any tumour below 10–12 cm requires a total mesorectal excision (TME). If mesorectum involved in tumour is breached during dissection, local recurrence is common. Originally, local recurrence was thought to be related both to residual tumour in the distal bowel wall remnant as a result of submucosal spread, and also to lymphatic drainage along both surfaces of the levator ani muscles and out into the ischiorectal fossae (Fig. 21.28). It is now known that neither route of spread is a significant issue. These, however, were the oncological justifications for the abdominoperineal resection which removed these tissues. In addition, before the advent of mechanical staplers the technical difficulty in hand-sewn anastomoses deep in the pelvis always discouraged anal preservation. An abdominoperineal approach can thus, at least in theory, be avoided in all rectal cancers except those which extend to the dentate line or invade the anal sphincters.[7] Excision of the very low rectal cancers is technically difficult, and as better results are achieved by surgeons

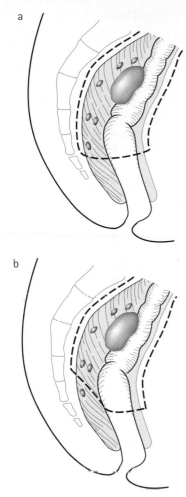

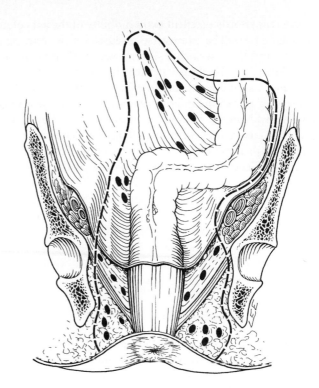

Figure 21.28 *The original hypothesis of the lymphatic drainage of the rectum, as described by Ernest Miles, which formed the oncological basis for the abdominoperineal excision of the rectum for cancer. It is now known that no lymphatic drainage occurs through the levator muscles into the ischiorectal fat from tumours above the dentate line.*

Figure 21.27 *The initial spread from a rectal tumour into the mesorectum is fan-shaped. Nodes up to a distance of 5 cm distal to the primary tumour may contain metastases. (a) A high anterior resection with mesorectal transection can only be oncologically sound if 5 cm of mesorectum distal to the primary tumour is removed. (b) An unsatisfactory cancer operation. The rectum has been divided at the same height, but the 'coning-in' through the mesorectum has cut across involved lymph nodes.*

with a special interest, referral should be considered. The preoperative assessment of these tumours is extremely important to the planning of surgery, and of any adjuvant therapy, and this is discussed further in Chapter 22. In addition to pelvic magnetic resonance imaging (MRI scan), a preoperative digital assessment and endo-anal ultrasound examination under anaesthesia can form an important part of the assessment of very low tumours.

Anterior resection

The patient is placed in a Lloyd–Davies position (see Fig. 12.1, page 200), and the operation commences with a digital rectal (and vaginal in women) assessment of the tumour. The abdomen and perineum are prepared for surgical access.

Postoperatively, there are advantages with suprapubic rather than urethral catheterization, and catheterization is therefore deferred until the abdomen is open (see Chapter 25). The initial mobilization and dissection for an anterior resection is identical to that for a left hemi-colectomy, unless there is a minor modification to avoid mobilization of the splenic flexure. This modification is dependent on the sigmoid colon proving suitable for reconstruction. If there is any diverticular thickening, the neorectum is rendered unsuitable due to reduced distensibility. In addition, the sigmoid colon may have a precarious blood supply after division of the inferior mesenteric artery. Vascularity of the sigmoid colon may be improved by retention of the ascending left colic artery, which arises as a branch of the inferior mesenteric within 2–3 cm of its origin (see Fig. 21.2). Radicality of the lymphadenectomy is probably not significantly reduced if, on skeletalization of the artery prior to clamping, all fat and lymphatic tissue is drawn into the specimen.

In most situations, however, the surgeon will have decided to mobilize the splenic flexure, and this is often most satisfactorily performed before the pelvic dissection. A single division of the inferior mesenteric vein still leaves the vein as a cord at the base of the mesentery, preventing the descending colon from reaching to the pelvic floor. A second higher ligation of the inferior mesenteric vein at the lower border of the pancreas affords excellent extra mobility of the left colon (see Fig. 21.3). The transverse mesocolon is retracted upwards, and the inferior mesenteric vein is then normally readily identified. The flimsy peritoneum is dissected on the left side of the duodenojejunal flexure to enter a bloodless plane, either side of the inferior mesenteric vein. The vein is then divided between artery forceps and ligated. Care must be taken to ensure that the proximal ligature is tied securely, with an adequate venous remnant beyond the ligature, since slippage will lead to troublesome bleeding, as the vein may retract underneath the pancreas. After this high division of the vein, the surgeon will encounter a large mesenteric window, extending between the ligated distal vein and the marginal artery. This can be divided to allow the left colon to be drawn down into the pelvis. This manoeuvre leaves an isolated segment of the inferior mesenteric vein in the mesentery.

POSTERIOR PELVIC DISSECTION

After full mobilization of the left colon, dissection of the posterolateral plane is then continued down into the pelvis. The rectum and mesorectum are lifted forwards, and upwards out of the concavity of the sacrum, with a St Marks retractor. It is this retraction which displays the plane for dissection. The mesorectum should appear as a smooth bi-lobar structure with a glistening surface suggestive of a 'capsule', and similar to that of a lipoma. The plane is between this and the thin fascia covering the structures of the pelvic side wall, and is crossed by fine strands of areolar tissue. The autonomic nerve plexi are located deep to the pelvic side wall fascia. If the areolar plane is opened by blunt dissection it does not separate accurately, and both the autonomic nerves and the mesorectum may tear. The incidence of postoperative urinary and sexual difficulties will be increased, and there is a greater risk of local tumour recurrence. Sharp dissection is either by scissors or diathermy. Diathermy dissection is more haemostatic, but more dangerous if the surgeon strays from the correct plane. Thermal damage to anatomically intact autonomic nerves is an additional concern. The 'wishbone' of the sympathetic hypogastric nerves will be visible at the pelvic brim posteriorly, and these nerves are easily injured if the dissection strays too far posteriorly. If the correct plane, on the front of the aorta between the back of the pelvic mesocolon and the superior hypogastric plexus, has been identified, this plane will lead the dissection into the pelvis in the correct plane medial to the hypogastric nerves. There is a second areolar plane outside the nerves, but this should only be followed for a tumour which is threatening circumferential excision margins at this site. This outer plane sacrifices autonomic nerves, and troublesome bleeding may occur from presacral veins. The final posterior dissection is in a forward direction under the end of the mesorectum along the surface of the levator muscles, but is completed only when mobility has been increased by the lateral and anterior dissection.

LATERAL PELVIC DISSECTION

The lateral plane on the surface of the mesorectum is best approached from the plane already developed posteriorly. It may be difficult to identify from above, and, therefore, early lateral division of the peritoneum may merely lead the surgeon into the wrong plane. The hypogastric nerves are easily damaged at this stage, but the correct plane of dissection on the lateral surface of the mesorectum will allow the hypogastric nerves, and then the inferior hypogastric plexi, to fall back safely onto the pelvic side wall. The small rectal branches from the plexi cross the plane of dissection and are divided. The original descriptions of lateral ligaments, which were clamped and ligated, were probably the hypogastric plexi tented away from the pelvic side wall by medial traction on the specimen. The middle rectal artery, if present, will also cross the areolar plane and requires diathermy coagulation or, occasionally, ligation. Earlier descriptions of large middle rectal vessels were almost certainly vessels of the mesorectum encountered when dissection was too medial and through, rather than around, the mesorectum. 'The pillar' of the erigent nerve, which is the parasympathetic outflow from S3 to the inferior hypogastric plexus, can be identified beneath the fascia of the pelvic sidewall. It is at risk of injury if the deep dissection strays too lateral. It is now known that the circumferential margin is important in preventing local recurrence in rectal cancer.[8] However, dissection in the correct plane will normally ensure adequate margins except in advanced tumours which have transgressed the confines of the mesorectum. In these circumstances the surgeon may be forced to sacrifice pelvic autonomic nerves to achieve adequate oncological clearance.

ANTERIOR PELVIC DISSECTION

Male patients

The anterior plane in the male pelvis lies between the thin anterior mesorectal tissue, and the prostate and seminal vesicles. It is entered by incising the peritoneum just anterior to the rectovesical pouch and entering an areolar plane which leads to the upper pole of the seminal vesicle. Alternatively, the lateral dissection, when carried forwards on the surface of the mesorectum, will lead round to the vesicles. An anterior tumour which has invaded the peritoneum and folded over with a malignant adhesion is easily disrupted at this point. The anterior pelvic peritoneal incision shown in Figure 21.25b, should be made more anteriorly in this situation. A forceps can then be applied to the divided peritoneum to hold it up, and hold this vulnerable area closed. This should help prevent traction disruption of the tumour during the deeper pelvic dissection. The dissection is kept on the posterior surface of the seminal vesicles. Denonvillier's fascia comes into view as a shiny white layer on the anterior surface of the distal anterior mesorectum. Dissection is continued down in front of Denonvillier's fascia. This thin fascial rectogenital septum forms a temporary barrier to anterior tumour invasion. Distally, Denonvillier's fascia curls forwards to fuse with the base of the prostate, and must therefore be divided at some stage during the rectal excision, and the plane directly on the anterior mesorectum re-entered. The final anterior dissection in front of Denonvillier's fascia puts the neurovascular bundles and the prostatic plexus at risk of injury. It is therefore safer to cut Denonvillier's fascia at a higher level and to continue any final dissection behind it. In very low anterior tumours, however, the risk of nerve damage must be balanced against tumour margins, and the dissection should proceed more distally before dividing Denonvillier's fascia.

Female patients

The anterior plane in the female pelvis lies between the thin anterior mesorectum and the posterior vaginal wall. Avoidance of nerve damage is also important, but until recently has been largely ignored. Denonvillier's fascia is a less well-developed structure, and an anterior tumour can breach the thin layer of anterior mesorectum relatively early. A cuff of posterior vagina should be included with the specimen if there is vaginal invasion, or any concern over circumferential tumour margins at this point.

Locally advanced tumours

These tumours may require a more radical excision, including the sacrifice of autonomic nerves with the removal of internal iliac nodes, an en-bloc hysterectomy, the excision of a seminal vesicle or a portion of involved prostate or bladder. A full anterior pelvic clearance with urinary diversion is occasionally justified (see also Chapters 25 and 26). These locally advanced tumours require careful preoperative assessment and multidisciplinary management with a combination of surgery, radiotherapy and chemotherapy for optimal results (see also Chapter 22).

FINAL PELVIC DISSECTION

The final dissection is important in very low tumours. A posterior condensation of fascia between the coccyx and the anorectum is released to display a bare rectal muscle tube below the mesorectum which passes through the puborectalis portion of the levator ani. Anteriorly, the dissection passes through Denonvillier's fascia onto the distal extremity of the thin anterior mesorectum and finally, below this, onto the bare rectal muscle tube. The anatomical plane between the visceral and somatic structures continues into the intersphincteric plane. A tumour at the anorectal junction which is still a T2 lesion can thus sometimes be adequately excised by following this plane. A T3 tumour, however, in this position has no mesorectum around it and will immediately breach the plane and invade the external sphincters (Fig. 21.29). An abdominoperineal resection then becomes essential for oncological clearance.

After completion of the dissection, the rectum should be sealed below the tumour to prevent further contamination from intraluminal malignant cells. The simplest technique is with a TA 30 or TA 45 (30 or 45 mm length), or with a similar

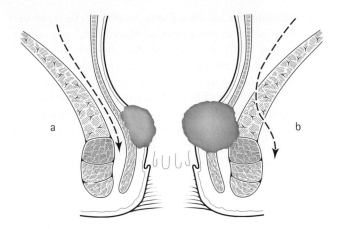

Figure 21.29 *A lower-third rectal cancer. (a) A T1 or T2 tumour which has not breached the plane between the visceral and somatic tissue can still be satisfactorily excised without sacrifice of the external sphincter. (b) A T3 tumour will breach this plane as there is no mesorectum surrounding the bowel at this level. An oncologically satisfactory excision is no longer possible without sacrifice of the external sphincters. The plane for an anterior resection must be abandoned before tumour is breached, and the plane for excision is through the levator ani muscles.*

linear stapler (see Chapter 13). This is a safer method of occlusion than with a right-angled clamp, which may slip and is difficult to position in a narrow pelvis. This staple line seals the distal end of the specimen to be removed. It must be below the tumour, but a margin of only a few millimetres does not compromise cure. The tumour is normally palpable through the rectal wall, but if there is any concern then an examination from below after the stapler is locked (but still not fired) can confirm the position. In a mid-rectal tumour, although a TME has been performed, the mesorectum is drawn up as the stapler is closed and a short cuff of distal rectum is left *in situ*. In a cancer of the distal rectum the stapler may have to be closed beyond the distal margin of the mesorectum in order to clear the tumour. The height of the anastomosis may therefore vary by 1–2 cm, even after a TME.

A proctoscope is inserted and the rectum washed with tumouricidal solution until the washings are clear of faecal residue. The TA 30 is then reloaded and placed distal to the first staple line and fired across the washed rectal stump. In very low tumours, this manoeuvre is easier if the TA 30 is left *in situ* after firing, to be used as a rectal retractor, and a new stapler used for the second staple line. The bowel is divided between the two lines of staples.

RECONSTRUCTION

The proximal bowel end is now re-assessed for reconstruction. It must reach with ease into the depths of the pelvis, and further mobilization may be required, especially if the original division of colon has had to be revised to a higher level to ensure a well-perfused bowel end. Further length can be obtained by dissection along the inferior border of the pancreas, releasing the left lateral attachment of the transverse mesocolon as far as the origin of the middle colic artery. There is frequently a small branch between the colonic mesentery and the inferior pole of the pancreas. This can be ligated and divided. Care must be taken with this manoeuvre as simple diathermy will often lead to troublesome bleeding from the pancreas. Where there is still inadequate length, the left branch of the middle colic artery is often smaller than the more centrally placed branch, and can be divided near its origin. Once again, a window up towards the marginal artery can be divided, and this can produce excellent length. If on completion of this mobilization it is still clear that there is insufficient length, then three options are available to the surgeon:

- The first is simply to transilluminate the mesentery and assess whether there are suitable points where vessels can be ligated.
- The second, which can often produce considerable improvement in mobility, is to mobilize the whole of the right colon. This is undertaken from the lower pole of the caecum around the hepatic flexure, such that the middle colic artery can be rotated downwards. The appendix and caecum will then frequently lie in the right

upper quadrant and considerable additional length can be achieved.

- If, following these two manoeuvres, there is still inadequate length, or the bowel does not appear of sufficient vascularity for a safe anastomosis, then the preferred option is to divide the origin of the middle colic artery. The mobilized caecum is moved downwards like a clock pendulum, such that the lower pole of the caecum sweeps an arc towards the left iliac fossa and then up into the left upper quadrant. This leaves a long, well-vascularized segment of bowel in the region of the hepatic flexure available for a tension-free coloanal anastomosis.

After a total mesorectal excision and a low anterior resection, bowel function and continence is better if a short colon pouch is created rather than forming a straight end-to-end coloanal anastomosis.[9] A short colon pouch (5×5 cm) is created with a GIA 60 linear stapling device. An enterotomy is made on the anti-mesenteric border about 6 cm from the closed end. The blades of the stapler are introduced, and a finger is swept between the blades to carry the mesentery out of the staple line before the device is closed. The instrument is then fired to anastomose the two limbs into a pouch (Fig. 21.30a). The head of the circular stapling device is intro-

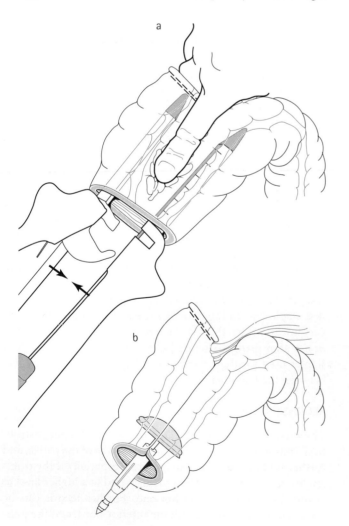

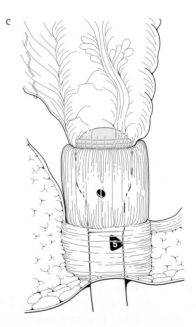

Figure 21.30 *A colon pouch is created with a linear stapling device introduced through an enterotomy about 6 cm from the closed bowel end. (a) The thick colonic mesentery must be swept out of the staple line with a finger before the device is closed and fired. (b) The head of the circular stapling device is then introduced into the colon pouch through the same enterotomy. (c) The anvil of the circular stapling gun is introduced through the anus, the two portions of the device are locked together, and the bowel ends approximated.*

duced into the pouch through the enterotomy made for the introduction of the linear stapler (Fig. 21.30b). A purse-string suture is inserted at the edge of the enterotomy and tightened to draw the bowel over the staples. The general principles of circular stapling techniques are described in Chapter 13. The main portion of the circular stapler is inserted through the anus. Care must be taken to cause minimal stretching of the anal sphincters, and gentleness and good lubrication are essential. The spike of the locking device is advanced through the anorectal stump, adjacent to the stapled closure. The bowel ends must then be orientated to exclude a twist before locking the two portions of the circular stapling device together. It is very easy to include the vagina in the staple line, and it must be securely retracted out of the way as the two bowel ends are apposed (Fig. 21.30c). The device is fired and removed. The 'doughnuts' of excised tissue from both bowel ends are removed from the stapler and checked to ensure that they are complete. The anastomosis is further checked for leaks by filling the pelvis with fluid, digitally occluding the bowel above the pouch and introducing about 200 mL of air per anum. Bubbles appearing in the fluid-filled pelvis indicate a leak.

The pouch fills the cavity of the sacrum, and reduces the pelvic dead space in which a haematoma can collect. This may reduce the incidence of anastomotic leak as the spontaneous discharge of infected collections of blood into the bowel lumen, through the anastomosis, is believed to be a factor in the aetiology of a leak. Low-pressure suction drains may also be of value. These should be liberally primed with washout fluid, which is left in the pelvis at the end of the operation in order to prevent occlusion of the drain with clots. Any anastomosis where there is technical concern, and probably all coloanal anastomoses, are safer if they are protected by a temporary defunctioning loop ileostomy or colostomy.[10] Preoperative chemotherapy and radiotherapy will also make this anastomosis more vulnerable, and should influence the decision reached regarding a temporary stoma. A stoma should not be closed until a water-soluble enema has shown the anastomosis to be sound, and a delay of 6–8 weeks is ideal (see page 389).

Variations

Some surgeons prefer to use a per-anal hand-sutured coloanal anastomosis in extremely low cases, and this technique is described in the section on ileo-anal pouches in Chapter 23. An alternative to a small colon pouch is a stapled end-to-side anastomosis (Fig. 21.31a). This also reduces faecal urgency when compared with a straight coloanal anastomosis, and the increased bulk in the pelvis during the immediate postoperative phase may also reduce postoperative pelvic collections and anastomotic leaks. Another alternative is a straight coloanal anastomosis with an anterior vertical enterotomy which is closed transversely (Fig. 21.31b). Both colon pouches and end-to-side anastomoses have the additional advantage that the better-perfused side, rather than the end, of the colon is used for the anastomosis.

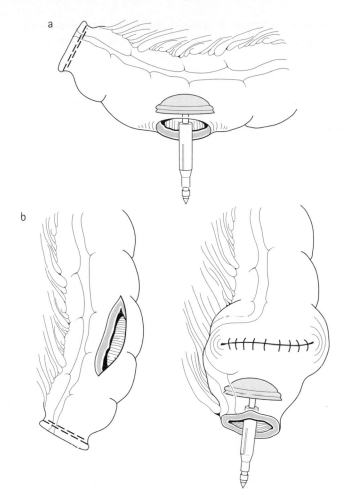

Figure 21.31 *(a) An end-to-side anastomosis. (b) An end-to-end anastomosis, but with a small colon pouch created by an anterior coloplasty.*

High anterior resection

This operation consists of transection of the mesorectum and preservation of the distal rectum. It may be performed in diverticular disease when a sigmoid loop is folded down and is adherent to the front of the rectum, and cannot be safely released. A distal sigmoid tumour, and the most proximal rectal tumours, are also appropriate indications for this operation. It is essential, however, that 5 cm of mesorectum is excised beyond any tumour, and the surgeon must avoid 'coning in' through the mesorectum as this results in compromised lymphatic clearance (see Fig. 21.27). It is therefore still necessary to mobilize the rectum, and the dissection is similar to that for a low anterior resection, except for the deepest parts of the dissection. The site of rectal division is chosen and, by dissection close to the lateral and then the posterior rectal wall of the bowel, a window is created between rectum and its mesentery. The mesentery with the terminal branches of the superior rectal artery are then divided between artery forceps and ligated. Access is difficult for a hand-sewn anastomosis, and a circular stapling device is usually preferred. A straight end-to-end or side-to-end colorectal anastomosis is satisfactory, but a colon pouch should not be used as this can lead to constipation. A defunctioning stoma is not usually indicated unless there is some specific concern about the anastomosis.

Hartmann's procedure

In this operation, following a large bowel resection, the distal bowel is closed and left *in situ*, and the proximal end is brought out as an end colostomy. After an anterior resection for rectal cancer the surgeon may decide that a permanent stoma is wiser in a patient with very poor anal sphincters. In this situation, only an anorectal stump, closed by staples, is left *in situ* (Fig. 21.32a). No later reconstruction is anticipated, but preservation of the anus avoids the additional morbidity associated with the perineal wound of an abdominoperineal excision of the rectum.

Although originally described as an operation for rectal cancer, a Hartmann's procedure is now employed more fre-

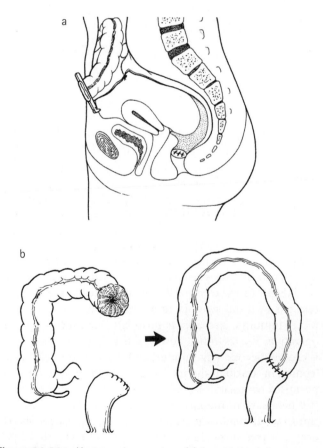

Figure 21.32 *Hartmann's procedure. (a) An end stoma is an alternative to restoration of bowel continuity after the anterior resection of a rectal cancer. Later restoration of continuity is then seldom undertaken. (b) After a sigmoid resection for diverticular disease a longer distal stump remains. If immediate anastomosis is contraindicated, later restorative surgery is usually considered.*

quently in conjunction with an emergency sigmoid resection for the complications of diverticular disease (see also Chapter 22). It has the advantage of shortening the operation and avoiding the risk of an anastomotic leak. However, restoration of continuity requires a second major laparotomy. The alternative of a primary anastomosis with a temporary defunctioning proximal loop stoma should therefore always be considered, as the loop stoma can be closed as a much more minor second procedure than the reversal of a Hartmann's.

When later restoration of bowel continuity after a Hartmann's procedure is anticipated, the distal bowel end should be left as long as possible. It can also be marked with a non-absorbable suture, with the ends cut long, to make subsequent identification easier.

REVERSAL OF A HARTMANN'S OPERATION

Reversal is often not appropriate. The reason for the original decision not to restore continuity, and the length of the rectal stump which has been left *in situ*, are both important factors in the decision. Reversal should be delayed for 3–6 months to allow all inflammation associated with the underlying pathology, and the original operation, to settle. A long stump which had been brought up to lie just beneath the lower end of the abdominal wound will be relatively easy to identify at laparotomy, and a hand-sewn anastomosis will be practical. More often, the stump includes very little rectum above the peritoneal reflection, and although the operation may be straightforward a number of difficulties may be encountered. The rectal stump must be identified, the end stoma dissected out and the two ends anastomosed (Fig. 21.32b). The stump may be difficult to identify, and access for a hand-sewn anastomosis can be limited without mobilization of the rectum. The use of the circular stapling device does not always solve this difficulty. It may not pass up the rectal stump until rectal folds have been straightened out by mobilization, and the defunctioned rectum may also have narrowed and be unable to accommodate the stapler without splitting. Restoration of continuity to a very short stump as shown in Figure 21.32(a), can be achieved relatively easily with a circular stapling device, but the empty pelvis may have adherent loops of small bowel and the initial dissection to free these can be tedious. In addition, function is often poor after a delayed anastomosis onto the distal rectum or anus.

The reversal of a Hartmann's operation is a procedure which is now often performed laparoscopically, and hence a major laparotomy wound is avoided. All the abdominal dissection is undertaken laparoscopically, and the anastomosis is performed with the circular stapling device. In the straightforward case this can make the procedure relatively minor for the patient, but unfortunately in some patients difficulties will be encountered and conversion to open surgery may prove necessary.

Abdominoperineal resection

This was the classic operation for both anal and rectal cancer, but the indications for this operation are dwindling. Squamous cell anal carcinoma is now managed by chemoradiotherapy, and abdominoperineal resection is reserved for the occasional salvage situation. In rectal cancer, an abdominoperineal resection removed all the tissue around the rectum which was believed to be at risk of lymphatic involvement (see Fig. 21.28), and in addition removed the anal stump which was thought to be at risk of intramural tumour spread. In the light of present knowledge, there is therefore no oncological benefit in sacrificing the anus in the majority of rectal cancers, and in specialized centres the percentage of rectal cancers requiring abdominoperineal excision continues to fall. There are, however, some low rectal adenocarcinomas which are invading the anal sphincters, or extending dangerously close to the plane of dissection at this level, and sacrifice of the anal sphincters becomes inevitable for a good oncological clearance (see Fig. 21.29).

A separate issue is that of restoration of continuity after a low anterior resection. Before the advent of the circular stapling devices, the difficulty of a hand-sewn anastomosis deep in the pelvis was a major deciding factor. Although it is now almost always technically possible to restore continuity after an anterior resection for an upper or mid-rectal tumour, it may still be inadvisable in a patient with very poor sphincter function. There is, however, no advantage in excising the anal canal and sphincters, and inflicting an additional perineal wound. This situation is an indication for a Hartmann's procedure. However, as the deep aspects of an anterior resection for a lower-third rectal cancer can be technically very difficult and unnecessarily close to tumour, the surgeon may opt for an abdominoperineal resection, if a restorative operation is felt to be contraindicated.

OPERATIVE PROCEDURE

An abdominoperineal resection is traditionally performed synchronously by an abdominal and a perineal operator. The initial abdominal dissection is very similar to that for a low anterior dissection. The plane immediately outside the mesorectum is developed to mobilize the upper and mid rectum. This plane, however, should not be followed as it cones in below the mesorectum, on the surface of the levators, or the circumferential margins will have been narrowed at the level of the tumour (see Fig. 21.29). Posteriorly, the dissection should stop when the pelvic floor musculature, with the overlying parietal pelvic (Waldeyer's) fascia, is first encountered. This is particularly important in those cases where the tumour was either too low, or too locally advanced, for an anterior resection ever to have been an option. These tumours are below the mesorectum and their main protective covering is the 'cradle' of the levators.

The perineal dissection commences with a purse-string suture, inserted just outside the anal verge, to seal the anus

and prevent any contamination of the perineal wound with mucus or blood from the tumour. The anus is then circumscribed with an elliptical incision, and laterally the dissection enters the ischiorectal fat. The dissection is deepened posteriorly towards the coccyx, which is a palpable landmark for the surgeon. The initial entry through the pelvic floor is a transverse incision immediately in front of the tip of the coccyx, although the alternative of excising the coccyx with the specimen has the advantage of leading the surgeon more naturally into a radical clearance of the lateral pelvic floor. The midline incision must go through Waldeyer's fascia to enable the surgeon to insert a finger into the supralevator compartment of the pelvis. This step can be recognized by the arrival of blood from the abdomen into the perineal wound. Failure to break through this fascia results in stripping of the parietal fascia, with subsequent tearing of pelvic veins and autonomic nerve damage. Rotation of the hand allows the levator muscle to be steadied, between finger above and thumb below, while it is divided near its attachment to the pelvic side wall, and well lateral to the tumour and the sphincter complex (Fig. 21.33a). The dissection is carried around on both sides.

Anteriorly in the male patient, the lower edge of the transverse peronei muscle is sought. The dissection should be immediately behind these muscles, to enter the embryological plane between the rectal and urogenital structures. This plane can be difficult to define, and the surgeon is concerned, particularly in the case of anterior tumours, about obtaining adequate oncological clearance, yet at the same time wishing to avoid damage to the urethral bulb. The urethral catheter is palpable and is a useful guide at this point. As the dissection is continued upwards, the abdominal surgeon can guide the perineal surgeon into the correct plane in the midline anteriorly, and finally the perineal surgeon breaks through into the supralevator compartment (Fig. 21.33b). It is important that the anterior plane has been dissected adequately from above. Only the anterior pillars of puborectalis still remain intact. A finger is hooked around them and they are divided as far forward as possible. During the final anterior dissection, delivery of the specimen out through the perineal wound may be helpful.

Anteriorly in the female patient, the plane between the vagina and rectum is difficult to follow, and part of the posterior wall of the vagina is often excised with the specimen. In anterior tumours this is a safer strategy oncologically.

Small bowel loops will tend to fill the empty pelvis, and late adhesion obstruction can be troublesome. The caecum can be mobilized, and allowed to drop into the pelvis to exclude the small bowel and reduce this complication. Alternatively, the uterus will often lie retroverted following an abdominoperineal rectal excision and will naturally fill some of the pelvis. Some surgeons favour mobilizing the omentum on a left gastroepiploic pedicle to bring it into the pelvis. Opinion is divided on the desirability of attempting to close the pelvic peritoneum, as closure may create a dead space below it. The problem of a dead space will be reduced if the fatty margins of the ischiorectal fossa can be drawn

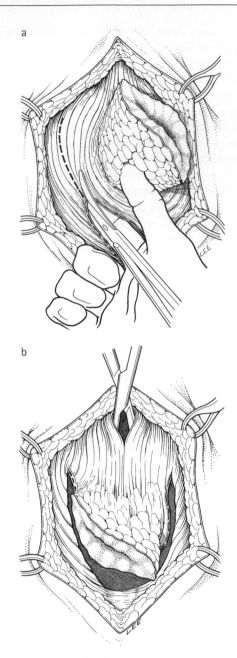

Figure 21.33 *The perineal dissection of an abdominoperineal excision of the rectum. (a) The fat of the ischiorectal fossa is entered and the incision deepened until the levator muscles are identified and incised well lateral to the bowel. (b) Anteriorly in the midline the perineal surgeon enters the supralevator compartment. Only the anterior pillars of puborectalis remain to be divided.*

together with a few absorbable sutures around a vacuum drain, but this may not be possible after a wide resection. Finally, the perineal wound is closed.

Variations

The surgeon performing the perineal dissection often has poor visibility anteriorly and, in addition, bleeding from above will pool in the pelvis further obscuring the planes. An alternative strategy to a synchronous combined approach is

to complete the abdominal dissection, close the abdomen and form the end colostomy. The patient is then turned into the prone jack-knife position for the perineal dissection under more favourable conditions. The surgeon operating from the perineum, however, can have no assistance from above in finding the right planes, and the operative time will be lengthened by turning of the patient.

A wide clearance of the perineal fat and skin may be necessary for an advanced tumour. Many of these patients have now routinely had preoperative radiotherapy or chemoradiotherapy, and there is substantial morbidity associated with delays in perineal wound healing. The wide surgical clearance may also predispose the patient to the development of a late perineal hernia. A flap, to bring well-vascularized muscle and skin into the perineum, may improve wound healing (see also Chapters 3, 12, 22 and 23). Rectus abdominis and gluteus maximus are both suitably placed for use in the perineum. The former is recommended when the perineal dissection has been performed without turning the patient, but a gluteus maximus myocutaneous rotation flap, either raised unilaterally or bilaterally, may be more appropriate when the perineal dissection has been performed in the prone jack-knife position. The involvement of a plastic surgical colleague is recommended.

LARGE BOWEL RESECTIONS FOR BENIGN DISEASE

Large bowel resections for benign disease do not require the extensive mobilization and resection of mesentery essential for colorectal cancer. The vessels may be ligated and divided adjacent to the bowel wall but, as multiple vessels are encountered at this level, a compromise is more often made (see Fig. 21.2). The surgical options in inflammatory bowel disease, diverticular disease and volvulus are discussed further in Chapter 22.

A **right hemi-colectomy** for benign disease of the caecum, or terminal ileum, requires a similar lateral peritoneal incision around the caecum, but mobilization of the hepatic flexure off the duodenum and head of the pancreas is not required. Mobilization need only be to a point where the relevant right colic and ileocolic vessels to the bowel to be excised can be isolated for ligation.

A **transverse colectomy** for benign disease does not require the excision of the omentum, which can be dissected off the colon and retained. However, this is an unsafe plane to develop if the bowel is distended, inflamed and friable, and in this situation it should be excised with the colon, as for a radical resection.

A **sigmoid colectomy** without a flush tie of the inferior mesenteric artery or a radical lymphadenectomy, may be performed for non-malignant pathology of the sigmoid colon. The initial dissection is similar to that for a radical left hemi-colectomy, except that mobilization of the splenic flexure is seldom necessary. The inferior mesenteric artery is identified. Its main trunk, and its continuation as the superior rectal artery, are preserved. The sigmoid mesentery is divided close to the bowel wall (see Fig. 21.2). The anastomosis is then fashioned between the distal descending colon and the rectosigmoid junction. The blood supply of the rectum is secure, and the distal resection line can be significantly above the peritoneal reflection. If, however, the resection is for diverticular disease the distal resection line must be at a level where the taeniae have spread out to form the continuous longitudinal muscle of the rectum.

A **total colectomy**, performed for ulcerative colitis or familial polyposis coli, is the combination of the segmental colonic resections for benign disease. An ileorectal anastomosis can be performed, or a terminal ileostomy fashioned. The rectal stump may then be closed or brought out as a mucous fistula at the lower end of the wound. Alternatively, the colectomy is combined with a rectal excision as a total proctocolectomy. Reconstruction with an ileoanal pouch is then possible.

A **proctectomy** for benign disease may be performed in a plane close to the rectal wall, leaving the mesorectum *in situ*. The potential for damage to the autonomic nerves is reduced, and the mesorectum retained in the pelvis is of value in filling the dead space. However, it is not a bloodless embryological plane, and many surgeons familiar with pelvic dissection prefer to follow the classic plane outside the mesorectum with only minor modifications to offer extra security to the autonomic nerves. These surgical options in inflammatory bowel disease are discussed in more detail in Chapter 22.

LAPAROSCOPIC LARGE BOWEL RESECTIONS

The entire dissection is completed laparoscopically, following similar principles to those employed in open surgery, except that a small incision is made for specimen retrieval. In some situations the anastomosis is also performed externally. These operations are therefore more accurately described as 'laparoscopically assisted resections'. Large bowel resections are increasingly performed laparoscopically by those colorectal surgeons who have the necessary expertise. Short-term measures of outcome indicate that it has some early advantages over open surgery. There is, however, still some concern that a laparoscopic resection could compromise the cure of colorectal cancer, and such surgery should be closely audited.

Right hemi–colectomy

This can be performed with an umbilical camera port, and three further ports established on the left side of the abdomen. A 12-mm suprapubic port, through which a bowel stapler can be passed if necessary, and two 5-mm ports, one in the left iliac fossa and the other low in the left hypochondrium, is a satisfactory arrangement. The exact position of the ports will depend on the preference of the individual surgeon, the underlying pathology, and whether a medial or lateral approach is planned. The principles of the dissection are essentially the same as for the open operation. In the lateral approach, the peritoneum is incised lateral to the right colon, and extended around the caecum and hepatic flexure. The right colon on its retroperitoneal mesentery is mobilized before the vessels are secured. However, the fully mobilized colon can obscure the operating field, and therefore a medial approach is usually preferred in malignancy, where a more extensive mobilization is required. In the medial approach a peritoneal incision is made below the caecal pole, and a tunnel created beneath the retroperitoneal mesentery. The dissection to mobilize the right colon is then completed, except for the incision of the lateral peritoneum, which is left until the right colic and ileocolic arteries have been secured and divided at their origins.

A small incision is then made, either at the umbilicus or in the right iliac fossa, for the delivery of the specimen. The edges of this wound must be protected from bacterial and malignant contamination. The proximal and distal bowel divisions and the ileocolic anastomosis can then all be completed outside the abdomen.

Sigmoid colectomy or high anterior resection

This can be performed with an umbilical camera port, a 12-mm main working port placed low and lateral in the right iliac fossa, and an additional 5-mm port in each flank.[11] Again, the arrangement of port sites will depend on the preference of individual surgeons and the approach planned. When a lateral approach is used to mobilize the sigmoid in a similar fashion to that normally employed in open surgery, the fully mobilized sigmoid colon can obscure the operative field. The alternative medial approach starts with a small incision in the peritoneum, lateral and below the distal sigmoid colon. A tunnel is created under the retroperitoneal mesentery of the left colon which is fully mobilized except for the release of the lateral peritoneum, which is left until the inferior mesenteric vessels have been secured and divided.

The dissection is carried into the pelvis to mobilize the upper rectum so that it can be drawn up into the abdomen. It is important to straighten out the rectal curves which otherwise may hamper advancement of the circular stapling device introduced from below. The rectum is divided with an endoscopic stapler, and the mesorectum is divided with a vascular reload of the same stapler. A small left iliac fossa muscle-splitting incision is made and the specimen delivered. The proximal bowel is then divided, with care being taken to ensure there is adequate length for it to reach for an anastomosis without tension. The anvil of the circular stapling device is then secured within the divided proximal bowel with a purse-string suture, and returned to the peritoneal cavity. The incision is closed, the pneumoperitoneum re-established, and the circular stapling device introduced per anum. The delivery of the spike through the stapled rectal stump, the locking of the anvil onto it and the approximation of the two portions of the stapler are all controlled laparoscopically.

REFERENCES

1. Lindsey I, Mortensen NJMcC. Iatrogenic impotence and rectal dissection. Leading article. *Br J Surg* 2002; **89**: 1493–4.
2. Deans GT, Spence RAJ. Neoplastic lesions of the appendix. Review. *Br J Surg* 1995; **82**: 299–306.
3. Sweeney KJ, Keane FBV. Moving from open to laparoscopic appendicectomy. Leading article. *Br J Surg* 2003; **90**: 257–8.
4. Cataldo PA. Intestinal stomas; 200 years of digging. *Dis Colon Rectum* 1999; **42**: 137–42.
5. Amin SN, Armitage NC, Abercrombie JF, *et al.* Lateral repair of parastomal hernia. *Ann R Coll Surg Engl* 2001; **83**: 206–8.
6. Lockhart-Mummery JP. Two hundred cases of cancer of the rectum treated by perineal excision. *Br J Surg* 1926; **14**: 110–24.
7. Heald RJ, Smedh RK, Kald A, *et al.* Abdominoperineal excision of the rectum – an endangered operation. *Dis Colon Rectum* 1997; **40**: 747–51.
8. Quirke P, Durdey P, Dixon MF, *et al.* Local recurrence of rectal adenocarcinoma due to inadequate surgical resection. Histopathological study of lateral tumour spread and surgical excision. *Lancet* 1986; **ii**: 996–9.
9. Hallböök O, Påhlman L, Krog M, *et al.* Randomised comparison of straight and colonic J pouch anastomosis after low anterior resection. *Ann Surg* 1996; **224**: 58–65.
10. Moran BJ, Heald RJ. Risk factors for, and management of anastomotic leakage in rectal surgery. *Colorectal Dis* 2001; **3**: 135–7.
11. Stevenson ARL, Sitz RW, Lumley JW, *et al.* Laparoscopically assisted anterior resection for diverticular disease. *Ann Surg* 1998; **227**: 335–42.

22

OPERATIVE MANAGEMENT OF SMALL AND LARGE BOWEL DISEASE

The standard techniques of intra-abdominal surgery, and the classical intestinal operations, have been described in the preceding chapters. There is often a range of surgical solutions available, and the ability to choose the most suitable procedure increases with the surgeon's experience. Most frequently surgeons choose the most appropriate of the classical operations relevant to the situation, but they should not be afraid of adaptations and modifications to standard procedures. It is extremely important, however, that any modifications are made within the framework of sound surgical principles.

SURGERY OF INTESTINAL OBSTRUCTION

The initial management of any patient with an intestinal obstruction is correction of the fluid and electrolyte deficit by intravenous fluids, combined, if possible, with deflation of the bowel (see Chapter 11). A nasogastric tube is passed and the contents of the distended stomach are aspirated. The nasogastric tube is then attached to a bag and left on free drainage, in addition to intermittent aspiration. The small bowel is progressively deflated as the obstructed intraluminal contents reflux back into the stomach and are aspirated. A patient with a distal large bowel obstruction may benefit from nasogastric aspiration if there is additional distension of the small bowel, but otherwise it is of little value.

The next phase in the management is the assessment of the patient and the decision as to whether emergency surgery is indicated. This decision hinges on the likelihood of an ischaemic or strangulated segment of bowel (see Chapter 14).

A firm diagnosis of the underlying pathology may be pos-

sible at this stage, but more often the surgeon continues with conservative treatment, or plans an emergency laparotomy, with only a tentative diagnosis. Preoperative erect and supine abdominal X-rays, however, should at least have helped to differentiate between small and large bowel obstruction. These are discussed separately as the issues differ.

Small bowel obstruction

EXTERNAL HERNIAE

An *irreducible* external hernia must be sought in any case of small bowel obstruction. A reducible hernia is an incidental finding, and not the cause of the obstruction. All hernial orifices must be checked, remembering that an irreducible femoral hernia is easily overlooked in the obese patient. A *strangulated* hernia is one in which the contents are constricted in such a way that the blood supply is impaired. An irreducible hernia causing a small bowel obstruction will usually quickly progress to a hernia with a strangulated loop of small bowel, and emergency surgery is indicated. A strangulated hernia in the absence of obstruction probably contains only omentum, but a *Richter's hernia* (Fig. 22.1), in which only part of the circumference of the gut is trapped and the lumen is still patent, is a possibility. Colon is less frequently obstructed, or strangulated, within a hernia than the small bowel.

The hernia may be a spontaneous groin, epigastric or para-umbilical hernia, or it may be an incisional or parastomal hernia. The surgical approach and initial dissection is similar to that in an elective hernia repair (see Chapters 12 and 24). The hernial sac is then opened. Blood-stained fluid confirms strangulation of the contents, and foul-smelling

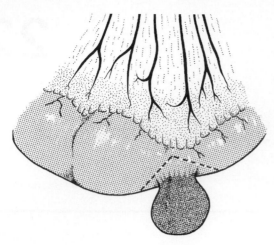

Figure 22.1   *A Richter's hernia. Only part of the circumference of the bowel is trapped, and strangulation can occur without obstruction.*

fluid suggests non-viable bowel. Contamination of the wound by this fluid should be minimized as it will be heavily colonized with faecal organisms. The strangulating constriction must then be released in order to restore perfusion to the compromised contents (Fig. 22.2). In an *indirect inguinal hernia* the constriction is usually the tight peritoneal neck of the sac, whilst in an incisional hernia it is more often the edge of the fascial defect, both of which are easily released. The strangulation in a *para-umbilical hernia* is frequently at the narrow neck of a loculus of the sac. A *femoral hernia* is constricted by the femoral ring itself; release is difficult and access poor from below. A minor release is possible by a medial incision into the lacunar ligament, but occasionally troublesome bleeding from an aberrant vessel is encoun-

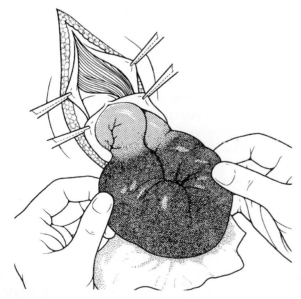

Figure 22.2   *A strangulated loop of small bowel in an inguinal hernia has been released by a peritoneal incision in the neck of the sac (after Hamilton Bailey).*

tered. If release is inadequate, and especially if there is any concern over the viability of bowel in the sac, access from above is also necessary. If a low approach to the hernia has been made, an additional abdominal incision is usually required; either a midline incision or a low iliac fossa incision (see Chapter 24). If the bowel still cannot be delivered out of the hernial sac it may be necessary to divide the inguinal ligament close to the pubic tubercle and re-attach it afterwards.

If on release of the constriction, the hernial contents quickly regain perfusion, a simple return to the peritoneal cavity and repair of the hernia is all that is required. The decision to resect is straightforward if no improvement occurs on releasing the constriction. If the surgeon is faced with doubtfully viable bowel and the abdomen is not open, it is unwise to replace the loop to aid recovery as it may be difficult to retrieve it again. Instead, it should be covered with a warm moist towel, and left undisturbed for a few minutes.

Occasionally, a strangulated hernia reduces spontaneously, early in an operation, before the sac is opened. If, on opening the sac, blood-stained fluid is encountered the surgeon must locate the bowel loop or omentum which had been trapped in order to check the viability of the strangulated tissue. A congested small bowel loop may be retrieved via the hernial neck, and drawn back into the operative field for inspection, but a small laparotomy incision is often required in this situation. In a ventral hernia, only an extension to the wound is required, but in a groin hernia a separate incision may be necessary.

Infarcted omentum is simply excised with a transfixion ligation just proximal to the termination of the viable tissue. A resection is mandatory for non-viable bowel, and may be difficult due to limited access. In an adult strangulated inguinal hernia a resection may be performed without opening the general peritoneal cavity. After completion of the anastomosis, the bowel is replaced within the abdomen and the peritoneum at the neck of the sac closed. If there is difficulty replacing the bulkier anastomosis through the deep ring, a lateral release of the ring may be necessary. This is a particular problem on the rare occasions when a bowel resection is necessary in a strangulated infantile inguinal hernia. A similar difficulty occurs after a resection for a strangulated femoral hernia approached through a low incision. This scenario should be anticipated and avoided by employing an additional separate abdominal incision for the resection and the anastomosis.

A non-viable loop of colon is fortunately relatively rare in a strangulated hernia, but if encountered will require a large bowel resection of obstructed colon, as discussed later in this chapter. A major laparotomy incision is mandatory for adequate access.

ADHESION OBSTRUCTION

The commonest cause of small bowel obstruction is an adhesion obstruction with a loop of small bowel compressed, kinked or twisted by an adhesion following previous surgery.

Any patient with an abdominal scar, or a history of a vaginal hysterectomy, can be presumed to have an adhesion obstruction of the small bowel in the first instance, provided that a strangulated external hernia has been excluded. Deflation with a nasogastric tube may be sufficient to allow the situation to resolve, and no surgery is then indicated.

Closed loop adhesion obstruction is a variant of the common small bowel obstruction. It may be a closed loop from the start if a small bowel loop has twisted around a band. Alternatively, it may start as a simple obstruction, but subsequent dilatation and displacement of bowel loops can cause a second more proximal obstruction. Once a closed loop obstruction has occurred, it cannot be decompressed from above by nasogastric aspiration. Distension increases and the bowel becomes ischaemic from excessive intramural pressure, even in the absence of a twist in the mesentery. The distended loop, however, often does rotate with resultant occlusion of the mesenteric vessels which then becomes the most important factor in the ischaemia of strangulation.

An ischaemic loop causes continuous abdominal pain in addition to the colic of obstruction. A careful history may elicit this symptom, and examination should demonstrate peritoneal irritation. It must be remembered, however, that in full-thickness inflammatory small bowel conditions causing obstruction (e.g. Crohn's disease) peritoneal inflammation does not necessarily indicate ischaemia, and continuing conservative management, despite local peritonism, may be appropriate. A rising pulse rate and a leucocytosis are markers of the systemic inflammatory response to an ischaemic loop of bowel, and are useful monitoring parameters during the conservative management of a small bowel obstruction. Urgent surgery is indicated whenever strangulation is suspected.

In a simple obstruction, with no indication of strangulation, conservative management may be continued for several days but, if no resolution is occurring, a laparotomy should be planned. A water-soluble small bowel contrast study has been reported by some to be valuable in distinguishing those obstructions which will resolve from those requiring surgery. For example, Urografin (40 mL in 40 mL of water) can be administered orally, or via a nasogastric tube, and the patient X-rayed 4-hourly to detect contrast medium reaching the caecum. The technique, however, often produces the answer without the need for X-rays, as the patient either passes flatus and diarrhoea, or becomes more distended and experiences increased pain.

A small bowel obstruction with no previous surgery is unlikely to be due to adhesions. Congenital adhesions, inflammatory adhesions from previous diverticulitis or gynaecological pelvic inflammatory disease and adhesions from blunt abdominal trauma remain a possibility, but some other intra-abdominal pathology, especially malignancy, is increasingly likely. In the absence of symptoms or signs of strangulation, an emergency laparotomy is not necessary and initial treatment can be conservative. A laparotomy is, however, usually required for diagnosis and should not be unnecessarily delayed.

A mixed picture of small bowel obstruction and ileus is sometimes encountered postoperatively. This was common after appendicectomy before antibiotics were used routinely, and often occurred after an initial return of bowel function. It is usually associated with intra-abdominal inflammation or abscess formation. If there is a significant collection of pus then drainage is required, but otherwise treatment should be conservative. The loops of oedematous small bowel involved in the inflammatory process will recover with rest and antibiotics. Intravenous feeding is often indicated if recovery is prolonged. Surgery should ideally be avoided as it carries a considerable risk of damage to friable bowel.

Prevention of adhesion obstruction

Adhesions are a major cause of late morbidity.[1] They may occur after any intraperitoneal intervention, but are unpredictable, as some patients have multiple operations and produce minimal adhesions. However, the risk does depend on the type of surgery, with a total colectomy carrying one of the highest risks of approximately 30 per cent incidence of small bowel obstruction within 10 years. Measures to prevent adhesions have included the elimination of talc from surgeons gloves and, more recently, various intraperitoneal applications of hyaluronidase and other chemicals. The results have so far been inconclusive. Intraperitoneal chemotherapy for malignancy appears to reduce adhesions, but the morbidity associated with routine use would be prohibitive. There is also concern that any agent that eliminates adhesions will also prevent serosal sealing of an anastomosis, with the potential to increase anastomotic leakage.

It has long been noted that many patients form extensive soft pliable adhesions between loops of small bowel. These adhesions prevent free mobility of the loops, without predisposing to obstruction. Surgical attempts to mimic this with plication techniques in patients experiencing repeat small bowel obstruction have not been generally successful.

Laparotomy for small bowel obstruction

Initial fluid and electrolyte resuscitation prior to surgery is important. General anaesthesia must be combined with protection of the airway from inhalation of vomit. On opening the peritoneum the cause of the obstruction may be immediately obvious, but more often nothing can be seen except distended loops of small bowel. In such cases the first step in the operation is to inspect the caecum. This can be done by retracting the right margin of the wound and by displacing distended loops of small bowel to the left.

A *collapsed caecum* confirms the presence of a small bowel obstruction. A search is made in the right iliac fossa and pelvis for a collapsed loop of bowel, and this is traced proximally until the obstruction is reached. Distended loops of bowel should, if possible, be retained within the abdomen but, if this is not possible, they should be covered with a warm moist pack and supported to prevent undue traction on the mesentery. The direction in which the small bowel should be traced can be determined in the following manner. The loop is held in the long axis of the body, and a finger is passed deeply along the left side of its mesentery. If the finger finds itself guided inevitably to the left iliac fossa, or to the left side of the vertebrae, the proximal end of the loop lies towards the thorax. If the finger is guided into the right iliac fossa, or to the right side of the vertebrae, the loop is inverted and the proximal end lies towards the feet.

Once the obstruction is located, the cause can be addressed. Occasionally, the release of a band adhesion may be all that is required. Alternatively, some other pathology or a loop of strangulated bowel may be encountered. Ashen grey, or black, bowel with a lustreless, flaccid sodden wall is obviously non-viable and must be resected. The mesenteric vessels to the loop should be clamped before any release of a constriction, or any untwisting of a volvulus, is undertaken. This prevents restoration of circulation through the dead tissue and the inevitable release of toxic metabolites into the circulation. (This is unfortunately seldom possible when infarcted bowel is found in a strangulated external hernia, as access to the mesentery is initially so limited.) More often, the viability of the strangulated loop is uncertain and perfusion must first be restored. The decision may then be easy if there is either a rapid recovery or no improvement, but if there is still doubt the loop should be returned to the peritoneal cavity and left undisturbed for 5 minutes before re-inspection. On occasion, the loop is viable except for two narrow non-viable bands at the site of the constriction; these can be safely invaginated with seromuscular sutures.

The situation may be very much more difficult if extensive dissection of adhesions is required to gain access to the obstruction, especially if loops of distended bowel are adherent in the pelvis. The operation may take several hours and the surgeon must proceed extremely gently. Tears in obstructed tethered small bowel loops, deep in the pelvis, make further mobilization increasingly difficult, especially as an inadvertent enterotomy often cannot be repaired, or even fully controlled, until the loop is freed.

Even if the obstruction has only required a simple release, closure of the abdomen may be difficult until further small bowel deflation has been achieved. This can be done by 'milking' back the small bowel contents into the stomach, from where they can be aspirated through the nasogastric tube by the anaesthetist (Fig. 22.3). Alternatively, a needle aspiration (see Chapter 13) may be a useful manoeuvre.

If there is a *collapsed caecum but no collapsed distal ileum*, the obstruction is very close to the ileocaecal valve and is almost certainly a carcinoma of the caecum. Unfortunately, this is frequently found to be the cause of a small bowel obstruction in an older patient. It may settle on conservative management, only to recur a week or two later.

If the *caecum is distended*, there is likely to be a large bowel obstruction.

A laparotomy which confirms a small bowel obstruction from adhesions requires only the release of the adhesions and

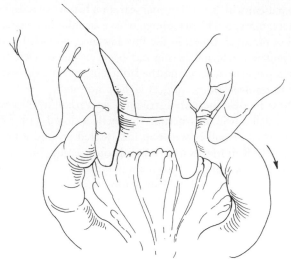

Figure 22.3 *Gastrointestinal contents can be 'milked' from a dilated segment of bowel into a segment from which they can be removed.*

the resection of any non-viable bowel. Alternatively, the obstruction may be shown to be secondary to some other underlying pathology which requires to be addressed in its own right.

INTRALUMINAL OBSTRUCTIONS

An impacted ingested foreign body, or gallstone, can be removed by simple enterotomy. In *gallstone ileus* this is adequate definitive treatment. The fistula between the biliary tract and the small intestine is serving a similar purpose to a therapeutic sphincterotomy and, as an associated cholecystectomy may be difficult and potentially dangerous, only an experienced biliary surgeon should consider proceeding further.

An *Ascaris* infestation can produce an obstruction from a bolus of worms. Management of the obstruction is conservative and de-worming postponed until the obstruction has resolved. If a laparotomy has been performed, an enterotomy is normally avoided for fear of migration of worms through the suture line; fortunately, it is usually possible to 'milk' the worm bolus through into the caecum.

BENIGN STRICTURES

The operative decisions in benign strictures depend on the aetiology. Fibrous strictures can be treated by stricturoplasty, or simple resection. Strictures associated with Crohn's disease and tuberculosis are discussed below. A radiotherapy stricture causing obstruction requires a resection that includes the adjacent bowel, which has inevitably also been damaged by the radiotherapy. If this is not done, the anastomosis will be performed with compromised tissue and there is a high risk of anastomotic breakdown.

INTERNAL HERNIAE

An internal hernia may involve only a partial circumference knuckle, or a short segment, of small bowel trapped beneath a peritoneal fold, or within an obturator defect. The bowel is released, resected if non-viable, and the space in which it was trapped obliterated or repaired. It may however represent a more serious form of the closed loop obstruction discussed above. The greater part of the small bowel may have herniated through a mesenteric defect. The anatomy is difficult to elucidate and release of the constriction must be cautious or mesenteric vessels at the edge of the defect will be damaged.

Strangulated stomach within an hiatus hernia, and strangulated colon through an old diaphragmatic laceration, are further potentially serious forms of internal herniation.

SMALL BOWEL VOLVULUS

A small bowel volvulus may endanger the perfusion of the whole small bowel. Those that occur in infancy are commonly associated with congenital malrotation. Adult small bowel volvulus is a common condition in some parts of the world, where it is sometimes encountered around the base of a sigmoid volvulus to produce a complicated 'sigmoid knot'.[2] The operation consists of the release of the constriction by derotation, first of the loops of small bowel, followed by the large bowel. Any non-viable portions are resected.

INTUSSUSCEPTIONS

The apex of an intussusception is usually lying in the ascending or transverse colon, and consists of an area of abnormal ileum. Operative reduction of an intussusception is by repetitive gentle squeezing of the bowel just distal to the apex, which moves progressively more proximal as the intussusception is reduced. Reduction by traction is liable to cause damage. If reduction is not possible a resection is necessary, most often in the form of a right hemi-colectomy. After a successful reduction, a resection may still be necessary if the bowel is infarcted, or if it has torn during reduction. In addition, in adult patients the apex is commonly a small bowel tumour which requires a resection with inclusion of its lymphatic drainage. The common infantile intussusception can usually be managed non-operatively, and is discussed further below.

SMALL BOWEL TUMOURS

The surgery of these relatively uncommon tumours is resection with a generous 'V' of mesentery in order to obtain a radical lymphadenectomy. The tumour may be an adenocarcinoma, a carcinoid or a lymphoma. It is important to check the whole small bowel carefully for additional tumours as carcinoids are frequently multiple (see Chapter 15).

MALIGNANT ADHESIONS AND PERITONEAL DEPOSITS

A patient presenting with a small bowel obstruction may have a loop of small bowel adherent to a previously undiagnosed intra-abdominal malignancy. If the primary tumour is resectable, the only chance of cure, and usually the best palliation, is achieved by a radical resection of the primary tumour en bloc with the involved loop of small bowel (see Fig. 15.2, page 248).

A patient with multiple peritoneal malignant deposits may present with a small bowel obstruction. One, or more, side-to-side anastomoses may relieve the obstruction, but often little can be achieved by surgery (see also Chapter 15).

Large bowel obstruction

Many large bowel obstructions pose no immediate threat to bowel wall viability. Urgent, rather than emergency, surgery is therefore indicated and a delay of 24–48 hours for further assessment can be beneficial. The rectum must be checked digitally, and by sigmoidoscopy, for an obstructing rectal cancer, and also for any synchronous pathology. On plain X-ray, a *pseudo-obstruction* cannot be differentiated from a mechanical distal large bowel obstruction. As pseudo-obstruction is almost always better managed conservatively, it must be excluded preoperatively. The level of a distal obstruction can also be difficult to interpret on preoperative X-ray as dilated loops of mobile sigmoid colon may be folded down into the pelvis. A water-soluble rectal contrast study is therefore advisable during this period of assessment, whether a distal large bowel obstruction is thought clinically to be mechanical, or not. This should differentiate a pseudo-obstruction from a mechanical obstruction, and should also indicate the level of the latter.

In some patients, who are only partially obstructed, conservative management may allow at least temporary resolution. An endoscopic, or contrast radiological, confirmation of the diagnosis is then possible, followed by surgery under more favourable elective conditions a week or two later. Recently, there has been interest in the use of temporary endoluminal stents, to relieve a malignant large bowel obstruction and allow definitive surgery to be undertaken in a truly elective situation after full investigations and bowel preparation. This technique may, however, cause peritoneal contamination with tumour cells if the dilatation causes serosal splits in the tumour. A stent, however, is an ideal solution for a patient with a malignant distal large bowel obstruction and inoperable intraperitoneal or hepatic metastases. If the diagnosis and staging can be established preoperatively, a major resection or a stoma can sometimes be avoided altogether.

In benign pathology, surgery can also occasionally be avoided. A sigmoid volvulus may be decompressed endoscopically and, in an unfit patient, an expectant policy may be a safer option than surgery to prevent possible recurrences. Sigmoid diverticulitis may cause an obstruction which is difficult to differentiate from one caused by a sigmoid cancer. When an obstruction is incomplete and there is evidence of inflammation in the left iliac fossa, a diagnosis of diverticulitis is favoured, and management is initially conservative with antibiotics. The obstruction will often settle, but further investigation, after the acute episode has settled, is important to exclude a cancer, as inflammation can also occur around a locally perforated tumour. An absence of inflammation does not exclude a simple fibrous diverticular stricture associated with long-standing disease. Most patients who have had an episode of obstruction associated with diverticular disease should be advised to have a resection, but in an unfit patient this may again be an unacceptable risk.

Occasionally, the surgeon may be forced to operate within a few hours of presentation when there is evidence of ischaemia developing in the obstructed colon. For example, in a large bowel volvulus there is a blind loop obstruction with additional torsion of mesenteric vessels. The risk of strangulation, with colonic infarction, is high, and urgent resolution is important, as discussed below. A simple distal large bowel obstruction can also develop into a dangerous closed-loop situation if the ileocaecal valve is competent, preventing reflux of intestinal contents into the ileum. Progressive large bowel distension is rapid, and the increasing intraluminal pressure and distension threatens the perfusion of the colonic wall (see Chapter 11). Caecal rupture finally ensues. This should not occur in a patient already in hospital as the deteriorating situation, with increasing distension and tenderness of the caecum, should have been noted.

Laparotomy for large bowel obstruction

If the obstruction is left-sided, the patient should be positioned with legs up to afford access to the anus. Supine positioning is satisfactory for a right-sided obstruction. The rectum must be assessed before laparotomy, by digital and rigid sigmoidoscopic examination, if this has not already been done. The abdominal gas pattern on plain X-ray, or a contrast study, may have indicated a more proximal obstruction, but the surgeon must exclude a small synchronous lesion in the rectum which will be difficult to exclude by palpation at laparotomy.

The abdomen is opened through a generous midline incision. If the ileocaecal valve is patent there may be gross small bowel distension in addition to large bowel distension, and deflation may be necessary before further exploration is possible. A sucker can be introduced into both the ileum, and the caecum, through a small incision in the distal ileum, controlled by a purse-string suture. This can be very helpful in reducing gaseous distension, but in the colon the sucker tends to block quickly with semi-solid faecal matter, and it is easy to cause gross peritoneal faecal contamination during this manoeuvre.

The operative strategy in a large bowel obstruction then depends on the underlying pathology and the site of the obstruction. At laparotomy, an obstruction in the pelvis can be mistaken for a pseudo-obstruction, and it is therefore essential to check that any distal bowel, to which access for inspection and palpation is difficult from above, has been fully examined from below.

MALIGNANT LARGE BOWEL OBSTRUCTION

Malignancy is the commonest cause of a large bowel obstruction in the Western world. Many of these tumours are still potentially curable, and a major radical resection, as described in Chapter 21, is required. When the tumour is irresectable, a proximal loop stoma may be the only practical solution, but a bypass should be considered as it avoids the distress of a stoma (see Figs 21.20, page 394 and 21.26, page 398).

Right hemi-colectomy

Right colon tumours are treated with a standard radical right hemi-colectomy. The presence of obstruction is seldom a major problem during mobilization, and the small bowel is deflated by intraluminal suction through the divided ileum prior to the anastomosis. The more distal colon is relatively empty, and an ileocolic anastomosis is safe in obstructed bowel. A transverse colectomy is unsuitable in an obstructed colon, and an obstructed transverse colon cancer should be treated with an extended right hemi-colectomy so that the ileum is anastomosed to the descending colon. In an attempt to use ileum in a safe anastomosis, this concept has been extended as a subtotal colectomy and ileorectal anastomosis for obstructing carcinomas of the descending colon or sigmoid. If this resection is chosen, the surgeon must keep in mind the segment of colon which requires the radical lymphadenectomy (see Fig. 21.2, page 378). This operation has great advantages if the viability of the caecum from distension is in any doubt. However, if the caecum is healthy a safer anastomosis has been created at the expense of the loss of a large proportion of healthy colon, and some patients will be left with troublesome diarrhoea.

Left colonic resections

Left colonic resections carry a high morbidity when undertaken for obstruction. The mobilization of left-sided tumours can be technically challenging with obstructed, dilated bowel. In addition, a primary anastomosis is compromised by an unprepared bowel and by alterations in the colonic wall secondary to distension. Local infection, or faecal peritonitis, will further increase the anastomotic vulnerability, as does the poor general state of an ill or elderly patient.

Previously, a simple defunctioning right transverse colostomy was recommended to relieve a left colonic obstruction and definitive surgery was undertaken at a later date. A primary resection is now considered preferable, but should not be performed by an inexperienced surgeon in sub-optimal conditions during the night. Fortunately, most surgery for malignant large bowel obstruction can be safely delayed for 24–48 hours and performed under more ideal circumstances. If intervention has proved unavoidable in difficult circumstances, there may still be a role for a simple defunctioning colostomy. For example, a tumour of the splenic flexure can be technically difficult to mobilize if the gut is distended. The surgeon may believe that it is in the best interests of the patient to bring out a defunctioning stoma and delay the resection so that it can be carried out under elective conditions by a surgeon with more colorectal experience. An advanced obstructed tumour of the upper rectum (as discussed later) should often not be excised as an emergency procedure, even by an experienced colorectal surgeon. A proximal loop colostomy, followed by full assessment and preoperative radiotherapy may give the patient a better prognosis.

In most situations, however, it is possible to perform an oncologically sound radical resection of the primary left colon tumour at the initial operation for obstruction and, if so, this is the ideal management. If the tumour is resected as an extended right hemi-colectomy, or a subtotal colectomy, a low-risk ileocolic or ileorectal anastomosis can be performed. However, if a standard radical left hemi-colectomy has been performed, the choice is between a Hartmann's operation or a high-risk anastomosis. The advantage of the speed and lower risk of a Hartmann's procedure is offset by the necessity of a further major operation to rejoin the bowel if the patient is unhappy with a permanent stoma.

When a reconstruction is planned after a left colonic resection for obstruction, the surgeon should consider the potential benefit of emptying the proximal colon prior to the anastomosis, and of protecting the anastomosis with a proximal loop stoma. Closure of this some 6 weeks later is a small procedure compared with the operation to reverse a Hartmann's operation.

On-table large bowel lavage This is the most satisfactory method of emptying the obstructed colon of faeces.[3] A catheter is inserted into the ileum through a purse-string suture and advanced through the ileocaecal valve into the caecum. (Alternatively, the appendix is removed and the catheter is inserted into the stump. The appendix stump is ligated when the irrigation is completed.) The colon is divided above the obstruction, and the end of the bowel is either placed outside the abdomen directly into a bowl, or connected to a length of tubing (as shown in Fig. 22.4) if there is insufficient length. Fluid is then run through the catheter until the bowel is empty of faecal material.

DIVERTICULAR OBSTRUCTION

When the diagnosis is certain at operation, the narrow area of bowel is excised by a sigmoid colectomy, and there is no need for a radical lymphadenectomy. However, a surgeon often has to operate for a sigmoid obstruction of uncertain aetiology, and the resection should follow the steps for a radical resection if cancer cannot be excluded. Following the resection, the same concerns exist regarding the re-establishment of colonic continuity.

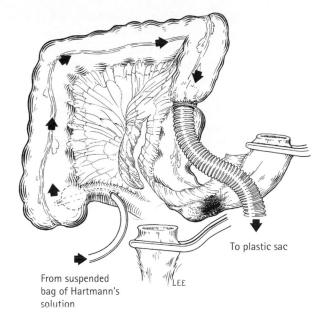

Figure 22.4 *An on-table colonic wash-out.*

VOLVULUS

Sigmoid volvulus

A sigmoid volvulus is the commonest cause of large bowel obstruction in parts of Africa and Asia, where it occurs in all age groups. In Europe and North America it is primarily a condition of the elderly. Diagnosis of sigmoid volvulus, and the less common caecal volvulus, is made on the classical X-ray appearances. A large bowel volvulus requires urgent release, and if the sigmoid is involved this can usually be achieved endoscopically. Recurrence is a problem, but major surgery in an elderly patient has been avoided. An endoscopic two-point fixation of the sigmoid loop using a percutaneous endoscopic gastrostomy (PEG) device is a compromise which may be worth considering in the elderly.[4]

If a sigmoid volvulus cannot be decompressed endoscopically, or if there is concern over sigmoid viability, then laparotomy is essential. A viable sigmoid may be simply untwisted but recurrence is likely. Attempts to fix the sigmoid to prevent recurrence are not always successful, nor are the ingenious attempts to plicate or widen the sigmoid mesentery.

However, the surgeon faced with a frail elderly patient wishes to avoid not only the risks of resection but also the danger of recurrent volvulus and the need for later elective surgery. It may then seem reasonable to attempt such a manoeuvre. By contrast, in the fit patient a sigmoid resection is the preferable option. A resection is also mandatory if the sigmoid has infarcted. Control of the vascular pedicle, before untwisting, will reduce the venous drainage of toxins into the circulation but may not be technically possible. A sigmoid colectomy is performed with preservation of the superior rectal artery. The surgeon then has three choices:

- On-table lavage and a primary anastomosis, which can be covered with a proximal loop stoma. Experience from Africa suggests that a primary anastomosis without a proximal temporary stoma is usually safe in young and otherwise fit patients.[5]
- The proximal end can be brought out as an end colostomy, and the distal end can be brought to the surface as a mucous fistula. If they are adjacent, re-anastomosis is then a more minor undertaking. However, there is seldom sufficient length in the distal limb to achieve this.
- The distal end can be closed as a Hartmann's operation and an end colostomy formed. A second laparotomy will be required if the patient wishes bowel continuity to be restored.

Caecal volvulus

A caecal volvulus is best treated with a right hemi-colectomy, even if the bowel is viable, as attempts at caecopexy seldom prevent a recurrence. If fixation is to be attempted the caecum can be sutured to parietal tissue, or it can be tethered by a caecostomy.

Pseudo-obstruction

Pseudo-obstruction is difficult to differentiate from a distal large bowel obstruction, and the diagnosis should not be made without a confirmatory distal contrast study to exclude a mechanical cause. Pseudo-obstruction occurs classically in the ill and elderly, and is particularly common in orthopaedic inpatients who have had recent hip surgery. There is an overlap with sigmoid volvulus, and some patients have a history of both conditions. It is thought that the colonic distension of a pseudo-obstruction may predispose to a volvulus.

Treatment

Surgery can usually be avoided. Endoscopic intervention, erythromycin, epidural blockade and neostigmine or guanethidine, may allow conservative management.[6] Neostigmine (2.5 mg dissolved in 50 mL saline) is given intravenously over 3–5 minutes. (If ineffective, the treatment can be repeated after 20 minutes.) A dramatic response is common, but the cardiovascular effects of the treatment must not be under-estimated and full resuscitation facilities should be available. Failure of these methods, or caecal distension which jeopardizes viability, will necessitate a laparotomy. More often, the abdomen has been opened on a preoperative diagnosis of a mechanical obstruction. The surgical options depend on the viability of the caecum, and the probable precipitating causes of the pseudo-obstruction.

If the caecum is gangrenous, a right hemi-colectomy with an ileocolic anastomosis is a possibility, but the back-pressure on the anastomosis is worrying if the pseudo-obstruction persists. The alternative of a right hemi-colectomy with a terminal ileostomy is safer, especially if the caecum has already ruptured. Distension of the distal bowel, however, may recur; this makes closure of the distal end hazardous, and it should be brought out as a mucous fistula (see Chapter 21). If the caecum is viable at laparotomy a tube caecostomy is a useful temporary solution in those patients who have a background of normal bowel function and an obvious precipitative cause of the episode of pseudo-obstruction. In patients with long-standing problems of bowel motility a caecostomy should be avoided, as it merely adds another complication to their already difficult long-term management.

CAECOSTOMY

A caecostomy does not provide adequate drainage of an obstructed colon, nor does it defunction the distal bowel sufficiently to afford useful protection of an anastomosis.[7] It is, however, occasionally a temporary life-saving solution which can even be performed under local anaesthetic in a very ill patient. The colonic deflation it provides should be sufficient to prevent caecal rupture. It may therefore be the only surgical intervention required in a pseudo-obstruction with a threatened caecum. A caecostomy may also occasionally be used as a temporary measure in a patient with a mechanical obstruction when decompression is urgent but the patient's general state precludes any more major intervention until further resuscitation is effective.

An appendix incision is made under local, or general, anaesthetic. The caecum presents on opening the peritoneum and the gaseous distension is relieved by needle puncture, with suction attached, through an anterior taenia. This portion of caecum can then be gently drawn out of the wound, and a soft clamp applied to isolate it. A purse-string suture is inserted around the needle, which is then withdrawn. An incision is then made in the caecal wall, the self-retaining catheter inserted, the purse-string suture tied, and the soft clamp removed. The best catheter for this purpose is a large *de Pezzer* catheter with the end excised (Fig. 22.5). A second purse-string suture provides added security as it is often not practical to tether the dilated caecum to the anterior abdominal wall. A separate stab incision is made in the right iliac fossa, artery forceps inserted and the caecostomy catheter withdrawn through this, separate from the main wound. A skin suture is then used to secure the catheter so that the caecum is held securely against the anterior abdominal wall.

Postoperatively, a caecostomy tends to block with faecal matter and must be flushed regularly if it is to be of any benefit. Hourly flushing with 50 mL of saline is recommended in the acute situation. After 2 weeks the tube can be removed without fear of peritoneal faecal contamination and, in the absence of a persisting distal anatomical or functional obstruction, the fistula heals within days.

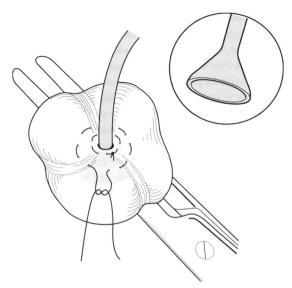

Figure 22.5 *A caecostomy still occasionally has a place in modern surgery. An amputated de Pezzer catheter is shown in the inset.*

SURGERY FOR LOWER GASTROINTESTINAL TRACT HAEMORRHAGE

Occasionally, the cause of a profuse lower gastrointestinal haemorrhage is obvious, as when the patient has severe colitis or had a haemorrhoidectomy 2 weeks previously. More often, the underlying pathology is obscure. The patient is classically middle-aged or elderly, and the most common source of the haemorrhage is either an eroded vessel at the neck of a sigmoid diverticulum or an ulcerated angiodysplastic lesion in the submucosa of the right colon. A spontaneous large haemorrhoidal bleed is another possibility. A major proximal gastrointestinal haemorrhage can also result in fresh blood at the anus, and must be excluded.

Treatment

The first priority is adequate resuscitation followed by gastroscopy to exclude upper gastrointestinal pathology. Any anti-coagulation must be reversed. Surgical intervention can usually be avoided as 90 per cent of patients with profuse lower gastrointestinal haemorrhage will stop bleeding spontaneously. The cause of the haemorrhage may never be elucidated, even after extensive investigations, but it seldom recurs.

A *colonoscopy* is of little help as the blood obscures the view. A *flexible sigmoidoscopy*, undertaken without a prior enema, can sometimes be helpful. If it passes beyond the blood to normal stool, it indicates that the bleeding is from the anus or rectum. This information has prevented the occasional inappropriate colectomy for severe haemorrhoidal bleeding.

If profuse bleeding continues and surgery seems inevitable, a preoperative angiogram should be performed to elucidate the site of the bleeding, as this often remains obscure even at laparotomy. Selective embolization of the bleeding vessel may also be possible at angiography, and surgical intervention avoided. Embolization must be precise and distal in the arterial tree, or there is an increased risk of a patch of non-viable colon developing, and rupturing several days later. Angiography will only be helpful if bleeding is occurring at a rate greater than 0.5–1.0 mL per minute. Unfortunately, although the bleeding is usually intermittently much faster than this, angiography performed between brisk bleeds will add no information.

If angiography is unavailable, or is unhelpful, the surgeon may be forced to operate without a diagnosis. Occasionally, a bleeding Meckel's diverticulum or other obvious pathology is identified, but more often there is no visible or palpable evidence of the site of bleeding. Mild diverticular disease of doubtful significance is noted, and the whole colon is full of blood. Blood in the right colon does not confirm a more proximal source of haemorrhage as it may have refluxed from the left side. The differential diagnosis is still between angiodysplastic bleeding which is more common from the right colon and diverticular bleeding from the left. A blind right or left hemi-colectomy leaves the patient at high risk of requiring a second major laparotomy within 48 hours. A subtotal colectomy and ileostomy is now the recommended procedure in this situation. The risk of further haemorrhage is significantly reduced, but at the expense of a more major initial resection. A second elective laparotomy is still required to restore intestinal continuity with an ileorectal anastomosis. In the meantime, however, if there is a further haemorrhage it will be obvious whether it is from the rectum, or from the proximal gastrointestinal tract.

A transverse 'split colostomy', in which the two ends of the divided transverse colon are brought out as separate stomas with an intact skin bridge between, can occasionally be a useful diagnostic measure in a patient who has temporarily stopped bleeding but in whom the aetiology remains obscure. It will then be obvious from which side of the colon the bleeding subsequently comes. A further laparotomy for a hemi-colectomy will probably be required, but the patient will not need to lose the whole colon.

ISCHAEMIC INTESTINAL CONDITIONS

The ischaemia secondary to the external compression of mesenteric vessels from a volvulus, and the strangulation of bowel within a hernia, have already been discussed, as has the intramural ischaemia of excessive dilatation. Ischaemia can also occur secondary to a mesenteric embolus or thrombus, or as a consequence of primary vascular pathology.

- *Chronic mesenteric ischaemia* due to an atheromatous stenosis of the superior mesenteric, or other visceral, artery may be amenable to angioplasty or surgical reconstruction as discussed in Chapter 6.
- *Acute mesenteric ischaemia* presents as an intra-abdominal intestinal emergency, and the mortality is

There are anecdotal long-term successes, but it is usually an unsatisfactory solution as the rectum is invariably involved to some degree, and often deteriorates rapidly during the months following the ileorectal anastomosis.

DYSPLASIA AND CANCER

These are significant risks in a patient with long-standing pancolitis of over 10 to 20 years' duration, and surgery should be considered. Many, however, are reluctant to consider surgery, and prefer regular colonoscopic surveillance with biopsies, and will only agree to colectomy when dysplasia has been demonstrated. A proctocolectomy, with formation of an ileal pouch, may be performed as a single operation in these generally fit patients.

Total colectomy with rectal preservation

This operation may be undertaken in the emergency setting, or as an elective procedure when, as discussed above, it may be combined with a proctectomy and even a pouch reconstruction. The whole colon is mobilized. The ascending, descending and sigmoid colon are elevated on their respective retroperitoneal mesenteries. The resection is then a combination of the right, transverse and left hemicolectomies, as described in Chapter 21. This is an operation for benign disease, and the resection does not have to include a radical lymphadenectomy. The mobilization can therefore be more conservative and need not extend to the mesenteric root. The superior rectal artery may be preserved, as it is in a sigmoid colectomy for diverticular disease, and this is important if the rectal stump is to be left long. Ligation of the mesentery can be close to the bowel wall but, as this requires ligation of multiple vessels, it is usually preferable to choose a somewhat more proximal site (see Fig. 21.2, page 378). If the colectomy is for long-standing colitis with dysplasia, the danger of an occult malignancy in the colon must be considered and in this situation a more radical lymphadenectomy, with vascular ligations at the mesenteric root, is advisable.

The omentum can be left *in situ* in a total colectomy for benign disease, but it has been implicated in the frequent adhesion obstructions to which these patients are prone. For this reason some surgeons prefer to excise it. In an emergency colectomy for severe ulcerative colitis, the colon is friable and will perforate easily, and therefore no attempt should be made to enter the plane between the transverse colon and the greater omentum. The greater omentum is separated instead from the greater curve of the stomach between ligatures, and removed en bloc with the colon.

The superior rectal artery is preserved and this enables the rectal stump to be left long. This is advantageous as an intraperitoneal closed rectal stump with severe disease may perforate, and it is safer to bring it out as a mucous fistula. An alternative is to attach the fascia at the lower end of the midline wound around the closed stump (Fig. 22.6) and

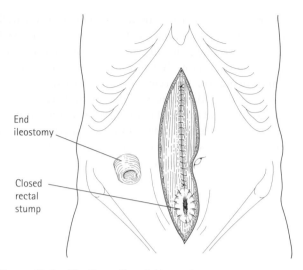

Figure 22.6 *The linea alba of this midline wound has been closed, except for the distal few centimetres, where the edges of the fascia have been sewn around the closed rectal stump. The skin directly over the stump is left open.*

leave the overlying skin open. This will heal over rapidly if the stump closure remains secure, avoiding the long-term inconvenience of a mucous fistula. However, if the stump blows, a mucous fistula should form without peritoneal contamination.

The terminal ileostomy is fashioned as described in Chapter 21.

Proctectomy

When a proctectomy is an extension of a total colectomy, the dissection planes around the mobilized sigmoid colon lead naturally into the plane around the mesorectum. Similar conditions prevail when a long rectal stump has been left under the abdominal wound, at an earlier total colectomy. Planes can be more difficult to define when a short rectal stump has been left deep in the pelvis. The operation to excise the rectum for rectal cancer is described in Chapter 21. When pelvic surgery is undertaken for benign disease there is considerable emphasis on preservation of the pelvic autonomic nerves. Many surgeons therefore favour a *close rectal dissection*, as the dissection will be kept well away from the nerves. This consists of excision of the rectum, leaving the mesorectum mainly *in situ*. Additional advantages include a smaller pelvic dead space into which small bowel may prolapse, and a supporting surround of fat for the pouch. Multiple ligations of mesorectal vessels on the rectal wall are required, and the access deep in the pelvis becomes progressively more difficult as the mesorectum is still filling the pelvis and tethering the remaining rectum into the hollow of the sacrum. Other surgeons therefore prefer to follow the same precise anatomical plane around the mesorectum that they would use for an anterior resection, carefully identifying and preserving the nerves. During the final dissection, however, they cone in through the distal mesorectum to reduce the risk of injury to the autonomic nerves. The dissection is more anatomically elegant with less bleeding, and, if there should be an unsuspected rectal cancer associated with the colitis, oncological clearance is more likely to have been achieved.

The dissection at the anus varies as to whether a pouch is planned, and whether a pouch-anal anastomosis is to be hand-sutured, or performed with a circular stapling device. In all situations, however, all columnar epithelium must be excised to eradicate the disease.

If the patient is to have a *permanent ileostomy*, the final dissection is completed from the perineum by dissection in the intersphincteric plane which is developed from the anal verge and followed proximally to join the pelvic dissection (see Chapter 23). The rectum and anus are removed but, in contrast to the abdominoperineal excision described in Chapter 21, there is no cuff of external sphincter, or ischiorectal fat, attached to the bowel, and there is no perineal wound.

When a pouch is planned with a *stapled anastomosis to the anus*, the final dissection for the proctectomy is a similar technique to that described in Chapter 21 for a very low anterior resection, but with the modifications already discussed above. It is important that a cuff of columnar epithelium is not left *in situ* as it may result in persistent inflammation, poor pouch function, and a continuing risk of malignant change. Transection of the anal canal, followed by a circular stapled anastomosis will result in a staple line at the dentate line and the final cuff of transitional mucosa will have been excised as the distal 'doughnut'. The final deep dissection to achieve this is technically difficult, especially in an obese male patient. A close rectal dissection technique may make access even more difficult. In addition, these very low stapled anastomoses are associated with the inevitable excision of the proximal part of the internal sphincter (see Chapter 23) which may prove crucial for the passive continence of the semi-liquid pouch effluent. For both these reasons some surgeons prefer a mucosectomy followed by a sutured pouch-anal anastomosis.

When a pouch is planned with a *hand-sutured anastomosis to the anus*, the rectum is divided several centimetres above the dentate line. The anorectal stump is retained, but is then denuded of all columnar epithelium. The surgeon, working from the perineum, inserts an anal retractor and injects 1:200 000 adrenaline submucosally to lift the mucosa off the muscle wall. The mucosa is then excised from just above the dentate line up to the rectal division. In severe colitis the mucosa is friable and haemorrhagic and will have to be excised in strips. It is very important to leave none behind and to obtain complete haemostasis.

Ileal pouch

The terminal loop of ileum is inspected for suitability, and in particular the apex of the loop must be able to reach to the

anus without tension. A J-pouch, formed by folding back the terminal ileum on itself, is the simplest. An anastomosis is formed between the two limbs of the loop, each of which should be between 15 and 20 cm in length. Thus, 30–40 cm of terminal ileum is needed for the pouch. The pouch can be constructed very simply with a mechanical stapling device introduced through a small enterotomy at the apex of the loop (Fig. 22.7a). Stay sutures to support the ileum are helpful, and a finger swept between the blades of the stapler, before it is closed, rotates the mesentery out of the staple line. A double firing of the GIA 80 stapler is necessary (Fig. 22.7b). Some surgeons prefer a hand-sewn pouch, although there appears to be little advantage and it is more time-consuming. A variety of different pouches have been tried, and hand-sutured W- and S-pouches were briefly popular, but have been largely abandoned as their function was inferior. The S-pouch in particular was associated with evacuatory difficulties.

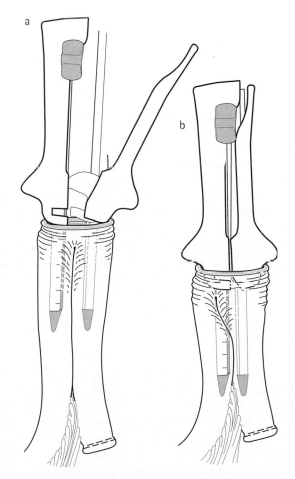

Figure 22.7 *Formation of an ileal pouch. (a) The blades of the stapler are introduced through an enterotomy at the apex of the ileal loop. One blade is inserted into each limb of the bowel, the two blades are locked together, the mesentery is rotated out of the line of the staples and the device closed and fired. (b) The stapler is reloaded, introduced into the pouch and then on into the remaining separate limbs. A second or third firing completes the pouch.*

Stapled ileal pouch–anal anastomoses

These are performed in a similar fashion to the coloanal anastomosis described in the section on anterior resection of the rectum in Chapter 21.

Hand-sutured ileal pouch–anal anastomoses

These are fashioned per-anally, after a mucosectomy. The orientation of the pouch is decided from above, and any rotation of the afferent ileum must be avoided. A suture is then passed through the distal opening of the pouch at the 3 o'clock position, and the needle passed through the pelvis to the perineal operator. This procedure is then repeated at the 9 o'clock position. The pouch is now guided down into the pelvis, and the surgeon passes the needles through the anal mucosa at the lower edge of the mucosectomy in the 3 and 9 o'clock positions. As these two sutures are ligated the pouch is fixed to the anus in the correct orientation, and lies within the internal and external sphincters. A small bite of internal sphincter should be included to avoid the suture tearing through the mucosa. The perineal operator then hand-sews the whole circumference of the pouch opening to the dentate line, using fine interrupted absorbable sutures. Access for per-anal surgery is always limited, and care must be exercised in anal retraction as excessive dilation will stretch or disrupt the sphincters.

Surgery for pouch complications

Ileoanal pouches are not trouble-free, and by 10 years about 20 per cent have either been removed, or have been defunctioned. Revision pouch surgery is often disappointing, but better results are obtained by referral to surgeons with a special interest in this work. A pouch may have to be revised if there are repeated episodes of inlet or outlet obstruction, or surgery may be undertaken for fistulous complications.[8] Pouch advancement may be performed from below for an outlet obstruction, but any more major pouch revision will require a pelvic dissection from above. The most feared complication is a fistula, which often means that the pouch is doomed. A fistula may occur during the immediate postoperative period in association with pelvic sepsis, but it may also occur years later in an otherwise trouble-free pouch. It is almost inevitable eventually if a pouch is constructed for Crohn's disease or an intermediate colitis. A fistula into the bladder or other intra-abdominal organ is repaired from above, and this is also the approach for the extrasphincteric fistula to the perineum. The more common intersphincteric and trans-sphincteric fistulae are also difficult to treat when associated with a pouch. Scarring from previous surgery makes any flap advancement technique less attractive, and the already precarious continence in these patients may be lost by any sphincter sacrifice. A drainage seton may be all that is wise, but a repair may have to be attempted for a symptomatic pouch vaginal fistula (see Chapter 23). Often, the pouch must be defunctioned again with a loop ileostomy while further attempts at pouch salvage are attempted. The

original histology should be reviewed, and if there were any features of Crohn's disease then further efforts to save the pouch will most likely prove futile.

A pouch may have to be excised for poor function, fistulous complications or intractable pouchitis. The latter is more common in pouches created for inflammatory bowel disease than in those for polyposis. The excision of a pouch is along similar lines to a proctectomy, but planes may be difficult to follow. If a replacement pouch has to be fashioned, a further 30–50 cm of small bowel has to be sacrificed. Occasionally, this will be contraindicated if it will leave inadequate small bowel length for absorption.

Crohn's disease

In contrast to ulcerative colitis, Crohn's disease can affect the gastrointestinal tract from the mouth to the anus, and therefore surgery can never guarantee its eradication. However, in those patients with localized pathology, excision of all symptomatic disease may provide long-term benefits. The involvement is classically patchy, with segments of inflamed bowel separated by lengths of normal bowel. The inflammation is transmural and, in addition to the mucosal ulceration and haemorrhage which is also seen in ulcerative colitis, deeper oedema or scarring can obstruct the bowel lumen. The inflamed serosal surface of an involved segment may also adhere to an adjacent organ with subsequent fistulation.

COLONIC CROHN'S DISEASE

This condition may present with very similar features to ulcerative colitis. A proctocolectomy can be indicated as an emergency in a fulminant case, or as an elective procedure when medical treatment fails to control symptoms. The long-term cancer risk was believed to be less than in ulcerative colitis, but is now understood to be similar. An ileoanal pouch carries an unacceptable risk of fistulous complications and should, in general, be avoided. Total proctocolectomy with a terminal ileostomy is the preferred option if the rectum or anus is also involved. A colectomy and ileorectal anastomosis may be a satisfactory alternative in Crohn's colitis with rectal sparing.

A defunctioning loop ileostomy can be an excellent temporary measure in severe Crohn's colitis. Intensive medical treatment is continued, and if remission is achieved then the ileostomy can be closed. In practice this is seldom recommended, as relapse is almost inevitable, but the patient has the opportunity to experience life with a temporary stoma before making a final decision regarding proctocolectomy.

TERMINAL ILEAL CROHN'S DISEASE

This is the most common form of the disease, and resection by a limited right hemi-colectomy may be preferable to long-term medical management with steroids and immunosuppression. This is particularly the situation in the adolescent in whom growth and development into adult life is stunted by postponing what is often inevitable surgery. There may be no evidence of other areas of gastrointestinal Crohn's disease, and 60 per cent of patients will have no further trouble. Even those who do develop further active disease may have several symptom-free years. Cessation of smoking and the continuation of treatment with mesalazine reduces the incidences of further problems, but there is now some evidence that surgical technique may also be important (see below).

Terminal ileal Crohn's disease coexistent with appendicitis is occasionally a difficult operative dilemma. An inflamed appendix with a normal caecum can be treated with a simple appendicectomy, whereas an inflamed appendix secondary to Crohn's inflammation of the caecal pole will require a right hemi-colectomy. More difficult to assess is the non-inflamed appendix and the surprise finding of a thickened inflamed terminal ileum, which although probably Crohn's disease could be a *Yersinia* ileitis, or a lymphoma. The presence of 'fat wrapping' supports a clinical diagnosis of Crohn's disease as it is not a feature of lymphoma or the acute ileitis of *Yersinia*.

A right hemi-colectomy for terminal ileal Crohn's disease is a more limited resection than that for a caecal cancer described in Chapter 21, as no lymphadenectomy is necessary. However, any loops of small bowel adherent to the inflammatory mass must also be excised. The terminal ileal involvement normally ends at the ileocaecal valve, and the aim of surgery is to remove only the diseased segment as recurrence proximal to the anastomosis is not prevented by a more radical excision of normal adjacent ileum. The method of anastomosis does however appear to influence recurrent disease, and a wide side-to-side stapled anastomosis may be preferable to the traditional sutured end-to-end anastomosis. It is uncertain whether the benefit is related to the width of the anastomosis and the avoidance of any hold-up, or whether staples are less irritant than sutures. Certainly, any sutured anastomosis in Crohn's disease should be created with absorbable sutures, and silk in particular should be avoided.

CROHN'S OBSTRUCTION

This may result from inflammatory oedema during an acute exacerbation. Clinical decisions are not easy, as the full-thickness inflammation inevitably produces localized signs of peritonism, and the exclusion of a strangulated loop is difficult. Surgery can usually be avoided: the obstruction is treated conservatively and the exacerbation of Crohn's inflammation managed with steroids. Chronic fibrous strictures causing partial obstruction of either the small or large bowel are better managed by limited resection, but consideration must be given both to preservation of adequate lengths of small bowel (see Chapter 11) and the inadvisability of performing an anastomosis with diseased bowel. Multiple small bowel strictures can sometimes be successfully managed by stricturoplasties, but endoscopic dilatation of these strictures is now another option.

CROHN'S FISTULAE

These may occur into another loop of bowel, or into the bladder or to the skin. Treatment is by resection of the fistula and repair through healthy tissue, if possible. The diversion of faecal contents may sometimes be the only practical surgical option.

CROHN'S DISEASE OF THE ANUS

This condition is discussed in Chapter 23.

SURGERY FOR INTESTINAL INFECTIONS AND INFESTATIONS

The treatment of all these conditions is medical, and surgery is only indicated for complications such as haemorrhage, obstruction or perforation. Often, however, the diagnosis has not been suspected preoperatively. Frequently, an ischaemic loop of bowel has been suspected, but at laparotomy the peritonism is found to be from the inflammatory process involving the peritoneum. No surgical intervention is indicated if there is no bowel loop, the integrity of which is in danger. The abdomen is closed, and appropriate medical treatment commenced. When there is no firm diagnosis the patient is in danger of inappropriately radical surgery. This may be inevitable, especially if malignancy is suspected, but the surgeon must always consider the possibility of infective pathology. On other occasions, there may be a preoperative diagnosis, but a complication of the infection requires surgical intervention.

Ascaris obstruction was discussed earlier in the chapter (see page 412).

Abdominal tuberculosis may cause obstruction either from a 'plastic peritonitis' or a mass of tuberculous glands to which bowel is adherent.[9] A side-to-side bypass is the most appropriate operative solution.

Amoebiasis can cause a toxic dilatation similar to that seen in ulcerative colitis. It can also produce a local inflammatory mass, or *amoeboma*, in the caecum and this can mimic a caecal malignancy. If a diagnosis of amoebiasis has been made, surgical resection is only indicated for a complication such as obstruction, perforation or toxic dilatation. These complications should be avoidable, unless the diagnosis and appropriate medical treatment have been delayed.

Typhoid ulcers form over the affected small bowel lymphatic tissue (Peyer's patches) during the third week of untreated typhoid fever. Intraluminal haemorrhage, a walled-off perforation with an associated intraperitoneal abscess, and free perforation with generalized peritonitis may all occur. Controversy persists with regard to the optimal management of a typhoid perforation. Simple over-sewing is recommended by some surgeons, and a resection by others.[10] It is probable that both approaches have their place, and the decision must be based on individual factors at the time of surgery.

Cytomegalovirus infection usually occurs in immuno-compromised patients, and may produce an acute inflammatory lesion which can bleed, perforate or obstruct. The commonest site is in the descending colon, just below the splenic flexure. Treatment is medical, unless a surgical complication ensues.

Pigbel is a necrotizing jejunitis, the underlying pathology of which is *Clostridium perfringens*. Treatment of mild cases is with antibiotics and fluid resuscitation but, when more severe, a laparotomy and resection of the necrotic bowel becomes unavoidable.

Yersinia causes an acute terminal ileitis which may be difficult to differentiate from the terminal ileitis of Crohn's disease. The short history, and the absence of the classical fat wrapping of Crohn's disease, may alert the surgeon to the correct diagnosis.

SURGERY FOR DIVERTICULAR DISEASE

Diverticulosis of the left colon is a common incidental finding on a barium enema. Diverticula are small and multiple, and occur predominantly in the sigmoid colon, although they may extend more proximally. Surgery is only indicated for those patients who develop complications of diverticular disease, or for those who have chronic symptoms of pain and disturbed bowel function. The symptoms and complications of diverticular disease are almost entirely confined to the sigmoid colon, and only the sigmoid colon need be excised, even when the diverticular process is extensive.

Elective resection

An elective resection may be undertaken for repeated attacks of diverticulitis, for a diverticular stricture, or for chronic low-grade symptoms. A *sigmoid colectomy* is the standard operation in the elective setting, and this was described in Chapter 21. For an open operation, a left iliac fossa muscle-cutting incision provides adequate access for a sigmoid colectomy, but it cannot be extended upwards as easily as a midline incision if more extensive access becomes necessary. The level of the proximal resection is chosen so that the colon reaches easily to the top of the rectum for an anastomosis. It should be above any narrow thickened sigmoid, but it does not need to be above all diverticula. A division at the level of the proximal sigmoid, or lower descending, colon is usually suitable. The superior rectal artery can be preserved and the sigmoid branches divided, as a radical lymphadenectomy is not necessary for benign disease. The distal resection is at the level where the taeniae have spread to form a continuous muscle coat (Fig. 22.8). Division at a more proximal level results in a high incidence of recurrent problems. A hand-sewn anastomosis just below the pelvic

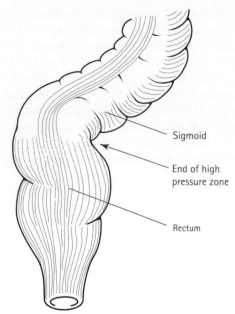

Figure 22.8 *The anastomosis after a sigmoid colectomy for diverticular disease must be to rectum distal to the high-pressure zone of the rectosigmoid junction. The surgical landmark is the spreading of the taeniae to form a continuous longitudinal muscle coat.*

brim is often easier than a stapled one, as the instrument may not pass easily up through the folds of the non-mobilized rectum. If the anastomosis is deeper into the pelvis a stapled anastomosis will be easier.

Unfortunately, even in the elective situation this classical sigmoid colectomy may not be possible. A shortened, thickened sigmoid colon and mesentery may make preservation of the superior rectal artery impossible, and the descending colon may not reach for a tension-free anastomosis without full mobilization of the splenic flexure. Occasionally, the proximal diverticula are so extensive that there is no suitable distal descending colon free of diverticula for a safe anastomosis, and a more proximal level for the transection becomes inevitable. The surgeon must therefore be prepared to carry out a left hemi-colectomy rather than a sigmoid colectomy if this is more appropriate.

Many surgeons prefer a left hemi-colectomy as their standard procedure for sigmoid diverticular disease, and argue that, in addition to avoiding the problems already discussed, it is a more anatomical dissection. Moreover, it is also oncologically sound if an unsuspected cancer is present within the diverticular segment. A more radical removal of diverticula may also improve the long-term outcome of surgery. In addition, straightening of the colon makes any subsequent endoscopic imaging less difficult. Unfortunately, it is also a more major procedure, requires the incision to be extended higher with a greater risk of postoperative respiratory complications, and splenic flexure mobilization may result in loss of the spleen as a result of iatrogenic trauma.

The dissection may also have to be carried down into the pelvis if the sigmoid loop is folded over and adherent. Dense adherence to the front of the rectum is best managed by converting the operation into an anterior resection. Dense adhesions to the bladder, uterus or vaginal vault can be pinched off by blunt dissection. If there is a fistulous opening into the dome of the bladder, or into the vagina, it is repaired. For both organs dissolvable sutures are mandatory and, as both are very vascular, a continuous haemostatic suture is to be recommended. It is advantageous to position the patient in the 'legs-up' position in anticipation of these problems, as it allows an assistant to retract from between the legs during any pelvic dissection. In addition, the anus is exposed should a stapled anastomosis prove preferable.

Urgent surgery

A more urgent operation may be necessary for an attack of acute diverticulitis which fails to resolve on medical treatment. Occasionally, surgery can be deferred if image-guided drainage of a pericolic abscess can be performed, after which the antibiotics are effective in treating the remaining infection. Surgery also has to be expedited in those patients who develop a frank colovaginal fistula or colovesical fistula. The operative conditions are worse during an active episode of inflammation than in the elective situation. The bowel is often partially obstructed, and certainly unprepared, and there is more likely to be doubt whether the underlying pathology is cancer or diverticular disease. The tissues are inflamed, friable with inflammation, and a pericolic abscess is common. The resection is similar to the elective case, but it may be technically more difficult. An anastomosis to restore continuity can usually be recommended, but consideration should be given to the advisability of a temporary proximal loop stoma to protect it.

EMERGENCY SURGERY

This will be necessary if there is generalized purulent peritonitis from the rupture of a pericolic abscess, or a faeculent peritonitis from the rupture of the inflamed sigmoid colon. Less commonly, emergency surgery is necessary for a diverticular obstruction, or haemorrhage, both of which can occur in the absence of an acute inflammatory episode. The surgery of these latter two complications has been discussed earlier in the chapter.

Emergency surgery for perforated diverticular disease carries a high mortality. Despite the poor condition of many of these patients when they come to surgery, a resection should be performed as simple drainage, combined with a defunctioning proximal stoma, has generally been shown to be associated with a worse outcome. Unless there is gross faecal soiling of the peritoneum, or the patient is so unwell that the operation cannot be safely prolonged, an anastomosis (after on-table lavage) is recommended. A temporary proximal stoma, however, is usually advisable. A loop stoma can be closed at a minor second operation, but after a Hartmann's procedure a major laparotomy is required to restore intestinal continuity.

When an anastomosis is contraindicated, a Hartmann's procedure is undertaken. The rectal stump is closed and marked with a nylon suture to make subsequent identification easier, and the proximal bowel end is brought out as an end stoma. Some surgeons recommend dividing the lower end more proximally, so that it can be brought out at the lower end of the wound as a mucous fistula to make the subsequent dissection for a rejoin easier. However, this is seldom a satisfactory solution, even when it is technically possible. A segment of distal sigmoid colon affected by diverticular disease has been retained, and must be resected at the subsequent operation before bowel continuity can be restored. In addition, if the inferior mesenteric artery has been ligated this distal colon brought out as a mucous fistula may be ischaemic.

A relatively mild diverticulitis is occasionally encountered at operation for a suspected appendicitis. The decision whether to proceed to a resection or to close the abdomen, with or without a left iliac fossa drain, and treat conservatively will depend on circumstances. These decisions were discussed in Chapter 14.

Differential diagnosis of sigmoid diverticular disease and sigmoid malignancy

Unfortunately, even at the start of an elective operation, preoperative endoscopy, barium studies and sophisticated imaging may have failed to elucidate whether the sigmoid pathology is diverticular disease or a cancer. Confirmation of the diagnosis by preoperative endoscopic biopsy is often frustrated by the angulation and fixity of the sigmoid loop. Paediatric scopes and brush biopsy techniques will shed further light in some patients, but these are not always successful. Today, CT and MRI scans now provide preoperative evidence of the 'invasion' of other organs, but they cannot differentiate between tumour invasion and the inflammatory involvement of adjacent tissue. If doubt remains after the abdomen is opened, and a sigmoid mass adherent to other organs is encountered, the surgery must be radical to prevent rupture into tumour planes. This requires not only a radical lymphadenectomy but also excision of the adherent disc of any other organ into which invasion is suspected. When this can only be achieved by an extended radical dissection, it is immediately apparent how important it was to have made every effort to differentiate between the two pathologies preoperatively. The difficulties in differentiating tumour adhesions from inflammatory adhesions, and in differentiating a diverticular mass from a sigmoid cancer at operation fall into several categories:

- *Desmoplastic or malignant adhesions.* An obvious cancer may be apparent which is adherent to surrounding structures. These adhesions may be malignant or a desmoplastic inflammatory reaction around the tumour. They cannot be distinguished clinically, and excision must include all such adhesions, with the assumption that they may contain viable tumour cells.

- *Inflammatory or malignant mass.* A mass may be encountered which is adherent to surrounding structures, but without any visible tumour. A diverticular inflammatory process is strongly suspected but cannot be proved and, in fear of performing an inadequate excision of a malignancy, a radical excision is undertaken. This may lead to the unnecessary sacrifice or damage to important structures.
- *Dual pathology.* A sigmoid diverticular mass may have within it a small unsuspected neoplasm as an incidental second pathology. The surrounding adhesions are inflammatory, but if a sigmoid colectomy without a high ligation of the inferior mesenteric vessels has been performed the lymphadenectomy may be inadequate.
- *Local perforation of a malignancy.* An inflammatory mass with surrounding inflammatory adhesions may be secondary to a ruptured malignancy. These adhesions will appear inflammatory in the acute phase and fibrous at a later stage, but they will also contain malignant cells. Unless a radical excision, including all adherent tissue, is undertaken, the tumour planes will be entered and local recurrence is almost inevitable. Tumour dissemination, however, usually will have already occurred at the time of the original tumour perforation, and the surgeon is unlikely to be able to offer the patient a cure.

Solitary giant diverticulum

This may occur anywhere throughout the colon, and excision is usually indicated. A caecal diverticulum with an inflammatory mass around it can mimic a caecal carcinoma. However, difficulties in differentiating a caecal inflammatory mass from a caecal malignancy are uncommon compared with the diagnostic difficulties in the sigmoid colon.

SURGERY FOR BOWEL CANCER

The principles of surgery for intra-abdominal malignancies are discussed in Chapter 15, and the standard radical large bowel resections are described in Chapter 21. However, the choice of operative management in large bowel cancer is not always straightforward, and some of the operative dilemmas are worth considering. Presentation as a surgical emergency, and with obstruction, has already been discussed in the relevant sections. The common problem of differentiation from sigmoid diverticular disease is discussed in the preceding section.

Locally advanced rectal cancer

Injudicious attempts to excise a locally advanced tumour may be counterproductive as tumour planes are entered, and

it is therefore important to assess all rectal tumours carefully preoperatively. A mid or low rectal tumour can be assessed fairly accurately by digital palpation for invasion into the sphincters, the prostate or the vagina, or for fixation to the pelvic side walls. Endo-anal ultrasound and MRI images provide superior information on the depth of invasion, and MRI in particular can also provide valuable information on tumours beyond the reach of the finger. In the light of all this information, the surgeon must then decide whether the surgical margins of excision will be adequate (Fig. 22.9). For those patients in whom the planes of excision are invaded, the options available include preoperative radiotherapy,

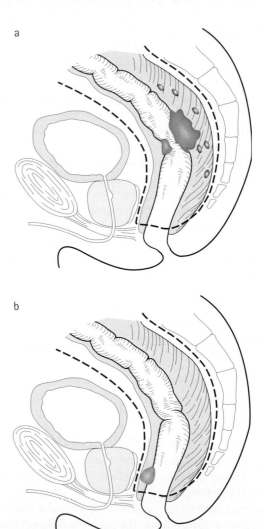

Figure 22.9 *Staging of rectal cancer by MRI scanning is valuable for showing the relationship of the tumour to the planes for excision. (a) A large tumour, which is invading for several centimetres into the posterior mesorectum. There are enlarged nodes which probably contain metastases. (b) A smaller, earlier tumour which extends only a few millimetres into the thin anterior mesorectum. There is no evidence of nodal involvement. Despite the more advanced staging of the tumour in (a) compared to the tumour in (b), the excision margin, shown as a dotted line, is well clear of tumour in (a) but very close in (b).*

chemotherapy or chemoradiotherapy to shrink the tumour, followed by a standard or extended resection, or palliative non-resectional local treatment. In addition, the presence of liver metastases, and their potential operability, should be established as this will influence operative management of the primary lesion.

PREOPERATIVE RADIOTHERAPY OR CHEMOTHERAPY

- *Radiotherapy with delay.* A long course of 45–50 Gy over 6 weeks will shrink and 'down-stage' an advanced tumour, and thus makes many fixed tumours resectable. A delay of 8 weeks after completion of the radiotherapy allows for maximum shrinkage of the tumour. Radiotherapy also kills the cells at the periphery of the remaining tumour mass, and reduces the likelihood of implantation of viable tumour cells in the event of the dissection entering a 'tumour plane'.
- *Chemoradiotherapy* sensitizes the tumour to the effects of radiotherapy and an enhanced response is achieved, but at the expense of a higher incidence of anastomotic breakdown and poorer final bowel function.
- *Chemotherapy* alone may be employed when there is also evidence of distant metastases. A dramatic response of both the primary and the liver secondaries can occasionally convert the situation into one which is potentially curable by surgery.
- *Short-course radiotherapy without delay*: a short, 5-day course of a total of 25 Gy radiotherapy immediately preoperatively may also 'sterilize' the tumour periphery, but no tumour shrinkage or down-staging is achieved with this regime. Increasingly, this approach is employed routinely to reduce the incidence of local recurrence, but late morbidity from short-course radiotherapy may be even higher than with the standard long-course regime. Many surgeons who have low rates of local recurrence therefore prefer to use radiotherapy selectively only in those patients in whom the tumour will be close to the excision margins.[11]

When a long course of radiotherapy is planned, a defunctioning stoma is often beneficial as local symptoms may intensify during treatment. This can be combined with a 'fold-down' technique to prevent loops of small bowel migrating into the pelvis and into the field of radiation. At laparotomy the sigmoid is divided so that the proximal sigmoid is brought out as a terminal colostomy, and the distal sigmoid is closed. The distal bowel is then allowed to fold back into the pelvis over the tumour and secured in this position with sutures. Some division of the sigmoid mesentery will be required before the distal end will fold into the pelvis. Great care must be taken not to traverse the lymphatic drainage of the tumour during this manoeuvre. Tissue diagnosis is essential before radiotherapy, and if this has not been successfully obtained preoperatively, Trucut biopsies can be taken from the depths of the mass *transluminally* from above after division of the bowel.

PELVIC EXENTERATION AND SACRECTOMY

Radiotherapy for an inoperable rectal primary tumour, or for a pelvic recurrence after surgery, may offer good short-term palliation. This can be invaluable in a patient with significant distant metastases and limited survival. Although good long-term control and occasional complete tumour response is possible, the results in general are inferior to those after surgery. In patients without obvious distant metastases and a longer life expectancy, local control, which is only temporary, has less to offer.

Recurrent symptoms associated with fistulae, and invasion of pelvic nerves, are very difficult to control. Radical and mutilating resections of advanced pelvic disease are therefore sometimes justified if the local tumour can be removed completely, and there is no evidence of distant spread. Anteriorly, the excision can include the bladder and prostate or, in a woman, the vagina, uterus and bladder. An end colostomy and urinary diversion, most commonly with an ileal conduit will then be required (see Chapter 25). Posterolaterally, the excision plane can be outside the autonomic nerves, which are intentionally sacrificed. In selected patients with posterior bony invasion, a portion of the sacrum can be excised with the specimen. Excision above S3 destabilizes the pelvic ring, but this is occasionally justified. The sacrectomy, and the mobilization of the tumour from below to remove it en bloc with the sacrum, is performed with the patient in a prone jack-knife position. Abdominal access is required for the mobilization from above, and for the urinary diversion. The patient must either be turned during surgery, or the procedure performed as two separate operations, with the abdominal phase being undertaken the day before the final excision of the tumour through the perineum.[12] This surgery should be performed only at centres with special expertise, or the results will be disappointing.

LOCAL PALLIATION

Excision of the primary tumour may still offer the best palliation in a fit patient with a resectable tumour and a small metastatic load. Radiotherapy has an important role in symptom control, and an end colostomy to divert the faecal stream away from a malignant fistula which has formed into bladder or vagina may relieve distressing symptoms. If the tumour is obstructing, a loop colostomy, rather than an end colostomy, is required, or the closed obstructed rectal stump may 'blow'. Intraluminal stents can be used to relieve an obstruction and may provide a better quality of life than a stoma. They are only a satisfactory solution for tumours above the mid rectum, as a lower stent increases local symptoms. Endoscopic debulking of a rectal cancer may decrease the discharge of blood and mucus, and reduce tenesmus. In addition to thermal ablative procedures, the malignant tissue can be resected via a cystoscope. A locally advanced tumour may obstruct the ureters and cause uraemia. Ureteric stents should be used selectively as it may not be in the patient's best interests to prevent a uraemic death when they are already terminally ill and have severe local symptoms from fistulae, nerve invasion or pelvic venous obstruction.

Local excision of superficial cancer

A small cancer confined to the mucosa and submucosa (T1) can often be easily removed by a local excision. This may already have been done at the stage when a cancer is identified histologically in a polyp snared at colonoscopy, or when a villous lesion excised per anum is shown to contain an early invasive malignancy. Malignant invasion of the submucosa, either beneath a flat lesion or beneath the stalk of a polyp, carries a risk of lymph node metastases of 5–10 per cent. The decision whether or not to recommend a major resection is difficult. T1 lesions which are poorly differentiated, or invade deeply into the submucosa (Japanese Sm 3), carry a higher risk of node involvement than Sm I well-differentiated tumours. MRI scans may identify nodes, but enlarged nodes may be reactive and normal small nodes may have microscopic deposits. The patient should be involved in the decision, and his or her age and fitness should also influence the decision reached, as the potential benefit of a more extensive resection must be balanced against operative mortality and morbidity.

On other occasions a decision is taken to excise a superficial rectal cancer per anum as a planned procedure. The same reservations regarding possible lymph node metastases remain unresolved. Endoluminal ultrasound and MRI scans are useful in this setting for estimating the depth of invasion, but they tend to overstage tumours, and their accuracy in detection or exclusion of small nodal metastases is poor. Deeper T2, and even T3, lesions may also be fully excised locally from below. The risk of involved nodes is higher, but a local excision is justified in patients in whom the risk of death from major surgery outweighs the risk of recurrence from undetected nodal deposits. Perineal and transanal operations, both conventional and with the *transanal endoscopic microsurgical* (TEM) technique, are considered in more detail in Chapter 23.

Multiple cancers and unstable mucosa

Synchronous and metachronous tumours should be treated on their merits, with each tumour receiving a radical excision. Most surgeons are prepared to leave the remaining colon *in situ* but insist on regular colonoscopic surveillance. A similar principle governs the treatment of a cancer in a patient who has additional polyps. An argument for a total colectomy and ileorectal anastomosis or even for a total proctocolectomy can be made especially in a young patient.

Patients with ulcerative colitis who develop a cancer should usually be considered for a total proctocolectomy which includes a radical lymphadenectomy of the segment of mesentery draining the tumour. Cancers in this condition arise more frequently from flat areas of dysplastic mucosa,

and regular surveillance is less satisfactory in identifying and removing further pre-cancerous lesions. The surgeon, however, will wish to avoid needless radical surgery, the difficulties of a permanent stoma or the uncertainties of a pouch when there are fears that a patient may have a limited life expectancy from a relatively advanced index tumour. A decision may therefore be made to limit the initial surgery to the treatment of the malignancy, and to accept that if the patient remains free of recurrence a second operation will then have to be considered.

Familial adenomatous polyposis (FAP)

Patients with this and other related genetic predispositions to colonic polyps and cancer should be managed according to the protocols of the specialist centres, if referral to such a centre for surveillance and surgery is impractical. Patients with FAP are also at risk of upper gastrointestinal polyps and malignancies, and intra-abdominal desmoid tumours. The polyps in patients with FAP are too numerous for their total endoscopic removal to be a practical long-term solution. The diagnosis is usually possible around puberty, and at this stage a total colectomy and ileorectal anastomosis is the best compromise in these asymptomatic patients who are understandably reluctant to accept a proctectomy. In addition, the formation of a pouch decreases fertility in female patients with both ulcerative colitis and FAP, and should be postponed until childbearing is complete.[13] Regular surveillance of the rectum and the removal of all rectal polyps is continued through adolescence and early adult life. A proctectomy, with ileostomy or an ileoanal pouch, should however be considered by the fourth or fifth decade of life, as even with regular surveillance almost 30 per cent will develop rectal cancer by the age of 60 years.

POSTOPERATIVE ANASTOMOTIC LEAKS AND FISTULAE

The management of leaks depends on whether they are early or late, whether they are from large or small bowel, and whether there is generalized peritoneal soiling, a localized collection or fistulation.

GENERALIZED PERITONITIS

An anastomotic leak which presents as a generalized peritonitis will require a laparotomy. The peritoneal cavity is cleared of small bowel contents or faeculent material. A simple repair of a defect is seldom practical as the tissues are friable and oedematous. Gastric and duodenal anastomotic leaks may sometimes be managed by over-sewing of the defect and diversional bypass. Other solutions include a more radical resection and re-anastomosis, or the use of a Roux loop brought up as the drainage conduit of an internal fistula. In an ileal or ileocolic anastomosis the safest management is to bring out an ileostomy with the proximal end. The distal end can be closed or brought out as a mucous fistula adjacent to the ileostomy. The latter is safer, and also makes the subsequent operation to restore intestinal continuity simpler. A leaking jejunal anastomosis is not so suitable for this management as the stoma will have a very high output. The situation may be better managed by resection and re-anastomosis. In colonic leaks, if the anastomosis is above the peritoneal reflection, the safest manoeuvre is to disrupt the anastomosis fully and bring out the proximal end as an end stoma. The distal end is safest if brought out as a mucous fistula, and if this is adjacent to the proximal stoma subsequent surgery to restore gastrointestinal continuity is less complex. Unfortunately, the distal end often has insufficient mobility to make this possible and instead it must be closed and returned to the peritoneal cavity. It is safer to wash out a closed colonic stump which is to be left *in situ*.

PELVIC PERITONITIS

Pelvic peritonitis after a leak from the anastomosis following an anterior resection requires intervention, even if the peritonitis is initially confined to the pelvis. Treatment by disruption of the anastomosis and an end stoma will almost certainly condemn the patient to a permanent colostomy, as any rejoin at a very low level is difficult and function is almost invariably poor. A better alternative is to select an area of the transverse colon which is suitable for a loop colostomy. A colostomy allows an on-table wash-out of the distal colon through the anastomosis. A proctoscope is inserted and the effluent is drained from the anus; washing is continued until the distal colon is empty. The colostomy is then used to create the defunctioning loop stoma. No further faecal material should then reach the disrupted anastomosis. If the anastomosis is partially intact, healing should occur and it should be possible to close the stoma some months later. A rectal contrast study should be performed before closure to confirm healing of the anastomosis and no residual connection with a pelvic abscess. Unfortunately, the final function is still often impaired.

SEALED LEAKS

A leak may seal and present as a localized intraperitoneal or pelvic collection with an associated ileus or small bowel obstruction. Conservative management with intravenous fluids and antibiotics will often suffice, but drainage of the collection may become necessary. A localized collection of infected gastrointestinal contents, walled off within the peritoneal cavity, may track into another viscus or to the exterior via the vagina or the surgical wound. When there is still a leak from the anastomosis into the walled off collection, a fistula will have been established.

WOUND FISTULAE

A fistula usually presents initially as a simple wound infection. It then becomes apparent that intestinal contents are draining through the wound. Immediate repair is not advisable, and the initial management is the maintenance of fluid and electrolyte balance, drainage of infection, maintenance of nutrition and the protection of the abdominal skin from intestinal juices. Ultrasound scans will show whether there is an intra-abdominal collection deep to the wound and, if there is, drainage of this should be improved. If defaecation, or a more distal stoma effluent continues, there is still continuity of the gastrointestinal tract and the fistula track may close spontaneously if there is no distal obstruction. When the fistula is from the duodenum or jejunum, parenteral feeding is preferable initially if spontaneous resolution seems probable as it will reduce the fistula losses and healing is more likely. There is little advantage in restricting oral intake in cases of colonic faecal fistulae.

A *persistent fistula* will require surgical repair. The dissection of a small bowel fistula and the anastomosis will be relatively straightforward if the fistula has been allowed to mature. A mature small bowel fistula starts to prolapse, similar to an ileostomy spout, as the peritoneal cavity reforms. This will usually require a delay of around 3 months, during which time it is important that nutrition is maintained. Unless the fistula is of very high output, enteral feeding is preferable to intravenous feeding during this period. The 'neo-stoma' of a faecal colonic fistula should also be allowed to mature before further surgery is undertaken to restore intestinal continuity.

RECTOVAGINAL FISTULAE

Rectovaginal fistulae may occur after the breakdown of a pelvic anastomosis. If the bowel was not already defunctioned prophylactically, this is now necessary. The fistula is then repaired as discussed in Chapter 23.

NEONATAL BOWEL SURGERY

Neonatal gastrointestinal surgical conditions should always be managed, if at all possible, by a paediatric surgeon working within a paediatric surgical unit. A successful outcome is dependent not only on surgical technique but also on specialist anaesthetic and intensive care. Unfortunately, any general surgeon who is unable to transfer a neonatal patient and is forced by circumstance to operate will be further hampered by inadequate facilities. It is with such a surgeon in mind that the following text is written and, although the ideal operative management is outlined and can be studied further in standard texts,[14] safer compromises in difficult circumstances are also covered briefly.

INCISIONS

An upper abdominal transverse incision provides good access to the whole neonatal abdomen and pelvis, and is described in Chapter 12. The surgery of congenital abdominal wall defects is also discussed in Chapter 12.

SMALL BOWEL ATRESIA

This condition presents with neonatal obstruction or, less commonly, with a neonatal perforation and peritonitis. An intrauterine perforation, occurring some days or weeks before birth, is another variant. The anastomosis of the dilated bowel, proximal to the atresia, to the hypoplastic bowel, distal to the atresia, is technically difficult due to discrepancies of size. A useful technique is shown in Figure 22.10. Unfortunately, atresias may be associated with other failures of mid gut development, including malrotation and a short small bowel. Those babies who have had an intrauterine perforation will have matted loops of small bowel, and the necessity for a prolonged period of intravenous feeding postoperatively should be anticipated.

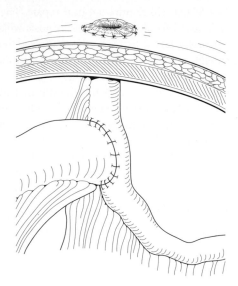

Figure 22.10 *In small-bowel atresia, an end-to-side anastomosis of the dilated proximal bowel to the distal hypoplastic bowel can be a useful manoeuvre. In this illustration it has been combined with a temporary end stoma of the distal limb (a Bishop Koop ileostomy). This stoma can protect the anastomosis if the distal segment is forming a functional obstruction. It can also be used for access to the distal bowel for treatment.*

FIBROCYSTIC DISEASE

This may present in the neonatal period with obstruction from the abnormally viscous meconium, and may initially be confused with the obstruction of an atresia. This condition of meconium ileus can usually be managed conservatively with dilute water-soluble enemata. If surgery becomes necessary, a Bishop Koop stoma (see Fig. 22.10) above the obstructed area allows postoperative pancreatin administration, or simple wash-outs, to be performed through the stoma.

NECROTIZING ENTEROCOLITIS

This condition is almost exclusively a disease of the premature neonate. Initial presentation is with general clinical deterioration and abdominal distension. Intestinal intramu-

ral gas, demonstrated on X-ray, confirms the diagnosis. Necrotizing enterocolitis is initially a mucosal disease, and at this stage conservative management, with cessation of enteral feeding and antibiotics, combined with fluid and electrolyte replacement, may be successful. Systemic complications can include endotoxic shock and disseminated intravascular coagulation, and the baby may require intensive support. The necrotic mucosa may slough and regenerate, but progression to full-thickness necrotic bowel will require a laparotomy and excision of non-viable bowel, which may already have perforated. It should be remembered when planning a resection that the mucosal disease will extend beyond the segment of bowel which appears affected from the appearance of the serosa. These premature, sick neonates, who already are frequently receiving ventilatory support, are unlikely to survive surgical intervention outside a specialist centre.

ANORECTAL ATRESIA

This condition is divided into 'high' and 'low' varieties. The abnormality is evident on examination at birth, and should be diagnosed before clinical obstruction becomes apparent. In both forms the bowel finishes as a blind end, with variable fistulous extensions forwards into the urogenital tract.

High anorectal atresia

In high anorectal atresia the bowel abnormality starts above the puborectalis sling, the pelvic floor anatomy and physiology is abnormal. Final continence, even after expert surgery, may therefore be disappointing. The fistulous track in the male is into the bladder or proximal urethra (Fig. 22.11), and in the female into the upper vagina. The high atresias require reconstruction by mobilization of the rectum from above. Any fistulous connection is ligated. The bowel is then drawn through the correct anatomical path anterior to the puborectalis sling and anastomosed to the skin of the perineum at the anal dimple. Until 25 years ago, this surgery was always

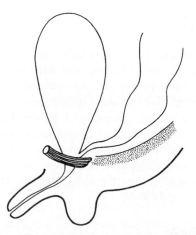

Figure 22.11 *A 'high' anorectal atresia in a male infant. The abnormality extends above the puborectalis sling, and there is an associated fistula into the bladder.*

delayed until the child was aged about 18 months and weighed at least 10 kg. The immediate neonatal problem was solved by a simple transverse defunctioning colostomy. A *split colostomy*, in which the bowel is divided and two stomas are formed, separated by a bridge of skin, was preferred. In a loop stoma there is greater potential for faecal material to be drawn down the efferent limb into the distal bowel, and thus a higher theoretical risk of recurrent urinary infections from the fistula. Recent advances in neonatal anaesthesia have made primary definitive surgery often the better option. However, any general surgeon who is unable to transfer such a neonate would be better advised to raise a stoma, and delay the more major procedure.

Low anorectal atresia

In low anorectal atresia the normal bowel extends through the puborectalis sling, and the abnormality is below this level. It may take the form of a covered anus with meconium visible beneath the thin covering, or an anal stenosis. A fistula in girls will be into the fourchette of the vagina (Fig. 22.12) and in boys the anterior extension is commonly as a track of meconium, visible under the median raphe of the scrotum. Another variety of the low anomaly is an anteriorly displaced anus. The primary surgery of the low lesions is by a perineal operation. This may only need to be an incision of a covered anus, but care must be taken not to damage the anal sphincters. Even all these apparently minor anomalies should be managed by those with a special interest, or results will be disappointing.

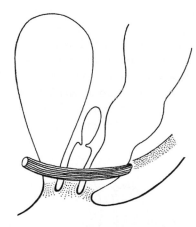

Figure 22.12 *A 'low' anorectal atresia, in a female infant. The atresia only affects the bowel beneath the puborectalis sling, and there is a fistulous opening into the fourchette.*

HIRSCHSPRUNG'S DISEASE

This disease is caused by a failure of development of the submucosal enteric ganglia. The length of the segment of affected bowel is variable, but distally it extends to the anal canal. Commonly, the rectum and sigmoid colon are both involved, but ultra-short segments extending only to the mid rectum, and cases in which the whole colon is affected, are also well recognized. Hirschsprung's disease may present either neonatally or later in infancy or childhood, with a large bowel obstruction or intractable constipation. The diagnosis is confirmed histologically by a rectal biopsy in which abnormal neural tissue and absent ganglia are demonstrated in the submucosa.

If a general surgeon has to operate on an infant presenting with a large bowel obstruction from Hirschsprung's disease, the immediate surgical management is the formation of a stoma and referral of the infant for assessment and definitive surgery. The stoma is formed in the dilated normal bowel, proximal to the non-dilated aganglionic segment which is forming a functional obstruction. A transverse colostomy is therefore usually the most appropriate stoma. Occasionally, the whole colon is aganglionic and an ileostomy will be necessary. In the very sick infant with late presentation, gangrenous enterocolitis may already have occurred in the dilated colon and a subtotal colectomy and terminal ileostomy is then the only surgical option.

Infants with very short segment Hirschsprung's disease, affecting only a few centimetres of rectum, have been managed successfully by an internal sphincterotomy, or anorectal myomectomy. Most patients, however, require a resection of the aganglionic segment, combined with restoration of continuity by a coloanal anastomosis. The small size of the neonatal anus makes a hand-sutured anastomosis per anum very difficult, and the standard stapling guns are too large. A variety of techniques for this anastomosis have been employed to overcome the difficulties in access. In adult coloproctology the application of the techniques described below is limited, but occasionally they have a place in benign disease.

Soave's anorectal pull-through

For this method, the abnormal muscle wall of the lower rectum is left in place. The deep pelvic dissection from above is taken to just above the pelvic floor, where a circular myotomy is made through the rectal wall, and the submucosal plane is entered. The dissection is then continued in the submucosal plane to the dentate line where the mucosa is divided. Normal bowel is then drawn through the denuded rectal muscle tube for a coloanal anastomosis. In the original descriptions of this technique a formal anastomosis was not attempted. The colon that had been drawn through the anus was left extruding by several centimetres. It became fixed by adhesions and finally sloughed, or was later excised. Soave's procedure has been used in adults for rectal strictures and extrasphincteric fistulae.[15] The mucosectomy may be performed either from above or below.

Swenson's operation

Here, the rectum is transected, and the rectal stump is inverted by drawing it out through the perineum by forceps introduced through the anal canal. Normal colon is drawn through the invaginated rectal stump, and the everted rectum is then excised. The anastomosis, performed just above the dentate line, is completed outside the anus and is then gently pushed back inside the sphincters (Fig. 22.13).

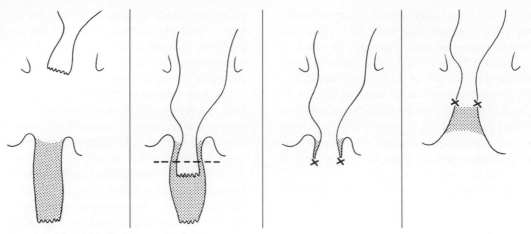

Figure 22.13 *In Swenson's operation the rectum is divided and the rectal stump everted. The proximal bowel is pulled through this, the remaining rectum excised, and the anastomosis performed outside the anus.*

Duhamel's operation

In this operation, a tunnel is created posterolateral to the rectum and opened into the posterior wall of the anal canal. Normal bowel, drawn through the tunnel, lies alongside the rectum. It is then anastomosed side-to-side to the native rectum with a linear cutting stapler, or a crushing clamp. The divided rectum is anastomosed end-to-side onto the normal colon above the level of the side-to-side amalgamation of the two lumens (Fig. 22.14).

BOWEL SURGERY IN INFANCY AND CHILDHOOD

Surgery in infancy

Hirschsprung's disease, and other congenital abnormalities, may present after the neonatal period. Intussusception and inguinal herniae are also common. It should be remembered that obstruction in the first year is most often caused by a strangulated inguinal hernia, which is discussed in Chapter 24.

Duplication of a segment of bowel results in a mucus-filled cyst which slowly expands and causes symptoms by pressure. Excision is indicated.

Malrotation describes the condition in which there is a failure of the normal embryological anticlockwise rotation of the gut. The most common presentation is with obstruction, which may be complete, or intermittent and partial. It may occur for the first time in the neonatal period, in infancy or in later childhood. A simple obstruction in malrotation may occur from a peritoneal band (Ladd's band) compressing the duodenum as it runs up to the superiorly displaced caecum. Alternatively, a volvulus can occur of the abnormally mobile midgut which is suspended on a narrow pedicle of mesentery. At laparotomy, a Ladd's band should be divided. If a volvulus has occurred, resection of non-viable bowel, and derotation of viable bowel, follows general principles. Any attempt at fixation of the mobile midgut, or correction of the malrotation, is seldom of any value.

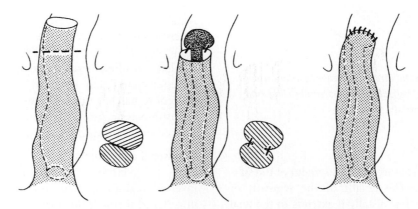

Figure 22.14 *In Duhamel's operation the rectum is transected, proximal aganglionic colon is resected and the normal colon is drawn down posterolateral to the rectum. After a side-to-side anastomosis, the neorectum has half of its circumference formed by normal colon and half by aganglionic rectum.*

Intussusception is a common cause of obstruction in a previously healthy older infant. The passage of bloody stools, or a right hypochondrial mass, aids diagnosis. Unless there is strangulation of the bowel, reduction can usually be achieved non-operatively, by air insufflation under ultrasound control, or barium insufflation under X-ray imaging. In contrast to intussusceptions in adults, the apex of the intussusception in infancy is almost exclusively a benign lymphadenopathy, and laparotomy is only indicated if reduction is not possible by non-operative means. For these techniques to be safe and effective, expertise is essential and transfer to a paediatric centre is indicated if ultrasound has confirmed the clinical diagnosis. If non-operative reduction has failed, surgical reduction at laparotomy is required, as described in the section on intussusception in adults. Resection is only necessary if there is non-viable bowel.

Surgery in childhood

Most congenital abnormalities will have presented in infancy, but malrotation, short segment Hirschsprung's disease and duplication cysts may have a late presentation. Inguinal herniae are common, but are less likely to strangulate in later childhood than in infancy. An adult range of pathologies starts to emerge with appendicitis and inflammatory bowel disease becoming more common. The surgical management of these conditions is similar to that in adults with only minor variations, and is discussed in the relevant sections.

A role for the appendix: paediatric urologists, and paediatric general surgeons, have developed techniques to avoid permanent stomas in children by utilizing the appendix as a narrow continent stoma which can be intermittently

catheterized. If the appendix is otherwise left undisturbed, a catheter can be passed into the caecum for antegrade enemeta. This technique has proved of great value in the management of children with faecal incontinence or intractable constipation. Alternatively, the appendix can be transferred to the bladder as a continent stoma which can be catheterized. This Mitrofanoff procedure can avoid the need for permanent catheterization, or urinary diversion, in children with spina bifida. The caecum is mobilized, and the appendix with its carefully preserved mesentery, is removed from the caecum and implanted into the bladder, with some form of invagination, or tunnelling, to prevent leakage.

Stenosis of the mucocutaneous interface of the stoma is troublesome, and a variety of flaps have been developed to create a partially skin-lined track and reduce this complication (Fig. 22.15).

REFERENCES

1. Ellis H, Moran BJ, Thompson JN, et al. Adhesion-related hospital readmissions after abdominal and pelvic surgery: a retrospective cohort study. Lancet 1999; 353: 1476–80.
2. Shepherd JJ. Ninety-two cases of ileosigmoid knotting in Uganda. Br J Surg 1967; 54: 561–6.
3. Dudley HAF, Radcliffe AG, McGeehan D. Intraoperative irrigation of the colon to permit primary anastomosis. Br J Surg 1980; 67: 80–1.
4. Daniels IR, Lamparelli MJ, Chave H, et al. Recurrent sigmoid volvulus treated by percutaneous endoscopic colostomy. Br J Surg 2000; 87: 1419.
5. Sule AZ, Iya D, Obekpa PO, et al. One-stage procedure in the management of acute sigmoid volvulus. J R Coll Surg Edinb 1999; 44: 164–6.
6. Hutchinson R, Griffiths C. Acute colonic pseudo-obstruction: a pharmacological approach. Ann R Coll Surg Engl 1992; 74: 364–7.
7. Thomson WHF, White S, O'Leary DP. Tube caecostomy to protect rectal anastomoses. Br J Surg 1998; 85: 1533–4.
8. Tulchinsky H, Cohen CRG, Nicholls RJ. Salvage surgery after restorative proctocolectomy. Review. Br J Surg 2003; 90: 909–21.
9. Kapoor VK. Abdominal tuberculosis. Postgrad Med J 1998; 74: 459–67.
10. Levy RD, Degiannis E, Saadia R. Management of intestinal typhoid perforation. S African J Surg 1996; 34: 138–41.
11. Simunovic M, Sexton R, Rempel E, et al. Optimal preoperative assessment and surgery for rectal cancer may greatly limit the need for radiotherapy. Br J Surg 2003; 90: 999–1003.
12. Wanebo HJ, Antoniuk P, Koness RJ, et al. Pelvic resection of recurrent rectal cancer. Dis Colon Rectum 1999; 42: 1438–48.
13. Olsen KØ, Juul S, Bülow S, et al. Female fecundity before and after operation for familial adenomatous polyposis. Br J Surg 2003; 90: 227–31.
14. Paediatric Surgery, J Atwell. London: Arnold, 1998.
15. Maxwell-Armstrong CA, Phillips RKS. Extrasphincteric rectal fistulas treated successfully by Soave's procedure despite marked local sepsis. Br J Surg 2003; 90: 237–8.

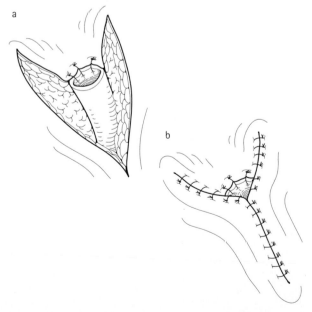

Figure 22.15 *The appendix as a continent catheterizable stoma is prone to stenosis. A partially skin-lined tract is less prone to stenosis and can be formed by a simple V-Y-plasty.*

SURGERY OF THE ANUS AND PERINEUM

Many patients present to the surgeon with anal symptoms. Discomfort, ranging from itching to severe pain, is common and may be associated with anal bleeding or minor prolapsing. More major problems include full-thickness prolapse, defaecatory difficulties and impaired continence. All patients require careful assessment to exclude serious pathology. Most, however, will be found to have minor anal pathology, the majority of which will require no surgery. Many patients only require reassurance that the symptoms are not caused by cancer. Others have troublesome symptoms related to haemorrhoids or fissures but medical treatment, or a minor procedure which can be undertaken in the outpatient clinic, may be all that is required. Many with defaecatory problems, or impaired continence, will require careful assessment of their problem, but only a minority will be helped by surgery.

ANATOMY AND PHYSIOLOGY

An understanding of the anatomy and physiology of the anal canal is of major importance to any surgeon undertaking even the most minor anal operation, as stretching of the sphincter muscles or partial division, whether inadvertently or in the treatment of a fissure or fistulae, may have a deleterious effect on continence.

Anatomy

The anal canal passes downwards, and backwards, for around 4 cm, as a direct but narrower extension of the rectum to end at the anal orifice, or *anal verge*. The anal verge is taken as the reference point when measuring the height of any rectal or distal colonic lesion. The *internal sphincter* is a condensation of the circular muscle of the bowel wall. When the external sphincter is relaxed, the distal edge of the internal sphincter can be felt at the anal verge (Fig. 23.1). However, as the subcutaneous fibres of the external sphincter contract they form a circle of muscle distal to, rather than outside, the internal sphincter. The *external sphincter* is a composite striated muscle. Its lower fibres encircle the anal canal and can be, somewhat arbitrarily, subdivided into deep, superficial and subcutaneous portions. Superiorly it blends with the puborectalis portion of the levator ani muscle of the pelvic floor. The puborectalis muscle sling does not encircle the anus and is deficient anteriorly (Fig. 23.2). The circular portion of the external sphincter is shorter in women, particularly anteriorly.

The lining of the anal canal changes at the *dentate line*. Below this line it is modified skin, or anoderm, consisting of squamous epithelium, but above the line the mucosa is a similar columnar epithelium to that of the remainder of the colon and rectum, except that there is a *junctional zone* extending for about 1 cm above the dentate line. This change in the mucosa is important, as malignant lesions arising in the distal anal canal are more likely to be squamous cell carcinomas than adenocarcinomas. The dentate line also marks the watershed for lymphatic drainage. The upper anal canal drains to the inferior mesenteric nodes, and the lower anal canal to the inguinal nodes. The dentate line is also the division between somatic and visceral sensation. Distal pathology in the anal canal may thus be extremely painful, whereas pain is a later feature of pathology at the anorectal junction. This is also the reason that it is possible for the surgeon to inject sclerosants, or place mucosal bands, *above* the dentate line with only minor discomfort. The dentate line can be identified visually, as the mucosa above is loosely attached and hangs in longitudinal folds, which are joined at the dentate line by crescentic folds, or *anal valves* (see Fig. 23.1). The *anal glands* lie partly in the submucosal plane and partly

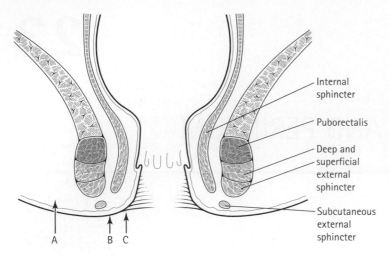

Figure 23.1 *Diagramatic coronal section of the anal canal. The longitudinal anal folds terminate in the anal valves at the dentate line. The extrasphincteric plane (A) is into the fat of the ischiorectal fossa beneath the levator ani muscles. In the relaxed anus the subcutaneous fibres of the external sphincter lie outside the internal sphincter and the intersphincteric groove (B) is palpable. The submucosal plane (C) is continuous with the subcutaneous plane beneath the anoderm.*

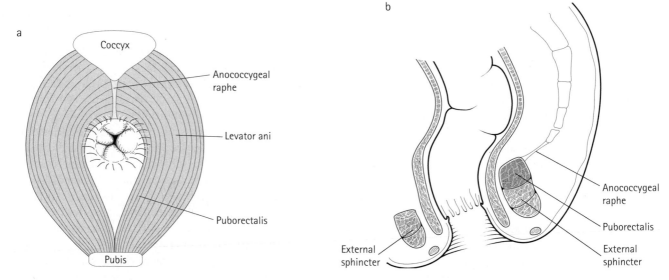

Figure 23.2 *(a) The pelvic floor musculature viewed from below. The puborectalis sling is the anteromedial free edge of the levator ani muscle and is of great importance in continence, although it does not encircle the anus. (b) The diagrammatic sagittal view of the anus demonstrates the absence of puborectalis anteriorly.*

between the sphincters in the intersphincteric plane; infection in these glands is thought to be the main cause of perianal sepsis and fistulae. The orifices of the glands open just above the anal valves and this is therefore the commonest site of the internal opening for a fistula (see below).

Vascular plexi lie beneath the mucosa of the anal canal. The main arterial inflow is from the terminal branches of the superior rectal artery which classically divides into a left lateral, a right anterolateral and a right posterolateral branch; they anastomose with branches of the inferior rectal artery. Three small swellings, or *anal cushions*, are associated with the underlying vascular plexi. A *haemorrhoid* is an excessive distension of a vascular plexus which stretches the overlying mucosa and anoderm, loosening their attachments to the muscle wall of the anal canal.

Physiology

DEFAECATION

Defaecation is a complex interaction of reflex sphincter and pelvic floor relaxation associated with a propulsive peristaltic wave. To this is often added voluntary straining to increase intra-abdominal pressure. Straining will overcome difficulties secondary to poor sphincter or pelvic floor relaxation, to an inadequate peristaltic wave or to a disproportionally large stool. However, straining also causes haemorrhoidal swelling which in itself partially obstructs the passage of stool. Minor defaecatory difficulties, often associated with bleeding and prolapse of haemorrhoidal tissue, may result. Some patients, however, develop more severe difficulties and present with a range of symptoms, collectively described as the 'obstructed defaecation syndrome'. These patients complain of incapacitating evacuatory problems often associated with tenesmus. The difficulty is thought, at least in part, to be due to failure of relaxation, or even inappropriate contraction, of the pelvic floor during defaecation. Trauma from straining can cause an ulcer, which is commonly in the lower anterior rectum (solitary rectal ulcer). Intra-rectal intussusception, and even full-thickness rectal prolapse, may also develop. Excessive perineal descent from straining can also stretch, and damage, the pudendal nerves. Surgery seldom has any place in the treatment of obstructed defaecation, and biofeedback[1] has proved to be the most promising line of management.

After rectal resection and the formation of a coloanal or ileal pouch-anal anastomosis there is inevitably a deficient afferent limb to any defaecatory reflex initiated by the presence of faeces above the sphincter. There was initial theoretical concern that evacuatory function would be poor, but this has not proved to be a major problem.

CONTINENCE

Continence is also complex as it is a balance between the effectiveness of the anal sphincters and the pressures which they have to withstand. Severe dysentery can cause incontinence, even in young men with excellent sphincters. Conversely, some elderly women with little measurable sphincter function may remain 'continent' due to a regular and constipated bowel habit, only to complain of incontinence when they develop some other large bowel pathology. Sphincter pressures naturally decline with age as muscle fibres in the sphincters are replaced with fibrous tissue. This natural deterioration also affects the muscles of the pelvic floor. The ability to detect flatus or faeces in the lower rectum or anal canal, and to differentiate between them, is another factor in the maintenance of continence. Deterioration in anorectal sensation also occurs with advancing age. However, partial sphincter denervation from pudendal nerve neuropathy is less important than was previously believed.

Resting anal pressure
Passive continence is the ability to prevent passive leakage of rectal contents. Leakage can occur without a major propulsive peristaltic wave, and is prevented by an effective anal seal and the resting anal pressure. The haemorrhoidal cushions form a soft seal to the anal canal, but the seal is mainly dependent on the activity of the unstriated muscle of the internal sphincter. Of equal importance is whether the lower rectum has faecal matter within it, and the consistency of that matter. Good passive continence is imperative in preventing the leakage of semi-formed ileal pouch contents during sleep and, as anal pressures decrease with advancing years, a pouch-anal reconstruction may not be a good solution for an elderly patient. A stapled anastomosis at the dentate line after a total proctocolectomy sacrifices the upper portion of the internal sphincter. For this reason, some surgeons prefer a mucosectomy and a hand-sewn per-anal anas-

tomosis to stapling in order to excise all the affected mucosa while still preserving the whole length of the internal sphincter (see Chapter 22). Blood and mucus in the lower rectum presents a similar challenge to continence, and an elderly patient with a rectal cancer or villous adenoma may present with passive incontinence. A patient with a very poor resting anal pressure who suffers from incomplete evacuation on defaecation may lose small pellets of solid faeces. This problem will be compounded if anorectal sensation is poor and the patient is unaware of the passage of stool.

Anal squeeze pressure
This is the maximum voluntary pressure which the patient can exert to close the anal canal, and is thus of more importance in delaying a call to stool than in maintaining passive continence. The voluntary increase in pressure is produced mainly by the external sphincter, but it is supplemented by other muscles of the pelvic floor, and even gluteal muscle contraction. These additional muscles of continence may be sufficient to compensate for a severely disrupted external sphincter after childbirth. The young woman may initially maintain acceptable continence, but present with impaired continence years later as other compensatory muscles atrophy with advancing age. The ability to delay defaecation is not solely related to sphincter integrity. The strength of the peristaltic waves in infective colitis, diverticular disease or inflammatory bowel disease may challenge even the normal sphincter. An additional factor is the volume and compliance of the rectum, or neorectum, to accommodate and store additional faecal material.

Anorectal physiology, including its investigation, and the maintenance of continence is a complex subject and further reading on this topic is recommended.[2]

GENERAL TECHNIQUE

Surgical approach

The importance of anal operations is often underestimated, and the surgery delegated to relatively inexperienced surgeons. However, unless this surgery is undertaken to a high standard, and with attention to detail, there is considerable potential for avoidable iatrogenic damage.

ACCESS

Anal surgery is difficult in the presence of faeces in the rectum. A preoperative enema is usually sufficient to clear the operative field, after which surgery can be performed in either the lithotomy or the prone jack-knife position (Fig. 23.3). A proctoscope holds the anus open and allows visualization of, and access to, the lower rectum. Unilateral anal retraction displays the opposite half of the anal canal, and the curved Sims retractor can be useful for this. However, a variety of bivalve retractors usually afford superior access with

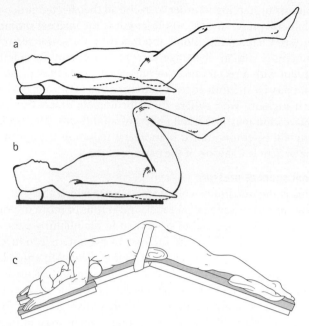

Figure 23.3 *(a) This is a suitable position for a lengthy procedure where only limited perineal access is required to perform a transanal stapled anastomosis. (b) This is a better position for any anal dissection, but the acute flexion of hips and knees is undesirable for any protracted period. The position of the thighs also restricts any simultaneous pelvic or abdominal access. (c) The prone jack-knife position with the buttocks strapped apart affords excellent access to the posterior perineum and anus with less venous congestion. The disadvantages are mainly in the turning and ventilation of an anaesthetized patient in this position, which makes it an unattractive option for a short minor procedure.*

visualization of, and surgical access to, the anus between the blades of the retractor. The self-retaining 'lone star' device gives excellent retraction with a series of disposable skin hooks which are inserted circumferentially. Each small hook is at the end of a long slim plastic-covered spring which is then fixed onto the circumference of the ring retractor encircling the anus. Prolonged or excessive anal retraction by any method can damage the internal sphincter however, and great care must be exercised.

ANAESTHESIA

Adequate anaesthesia, whether general, regional or local infiltrative, is essential for any procedure on the sensitive anoderm below the dentate line. The anaesthesia necessary for per-anal surgery on the relatively insensitive rectum is to relax the anal sphincters to facilitate access.

INITIAL PROCEDURE

Anal operations should commence with a digital rectal examination and proctoscopy. A rigid sigmoidoscopy is performed to exclude any other previously undetected pathology. If there is to be any open external wound, the perianal

skin should be shaved at the start of the procedure, as hair matted with blood will become adherent postoperatively, and greatly increase patient discomfort.

DISSECTION

Precise dissection in anatomical planes, and the identification of the sphincters is the key to successful anal surgery (see Fig. 23.1). Uncontrolled haemorrhage during dissection obscures vision and must be avoided. Diathermy dissection is associated with less bleeding than scissor dissection, but alternatively scissor or scalpel dissection can be combined with diathermy coagulation of bleeding points. External sphincter fibres twitch when stimulated by diathermy current, and this observation can aid identification during dissection. Injection of a dilute solution of adrenaline (1:400 000) before commencing surgery will reduce haemorrhage and, if injected into the plane to be followed, can make the dissection easier. While some surgeons favour this technique, others find that it distorts the anatomy and is unhelpful.

- The *submucosal plane* for a haemorrhoidectomy is entered outside the anal verge; for a mucosectomy it is entered at the dentate line; for a Delormes' procedure it is entered 1–2 cm above the dentate line, and for a transanal excision of a villous adenoma close to the base of the tumour.
- The *intersphincteric plane* is the key to anal sepsis and fistulae. It is also the plane through which the rectum can be excised either from above or from below for benign conditions. It is entered from below at the palpable intersphincteric groove at the anal verge.
- The *extrasphincteric plane*, which is entered when draining an ischiorectal abscess, ends blindly at the pelvic floor musculature. This is also the plane for a radical abdominoperineal excision of the rectum for a very low cancer in which the pelvic floor muscles are then divided (see Chapter 22). A rectocoele can be approached through the extrasphincteric plane between the circumferential portion of the external sphincter and the vaginal mucosa as there is an anatomical window through the pelvic floor in the midline anteriorly (see Fig. 23.2). To enter the extrasphincteric plane from the perineum, the surgeon must be confident of the position of the external sphincter. The perianal skin is lightly pigmented for a few centimetres outside the anal verge, and the change to normal pigmentation is the surface landmark of the external sphincter.

THE ANAL WOUND

Any bleeding from a raw surface should be stopped by diathermy coagulation. The traditional large anal pack is almost always unnecessary and causes significant postoperative pain. A small absorbable haemostatic pack is favoured by some surgeons, but is expensive. Local infiltration of bupivicaine with adrenaline is effective in arresting minor ooze and will also reduce early postoperative pain. Anal skin wounds are often left open, and a greased dressing will prevent adherence to clothes or pads, and reduce discomfort. Absorbable sutures should be used in the anal mucosa and in the anal verge skin.

Faecal contamination of an anal wound seldom gives rise to major local or systemic sepsis. It is even safe to use non-absorbable material for suturing the anal sphincters, although the use of non-absorbable mesh should generally be avoided. Minor infection is, however, probably common, and is now believed to be the cause of the increase in postoperative pain at about 3–5 days after a haemorrhoidectomy.[3] The early passage of hard faeces causes pain, and even mechanical disruption of a repair. Postoperatively, stool softeners are used routinely to encourage an early soft motion. The addition of a course of preoperative stool softeners will be more effective in achieving this, and a full bowel preparation should be considered for more major surgery. The old practice of confining the bowels after anal surgery is generally harmful, as the eventual first stool will be large and hard. If there is an overwhelming desire to avoid early passage of stool a temporary defunctioning stoma should be considered.

Postoperative complications

- *Urinary retention* is common after anal procedures, and in more major perineal operations anterior to the anus prophylactic urethral catheterization should be considered.
- *Early haemorrhage* after anal surgery is usually best treated by a return to the operating theatre, an examination under anaesthesia and coagulation or ligation of the bleeding point.
- *Secondary haemorrhage* at 10–14 days may be profuse. As neither sutures nor diathermy are likely to arrest the bleeding from friable infected granulation tissue, it is initially treated conservatively with blood replacement and antibiotics. A balloon catheter introduced into the rectum, followed by inflation of the balloon for local pressure on the bleeding area, can be an effective manoeuvre.
- *Anal stenosis* and *anal mucosal ectropion* are complications of anal surgery where too much anoderm has been sacrificed, and they occur mainly after haemorrhoidal surgery. For many mild forms conservative management with anal dilators, stool softeners and the protection of the perianal skin from minor discharge often suffices. More severe symptoms may justify surgery. A simple Y-V advancement flap may help (see Fig. 23.7a).

HAEMORRHOIDS

Haemorrhoids are a distension of the normal vascular haemorrhoidal cushions. *Internal haemorrhoids* are submucosal

and above the dentate line. Initially, symptoms are confined to bleeding, during or after, defaecation (1st degree). The lax mucosa, which is separated from the underlying muscle wall by the distended vascular plexus, later prolapses along with the haemorrhoidal tissue during defaecation, but reduces spontaneously after defaecation (2nd degree). Haemorrhoids which no longer reduce spontaneously (3rd degree) require digital replacement. Failure of replacement may progress to *thrombosed prolapsed internal haemorrhoids* which are also described as *strangulated piles*, although the strangulating effect of the sphincters is variable.

There is frequently some extension of haemorrhoidal tissue below the dentate line, and the distension of this, combined with prolapsing from above, separates the entire anal canal epithelium from the underlying muscle wall. The anus becomes protuberant with the external component of the haemorrhoids visible as broad-based tags at the anal verge. These are predominantly skin-covered, although there may be mucosa visible on eversion of the tag. Permanently prolapsed haemorrhoids (4th degree) have traumatized exposed mucosa which produces a mucous discharge.

External haemorrhoids are at the anal verge and are covered with skin rather than mucosa. They may occur in isolation, but more frequently are associated with internal haemorrhoids. Thrombosis of an external haemorrhoid is extremely painful but resolves spontaneously in a few days, often with the formation of a perianal skin tag.

Many patients with minimally symptomatic haemorrhoids require no intervention other than the exclusion of a rectal neoplasm or other serious pathology. Treatment, to be effective, must either reduce the size and vascularity of the haemorrhoidal cushions or reduce the laxity between the anal canal epithelium and the muscle to prevent the mucosal prolapse. These objectives can often be achieved by conservative treatments and surgical haemorrhoidectomy avoided.

Conservative treatment of haemorrhoids

SCLEROTHERAPY

Sclerotherapy initiates thrombosis of the proximal haemorrhoidal plexus, and promotes a localized fibrosis which leads to retraction and tethering of the lax mucosa. It can be performed through a proctoscope and, as the injection is at the upper limit of the haemorrhoid and well above the dentate line, discomfort is minimal and no anaesthesia is needed. The solution advocated is 5 per cent phenol in almond oil, and up to 5 mL may be injected at one site. More commonly, 2–3 mL are injected above each of the three main haemorrhoids. The injection should be seen to raise a pale swelling which spreads immediately deep to the mucosa. A white wheal indicates too superficial an injection and the risk of mucosal sloughing, but too deep an injection anteriorly may have more serious consequences; in men, chemical prostatitis and impotence are rare but well-recognized complications, and anovaginal fistulae have been reported in women. Minor 'septic' reactions are not uncommon and occasionally severe sepsis can occur. Sclerotherapy is often successful for 1st and 2nd degree haemorrhoids, and may be successful for 3rd degree haemorrhoids if there is no significant skin or external component. Treatment often requires a series of two or three injections at 6-weekly intervals.

BANDING

Banding of haemorrhoids can also be carried out in outpatients without anaesthesia. The mucosa above a haemorrhoid is drawn into a suction device and a rubber band delivered over it. The contained mucosa and vascular plexus are strangulated, and separate at around 10–12 days. Banding is more effective for prolapsing (2nd and 3rd degree) haemorrhoids than sclerotherapy but, even when the band is safely above the dentate line, the occasional patient experiences severe pain a few hours later and, in general, discomfort is more common than after sclerotherapy. A secondary haemorrhage, which is occasionally profuse, may occur as the strangulated tissue separates.

CIRCULAR STAPLING OR ANOPEXY

This method is a relatively recent addition to treatment. It has the disadvantage of the high cost of a disposable stapling device. It is normally performed under general anaesthetic, but postoperative pain is usually minimal as there is no wound below the dentate line. A circumferential mucosal purse-string suture is first placed per anum 3–5 cm above the dentate line, so that tightening of this purse-string will draw mucosa and submucosa into the stapler. When the stapler is closed and fired, a ring of staples is delivered and a 'doughnut' of mucosa and submucosa is excised which includes the arterial inflow to the upper end of the haemorrhoids. Vascularity is reduced, and prolapsing haemorrhoidal mucosa is drawn back up into the anal canal. More widespread use is limited by cost and is also related to concern over complications. Too low a purse-string results in severe pain, while a purse-string which is too deep and incorporates muscle results in a full-thickness circular excision with the potential to cause pelvic sepsis or a rectovaginal fistula.

Haemorrhoidectomy

MILLIGAN MORGAN HAEMORRHOIDECTOMY[4]

This is still the 'gold standard' of haemorrhoid treatment. Haemorrhoidal tissue is excised radially at one or more sites, and each excision includes the external skin component of the haemorrhoidal complex in continuity with a strip of anal canal mucosa and the underlying haemorrhoidal plexus (Fig. 23.4). Adequate bridges of skin and mucosa must be left intact between the excisions to prevent anal stenosis developing during healing. This is particularly important in the anal canal below the dentate line and at the anal verge (Fig. 23.5).

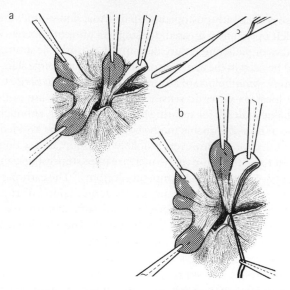

Figure 23.4 *A Milligan Morgan haemorrhoidectomy. (a) An artery forceps has been applied to the skin and to the mucosal elements of each haemorrhoid. A V-shaped incision is made beneath the external skin element of the haemorrhoid and the haemorrhoid is dissected off the underlying internal sphincter. (b) The mucosal and submucosal pedicle at the proximal extremity of the haemorrhoid is transfixed and ligated, or sealed by diathermy coagulation, before division.*

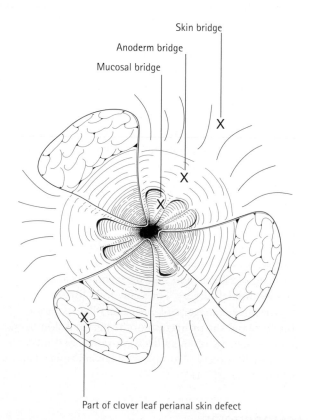

Figure 23.5 *A clover leaf-shaped defect in the anal canal and perianal skin will be left after a haemorrhoidectomy. It is important that intact bridges of mucosa, anoderm and perianal skin are retained.*

The dissection is in a deep submucosal plane between the haemorrhoidal plexus and the internal sphincter muscle, which must be identified and preserved. An anal retractor to retract, but not over-stretch the anus, can make the identification of the internal sphincter easier. It will also hold the other haemorrhoids out of the operative field, and it is rotated to display each haemorrhoid in turn.

Operative procedure

The operation commences with an examination of the anus and rectum, including sigmoidoscopy. A proctoscope is inserted and, when slowly withdrawn, allows the haemorrhoids to prolapse. An artery forceps is applied to the skin element of each haemorrhoid and a second forceps applied to its prolapsing mucosa. These artery forceps hold the haemorrhoid for dissection, but can also be used to retract the others out of the operative field if an anal retractor is not employed. It is often easier to mark all the incisions in the anal canal, to ensure adequate skin and mucosal bridges between the excisions, before proceeding with the removal of the first haemorrhoid. A fine diathermy point is ideal for this, and incises the anoderm and mucosa with minimal bleeding. Excision of the first haemorrhoid is then commenced by a V-shaped incision through the skin at the base of the external component (Fig. 23.4a). The V-incision is extended across the anal verge to join the preliminary superficial marking incisions and defines the tissue to be excised. The dissection is deepened under the V to develop the plane outside the haemorrhoidal tissue, but great care must be exercised to ensure that this dissection is *inside* the internal sphincter. The muscle fibres should be clearly visualized and preserved. The haemorrhoidal tissue is dissected off the underlying internal sphincter up into the anal canal until it is only attached by its pedicle of mucosa, and the feeding vessels of the plexus. A transfixion suture is then placed through the pedicle and the haemorrhoid excised (Fig. 23.4b). Haemostasis with diathermy coagulation avoids the painful anal pack. The wounds are left open. The surgeon is often concerned by the residual haemorrhoidal tissue left *in situ* under the bridges of stretched and prolapsed mucosa and anoderm. In almost every patient healing with scar contraction draws this tissue back into the anal canal and reattaches it to the muscle coat.

Later modifications

Modifications of the procedure include:

- *Diathermy dissection*: this is very effective, and many surgeons who routinely use it have abandoned any transfixion of the pedicle.
- *Closed Ferguson haemorrhoidectomy*: on completion of the operation the mucosa and skin can be closed with absorbable sutures. Haemostasis must be meticulous or an infected haematoma will form deep to the closure and disrupt it.
- *Park's submucosal excision* differs in that a linear radial incision is made over the haemorrhoidal tissue, which is

then dissected out from beneath the anoderm and mucosa. No epithelium is excised and the wound is closed. This method can also be used to retrieve haemorrhoidal tissue, left behind beneath an intact skin-mucosal bridge, at the end of a Milligan Morgan haemorrhoidectomy.

- *Radial clamps or staples* can be used to remove the lax, stretched anal mucosa and anoderm with the underlying haemorrhoidal plexus. Both the linear stapler and the 'Ligasure' technique follow similar principles to the traditional clamp and cautery favoured by Eric Farquharson (Fig. 23.6).

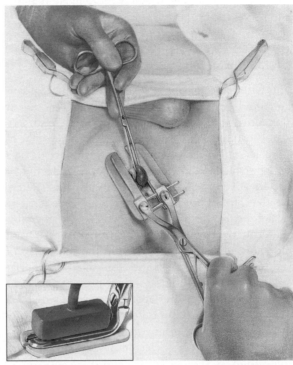

Figure 23.6   *A photograph from the original 1954 edition of a clamp and cautery haemorrhoidectomy in Eric Farquharson's unit.*

WHITEHEAD HAEMORRHOIDECTOMY

This procedure consists of a circumferential, rather than a radial, excision of haemorrhoidal tissue and is superficially a more attractive option when the haemorrhoids are circumferential. A new mucosa-anoderm junction is fashioned. It is essential to tether this to the muscle of the anal canal at the site of the normal dentate line. Unfortunately, if this last step is unsuccessful a mucosal ectropion develops and is a sufficiently common complication to be named the *Whitehead deformity*. The same considerations are important if a decision is taken to excise and resuture a portion of a skin-mucosal bridge during an otherwise standard haemorrhoidectomy.

THROMBOSED EXTERNAL HAEMORRHOIDS

Evacuation of the haematoma through a cruciate incision, as for the drainage of a perianal abscess, may shorten the natural history, but conservative management is usually equally satisfactory.

ANAL TAGS

These may cause irritation, and difficulties with hygiene, and a patient may request excision. The removal of small tags can be disappointing as a new tag sometimes forms on healing. Narrow-stalked tags can be simply excised under local anaesthesia, but careful preoperative assessment is important. The tag may be a sentinel pile marking an underlying anal fissure, or it may be the broad-based external component of an associated internal haemorrhoid. Treatment should then be of the underlying pathology, which is more likely than the tag itself to be the cause of the symptoms.

THROMBOSED PROLAPSED (STRANGULATED) HAEMORRHOIDS

Patients with these prolapsed, thrombosed, mucosal-covered haemorrhoids are often in severe pain. Conservative treatment is aimed at the relief of pain, and definitive surgery can then be postponed for some weeks until after the acute episode has settled. Local applications, whether of sugar or salt which reduce swelling by osmosis, or of hyaluronidase or ice, are effective in relieving symptoms. An anal stretch also relieves symptoms, but only because it abolishes anal spasm by partial disruption of the sphincters, and is therefore no longer recommended. Earlier concerns regarding infection if haemorrhoidectomy is undertaken in the acute phase have proved unfounded, and it is therefore often appropriate to proceed with haemorrhoidectomy at presentation. In general, it is better to excise the largest, or at most two, haemorrhoidal areas as attempts to perform a definitive haemorrhoidectomy as an emergency can result in complications, particularly stenosis. Decompression by single haemorrhoidectomy is very successful and often gives excellent long-term results. An inexperienced surgeon may, however, be at increased risk of inflicting sphincter damage, and great care must be exercised.

ANAL FISSURES

Simple anal fissures occur almost exclusively in the midline, both anteriorly and posteriorly. The acute anal fissure is a radial split in the anoderm extending from the anal verge for a variable distance proximally towards the dentate line. These fissures are seen in association with constipation, childbirth and severe diarrhoea, and may be caused by the passage of a large hard stool, though straining with failure of relaxation of the internal sphincter may also be implicated. Chronic anal fissures are those which fail to heal and form a linear, indurated chronic ulcer. Patients request treatment for defaecatory bleeding and severe post-defaecatory pain. There is considerable evidence that the failure to heal is, at least in part, due to localized tissue ischaemia from a high anal pressure. A permanent surgical, or temporary pharmacological, reduction in resting anal pressure is the mainstay of treatment.

A partial internal anal sphincter release is very effective in reducing resting tone, relieving the symptoms and healing the fissure. Many patients, however, will have a minor deterioration in continence, and a few will have significant problems. The knowledge that women with childbirth sphincter damage often compensate for many years and present in later life with incontinence has also raised surgical awareness of late morbidity from partial division of the sphincters. Conservative treatment has therefore become more popular, and internal sphincterotomy is now used selectively and only when conservative measures have failed. These treatments include stool softeners and local anaesthetic or steroid ointments, but the most effective treatment is with topical agents which reduce smooth muscle tone. Glyceryl trinitrate (GTN) ointment (0.2%) is the most widely used, but this often causes unacceptable headaches. Calcium antagonist ointments are proving equally effective but with fewer side effects. Botulinum toxin injection into the internal sphincter has provided good results in some small studies.[5] However, although healing of a chronic fissure may be achieved, when the treatment is discontinued and the anal resting pressures return to pretreatment levels, recurrence is not uncommon.

Subcutaneous lateral internal sphincterotomy (SLIS)

This procedure consists of the division of the internal sphincter. Originally, the whole length of the sphincter was divided, but even release to the dentate line is now considered excessive in most situations. The length of the fissure may be a good guide to the length of the release indicated. Inadequate release results in treatment failure, and too generous a release increases the likelihood of passive incontinence. An anal stretch is also effective but is a less-controlled method of disrupting the internal sphincter; there is also a greater danger of additional damage to the external sphincter. Historically, the practice of incising the base of a fissure, or of excising the whole fissure, was effective as these operations divided the internal sphincter, the fibres of which are visible in the floor of a chronic fissure. However, these operations create a keyhole deformity of the anal canal which is less effectively sealed by the haemorrhoidal cushions and may be detrimental to passive continence. A lateral release of the internal sphincter, separate from the fissure, is therefore preferable.

Operative procedure

With the patient anaesthetized, the intersphincteric groove is palpable at the anal verge (see Fig. 23.1). If the *open method* is to be employed, a 1- to 2-cm circumferential incision is made at the anal verge over the free edge of the internal sphincter. Blunt scissor dissection opens the plane inside, and outside, the internal sphincter to free it. The free lower edge of the internal sphincter is then grasped, drawn into the wound and its distal portion divided. In the *closed method*, a pointed no. 11 blade is introduced between the internal sphincter and the anoderm, with the blade orientated so that it lies parallel to the anal skin. It is then rotated to face outwards and gently pressed against the distal portion of the internal sphincter, which is held taut with a bi-valve retractor. Alternatively, the scalpel can be introduced into the inter-sphincteric plane and the internal sphincter incised from without. The scalpel is withdrawn and on digital palpation the tight band of the distal internal sphincter can be felt to have released. Any residual band will 'give way' on gentle digital pressure on the anoderm over the area of the release. This is safer than reintroducing the scalpel. There is often an associated sentinel skin tag at the outer end of the fissure, and sometimes a fibroepithelial polyp at the inner end. These should be excised. The wounds are left open.

Advancement flaps

A chronic fissure, which has not healed on conservative management, may also be unsuitable for any form of sphincterotomy. For example, the patient may already have some impairment of continence or is known to have had external sphincter damage during a forceps delivery. Excision of the fissure and sentinel pile with preservation of the integrity of the internal sphincter can be followed by a diamond-shaped anal advancement flap to bring healthy, well-vascularized tissue into the fissure bed (Fig. 23.7b).

Fissures associated with Crohn's disease are often multiple, atypical, and not in the midline. In general, surgery should be avoided. The surgeon must also be aware of other chronic ulcers in the anus including anal carcinoma, and ulcers secondary to infection with cytomegalovirus (CMV) or syphilis.[2] If the aetiology is in doubt, the patient should be examined under anaesthesia, the fissure assessed, a swab taken for bacteriological investigations, and a biopsy sent for histology.

ANAL SEPSIS

Anal and perianal sepsis are commonly confined to a compartment defined by muscle and fascial attachments (see Fig. 23.1). These compartments are all circumferential and pus may therefore track around the anus in any plane (Fig. 23.8). The circumferential tracking of pus is more frequent posteriorly, and has implications in the treatment of fistulae.

Intersphincteric abscess

Most perianal sepsis starts in this space in association with infection within an anal gland. Occasionally, an intersphinc-

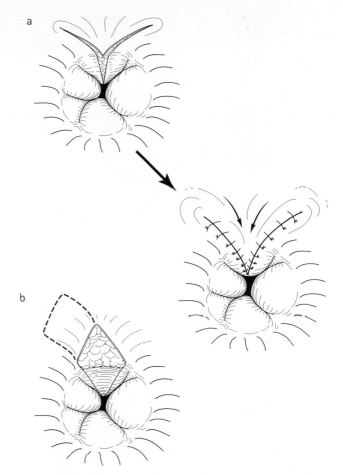

Figure 23.7 *(a) A Y–V anal advancement flap is a simple procedure for an anal stenosis. The Y incision at the anterior anal verge has been closed as a V, bringing extra tissue into the stenosed anus. (b) A chronic anal fissure can be excised and a local flap of healthy perianal skin and subcutaneous tissue brought in to fill the defect. The excision of this posterior fissure has left a diamond-shaped defect. The flap has been marked. It will be left attached to the underlying tissue from which it obtains its blood supply. The resultant donor defect can be closed or left to granulate.*

teric infection will fail to point, and presents with severe anal pain without an obvious explanation. An endo-anal ultrasound under anaesthesia will elucidate the underlying pathology. On other occasions the pus discharges spontaneously into the anal canal. If the patient is first seen at this stage, the atypical ragged ulceration can mimic more serious pathology. More frequently, the pus tracks down to the anal verge to present as a perianal abscess, or tracks through the external sphincter to form an ischiorectal abscess. Pus in these abscesses has a potential, or established track, to the lumen of the anal canal along the duct of the anal gland in which the infection originated.

Perianal abscess
This presents as a painful superficial swelling which distorts the anal verge (Fig. 23.9a). There may be a considerable collection of pus extending both cranially and caudally in the

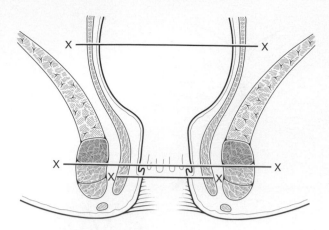

Figure 23.8   *Pus can track circumferentially in any perianal plane.*

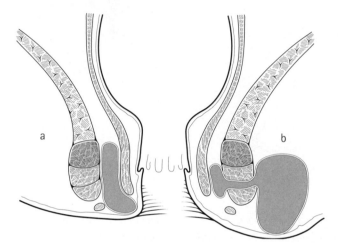

Figure 23.9   *Pus in the intersphincteric plane may track down to point as a perianal abscess (a) which distorts the anal verge. Alternatively, it may track through the external sphincter to form an ischiorectal abscess (b) which is deeper and points late to an area a few centimetres lateral to the anal verge.*

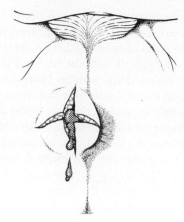

Figure 23.10   *A perianal abscess is drained via a cruciate incision at the anal verge.*

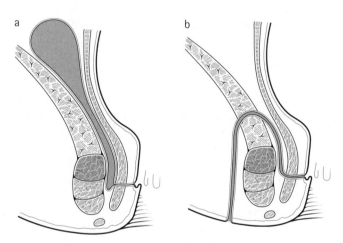

Figure 23.11   *(a) Intersphincteric sepsis can track up into the supralevator compartment. (b) Drainage of such an abscess through the levators will result in a suprasphincteric fistula. This is a high fistula despite an internal opening at the dentate line.*

intersphincteric plane, and pus may even track up into the supralevator space (see Fig. 23.11). Drainage is achieved with a cruciate incision over the swelling at the anal verge. The cavity is then deroofed, by the excision of the four flaps created by the initial cruciate incision, to allow good drainage (Fig. 23.10). Any associated intersphincteric anal fistula should not be explored in the acute phase.

Ischiorectal abscess

This presents with evidence of deep pus in the fat of the ischiorectal fossa, and the swelling is a few centimetres away from the anus (Fig. 23.9b). In the early stages, fluctuation and erythema of the overlying skin may be absent. Treatment again consists of drainage of the abscess through a cruciate incision. Deroofing of this deep abscess is essential if drains or packs are to be avoided. The incision must be sufficiently large to allow continued drainage of any residual pus, and to prevent premature closure of the skin. A drain into the depths of the abscess is then often superfluous and increases

discomfort. A temporary pack can be useful as a means of achieving postoperative haemostasis. Repeat packing is not recommended as it merely delays healing. The majority of ischiorectal abscesses are associated with an underlying trans-sphincteric fistula, following intersphincteric sepsis which has burst through the external sphincter. The fistula should not be explored, however, until the acute inflammation has settled.

Supralevator pus

Pus may extend cranially in the intersphincteric plane into the supralevator compartment (Fig. 23.11). However, pus can also track to this compartment from an ischiorectal abscess with a blind cranial extension penetrating the levator ani muscle. In addition, supralevator pus can be secondary to deep pelvic sepsis, and this pus may even track spontaneously down through the levators into the ischiorectal fossa. Pus above the levator ani muscles must therefore be carefully assessed, as inappropriate drainage from below can create a suprasphincteric or an extrasphincteric fistula. In Figure 23.11, supralevator pus from a large intersphincteric abscess has been drained through the levator ani with a resultant suprasphincteric fistula. When the primary pathology is pelvic, associated with a paracolic abscess, an iatrogenic extrasphincteric fistula may result unless the sepsis is drained from the abdomen.

Severe perianal sepsis with spreading cellulitis

This is a life-threatening condition that is encountered almost exclusively in immunocompromised and diabetic patients. The infection is no longer confined to one compartment, and may be a spreading cellulitis or a necrotizing soft tissue infection (see Chapters 1 and 3). Successful treatment depends on drainage of pus and excision of all dead tissue, combined with aggressive antibiotic therapy. Repeated examinations under anaesthesia are necessary to drain, or excise, areas which were previously deemed healthy but which have subsequently become involved. Faecal diversion by a colostomy is frequently necessary.[6]

In the elderly debilitated patient an indolent variant of severe perianal sepsis is occasionally seen. An apparently minor infection is drained, but healing does not occur. Although there is minimal cellulitis or necrosis the wound slowly extends and the sphincter muscles, lying exposed within it, are progressively destroyed. This distressing condition may occur during the last few days of life when pain relief is the only appropriate intervention. If more prolonged survival is likely, and the patient is fit for surgery, a defunctioning colostomy can be the best solution, both for the control of the pain and for the management of the incontinence.

ANAL FISTULAE

Anal fistulae are classified on the relationship of the track to the sphincters. The definition of *high* or *low* describes the height of the track as it traverses the sphincter muscles, and not the position of the internal opening which is, almost without exception, at the dentate line. More accurate classification defines the relationship of the track to the internal and external sphincters separately, and it is on this information, and the underlying pathology, that surgical treatment is based.[7] Most fistulae are either *intersphincteric* or *transsphincteric*. Preoperative MRI scans are valuable, but sinograms and CT scans have not proved helpful. Intraoperative endoanal ultrasound is a valuable diagnostic tool for those experienced in its interpretation.

FISTULAE SECONDARY TO INTERSPHINCTERIC SEPSIS

The commonest anal fistulae are secondary to infection in an anal gland. Pus collects initially in the intersphincteric plane. It may track to the anal verge to present as a perianal abscess, or break through the external sphincter into the ischiorectal fossa (see Fig. 23.9). The fistula is formed by spontaneous or surgical drainage which creates another channel into the abscess in addition to the opening of the anal gland at the dentate line. A primary track has been formed, and continuing sepsis and poor drainage prevent healing. Bilateral circumferential tracking in a variety of planes (see Fig. 23.8) is the aetiology of the posterior horseshoe fistula, with bilateral posterolateral tracks and external openings from a single internal opening (Fig. 23.12). The blind extensions and secondary tracks of complex fistulae are created by the tracking of pus, and the spontaneous or surgical drainage of these collections. The assessment of the anatomy is difficult, and previous failed attempts at surgery for these fistulae result in increasing complexity. Referral of patients with high, and complex, fistulae to colorectal surgeons with a special interest is advisable.

FISTULAE SECONDARY TO OTHER PATHOLOGY

Anal fistulae can develop secondary to other infective, inflammatory and malignant pathologies. They are common in tuberculosis and Crohn's disease. They also occur as a late complication of ileoanal pouch reconstruction surgery for inflammatory bowel disease (IBD).

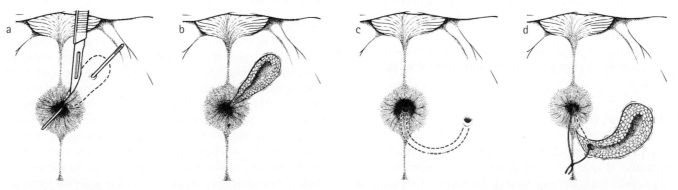

Figure 23.12   *(a) An anterior track is usually straight and radial. (b) The low anterior fistula has been laid open. (c) A posterior fistula is often curved and may have bilateral posterolateral external openings from a single midline internal opening. (d) The external portion of the track has been laid open, and the decision must now be made as to whether it is safe to lay open the part of the track which passes through the sphincter muscles.*

Rectovaginal and anovaginal fistulae

These are a subdivision of anal fistulae which have a different spectrum of aetiology and management. They are short and lined with epithelium, and therefore resolution is unlikely without surgical repair. The fistula is often wider than other anal fistulae, allowing significant faecal contamination of the vagina. Excoriation of the vaginal mucosa is a major symptom even if faecal incontinence appears minimal. A rectovaginal fistula is extrasphincteric, and an anovaginal fistulae is either extrasphincteric or trans-sphincteric. A large anovaginal fistula is usually associated with a significant anterior sphincter defect. Rectovaginal and anovaginal fistulae may be secondary to intersphincteric anal gland sepsis, but more often are secondary to other pathology:

- Mechanical and ischaemic: These factors are often linked. In obstetric trauma, which is globally the commonest cause of rectovaginal fistula, the damage may be from direct tissue disruption or ischaemic pressure necrosis induced by foetal head. Spontaneous stercoral perforation has a similar ischaemic aetiology. Radionecrosis, which is partially an ischaemic problem, can result in a fistula which may be difficult to differentiate from tumour recurrence. Pure mechanical causes include the incorporation of the vagina in the staple line of a coloanal anastomosis.
- Chronic inflammation: Fistulae are associated with Crohn's disease and with tuberculosis. A late pouch vaginal fistula is common if a pouch has been created in Crohn's disease and represents continuing Crohn's inflammation. However, late pouch vaginal fistulae may occur secondary to simple cryptoglandular sepsis, deep pelvic sepsis, or mechanical and ischaemic factors.
- Pelvic sepsis: An anastomotic break down of a coloanal or ileal-pouch-anal anastomosis may present with a rectovaginal fistula. The initial anastomotic leak results in a pelvic collection which then discharges into the vagina, or an infected haematoma discharges both into the vagina, and into the lumen of the bowel through the anastomosis.
- Malignancy: A locally invasive, or recurrent, rectal or gynaecological malignancy may cause a rectovaginal fistula.

Colovaginal fistulae

These fistulae occur when a pericolic abscess secondary to diverticular disease, Crohn's disease or a malignancy discharges into both the vagina and the segment of diseased colon. A sigmoid cancer lying folded down in the pouch of Douglas may form a colovaginal fistula by direct invasion of the vaginal vault. Colovaginal fistulae are more common in those patients who have had a previous hysterectomy.

Surgery of anal fistulae

Examination under anaesthetic, with gentle insertion of probes to define the tracks, remains an important manoeuvre, despite increasing sophistication of preoperative and intraoperative imaging. Care must be taken not to create an additional internal opening by forcing the probe from a blind extension through the muscle and mucosa in the belief that there must be an opening in that position (Fig. 23.13). The knowledge that anterior tracks are commonly radial, whereas posterior ones are more often curved, and may be horseshoe in configuration, arising from a midline posterior opening (Fig. 23.12), will make it easier to follow a track. Hydrogen peroxide, or dye, injected into the external opening to produce a bubble, or staining of the mucosa with dye, at the internal opening are still useful additional manoeuvres.

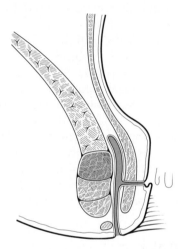

Figure 23.13 *This low intersphincteric fistula has a secondary blind extension up into the supralevator compartment. The probe may miss the internal opening and enter this extension. The probe must not then be forced through the bowel wall at the blind end on the assumption that there must be an internal opening at this point.*

LAYING–OPEN

Laying-open of the track is the simplest definitive surgical treatment of a fistula. A grooved probe is passed along the track, onto which the incision is made through anoderm, skin, fat and distal sphincter musculature to the track itself. The edges are trimmed to marsupialize the track and prevent bridging over during healing. Haemostasis is secured and the wound left open to granulate. This method is only suitable for those situations where an *insignificant* proportion of the anal sphincters will be sacrificed. 'Insignificant' is difficult to define, but the old concept that it was safe to sacrifice the entire internal sphincter, and all of the external sphincter below the anorectal ring, without impairment of continence is no longer accepted. It remains a suitable technique, however, for all subcutaneous fistulae in which no sphincter muscle is cut and for most intersphincteric fistulae, in which the distal internal sphincter will have to be divided but the proximal internal sphincter and the whole external sphincter can be preserved. Laying open is also applicable for a very low trans-sphincteric fistula in which under one-third of the external sphincter is divided, but other techniques should be considered if a greater proportion of the external sphincter will need to be sacrificed. Patients must be warned preoperatively that there may be some deterioration in continence even when only a small portion of the sphincter is divided.

SETONS

A seton is a thread which is introduced along the track of a fistula and left *in situ*. This is a very old method of treatment both in Western, and in traditional Indian, medicine and setons have been used in a variety of different ways which determine the effect they have on the fistula track.[8] Setons have regained popularity recently and are currently used either as a loose draining seton or as a tighter cutting seton.

A fistula probe is first passed through the track. When a grooved fistula probe is used, a slippery thread such as Prolene can be threaded along the groove through the whole track of the fistula. Suture material which will not slide along the groove can be delivered into position by first passing a Prolene suture. The chosen thread is then tied to the Prolene and drawn through the track. Alternatively, a probe with an eye is passed through the track, the seton is threaded through the eye and drawn through the track as the probe is removed.

Loose seton

A loose seton ensures continuous drainage of any discharge and prevents premature closure of the external opening, which is the forerunner of recurrent sepsis. It is frequently a temporary measure to render a track more suitable for definitive treatment. A permanent loose, long-term seton may be the best treatment in some patients in whom more definitive surgery is likely to result in incontinence. Any portion of the primary track, or extensions, outside the sphincters are extensively laid open (Fig. 23.12). Soft braided nylon (e.g. Ethibond) is a suitable material, and is passed through the track as described above, after which the two ends are knotted together outside the anus to form a loose encirclement (Fig. 23.14a). Simple removal of a loose seton after some months of good drainage will result in definitive healing in some patients.

Fibrin glue can increase the percentage of fistulae which will heal after removal of a seton to around 60 per cent. All sepsis must have been eradicated, and therefore a period of loose seton drainage should always precede treatment if there is any significant sepsis. The seton is removed and granulation tissue curetted from the track. The nozzle of the injection kit is introduced into the external opening, and the two solutions of fibrinogen and thrombin are injected simultaneously until a bleb appears at the internal opening. The two solutions mix within the fistulous track and set. The anal retractor should be left in place for around 10 minutes until the bleb solidifies, as it is this plug at the internal open-

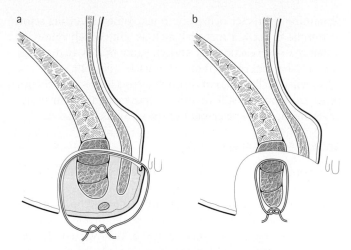

Figure 23.14 *A trans-sphincteric fistula which is not suitable for a simple laying open of the track. (a) A loose seton through the fistula secures good drainage of the sepsis. (b) The fistula can then be treated with a cutting seton. The internal sphincter, anoderm and perianal skin below the track have all been divided and the seton has been tied snug around the external sphincter.*

ing which is critical for success. If treatment is unsuccessful and the fistula recurs, the procedure can be repeated.

Cutting seton

A cutting seton is a definitive treatment of a fistula. A cutting seton works by the slow division of the sphincters which it encircles, and the fistulous track becomes progressively 'lower', until finally the seton falls out. The advantage of the slow division of the sphincter is that only a small length of sphincter is divided at any instance and is prevented from retraction by the intact sphincter above and below. In addition, there is inflammatory tethering of the cut ends of the sphincter muscle. Healing occurs sequentially from above downwards with a narrow fibrous scar which in turn prevents retraction of the fibres of the next portion that is divided. There are, therefore, theoretical advantages over simple surgical laying-open of any trans-sphincteric track in which a significant portion of the sphincter mechanism must be divided. However, some surgeons argue that it merely prolongs the treatment in those in whom laying-open was safe from the onset, and that in those in whom it was unsafe incontinence will not have been avoided.

A period of loose seton drainage should be employed first if there is significant sepsis. The patient is then re-examined under anaesthesia, and the skin, subcutaneous ischiorectal fat and anoderm overlying the track are divided. The internal sphincter is usually divided, although a seton can also be used around the internal sphincter. The track has now been laid open except where it passes through the external sphincter. The surgeon re-assesses what proportion of the external sphincter would be sacrificed if laying-open is to be completed, and makes a final decision on management. As some distal migration of the track is seen even with a loose seton, it may occasionally be judged to have become safe to divide the remaining sphincter below the track. When a cutting seton technique is used, a material such as silk (which causes an inflammatory reaction) is chosen, and this is tied snugly around the external sphincter muscle (Fig. 23.14b). The seton will usually have cut through by 6–8 weeks. If, after this time, the seton is still *in situ* a repeat examination under anaesthesia, and replacement of the seton, is indicated.

ADVANCEMENT FLAPS

These obliterate the internal opening, and allow the fistula to heal. The surgery is technically demanding and performed through the anus. The position of the internal opening dictates the optimal position for surgery; the prone jack-knife position is the more suitable for a rectovaginal fistula, and the lithotomy position the more suitable for a posterior fistula. A flap of mucosa with underlying internal sphincter, which ensures both blood supply and strength, is mobilized and advanced down to cover the internal opening (Fig. 23.15). An alternative is a flap advanced up rather than down. Excellent results can be obtained, but often only by those surgeons performing these operations frequently.

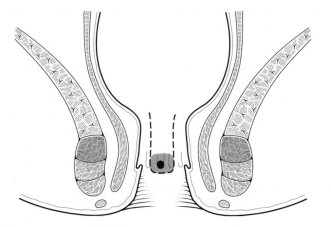

Figure 23.15 *A flap of mucosa, with the underlying internal sphincter, is mobilized and brought down to cover the proximal track The shaded area which includes the internal opening is excised.*

TRACK EXCISION

A variety of techniques are based on the concept of excision of part, or the whole length, of the mature fistula tract, removing just the core of sphincter muscles through which it passes. This is a difficult operation, and the approach can be either from outside the sphincters or via the intersphincteric plane. Success is probably dependent on the obliteration of the internal opening and the eradication of residual intersphincteric sepsis, rather than the complete excision of the track.

Surgery of rectovaginal fistulae

The true rectovaginal fistula is extrasphincteric, and the anovaginal fistula is either extrasphincteric or trans-sphinc-teric. Simple laying-open techniques are therefore seldom satisfactory, and some form of surgical repair is usually indicated. However, repair is not always possible or is doomed to failure. The surrounding tissue may be either scarred or ischaemic, whether compromised by previous infections, surgery or radiotherapy. There may be malignant invasion. Anovaginal fistulae associated with Crohn's disease are also prone to recur, even after seemingly successful surgery. Long-term loose seton drainage is sometimes of benefit, but has little to offer in a short, wide track with symptoms from faecal contamination of the vagina. Fibrin glue is also less successful in short, wide fistulae. Not infrequently, a patient with a rectovaginal or anovaginal fistula which cannot be repaired has to decide whether their symptoms are sufficiently severe that they would prefer to have a colostomy.

If repair is to be undertaken, an anal advancement flap, performed in the prone jack-knife position, is suitable for most small anovaginal fistulae. Larger, higher, true rectovaginal fistulae above the sphincters are more easily approached per vaginum or from the perineum, with the patient in lithotomy. Very high rectovaginal fistulae, and colovaginal fistulae, are approached from the abdomen. There are several planes between the vaginal and the rectal mucosa which can be entered from the perineum. For all surgery in this area surgeons must understand in which planes they are working, or damage to sphincters is inevitable. An intersphincteric dissection is appropriate for a small low fistula, but it is easier to extend the dissection more proximally for a higher fistula if an extrasphincteric approach is chosen. The choice of approach depends on access, the size and height of the fistula, the condition of local tissues and often, most importantly, the plane in which the surgeon feels most confident.

Post–partum anovaginal and rectovaginal fistulae

These are common in the developing world. They are mostly associated with prolonged or difficult deliveries, but they fall into three distinct categories:

- The first is the result of a 4th degree perineal tear, and the anal sphincters are also disrupted. The emergency sphincter repair (described below) is combined with repair of the anal and vaginal mucosa. The tissue is healthy, and immediate repair has a good chance of success. However, if the deeper aspects of such a repair fail the patient may be left with healed perineal skin between the anal and vaginal orifices but an anovaginal fistula above, which is usually associated with significant anterior sphincter disruption.

- The second is a tear above an intact perineum. The anal sphincters may be damaged or intact, and there may have been no significant perineal skin tear to alert the birth attender to the significant deeper damage. These fistulae are usually diagnosed a few days after delivery at the time of the first bowel movement.

- The third variety is encountered almost exclusively in areas remote from obstetric intervention. A woman has laboured unsuccessfully for days with a deeply engaged head and pelvic outlet disproportion. Eventually, a stillborn child is delivered but only after ischaemic pressure necrosis has occurred within the maternal pelvis. The most common damage is to the bladder against the pubis, and a vesicovaginal fistula forms (see Chapter 26). In more severe cases there is additional ischaemic pressure necrosis of the posterior vaginal and the anterior rectal wall, and a rectovaginal fistula develops. The perineal skin and anal sphincters are frequently undamaged. The diagnosis may be delayed for a week or more and only become apparent as necrotic tissue sloughs.

The repair of these fistulae depends on the time of presentation and whether a sphincter repair is also required. Unless the repair can be performed within 24 hours of delivery, a delay of 2–3 months will be advisable, and a defunctioning stoma may be required in the interim. A small fistula associated with a disrupted sphincter is best approached from the perineum, and a ring retractor to which skin hooks are attached is invaluable. A larger, higher fistula is easier to repair per vaginum. The edges are excised and then each layer repaired separately starting with the rectal mucosa. Extensive dissection above the fistula, and laterally in the plane between the vagina and rectum, increases tissue mobility and enhances the chance of success. The vaginal suture line should be positioned, if possible, so that it lies to one side of the rectal closure. Interposition of tissue between the mucosal suture lines is highly desirable. An anterior levatorplasty will achieve this, or alternatively a Martius flap can be used. In the injuries following pressure necrosis tissue loss may be extensive and an abdominal approach may be necessary to bring down colon to form a neorectum.

LOCAL FLAPS

These provide tissue for interposition in the closure of rectovaginal fistulae. A *Martius flap* consists of the fat pad of a labium majus with the underlying bulbocavernosa muscle, mobilized on a posterior pedicle containing the perineal branch of the pudendal artery. It is dissected out through a labial incision with the patient in lithotomy. It is swung through a subcutaneous tunnel to lie over the rectal closure (Fig. 23.16). Alternatively, an island of skin with underlying fat, fascia and muscle can be cut from the perineal groin crease. Its deep attachment is preserved to maintain blood supply, and it is then tunnelled under the lateral perineal skin to lie between the anus and vagina as a spacer (Fig. 23.16). These techniques are particularly important when there is a large fistula with associated tissue loss from pressure necrosis, or when the blood supply of the tissues is poor from previous surgery or radiotherapy. Flap operations will be disappointing in the hands of the occasional operator, and referral to those with a special interest is recommended.

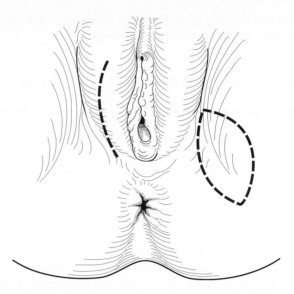

Figure 23.16 *Separation of the suture lines is desirable in the repair of vaginal fistulae. Local flaps can be utilized. A Martius flap consists of the bulbocavernosa muscle and fat elevated from the labium majus. The posterior pedicle is retained. This flap reaches with ease for a vesicovaginal fistula repair but can also reach for a rectovaginal fistula repair. An alternative flap can be obtained from the perineal groin crease.*

CROHN'S ANUS

Anal tags and fissures, recurrent anal sepsis and fistulae-in-ano are common in patients with Crohn's disease. In some patients, the anal pathology is incidental to their Crohn's disease, and no histological evidence of Crohn's inflammation is found in anal biopsies. Treatment follows the same principles as outlined above. In other patients the anus is involved in the Crohn's disease, and in these cases there may be associated Crohn's proctitis or the rectum may be spared. Intensive medical treatment, with antibiotics and immune modulation, is frequently very effective, at least in the short term. Surgical treatment of these fissures and fistulae should be as conservative as possible, and the underlying pathology must not be ignored. For example, a Crohn's fissure is a deep inflammatory ulcer and not a mechanical tear, and a Crohn's fistula has granulomatous inflammation along it in addition to bacterial infection. Attempts at flap advancement techniques will usually fail, and great reliance is placed on loose setons to prevent recurrent sepsis.

A colostomy diversion may bring some temporary relief but seldom long-term gain after reversal. A permanent colostomy without proctectomy does not prevent the continuing perineal sepsis. Many patients eventually require proctectomy, either for recurrent sepsis, or for incontinence which may in part be due to iatrogenic sphincter damage during attempts at surgical treatment. The prognosis is worse in those patients who have rectal involvement, particularly if there is an anorectal stricture or supralevator induration. Healing of the perineum after a proctectomy for anorectal Crohn's may be very protracted.

SURGERY OF THE SPHINCTERS AND PELVIC FLOOR

Careful preoperative sphincter assessment, both anatomical and physiological, is essential prior to any surgery for incontinence. Anatomical disruption of the external sphincter can be repaired with good short-term results, but longer follow-up shows deterioration in continence over time. Surgical repair of the internal sphincter is less satisfactory. Poorly functioning, but intact, sphincters are also a common cause of incontinence. Operations to shorten lax sphincters by plication, or to increase pelvic floor support by approximation of the levator muscles, have generally been disappointing. Plication of the levators behind the anus has the added theoretical advantage of restoring the anorectal angle, but the functional benefit is often only temporary.

The decision to operate is relatively straightforward if the patient has a complete external sphincter disruption and major incontinence. Many, however, have only impaired continence, and investigations confirm a partial tear. If a surgical repair is undertaken, but breaks down, the patient may have continence inferior to the preoperative level. The patient must therefore be aware of the risks and limitations of surgery.

The surgery is precise, and good operative conditions are essential with the patient positioned in either the lithotomy or prone jack-knife position. Access for an assistant is often limited, especially in lithotomy, and some form of mechanical retraction is often superior. A ring retractor to which tissue hooks can be fixed at multiple sites on the circumference with varying degrees of tension is ideal. However, the hooks are designed for single usage and this method of retraction is thus expensive.

Emergency sphincter repairs

These are most commonly performed by gynaecologists as part of the deeper perineal muscle repair of an episiotomy or tear in childbirth. Operative conditions are seldom ideal, and the extent of the damage to the external sphincter may not be appreciated. Despite this, many heal satisfactorily.

When major sphincter damage is associated with a perineal tear that extends to the anal verge and into the anorectum, the severity of the injury is recognized at delivery. A general surgeon with experience in perineal surgery should be involved in the primary repair whenever possible. The repair should be undertaken under optimal operative conditions some hours after delivery. Working from the vagina, with the patient in the lithotomy position, all layers starting with the anorectal mucosa are identified, cleaned of faecal contamination and anatomically approximated. A defunc-

tioning stoma will give the best chance of good healing if the anorectal mucosa is torn, but the patient may be reluctant to consider this. Similar principles apply to traumatic sphincter damage from perineal impalement injuries.

The occasional patient presents several days or weeks after delivery with an obvious sphincter disruption as part of an episiotomy which has broken down, and this may even be associated with the development of an anovaginal or rectovaginal fistula. Secondary repair should be delayed for some months as all tissue will be too friable for a satisfactory repair at this stage. If there is a significant rectovaginal fistula or complete incontinence, faecal diversion with a temporary colostomy may be required in the interim.

Elective sphincter repair

Elective repair of an external sphincter defect is most often undertaken months or years after major sphincter damage sustained in childbirth or during anal surgery. The incision is made just outside and parallel to the anal sphincters at the site of the defect (Fig. 23.17). Dissection proceeds in the

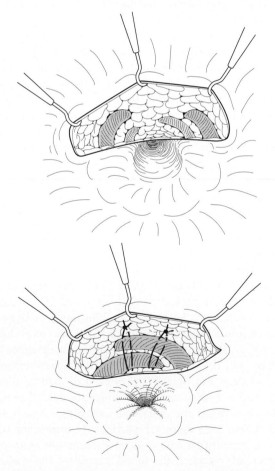

Figure 23.17 *External sphincter repair. A curved incision is made just outside the pigmented perianal skin. The ruptured ends of the sphincter are identified in the fat, mobilized and repaired with overlap.*

extrasphincteric plane until the sphincters are defined. The divided sphincter ends will have retracted circumferentially, but will also be displaced laterally from their normal position. The external sphincter twitches when touched with diathermy, whereas there is no response from perineal scar tissue nor the internal sphincter. This sign can be very useful in a difficult operation. Dissection is continued to mobilize the external sphincter over about one-third of its circumference. Any fibrous connection between the disrupted muscle fibres is divided, but not excised. An overlap repair is then performed with non-absorbable Prolene or a long-acting dissolvable suture (Fig. 23.17). An infected haematoma is a potential cause of breakdown of the repair, and both meticulous haemostasis and antibiotic prophylaxis are important. A repair will often have changed the orientation of the skin incision from transverse to longitudinal, as the anatomical configuration of the perineum is restored, and the skin should be closed in the axis in which it lies most naturally. A small portion of the wound should be left open to facilitate free drainage of any serosanguinous collection. Postoperatively, antibiotics and stool softeners are continued.

Lateral defects in the external sphincter are less common than anterior defects, and are more often iatrogenic in aetiology. Repair is complicated by the lateral innervation of the sphincters and nerve damage during the dissection is a risk. A nerve stimulator to identify the neurovascular bundle may be helpful.

INTERNAL SPHINCTER REPAIR

This is often unsatisfactory and is seldom attempted in isolation. In major disruption of both sphincters the whole sphincter complex may be overlapped as a single unit. It is, however, usually possible to identify the internal sphincter as a separate entity and it is then preferable to repair it separately. It is a thin sheet of muscle which can be sewn with a continuous suture. Prolene sutures so close to the anoderm cause irritation, and a long-acting absorbable suture is preferable.

Collagen injections deep to the internal sphincter are a simple method of producing an anal cushion and improving resting anal tone in passive incontinence associated with a poor internal sphincter.[9]

Further perineal repairs

LEVATORPLASTY

Levatorplasty consists of the plication of the levator muscles either behind (*posterior levatorplasty*) or in front (*anterior levatorplasty*) of the anus. The approach is through the extrasphincteric plane. Two or three non-absorbable interrupted sutures are placed to approximate the muscle. The operation in isolation is generally disappointing in the long term, and is now most often employed in combination with a sphincter repair.

RECTOCELE REPAIR

This surgery is carried out both by gynaecologists and coloproctologists. There is a defect in the rectovaginal septum, and the rectum herniates into the vagina above the sphincters. The initial disruption is almost exclusively associated with childbirth, and although it occurs in isolation it is also seen in association with a complete, or partial, anterior sphincter disruption. Many large defects are symptomless, but some patients complain of a lump in the vagina on straining, and symptoms of obstructive defaecation. Surgical opinion varies as to the benefit of repair. Repair can be undertaken transvaginally, transanally or through the perineum. A satisfactory approach with good exposure is illustrated in Figure 23.18. A transverse perineal incision is made immediately posterior to the vagina, and the plane dissected deep to the posterior vaginal wall as far as the upper extent of the rectocoele. The vaginal wall is then divided vertically and the dissection carried laterally to expose the extent of the rectocoele. Great care must be taken not to enter the rectum which has to be pushed posteriorly.

Some surgeons have good long-term results with either simple plication of the posterior vaginal musculature or rectal wall plication. Most, however, favour some form of additional support between the rectum and vagina to prevent recurrence. Ideally, the rectovaginal septal defect is defined and repaired. Unfortunately, the rectovaginal septum cannot normally be identified as a layer suitable for a strong sutured repair, and extra strength can only be obtained by deep sutures to draw the levator muscles into the midline from

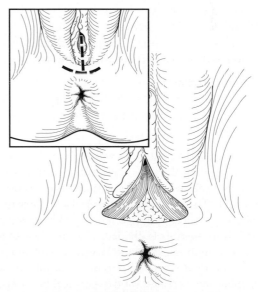

Figure 23.18 *Repair of a rectocele. A transverse incision just posterior to the vagina is later extended by a vertical division of the posterior vaginal wall. The rectum is pushed posteriorly, and deep sutures are used to draw the puborectalis portion of the levators across between the vagina and rectum. The muscle is easier to feel than see as it is covered with fascia and lying within fibro-fatty tissue.*

either side (Fig. 23.18). A vaginal ridge, or undue narrowing of the vagina, can be caused by this levatorplasty if too much tissue is drawn in. Care must be taken to avoid this as it results in dyspareunia. The vaginal mucosa and perineal wound are then closed and a vaginal pack for local pressure reduces the risk of a haematoma. A mesh repair would be ideal, but the infective complications of mesh introduced through the perineum are prohibitive. A mesh can, however, be used in the rectovaginal septum for support on the occasions where additional pathology has made it more appropriate to perform the rectocele repair from above.

The irreparable sphincter

Unfortunately, many patients with incontinence cannot be helped by sphincter surgery. Sphincter damage may be too extensive, previous repairs may have failed, or the underlying cause may be denervation from a pudendal neuropathy or a spinal injury. An anus with no functioning sphincter is in essence a perineal colostomy to which no stoma bag can be attached, and unless the patient has a very predictable bowel pattern they will almost all be better served by an end colostomy. Antegrade enemas via a continent Malone stoma (see Chapter 22, page 433) is a preferable alternative for some patients,[10] and others may wish to explore the still mainly experimental options outlined below. These procedures should only be performed by those with a special interest and expertise.

Permanent sacral nerve stimulation

This procedure is showing promise. It is the least invasive alternative, and success can be predicted by trial of temporary stimulation.[11] The technique is probably only suitable for those patients with some demonstrable pudendal nerve conduction and at least partially intact sphincters.

Artificial anal sphincters

These are associated with both defaecatory difficulties and late failure, but they should be considered for patients to whom a stoma is abhorrent:[12]

- *A stimulated gracioplasty*, in which a gracilis muscle is wrapped around the anus, can restore continence. An implantable electric stimulator is necessary as otherwise the wrap of fast twitch fatiguable muscle fibres functions merely as a stenosing device. The distal insertion of gracilis into the tibia is divided. The muscle is mobilized through a thigh incision, and swung up subcutaneously into the perineum, where a circum-anal subcutaneous tunnel has been created via two perineal incisions. It is then wrapped around the anal canal and fixed to the contralateral ischial tuberoscity. A similar operation has been tried using gluteus maximus.
- *Artificial implantable mechanical sphincters* may be a valuable future modality, but they are still beset with problems. Infection and extrusion occur and, in addition, high pressures, which can cause ischaemic

damage to the anorectal mucosa, are required to maintain continence.

RECTAL PROLAPSE

The number of operations designed to treat rectal prolapse is a reflection of the difficulties that surgeons experience in securing good long-term results. Both abdominal and perineal approaches to this condition have been extensively explored.

Abdominal rectopexy

This procedure was considered to be the 'gold standard' for the treatment of full-thickness rectal prolapse. The rectum is mobilized out of the sacral hollow and fixed to the pelvic brim with non-absorbable sutures. Success is increased by adding a high anterior resection to the operation – a *resection rectopexy*. Mesh placed behind the rectum, or as a sling around the rectum, has generally fallen out of favour due to infectious complications and evacuatory dysfunction. Enthusiasm for the abdominal approach is waning as it is a major procedure for a benign condition, especially as most patients are elderly and frail. Many surgeons who favour an abdominal approach are now performing the surgery laparoscopically. Rectal prolapse is uncommon in young patients, but when surgery is indicated an abdominal rectopexy probably places the autonomic nerves and sexual function in unnecessary danger, which is difficult to justify for benign pathology.

Perineal approaches

Perineal approaches for rectal prolapse are regaining popularity. The postoperative pain is minimal and the surgery is well tolerated, even by the very elderly who are often fit for discharge home within a few days. The simplest operation of placing a circumferential subcutaneous *Thiersch wire* around the anus to narrow it was extremely successful in preventing prolapse, but faecal impaction above the iatrogenic anal stenosis was a major problem, and the operation was largely abandoned. The *Altmeier* and *Delormes* operations are now the standard perineal procedures for rectal prolapse.

Both operations are performed in the lithotomy position. The prolapse is encouraged to prolapse to its full extent by gentle retraction of the rectal wall out through the anus. A series of six to eight sutures are passed both through the skin at the anal verge and through more distant perineal skin. Once tied, they will evert the anal canal and form a simple means of retraction. Alternatively, a self-retaining ring retractor with skin hooks as described above may be preferable. A dilute solution of adrenaline (1:400 000) is injected submucosally into the outer tube of the prolapse and the mucosa incised circumferentially with diathermy 1–2 cm above the dentate line for a Delormes' operation, and 1 cm or so higher for an Altmeier's operation.

DELORMES' OPERATION

This consists of removing the mucosa from the whole prolapsed segment of bowel, followed by re-attachment of the proximal mucosal edge, with the underlying muscle of the bowel wall, to the initial circumferential incision just above the dentate line. Diathermy dissection in the adrenaline-filled submucosal plane can be relatively bloodless. Initially, the detached mucosa is lifted in forceps, or rolled over a finger, to display the plane for dissection (Fig. 23.19a). The dissection is usually commenced anteriorly and the plane followed around each side to the posterior aspect of the prolapse. Difficulty will be encountered if the initial circumferential incision was not completed posteriorly as the tethered mucosa will fail to lift and will tear. As the dissection reaches the apex of the prolapse, the mucosa forms a sleeve which can be retracted to facilitate dissection on the inner surface of the prolapse (Fig. 23.19b). Further adrenaline can now be injected into the submucosal plane of the inner tube. When no further mucosa can be prolapsed, the dissection is complete.

Some form of plication suture should be placed in the denuded muscle of the bowel wall. This may be done by sep-arate deep sutures before mucosal apposition, but it is also satisfactorily achieved if the first four sutures for mucosal apposition also pass through multiple points in the muscle (Fig. 23.19c). It is important that mucosa does not retract, and the first three sutures should be in place before the mucosal tube is completely divided. Once all four sutures are in place they are tied, and the muscle tube is reduced back inside the anus as a bulky ring. The ends of these initial sutures are left long and held in forceps so that retraction can facilitate the positioning of later sutures. A further 8–12 sutures completes the mucosal apposition. Each suture should include the muscle immediately deep to the mucosa for adequate strength, but no further deep plication is attempted. An absorbable suture which retains tensile strength for a few weeks is suitable, and Vicryl is commonly used. The first sutures, which include the muscle plication, need to be heavier and stronger than the subsequent sutures, which are solely for mucosal apposition. The anal verge retraction sutures are cut, or the skin hooks detached, and the suture line retracts within the anus.

ALTMEIER'S OPERATION

This is a perineal rectosigmoidectomy. The initial steps of the operation are similar to the Delormes' operation, but the circumferential mucosal incision is a little higher and is

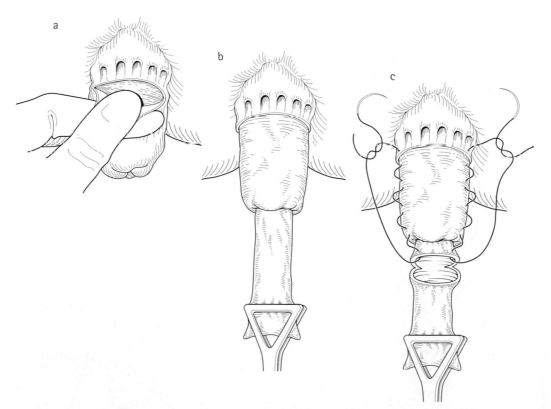

Figure 23.19 *Delormes' procedure. (a) A circumferential incision is made through the mucosa 1–2 cm above the dentate line. The mucosa is separated off the underlying bowel wall. It is easily torn, and rolling it over a finger may be gentler than holding it with forceps. (b) The mucosa forms a tube once the dissection reaches the apex of the prolapse. (c) The lateral plication sutures include several bites of prolapsed muscle wall. In this diagram they are also forming the initial mucosal apposition sutures. (The anterior suture has been omitted from the drawing.)*

deepened through the full thickness of the bowel wall. This division is safely above the anal sphincters if the initial mucosal incision is placed correctly 2–3 cm above the dentate line. The prolapsed rectum then unfolds and is drawn out further through the anus as a single full-thickness tube along with its mesorectum. Anteriorly, a pocket of peritoneum in the rectovaginal pouch is also prolapsed (Fig. 23.20). In a Delormes' operation the surgeon is not specifically aware of this but in an Altmeier's operation it must be entered and any small bowel loops replaced into the abdomen. Posteriorly, the mesorectum is drawn down with the rectum, and is separated from it by multiple ligations of mesorectal vessels close to the rectal wall. The dissection is continued until further bowel is reluctant to prolapse. An initial division of part of the circumference of the bowel allows the first sutures of the anastomosis to be secured as it is important at this stage that the bowel does not retract up into the pelvis. The initial four sutures can be left long and used for retraction to facilitate the placement of the remaining sutures. In contrast to a Delormes' operation, the sutures are not merely to achieve a mucosal apposition but to form a full-thickness low coloanal anastomosis, and a defect in it could result in leakage and pelvic sepsis. However, the frequent leaks, and major associated morbidity, encountered in coloanal anastomosis after an abdominal resection of the rectum for cancer are not a feature of Altmeier's procedure, possibly due to the retained mesorectum filling the pelvis.

Post-operative prognosis

Patients with rectal prolapse often have poor anal sphincters. The prolapse itself causes further stretching and laxity, and most patients are at least partially incontinent preoperatively. Some improvement can be expected with surgery, but the increased perianal muscle bulk after a Delormes' operation is an added advantage. A perineal operation can only deal with bowel that is already able to prolapse, and a high recurrence rate has disheartened some surgeons. However, the operation can simply be repeated a few years later, and this may be preferable to a major abdominal operation.

PERINEAL APPROACHES TO THE ANUS AND RECTUM

The surgery for primary pathology of the anus is almost exclusively performed from below, either transanally or through the perineum, and has already been described. However, the anus may have to be excised for a low rectal carcinoma, and abdominoperineal resection is described in Chapter 21. When restorative surgery is possible, a hand-sewn coloanal anastomosis may be required. In a proctocolectomy for ulcerative colitis, the mucosectomy and hand-sewn ileal pouch-anal anastomosis is performed transanally. These procedures are described in Chapter 22.

The rectum may also be approached surgically solely from below.

TRANSANAL APPROACHES

A transanal approach is routinely used for endoscopic snare removal of benign polyps throughout the colon. In addition, direct surgical access through the anus allows surgical excision of benign tumours in the rectum. It may be possible to deliver a mobile polyp out through the anal sphincters (Fig. 23.21). A higher, more broad-based villous lesion will have to be removed *in situ* through a proctoscope, or anal bivalve retractor. Access is inevitably restricted as excessive anal dilation must be avoided. Elevation of the lesion off the underlying muscle by a submucosal injection of 1 in 400 000 adrenaline may be helpful in reducing bleeding and in identifying the optimal plane. A full-thickness excision can achieve complete removal of even a T2 rectal cancer, but the possibility of lymph node metastases will not have been

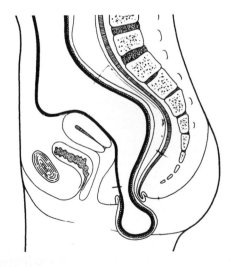

Figure 23.20 *Anteriorly a rectal prolapse includes a prolapsed Pouch of Douglas. An understanding of this is essential in an Altmeier's operation.*

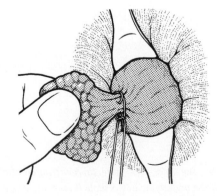

Figure 23.21 *Excision of a rectal polyp. It may be possible to prolapse a polyp on a stalk out of the anus for resection.*

addressed. This makes the technique unsuitable except in the limited circumstances that are discussed in more detail in Chapter 22. A mucosal defect is usually closed with absorbable sutures, and it was believed that this was mandatory if a full-thickness excision had been performed. However, it has now been shown that even a full-thickness defect below the peritoneal reflection can safely be left unsutured.[13]

Transanal endoscopic microsurgery (TEM)

This is a recent technical advance which enables more precise surgery to be undertaken up to around 15 cm from the anal verge. Specially designed small instruments are manipulated through the ports of an operating sigmoidoscope.[14]

York Mason approach

The York Mason approach to the rectum combines transanal access with a posterolateral approach. The patient is placed in the prone jack-knife position and a posterolateral incision is extended up from the anal verge. The bowel is incised in line with the skin incision from the anal verge upwards so that the anus and lower rectum can be opened out. The divided anal sphincters and the bowel wall are re-sutured on completion of the procedure. Excellent exposure of the anterior rectum is obtained, but the damage to the sphincters is rarely justified.

POSTERIOR APPROACHES

The posterior approaches to the rectum, the posterior pelvic floor and the retrorectal space may be posterolateral between the sacrum and the pelvis, transverse between anus and coccyx or through the midline posteriorly. All of these approaches share the problem of limited access to the rectum itself, but afford good access to the retrorectal space, as may be required for the excision of a benign developmental cyst. If the anococcygeal ligament is divided to improve access, it should be re-attached at the end of the operation or the contractions of the puborectalis sling will simply displace the anus forwards and be less effective. When a posterior incision is used for rectal access there is the additional problem that the approach is through the mesorectum and the lymphatic fields of drainage of any malignancy will be traversed.

The Kraske or sacral approach

This is a midline posterior approach to the rectum. The skin incision is deepened onto the surface of the coccyx and lower sacrum. The muscle attachments to the sides of the coccyx are freed, and the anococcygeal raphe incised in the midline from the tip of the coccyx to the external sphincter (Fig. 23.22). The coccyx is excised, and if access is still insufficient, the 5th and 4th sacral vertebrae can be partially nibbled away in the midline. The 3rd sacral nerve should be preserved. Waldeyer's fascia is then incised and the posterior mesorectum exposed. After completion of surgery, Waldeyer's fascia is closed and the anococcygeal ligament and the muscular attachments to the coccyx approximated.

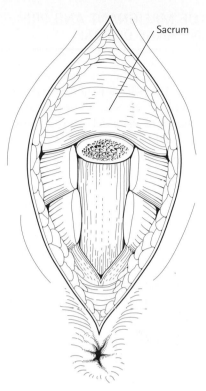

Figure 23.22 *The Kraske posterior approach. The muscles have been separated from their attachments to the coccyx, the anococcygeal raphe has been incised in the midline and the coccyx removed. Waldeyer's fascia is exposed.*

PERINEAL EXCISION OF THE RECTUM

This is now considered to be an inappropriate operation for any malignant rectal lesion, as adequate excision of the lymphatic drainage is not possible without abdominal access. In the standard abdominoperineal resection for a low rectal cancer, a variable portion of the dissection is undertaken from below in a plane outside the anal sphincters. However, the radical lymphadenectomy is performed from above (see Chapter 21).

Rectal excision for benign disease can be undertaken solely from the perineum when, for example, the colon has already been excised, the patient has an end colostomy, and there is no other reason to re-enter the abdomen. The intersphincteric plane is entered at the anal verge, and the mobilization continued as a close rectal dissection to remove the bowel tube but to leave the anal verge skin, the external sphincter and the pelvic floor musculature intact, in addition to retaining the mesorectum *in situ*. This approach is suitable for a short rectal stump, but there is a risk of damage to small bowel loops adherent within the pelvis. The Altmeier operation is in effect a 'close' rectal excision from below, but the intersphincteric plane is entered above the sphincter mechanism, and not in the intersphincteric groove at the anal verge.

SURGERY OF MALIGNANT AND PRE-MALIGNANT ANAL DISEASE

An anal cancer may be either an adenocarcinoma or a squamous carcinoma. The behaviour and management of the two tumours are very different. A preoperative biopsy for histology is therefore essential prior to any planning as differentiation is not possible clinically.

An **adenocarcinoma** arising in the mucosa of the upper anal canal and anorectal junction behaves like an adenocarcinoma of the rectum and the treatment is primarily surgical. Direct extension, however, will occur early into the sphincter muscles and to obtain adequate clearance an abdominoperineal excision is usually inevitable except in very early tumours which are still mobile on the external sphincter (see Chapter 21).

Squamous carcinomas arising from the squamous epithelium of the lower anal canal have a different behaviour and pattern of spread. Treatment is now primarily by chemoradiotherapy, and surgery is confined to a diagnostic biopsy, and possibly a defunctioning stoma during treatment if local symptoms are severe. Those that show only a partial response to chemoradiotherapy, or relapse after completion of treatment, may come to salvage surgery consisting of an abdominoperineal excision. An inguinal node clearance may also be indicated as a salvage procedure. The disease, or the treatment, may destroy the anal sphincters and in these patients a permanent left iliac fossa end colostomy is usually the best solution.

Anal intraepithelial neoplasia (AIN) appears as a patch of abnormal epithelium at the anal verge, or in the perianal skin. Clinical suspicion is confirmed by biopsy, or complete excision if the area is small. Mild degrees of dysplasia can be watched, but severe dysplasia amounting to carcinoma *in situ* should be excised, as progression to invasive carcinoma is a significant risk.

PILONIDAL SINUS SURGERY

This apparently minor condition can present the surgeon with major challenges. Many of the standard surgical procedures are associated with a significant risk both of delayed healing and of recurrent disease. The initial pathology is of one, or more, tiny deep midline pits in the natal cleft which connect with a granulation tissue lined cavity, lying in the subcutaneous fat and containing loose hairs. Recurrent infections occur in this cavity which later extends under apparently normal skin, both in the natal cleft and laterally into one or both buttocks. Minor infections may settle on antibiotics but if an abscess develops it will discharge or require drainage. The underlying disease remains however and repeated episodes of infection are likely.

When the disease is confined to the midline, one option is to *excise* the affected area and close it in an attempt to achieve primary healing. When this fails a large wound then has to granulate. Even if primary healing is successful, the patient remains at great risk of recurrent disease as there is now a midline scar deep within the natal cleft through which hairs may penetrate with greater ease than through undamaged skin.

The alternative of *deroofing* all sinuses, clearing hairs and granulation tissue and leaving the wound open for secondary healing has the advantage that the total tissue defect is smaller than that where an excision and primary repair has broken down. It is also a feasible operation when the disease extends laterally and primary closure would not be possible. The disadvantages though are of slow healing and, even if this proceeds without complication, it will be at least 6 weeks before the wound has filled and epithelialized. During the healing period the granulating wound must be kept clean, any loose hairs must be removed, and the surrounding skin kept shaved. All heal with a wide midline scar which is vulnerable to recurrent disease, and despite meticulous postoperative attention the occasional patient develops a persistently unhealed midline wound.

Recent advances in treatment have focused on the avoidance of a midline scar.[15,16] The two flap techniques described below have proved very successful for advanced pilonidal disease, but are unnecessarily extensive for the early minor disease for which the authors favour a modification and simplification of the original Bascom procedure.

MODIFIED BASCOM PROCEDURE

This is an ideal operation when there are no midline unhealed wounds, abscesses or scars. The patient lies prone and local infiltrative anaesthesia is satisfactory. The buttocks are strapped apart. Each pit is excised with the pointed no. 11 blade, removing a diamond-shaped piece of skin no larger than a rice grain, but to include the epithelialized portion of the pit which extends down for 2–3 mm. An incision of 2–3 cm in length is then made approximately 2 cm from the midline. A probe introduced into a pit may act as a guide as to which side to make this lateral incision if there is no other evidence of previous lateral infection. The incision is positioned so that it is alongside the area of the cleft in which the puncti are present (Fig. 23.23). This incision serves three functions. First, it is used to enter the sinus system and curette out all hairs and infective granulation tissue. Second, through it the midline skin is released from its tethering to the post sacral fascia, and the depth of the natal cleft is reduced. Third, as the incision is left open, it relieves any tension on the subsequent closure of the pits.

The buttock strapping is then removed to relieve tension and each pit excision closed with a 5/0 subcuticular nylon suture. The remaining steps described in the original Bascom procedure are omitted, in which a fibro-fatty flap is rotated under the midline skin. A wick soaked in iodine is simply tucked into the lateral wound so that it lies under the midline, and is removed after 48 hours. A course of antibiotics is

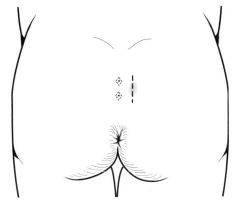

Figure 23.23   *A Bascom procedure. The lateral incision is alongside the midline clefts, and is over the scar of any previous lateral abscess. Each pit is excised with a 'diamond' of skin which must include all the epithelialized portion of the pit. The pit excisions are closed with fine subcuticular sutures and the lateral incision is left open.*

given, the pit closure sutures are removed at 1 week, and healing of the lateral wound is usually complete by 2 weeks. Obliteration of the pits is achieved and each leaves only a midline wound of a couple of millimetres in length. If there is recurrence and more radical surgery is indicated, the scars are within the area of skin which will be excised in either of the flap procedures described below.

KARYDAKIS FLAP

In this procedure an ellipse of skin and underlying fat down to the deep fascia is excised. The ellipse is parallel to, but 2 cm from, the midline. It must be at least 5 cm in length as there is increased tension on closure of a short ellipse. The medial side of the incision should just cross the midline and should encompass all the diseased midline tissue (Fig. 23.24a). In extensive natal cleft disease a very long ellipse may thus be required, but this does not create any problem. However, when there are bilateral sinus extensions it may not be possible to excise all diseased tissue with this technique. The ellipse must be symmetrical, and the surgeon must resist the temptation to cut the lateral part of the ellipse less generously in an attempt to remove less tissue, as this only results in the scar failing to lie away from the midline. The whole length of the medial side of the incision is then mobilized by undercutting a distance of 2 cm at a depth of 1 cm (Fig. 23.24b). In thin patients the undercutting incision is at the junction of the fat and deep fascia. Any strapping to distract the buttocks is now removed. The first sutures are placed between the limit of the undercutting incision and the deep fascia in the midline (Fig. 23.24c). These draw the flap over and recreate a new shallow midline sulcus. Pressure from an assistant to unroll the flap as the sutures are tied will reduce tension. A vacuum drain and a second layer of more superficial fat sutures are then inserted, and finally the skin is apposed with interrupted non-

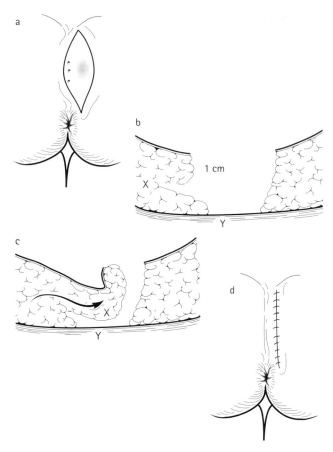

Figure 23.24   *Karydakis flap. (a) The long axis of the ellipse is parallel to the midline and 2 cm from it. The length of the ellipse must be such that the medial side of the ellipse crosses the midline to include all diseased midline tissue. The lateral side of the incision must be planned so that the ellipse is symmetrical. (b) An undercutting incision is made along the whole length of the medial side, 1 cm below the skin surface. This undercut should be extended out for 2 cm. (c) The medial flap is unrolled and advanced over the midline. Deep sutures are placed between points X and Y. (d) The final scar is not in the midline.*

absorbable sutures. The wound lies a few centimetres from the midline, and the patient has a new shallow natal cleft with healthy unscarred skin (Fig. 23.24d).

LIMBERG FLAP

For this operation the patient is placed prone and the buttocks are strapped apart. A rhombic area of skin and subcutaneous fat is excised which includes both the midline pits and any lateral sinus extensions (Fig. 23.25). The long axis of the rhomboid is in the midline and its shape determined by angles of 60 degrees at **A** and **C** and 120 degrees at **B** and **D**. Accuracy is essential for success, and the rhomboid of tissue to be excised and the flap must be measured and marked with indelible pen at the start of surgery. Planning with angles is difficult and the following linear measurements will portionally shorter and less oblique than in the adult. The testis is commonly retractile in childhood, and may be withdrawn intermittently into the inguinal canal or even into the abdomen by cremasteric muscle contraction.

INDIRECT INGUINAL HERNIAE

The *sac,* or peritoneal tube through which the abdominal contents protrude, accompanies the spermatic cord in its oblique course through the inguinal canal. The neck of the sac, which is often constricted, lies at the deep inguinal ring, lateral to the inferior epigastric vessels (Fig. 24.1a). The sac is enclosed within the coverings of the cord and lies anterior to the vas and testicular vessels. Many of these herniae are congenital, but may remain as an empty sac for many years and present in adult life. Sliding indirect herniae also occur where a variable portion of the herniated tissue is extraperitoneal (see Chapter 12).

DIRECT INGUINAL HERNIAE

A direct inguinal hernia traverses only the medial part of the inguinal canal, and does not, therefore, pursue the oblique course taken by the spermatic cord. It protrudes from the abdominal cavity through the posterior wall of the inguinal canal medial to the inferior epigastric vessels (Fig. 24.1b). It seldom descends completely into the scrotum. The sac may be narrow-necked and protrude through a small posterior wall defect. More often, it is wider at its neck than at its fundus, and is little more than a bulging of the peritoneum as it protrudes through a wide defect. The hernia lies behind the spermatic cord and is covered by a thin stretched fascial layer derived from the edges of the defect.

SELECTION FOR SURGERY

Treatment of inguinal herniae should be advised for all that carry a significant risk of strangulation. Herniae which are difficult to reduce, and all herniae in infancy are in this category.

Wide-necked direct herniae which reduce spontaneously, immediately on lying down, are very unlikely to strangulate. Many of these herniae are asymptomatic and, if the patient is elderly and an operation would entail a significant risk, there is little justification for surgery. Repair is, however, recommended for the majority of herniae in younger people, as, even if they are asymptomatic and unlikely to strangulate, the natural history is of increase in size.

Incarcerated (irreducible) herniae should always be considered for repair unless the risks of surgery are exceptional. Certainly any hernia which has only recently become irreducible is at high risk of progression to strangulation. Some long-standing but uncomplicated irreducible herniae may be left alone if not symptomatic.

Herniotomy

This involves simple ligation and division of the neck of the sac. It is a satisfactory procedure for the congenital indirect

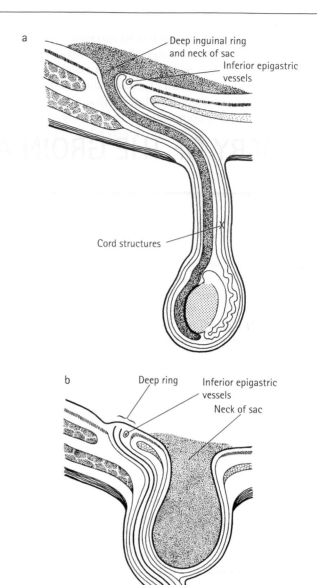

Figure 24.1 *(a) An indirect inguinal hernial sac traverses the oblique lie of the inguinal canal which it enters through the deep ring lateral to the inferior epigastric vessels. It lies within the coverings of the cord anterior to the vas and vessels. Note the narrow neck of the sac. (b) A direct inguinal hernia enters the inguinal canal through a posterior wall defect medial to the inferior epigastric vessels. It lies behind the cord and its coverings. Note the wide-necked sac.*

sacs encountered in infancy, childhood and adolescence. It is also probably all that is required in some young adults with a congenital indirect sac and good inguinal canal musculature. Most surgeons, however, favour some form of posterior wall repair even in young adults, and all would agree that the risk of recurrence after simple herniotomy is unacceptably high in the middle-aged and elderly. A recurrent inguinal hernia is almost always direct whether the initial hernia was direct or indirect. Although the deep inguinal ring remains a point of potential weakness, as it cannot be closed unless the testis is removed, a recurrent indirect hernia is rare.

Herniorrhaphy

This implies some form of repair or re-enforcement of the posterior wall of the inguinal canal. The posterior wall of the inguinal canal can be approached through the canal, and this is the most common route for repair. A pre-peritoneal approach from above the inguinal canal is preferred by some surgeons for bilateral repairs, and for recurrences. This is now the favoured approach for a repair by minimal access techniques and is considered superior to the transperitoneal laparoscopic herniorrhaphy.

A great number of methods of repair of the inguinal canal have been employed over the past 120 years. Hernia recurrence appeared to be related more to the individual surgeon than to the method of repair employed, and only recently have large multi-centre trials established that the most secure method, independent of surgeon bias, is either the *Lichenstein mesh* repair or the *Shouldice* repair if an open method is used.[1]

Extraperitoneal laparoscopic hernia repair compares favourably with open repair and the debate continues as to whether it should replace open herniorrhaphy as the treatment of choice.[2,3] In expert hands the complications and recurrence rates are comparable with standard open-groin repairs, but postoperative pain is reduced. It requires a general anaesthetic, a high level of laparoscopic expertise, and the cost of disposable laparoscopic instruments is high. It is, however, a particularly useful technique for bilateral and recurrent herniae.[4]

Adult inguinal herniotomy

This may be a simple herniotomy, or the first stage of a herniorrhaphy. General, regional or local infiltrative anaesthesia is suitable.

The classic incision is made 2.5 cm above and parallel to the medial three-fifths of the inguinal ligament, but a more horizontally placed skin-crease incision will produce a more acceptable scar. One or more superficial epigastric veins cross the line of incision in the subcutaneous fat and require ligation. Diathermy coagulation may be sufficient, but there is possibly a risk of haemorrhage a few hours later. The incision is deepened until the aponeurosis of external oblique is exposed. The superficial inguinal ring, through which the cord emerges, is identified. The external oblique aponeurosis is divided in line with its fibres, the incision being placed so that it opens into the upper part of the superficial ring (Fig. 24.2a). Forceps are applied to the two cut edges, and both leaves elevated. The ilio-inguinal nerve can usually be identified and preserved.

The cord, with its coverings, is lifted up from the medial part of the incision, and spread out on the finger (Fig. 24.2b). The coverings are incised longitudinally, and separated off the underlying cord. The sac appears as a pearly-white structure, lying anterior to the main components of the cord. It is most easily identified at the fundus, the crescentic border of which lies transversely across the cord, and is picked up and held in artery forceps (Fig. 24.2c). The cord must also be inspected in this way when a direct hernia is repaired as an additional indirect sac is not infrequently present. The cord structures are then separated from the sac as far as the neck. Sharp dissection, with scissors or diathermy, or blunt stripping with a swab are acceptable techniques. Care must be taken in all methods to avoid injury to the testicular vessels. The vas is also vulnerable to inadvertent division as it often lies separate from the other cord structures, closely applied to the sac. A Lane's forceps around the cord structures is useful both to safeguard them and to provide counter-traction (Fig. 24.2d). Dissection continues until the neck of the sac is exposed.

The sac should then be opened, some distance from the neck, to ensure that it is empty. A finger inside the sac can also be used to feel for an excessively thick medial or lateral wall which could represent an additional sliding component to the hernia. Tension on the sac then allows a transfixion suture to be placed immediately above the neck (Fig. 24.2e). Care must be taken that underlying bowel is not transfixed. The sac is then amputated 1 cm distal to the ligature and, if the dissection has been adequate, it will retract inside the deep ring. If no repair is deemed necessary the external oblique is closed, and the skin sutured.

The alternative approach to the cord for a simple herniotomy is through an incision in the external oblique which leaves the superficial ring intact. Access is more limited, but the advantage is less disturbance to the anatomy and function of the inguinal canal. This approach is particularly favoured by paediatric surgeons, and is described below.

Scrotal hernia

In a scrotal hernia, where the fundus of the sac may not come easily into view, there is no contraindication to leaving the distal part of the sac *in situ*. The sac is separated for a short distance from the cord structures, and is then divided transversely. The distal part is dropped back, while the proximal part is cleared up to its neck and removed in the usual fashion. This method obviates the dissection required to deliver the sac from the depths of the scrotum, and greatly reduces the risk of postoperative haematoma.

Sliding hernia

A sliding hernia contains tissue which lies outside the peritoneal sac. This may be extraperitoneal fat, sigmoid colon, caecum or bladder. If the associated sac is small and the situation is fairly obvious, there is no necessity to excise the sac and the abdominal contents are merely replaced before repair of the hernial defect. On other occasions, the bowel or bladder forms one wall at the neck of a large sac, and is in danger of injury if not recognized. Only a partial sac excision is then possible, the remaining extraperitoneal tissue being simply replaced into the abdominal cavity before the posterior wall repair. However, it is sometimes possible to release whole posterior wall of the canal and extend around the deep ring. There is no tension, and sutures are only used to prevent early displacement before tissue ingrowth secures it in position. A Prolene running suture holds the lower edge of the mesh to the inguinal ligament. An additional four to five sutures will prevent rolling of the edges of the mesh, and can hold the cut edges of the mesh together again around the cord at the deep ring (Fig. 24.4). No suture should be placed through the periosteum of the pubic tubercle. Previously, when repairs commonly included this stitch it was a frequent cause of late groin pain.

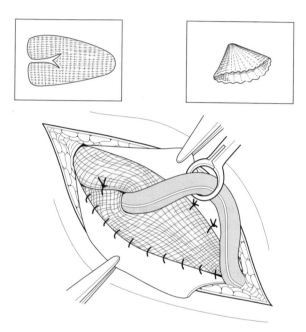

Figure 24.4   *A right mesh herniorrhaphy. The mesh is cut to the shape of the posterior wall. It should extend medially beyond the pubic tubercle, and laterally beyond the deep ring. A continuous suture attaches the mesh to the inguinal ligament. A few additional sutures prevent rolling up of the edges. The insets show a mesh plug and the shape of mesh required to cover the whole posterior wall. Note the slit to allow the mesh to be lain around the deep ring.*

BASSINI REPAIR

The original repair developed by Bassini during the 1880s emphasized the importance of the reconstitution of the transversalis fascial layer of the posterior wall of the inguinal canal. However, the modified operations which bore his name had a high recurrence rate.[6] Often, the repair was performed too superficially and failed to repair the transversalis fascia, the sutures merely opposing the muscle fibres of internal oblique to the inguinal ligament. Tension was recognized as a potential problem when a true transversalis fascia repair was performed. The vertical release of the anterior rectus sheath, the *Tanner slide*, was a useful later modification which reduced tension on the repair (Fig. 24.5).

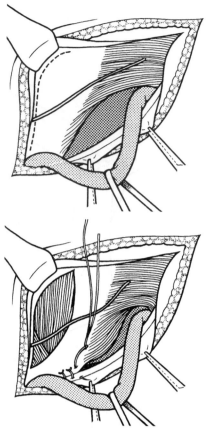

Figure 24.5   *A left herniorrhaphy in which a Tanner slide is illustrated. A vertical incision has been made in the anterior rectus sheath to reduce tension in a Bassini repair.*

SHOULDICE REPAIR

This repair is a development and refinement of the repair described by Bassini in which a reconstruction of the posterior wall is performed.[7] Recurrence rates of under 1 per cent are reported. It is a difficult repair to perform to the original specifications, and modifications are often associated with poor results. After the posterior wall has been cleared of the cremaster muscle, the wall is divided medially from the deep ring throughout its length. The posterior wall is then closed with a four-layer overlapping technique, but a modification to two layers is simpler and is also satisfactory. The overlapping closure both strengthens the posterior wall and tightens the internal ring. Continuous non-absorbable sutures are used, and although it is not a tension-free repair any tension is widely distributed.

NYLON DARN REPAIR

After the posterior wall has been cleared and any direct defect closed, an alternative to a mesh is a re-enforcement of the posterior wall with a monofilament nylon darn. The darn should be loosely laid in the muscle and must not draw the tissue together. It must cover the whole posterior wall, and no significant gaps should be left between fibres, or small narrow-necked direct herniae may occur between strands of the darn. Recurrence rates overall are high except for those surgeons whose darns are so dense that they resemble a mesh. The technique has been generally abandoned in favour of mesh repairs.

Pre-peritoneal inguinal hernia repair

This approach is particularly useful for bilateral herniae when a double incision can thus be avoided, and for recurrent herniae where it avoids the necessity of dissection within a scarred inguinal canal. The sac is approached at its neck where it is ligated and divided. The remainder of the sac can be left *in situ* if it does not deliver easily. A fascial defect can be satisfactorily repaired from within, but this is not always necessary as any mesh will be in the ideal position between the peritoneum and the muscle wall, against which it is held by intra-abdominal pressure. Some sutures or staples are, however, usually still employed to prevent rolling or displacement of the mesh in the immediate postoperative period. A pre-peritoneal approach can be either open or laparoscopic.

OPEN APPROACH

A transverse incision is made two finger-breadths above the pubic tubercle and deepened through the anterior rectus sheath. The rectus muscle is then retracted laterally to expose the inferior epigastric vessels, which are ligated and divided. After division of these vessels it is possible to enter the correct plane on the peritoneum and sweep this up to deliver the tongue of peritoneum which is entering the hernial orifice. The hernial sac is ligated at its neck, and the mesh is then laid across the defect. It can be easily tethered anteriorly before the peritoneum is allowed to return to its normal position supporting the mesh against the undersurface of the abdominal wall.

LAPAROSCOPIC TOTAL EXTRAPERITONEAL PROCEDURE (TEP)

A pre-peritoneal workspace is created with balloon distension, after which the further deperitonealization of the abdominal wall is continued by dissection. The initial entry into the pre-peritoneal space can be made by open entry into the medial edge of the ipsilateral rectus sheath just below the umbilicus. The rectus muscle is displaced laterally to enter the plane between the rectus muscle and the posterior sheath. The balloon trocar is introduced and advanced. At the lower edge of the rectus sheath it enters the pre-peritoneal plane. Two secondary ports are introduced and dissection continued until the neck of the sac is exposed. The inferior epigastric vessels are visible and are a useful landmark. After the inversion of the peritoneal sac of a wide direct defect, or the ligation of the neck of a narrow indirect sac, the dissection continues until a sheet of mesh can be laid behind both the inguinal and femoral canal. The mesh is introduced through a port, unrolled into position and most surgeons elect to tether the mesh with sutures or staples. There is the potential for injury to the inferior epigastric, the testicular and the external iliac vessels. This is now the standard laparoscopic technique and has virtually replaced the earlier transabdominal pre-peritoneal procedure (TAPP).

Inguinal hernia repair in specific circumstances

EMERGENCY INGUINAL HERNIA REPAIR

Emergency repair is necessary when strangulation is present or imminent. An irreducible hernia is always suspect, and if it has become irreducible only in recent days it should be considered in danger of strangulation and treated urgently. The issues involved in strangulated herniae in general are discussed in Chapter 22. A strangulated inguinal hernia should be approached through the groin. The first priority is the release of the strangulated contents, and their resection if they are infarcted. An indirect hernia is strangulated by the narrow peritoneal tunnel at the neck of the sac (see Fig. 22.2, page 410). A direct hernia is constricted by the edge of the transversalis fascial defect. The hernia is then repaired by one of the methods described above. In the presence of strangulated bowel the operation field is inevitably contaminated with bacteria. A mesh is at increased risk of becoming infected, and surgical opinion is divided as to whether mesh should be avoided in these circumstances.

RECURRENT INGUINAL HERNIAL REPAIR

The dissection in the inguinal canal may be straightforward or very difficult due to the presence of dense adhesions. The surgeon must be aware that the cord will lie very superficially if the external oblique was closed behind the cord. This was a common technique at one time to increase the strength of the posterior wall. Damage to the cord is much more likely in a recurrent repair, and possible orchidectomy, or late loss of the testis, should be discussed with the patient preoperatively. A mesh repair is almost mandatory in a recurrent hernia. The pre-peritoneal approach – either open or laparoscopic – should be considered, as it avoids the scarring within the inguinal canal.

A recurrent hernia occasionally occurs through the prevascular space in front of the femoral artery and vein. Safe dissection may require the division of the medial end of the inguinal ligament. It is reattached after the sac has been dissected off the vessels and the peritoneum closed.

INGUINAL HERNIA REPAIR IN THE FEMALE

The operation in the female is essentially the same as in the male, except that the round ligament can be divided and the internal ring obliterated during the repair.

AMBULATORY SURGERY

Eric Farquharson had a particular interest in ambulatory hernia surgery. This followed a more general interest in groin herniae and the mechanical and biological principles of repair. He believed in the importance of a strong external oblique and the obliquity of the inguinal canal to allow intra-abdominal pressure to hold the canal closed. He therefore condemned the then common practice of closing the external oblique behind the cord to give extra strength to the posterior wall. Instead, he performed a double-breasted external oblique repair to take up any laxity in the stretched aponeurosis. When a Bassini repair could not be performed without tension, he employed a darn using a strip of fascia lata, or a skin ribbon cut from the wound edges. Many of these techniques are now only of historical interest, and although described in detail in early editions must now be omitted.

Eric Farquharson's interest in ambulatory hernia surgery[8] was revolutionary at a time when patients were confined to bed for between 2 and 4 weeks after hernia repair. Same-day discharge after surgery during the 1950s was only practical after local anaesthetic techniques, but is now equally appropriate after general anaesthesia. All of the groin repairs described above can be performed on adult patients under local anaesthesia.

Local anaesthetic hernia repair

This is specifically indicated when a general anaesthetic is believed to carry a significant risk, and it is particularly well tolerated in the elderly. Diathermy and blunt dissection are more likely to cause pain than sharp scissor dissection, and care should be taken to avoid traction on the cord, or peritoneum, which can provoke bradycardia and arrhythmias. The incision should always be of adequate length to avoid excessive retraction, and gentleness is essential. A variety of anaesthetic agents and techniques are in use but the formula described below is satisfactory.

A solution of 0.5 per cent lignocaine with adrenaline is first prepared using the standard 1 per cent solution of lignocaine with 1 in 200 000 adrenaline. This is mixed with equal volumes of normal saline. Initially, 5–10 mL of this dilute solution is injected immediately under the intended skin incision, and a further 5 mL into the deeper subcutaneous fat in the lateral third of the wound. Anaesthesia occurs almost immediately, and the skin incision is made and extended down to the external oblique at the lateral end of the incision. A further 5 mL of the local anaesthetic is injected just deep to the external oblique aponeurosis at this point and left while the rest of the wound is extended down to external oblique. Small nerves run alongside the veins which have to be ligated in the subcutaneous fat, and before clamping these a further 1 mL of local anaesthetic may be required. The external oblique is then opened and the operation continued in the normal manner. The peritoneum is sensitive, and a few millilitres of anaesthetic should be injected at the neck of the sac before transfixion. Further local anaesthesia is also often required around cremasteric vessels. Bupivicaine can be mixed with lignocaine for postoperative pain relief or injected separately towards the end of the operation. When bupivicaine is used on its own, the delay in action has disadvantages.

Bupivicaine injected during surgery under general anaesthesia provides excellent postoperative analgesia for the ambulatory patient. Effectiveness is improved by injecting the bupivicaine at the start rather than after completion of surgery.

Inguinal herniotomy in a child

Surgery of infantile herniae should not be delayed as the risk of incarceration and subsequent strangulation is high.[9] The risk is highest in babies aged under 6 months, and at this age the initial presentation may be with a strangulated hernia. In infants and children an inguinal herniotomy is sufficient and no repair is necessary. The herniotomy can be performed as described above for an adult hernia, but as no repair is to be performed, there is an argument for disturbing the shutter mechanism of the inguinal canal as little as possible and preserving an unscarred superficial ring. Three approaches to the neck of an indirect sac which do not divide the superficial inguinal ring are described below.

Hydroceles are common in infancy, and many resolve by spontaneous obliteration of the processus vaginalis. Surgery is therefore normally postponed until the child is 2 years old. Encysted hydroceles of the cord are less common and seldom resolve spontaneously. The operation for an infantile hydrocele is the ligation and division of the proximal end of the processus vaginalis, and is thus the same operation as that for an infantile hernia.

THE LOW OPERATION

The cord is approached outside the superficial ring. A skin crease incision 2–3 cm in length is made just above the pubic tubercle (Fig. 24.6a). The incision is deepened through the membranous layer of superficial fascia, which is a significant layer at this age and may cause confusion if it is mistaken for the external oblique. Veins in the fat can be safely coagulated. Once the external oblique aponeurosis is defined, the lower edge of the wound is retracted and the cord identified just outside the superficial ring. If difficulty is encountered, traction and release of the testis will usually help to identify the cord moving in the fat. The cord is then gently delivered into the wound along with its coverings. An artery forceps passed beneath it will hold it securely on the surface under light traction. Alternatively, a vascular sling can be passed under the cord, as shown in Figure 24.6(b). The coverings are incised longitudinally. These include the cremaster muscle, which is frequently thick and hypertrophied in association with an infantile hernia. Artery forceps are placed on both cut edges and act as retractors to enable the surgeon to enlarge this incision in the correct plane and to separate the cord from its coverings. It is then possible to lift the cord free and pass another artery forceps under the isolated cord and

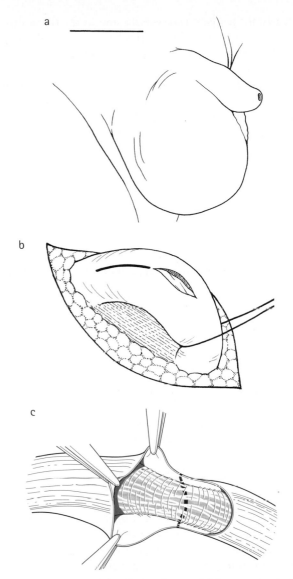

Figure 24.6 *A right infantile herniotomy. (a) A transverse incision above the pubic tubercle. (b) The cord and coverings are identified outside the superficial ring and delivered up into the wound. The coverings are incised and lifted off the cord structures. (c) A thin, wide-necked sac may have to be dissected from within. The vas and vessels are visible through the undivided segment of sac, which must be separated from them very gently.*

allow the coverings of the cord to fall back into the wound. It is important to have haemostasis assured before allowing this tissue to retract.

The sac is then identified. A short sac is lifted in its entirety off the vas and vessels. A long scrotal sac is separated from the vas and vessels sufficiently to allow transection. The distal sac is left *in situ* and the dissection restricted to the proximal portion of the sac. The isolation of an *infantile hernial sac* may be extremely difficult as it is often wide and gossamer thin, with the cord structures spread over the surface. Delicate unhurried dissection with fine instruments and good light is essential. Ideally, the cord structures are teased

off the unopened sac which can be held between finger and thumb. However, this is not always possible and the surgeon may find that the sac has been entered and that the dissection has to be completed from within. In this situation, two-thirds of the diameter of the sac is free of cord structures and is divided transversely, with fine artery forceps being applied to the proximal cut edge. The remaining third has to be dissected off the underlying cord structures. This is difficult due to the extreme delicacy of the thin-walled sac (Fig. 24.6c). Once the circumferential division is complete, the proximal sac is ready for dissection off the cord.

A single artery forceps can now be placed on the isolated proximal sac and gently retracted away from the cord structures. An Allis forceps around the vas and vessels provides useful counter-traction. Fine areolar strands are divided and the sac separated from the cord as far proximally as is possible. The dissection can be carried up to the neck of the sac without opening the short inguinal canal of a pre-school child. When the sac is transfixed, divided and released it will retract through the canal to lie inside the deep ring. Great care must be taken to avoid inclusion of vas or vessels in the transfixion stitch.

The identification and isolation of a *narrow persistent processus vaginalis* is usually straightforward. It appears as a pale, thin-walled, translucent tube of 1–2 mm diameter. The testicular vessels appear blue and the vas, although of similar diameter, can be identified as a palpable cord. The processus is picked up and divided. Hydrocele fluid empties from the distal cut end. In the less common encysted hydrocele of the cord it is preferable to follow the distal cut end and excise the cystic swelling, but in the more common hydroceles around the testes the distal end is simply dropped back into the wound and left *in situ*. The proximal end of the patent processus is transfixed after the same dissection as for an infantile hernia.

THE 'HIGH' OPERATION

The cord is approached within the inguinal canal through an incision in external oblique. A skin crease incision is made over the deep inguinal ring and the external oblique is opened in the same line. This incision is only 1–2 cm in length, and is not extended to the superficial ring. The internal oblique is then split at its junction with the cremaster muscle. The cremaster muscle and the internal spermatic fascia are then opened to expose the sac and the structures of the cord which are lifted forwards into the wound. Thereafter, the dissection is similar to that in the low operation.

THE PRE-PERITONEAL OPERATION

The skin incision can still be placed inconspicuously as for the low operation but must be longer. After incision through Scarpa's fascia the upper flap is raised off the external oblique for 2–3 cm. A transverse muscle-splitting incision is then made through external oblique, internal oblique and transversus. The neck of the sac is then approached from above, by dissection deep to the abdominal wall muscles. The transversalis fascia must be divided to ligate the sac flush with the parietal peritoneum. It can either be divided before the dissection, and lifted with the rest of the abdominal wall, or left to support the thin peritoneum during dissection and divided only once the sac has been identified in a more superficial plane.

INGUINAL HERNIOTOMY IN THE FEMALE CHILD

In the young girl, or baby, an ovary or the fimbrial end of a fallopian tube can prolapse into the sac. The ovary is frequently irreducible and may be mistaken preoperatively for a lymph node. Inguinal herniae are common in testicular feminisation syndrome, and sex chromosomes should be checked in female children with inguinal herniae. The operation is similar to that in the male, but the sac is easier to dissect in the absence of fine cord vessels to be safeguarded. Care must still be taken to avoid injury to a herniated ovary or tube, which must be returned into the peritoneal cavity.

INCARCERATED INFANTILE INGUINAL HERNIAE

An incarcerated hernia can usually be reduced by sedation of the baby, followed by gentle manual reduction. The contents are most commonly loops of small bowel, or an ovary. If non-operative reduction is achieved surgery should ideally be delayed for 48–72 hours to allow the oedema to settle. Further delay risks recurrent strangulation. A pre-peritoneal approach may be preferable when there has been a recent episode of strangulation as it avoids the need to dissect a friable oedematous sac. Emergency herniotomy is essential if reduction is not achieved. At operation, the reduction is usually straightforward and a simple herniotomy is all that is required. The infantile gonad is more vulnerable to strangulation than the bowel and subsequent testicular infarction is not uncommon. Infarcted bowel requiring resection is rare. When bowel cannot be reduced at operation and viability is in doubt, it is very difficult to release and repair the neck of the peritoneal sac in the same fashion as in an adult. An additional separate laparotomy approach may be the safer option (see Chapter 22). If a resection and anastomosis is indicated, it can also be performed more satisfactorily by this approach, as it is difficult to return an anastomosis through the small deep ring.

FEMORAL HERNIAE

Femoral herniae occur almost exclusively in adult women in whom the femoral ring is wider. They are rare in men and in children. However, in both sexes and at all ages, femoral herniae are less common than inguinal herniae.

Anatomy

The *femoral canal* is the medial of the three compartments of the femoral sheath which is formed by a prolongation into the thigh of the fascia transversalis and of the fascia iliaca, which line respectively the anterior and posterior abdominal walls. The lateral compartment of the sheath contains the femoral artery, and the intermediate one the femoral vein. The internal orifice of the femoral canal is the *femoral ring*. It is relatively rigid as it is bounded anteriorly by the inguinal ligament, posteriorly by the pectineal line of the pubis and the pectineal ligament which lies along it, and medially by the free edge of the lacunar ligament. Laterally, it is bounded by the femoral vein. The ring is normally occluded by a pad of fat containing lymphatic tissue.

The hernia descends through the femoral canal and then turns forwards through the saphenous opening in the fascia. The cribriform fascia, which covers the opening, is thinned-out in front of it. The hernia may then turn upwards and laterally to overlie the inguinal canal. The femoral ring is narrow and many herniae are irreducible from the time of presentation. Potential for strangulation is high and surgery should be advised.

The 'low' operation

The incision is made 1 cm below and parallel to the medial portion of the inguinal ligament. A lipoma-like swelling is immediately encountered covered with thin fascia (Fig. 24.7). Dissection around this leads to the femoral canal, and confirms that it is a femoral hernia and not a lipoma. The actual sac is often surprisingly small and is deeply embedded in the condensed fatty tissue contained within the stretched cribriform fascia. The sac is isolated by incision into these tissues. It is freed to its neck, then opened at the fundus and any viable contents returned to the abdominal cavity. Omentum is often adherent to the sac and requires to be separated. Alternatively, if it is free at the neck but adherent at the fundus, the adherent portion can be removed with the sac. When the neck of the sac is constricted by a tight femoral ring, so that the return of contents is difficult, the ring may be gently dilated by a finger passed upwards outside the sac. The ring can be released by an incision medially into the lacunar ligament but an aberrant vessel on its surface will occasionally cause troublesome bleeding. Temporary division of the medial end of the inguinal ligament is occasionally justified in very difficult circumstances. The neck of the sac is freed from the margins of the canal, and then transfixed and ligated as high as possible so that it retracts above the canal.

The femoral ring palpated from below feels triangular with a semi-rigid anterior and posterior wall which meet at a very short medial wall. The femoral vein forms the soft lateral wall of the triangle. Complete closure of the femoral ring itself with sutures is seldom possible, as even if the anterior and posterior walls can be pulled into apposition the femoral vein will be compressed and partially occluded. A compromise is the placement of two to four sutures across the ring from the fascia over pectineus muscle posteriorly to the inguinal ligament anteriorly, avoiding sutures in the rigid

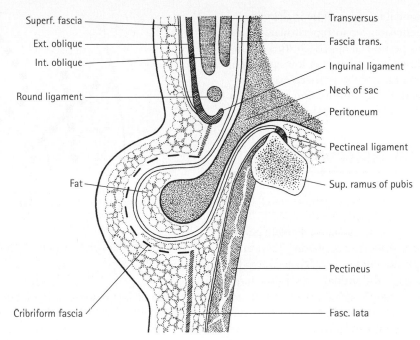

Figure 24.7 *The anatomy of a femoral hernia. The fat beneath the thin cribriform fascia presents at operation as a lipoma-like swelling.*

pectineal ligament itself. A J-shaped needle makes the placement of these sutures easier, and the femoral vein is protected throughout by a finger placed over it. The sutures are all inserted before any are tied, the most medial is then tied first and ligation is continued laterally until it is judged that tying the next suture would compress the femoral vein (Fig. 24.8). Any remaining untied sutures are then removed. A small plug of mesh inserted after transfixion of the sac and before these sutures are placed will give extra security, but recurrence of femoral herniae is surprisingly uncommon.

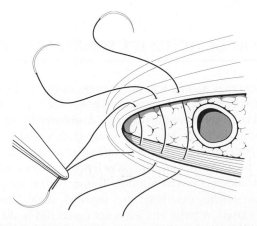

Figure 24.8 *Left femoral hernia repair. Sutures placed between the inguinal ligament and the fascia overlying the pectineus muscle close to its attachment to the pubic bone can be used to obliterate the femoral ring.*

The 'high' operations

There are several operations described which all involve approaching the neck of the sac from above, through the pre-peritoneal plane. The advantages include a higher transfixion of the peritoneum and better access for closure of the femoral ring. It is therefore a better approach for a recurrent hernia and a sheet of mesh can be used to occlude the ring. The pre-peritoneal approach described above for inguinal hernia repair is suitable. The two older classical approaches both have major disadvantages.

- The *Lotheisen* approach is through the conjoint tendon in the medial part of the inguinal canal, which is inevitably weakened.
- The *McEvedy* approach is via a vertical skin incision which is deepened through the lower part of the anterior rectus sheath near its lateral border. The rectus muscle is displaced medially. Superficial wound healing across the groin crease may be troublesome.

Proponents of the 'high' approaches claim they are superior in the strangulated case. However, viable bowel can be released from within the sac from below and returned to the abdomen, and infarcted omentum can be excised from below. When infarcted bowel is encountered it may not be possible to draw healthy tissue down through the femoral ring for the resection. It is therefore usually necessary to divide the strangulated loop within the peritoneal cavity and then to remove the gangrenous loop from below. Even if a resection and anastomosis has been achieved from below, the bulky anastomosis may be impossible to replace through the femoral ring. An additional lower midline incision or an iliac fossa muscle-cutting incision for intraperitoneal access is satisfactory. A 'high' pre-peritoneal approach thus has little benefit unless the peritoneum is opened. A low approach, even in a strangulated femoral hernia, is therefore recommended. In a difficult situation the combination of this with a small laparotomy incision will provide optimum access.

INGUINAL LYMPH NODE DISSECTION

Anatomy

The *superficial inguinal nodes* form a horizontal group below the inguinal ligament and a vertical group along the upper 5–8 cm of the great (long) saphenous vein. They drain the superficial tissues of the lower abdominal wall, lower limb and perineum. The *deep inguinal nodes*, three or four in number, lie along the proximal end of the femoral vein and in the femoral canal; they drain the deep tissues of the lower limb. The superficial and deep nodes drain into the external iliac nodes.

Excision biopsy

An excision biopsy of an inguinal node is undertaken for histological diagnosis. An enlarged node may be selected, or a *sentinel node* identification technique may be employed, as described in the section on malignant melanomas in Chapter 1.

Inguinal node dissection

This is undertaken as a potentially curative operation when malignant spread is believed to be only to these nodes. It can also be used as a palliative procedure to gain local control of a malignancy. It must be remembered in both scenarios that the division between inguinal and external iliac nodes, which are in direct continuity, is artificial. Malignant melanoma and squamous cell carcinoma of the anus, vulva and penis are tumours in which this operation is most likely to be considered. There is significant morbidity following radical inguinal node excision. Complications include skin breakdown because of poor blood supply to skin flaps, subcuticular lymph collection despite postoperative vacuum drainage, and late lymphatic oedema of the lower limb.

Operative procedure
The skin incision may be oblique, vertical or curved (Fig. 24.9). Skin flaps must then be elevated so that all but the most superficial subcutaneous fat can be excised from the groin. The upper limit of this excision is 5 cm above the inguinal ligament, where a transverse incision is made through the fat to expose the external oblique. All fatty, fascial and nodal tissue is then stripped off the aponeurosis down to the level of

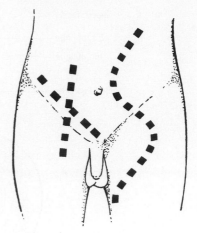

Figure 24.9 *Incisions for a radical inguinal node dissection.*

the inguinal ligament, securing superficial vessels crossing the field. Distally, a skin flap is raised so that the long saphenous vein is exposed. If the saphenous vein is to be removed with the nodes, it is ligated and divided between ligatures at least 10 cm below the inguinal ligament. Its stump is then turned upwards together with all the surrounding fat and lymph nodes. Some surgeons preserve the vein in an attempt to reduce lower-limb oedema, but the subcutaneous tissue must still be divided at the same level to remove all the fat and lymph nodes. The partially separated tissue is then stripped from the inguinal ligament from the lateral to the medial side. If the long saphenous vein has been divided, it is divided again at its junction with the femoral vein, and small arteries arising from the femoral artery are also divided. The femoral vessels are exposed and all fatty and nodal tissue is cleared away from the medial side of the femoral vein and from the femoral canal. Haemostasis is secured and the skin flaps closed over vacuum drains through which lymphatic drainage is usually substantial and may persist for some weeks. The operation may be combined with a further dissection of the iliac nodes, as discussed in Chapter 15.

SURGERY OF THE TESTES, SCROTUM AND CORD

This surgery is mainly within the remit of the urologist, or paediatric surgeon, but some overlap between specialists is inevitable. In children, the surgery is dominated by the treatment of testicular maldescent. A truly *undescended testis* lies in the path of descent; in the abdomen, inguinal canal or scrotal neck. An *ectopic testis* has left the normal path of descent and is most commonly found in the superficial inguinal pouch, overlying the inguinal canal, deep to Scarpa's fascia. A testis which has not descended to the scrotum rarely has satisfactory spermatogenesis, and histological deterioration can be demonstrated from early childhood. If the baby is full term it is unlikely that spontaneous descent will occur after 2 months of age, and surgical correction should be undertaken as soon as it is reasonable to do so. The surgeon should, however, be aware that the incidence of testicular atrophy after an orchidopexy may be higher when the operation is carried out at a younger age. The age for operation will also depend on the local provision for paediatric anaesthesia, but where facilities are good, operation is often undertaken before 2 years of age. By 1 year of age all but 0.9 per cent of testes are in the scrotum, but after that time the cremasteric reflex develops and care must be taken to distinguish a normally descended, but retractile, testis for which no treatment is indicated.

Orchidopexy

This is the operation to mobilize a maldescended testis and bring it into the scrotum. A groin exploration is suitable when the testis is palpable. The incision is made over the inguinal canal and deepened to expose the external oblique. Retraction allows identification of the external ring. An ectopic testis, or one in the scrotal neck, can be delivered into the wound and held between finger and thumb. This may also be possible at this stage for a testis which can be milked along the inguinal canal and held as it emerges from the superficial ring. However, a small high testis, lying near the deep ring, may only become apparent once the canal is opened. A gubernacular attachment down to the scrotum may be an obvious band, and the testis must be released from this. The external oblique is divided in a similar manner as for a hernia repair but the incision must be carried 1–2 cm lateral to the deep ring to allow sufficient access for the later dissection. Gentle traction on the testis demonstrates the fibres of cremaster which are holding it and release of these usually gives significant extra length (Fig. 24.10a). The testis is now free except for its attachments through the internal ring – the vas, testicular vessels and a hernial sac, if present.

The peritoneum must now be dissected off the cord. On occasion, it is only a small thick-walled knuckle lying on the anterior surface of the cord. Artery forceps are applied to it and as it is lifted forwards, the plane is developed behind it (Fig. 24.10b). This plane is essential for the final dissection behind the deep ring. This small sac is then transfixed and excised. Unfortunately, this surgically easy hernia is usually only encountered at orchidopexy in children aged over 4 years, and orchidopexy is now recommended between the ages of 1 and 3 years. A wide, thin-walled sac extending as far

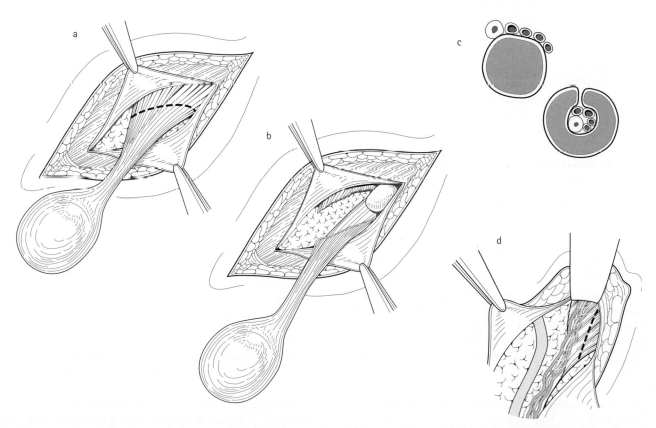

Figure 24.10 *Left orchidopexy. (a) The external oblique is incised. The testis is retracted anteriorly and the cremasteric fibres divided. (b) The small knuckle of peritoneum on the surface of the cord at the deep inguinal ring must be lifted and dissected off the cord. (c) The sac is commonly thin-walled and wide-necked. The cord structures may be spread out over its surface or even enclosed within a peritoneal fold. (d) Retraction of the deep ring displays the avascular lateral bands to the testicular vessels which must be released. Insufficient lateral release of the external oblique will restrict access. The vas can be seen to be turning medially away from the vessels.*

as the testis, and often further into the scrotum, is common at this earlier age. The cord structures may be spread out over it, as described in the surgery of infantile herniotomy above. Alternatively, the cord appears to be running in the free edge of a testicular mesentery (Fig. 24.10c). In both of these situations delicate dissection to isolate and close the sac, whilst preserving the gonadal vessels and vas, is essential.

Once the peritoneum, or sac, has been released from the cord, lateral retraction of the deep ring, as the testis is held medially under gentle tension, will demonstrate avascular filmy bands of tissue lateral to the testicular vessels (Fig. 24.10d). Division of these strands produces a significant increase in length, and it is then usually possible for the testis to reach a normal position in the scrotum. Any limiting factor is almost always insufficient testicular vessel length and therefore the manoeuvre described of division of the inferior epigastric vessels to allow a straighter course for the vas is usually unhelpful.

A subcutaneous tunnel to the scrotal skin is created by the surgeon's finger, or a small swab held in forceps; a scrotal skin incision is made and a pocket created between the dartos muscle and the skin (Fig. 24.11a, b). An artery forceps is then passed up through the otherwise intact dartos into the main wound, and is used to draw the testis down. Care must be taken to avoid torsion. The testis is eased through the small hole in the dartos muscle which will prevent postoperative displacement of the testis out of the scrotum. The scrotal skin is then drawn over the testis and closed with absorbable sutures. One suture can be passed through the capsule of the testis if the dartos is not forming a snug hold on the testis, but this manoeuvre is no longer recommended as it may be associated with a higher incidence of infertility and testicular malignancy.[10,11] A testis which cannot be brought down fully can still be placed in a dartos pouch. The scrotum will pucker upwards, but no damaging traction on the vessels will occur. Improvement in position will continue for at least a year and a further exploration after this time may be beneficial if the testis is still high.

Alternative approaches for orchidopexy are similar to those described for herniotomy in childhood. A high approach through the external oblique directly onto the deep ring, with preservation of the superficial ring, is favoured by some surgeons. The cord is lifted upwards and an incision through the transversalis fascia at the deep ring brings the dissection directly onto the testicular vessels and vas, making separation from the hernial sac easier. After full mobilization, the testis is guided into the scrotum through the intact superficial inguinal ring. A retroperitoneal approach can similarly be used for the testicular mobilization and may provide better access when extensive retroperitoneal dissection is required for a high testis.

The intra-abdominal testis

When the testis is impalpable there is often doubt as to whether the testis is absent or intra-abdominal. Groin exploration is contraindicated until there is clarification. An ultra-

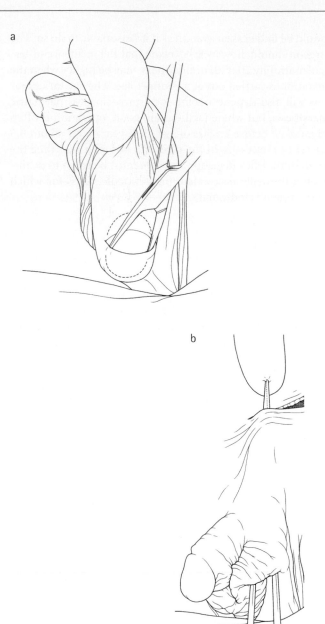

Figure 24.11 *(a) A tunnel has been created from the main wound through to the empty scrotum by the surgeon's finger. A scrotal incision through skin alone is made and a pocket created between the skin and the dartos muscle. (b) An artery forceps is guided up by contact with the surgeon's finger. It passes from the scrotal incision through the dartos muscle and through the scrotum to the main wound. It is then used to draw the testis down into the dartos pouch.*

sound scan may be of value but diagnostic laparoscopy is the most helpful investigation, as it will show testicular vessels and vas entering the deep ring if there is an impalpable atrophic testis in the groin. Alternatively, it will confirm or refute the presence of an intra-abdominal testis. These high testes will seldom reach the scrotum due to short vessels. Preservation of the testicular vessels is not essential to testicular survival as there are anastomotic channels, predominantly with the artery to the vas. Division of testicular vessels above the pelvic brim is a more minor ischaemic insult than division within the inguinal canal. A laparoscopic high division of the testicular vessels can be undertaken at the same time as the diagnostic laparoscopy (*Fowler–Stephens operation*). The testis is left undisturbed for the collateral blood supply to improve, and some weeks later the orchidopexy is performed. Even in expert hands, a Fowler–Stephens operation is still associated with disappointing results. Around 50 per cent rates of testicular atrophy are reported and spermatogenic function may be even worse. Results from microvascular techniques in which, after high mobilization and division of the testicular vessels, they are anastomosed to the epigastric artery and vein, show some promise. General surgeons who operate on children with undescended testes must be aware of the potential of these specialist techniques so that cases which are not suitable for groin exploration by them can be identified and referred to the appropriate specialist.

A testis which cannot be brought into the scrotum should be removed after puberty is complete as the risk of malignant change is significant. In cases of bilateral intra-abdominal testes, gonadal dysgenesis should be considered and karyotype analysis undertaken. Because of the high risk of malignancy in these cases, bilateral orchidectomy may need to be considered.

Torsion

Torsion may occur when there is an abnormal insertion of the tunica vaginalis high up on the cord, allowing the testis to rotate. This abnormality is frequently bilateral and the testes lie horizontally. The twisting of the cord occludes the blood flow. As a testis can only survive around 6 hours of total ischaemia, the management of a suspected testicular torsion is urgent exploration of the scrotum. The diagnosis is mainly clinical but, if torsion is considered clinically to be unlikely, a normal Doppler ultrasound investigation will strengthen the grounds for exclusion and may prevent unnecessary surgery. It must be remembered, however, that an unnecessary exploration for orchitis, or for idiopathic scrotal oedema, is preferable to a missed diagnosis of torsion. At exploration an infarcted testis, if encountered, is removed and a viable testis is untwisted and fixed. The use of absorbable suture has been associated with recurrent torsion, and fixation at three points of the tunica albuginea to the tunica vaginalis with fine Prolene sutures has been recommended. However, there is now concern regarding any adverse effects of such sutures.[12] An alternative method of fixation is to place the testis in a dartos pouch. The opposite testis should also be fixed as the anatomical variants which predispose to torsion are commonly bilateral. On occasion, repeated episodes of testicular pain are suspected to be due to recurrent partial torsion. An elective bilateral fixation is undertaken. In early childhood a variant of the classical torsion may occur in which the body of a testis, abnormally separate from the epididymis, twists on its own.

At exploration for a suspected torsion, a torted small cyst on the head of the testis (*cyst of Morgagni*) may be the only finding and it is simply excised. If a confident diagnosis can be made preoperatively an operation can be avoided, but if in doubt it is always better to explore.

Orchidectomy for testicular cancer

Testicular cancer is the commonest cancer in young men. Scrotal ultrasound is very accurate in the diagnosis of testicular cancer as a cause of a scrotal swelling. Once the diagnosis is suspected, and before operation, blood should be sent for tumour markers. Also, where it is available, consideration should be given to cryopreservation of sperm and again this should, whenever possible, be done before orchidectomy. The traditional operation for testicular cancer includes removal of the testis and spermatic cord up to the deep inguinal ring. An inguinal incision is made and a non-crushing clamp is placed across the cord at the deep ring. The testis is then delivered out of the scrotum for inspection and palpation. When any doubt still remains, and intraoperative histology is required, the testis is isolated from the rest of the wound to prevent malignant contamination. The testis is then opened and a biopsy is taken from the appropriate area for frozen-section examination. If there is no malignancy, the soft clamp is released, haemostasis obtained and the testis reconstituted and returned to the scrotum. If malignancy is confirmed, the testicular vessels and the vas are ligated and divided at the deep ring, which is then closed. Some surgeons recommend a vacuum drain to prevent a scrotal haematoma.

When a testicular tumour is unexpectedly discovered during a scrotal operation, then the testis can be removed through the scrotal incision. It is not necessary to make a separate inguinal incision in order to excise more of the spermatic cord. Blood should be sent from theatre for tumour markers.

Current UK guidelines on the management of testicular cancer advise that all young men who are about to have an orchidectomy should be offered a testicular prosthesis. Consideration should also be given to biopsy of the contralateral testis. This is indicated if the ultrasound shows microcalcification, if the contralateral testis is small and soft, or if there is a history of maldescent of the contralateral testis. However, contralateral testicular biopsies should only be undertaken when there is the appropriate pathological expertise available for their interpretation.

Orchidectomy for benign conditions

The removal of a testis for *benign* pathology is through the incision from which the testis is most accessible. For a normally placed scrotal organ, an incision in the upper scrotum allows the testis to be delivered out of the wound. The coverings of the cord are divided and the vas and vessels isolated. In some chronic inflammatory situations *an epididymectomy* alone may be considered, although it must be remembered that epididymectomy for testicular pain is often ineffective and may make any pain worse.

Vasectomy

Vasectomy for male contraception is one of the most commonly performed surgical procedures in the world. The principle is to use a technique which is minimal but effective, so that complications are minimized and so that it can be performed on an outpatient basis under local anaesthesia. Using finger manipulation, first one vas then the other is brought to lie in the midline just under the scrotal skin. Access to the vas can be through a single midline scrotal puncture, using the sharp-pointed artery forceps from the 'no-scalpel instrument set', or by a scalpel incision of 1 cm or less in length. There are various techniques to fix and deliver the vas through the wound, including the use of a special ring forceps in the no-scalpel set, or alternatively an Allis forceps. The next step is to ensure that the vas is cleanly separated from its coverings. This is done by puncturing or incising down onto the vas and reapplying the ring or Allis forceps, allowing the coverings to drop back; care must be taken never to let go of the vas. The next step is to divide the vas and tie both ends. Most surgeons use Vicryl, although clips can also be used. Silk ties have been abandoned because of problems with sinus development. Some surgeons leave the testicular ends open as this has been shown to reduce granulomata. However, whether or not the testicular ends are left open, it is important to use a technique to prevent recanalization. The most effective options are either to separate the ends within different tissue planes, or to cauterize the vas lumen. The patient must still be warned that both early and late recanalization can occur.

Epydidymal cysts

These thin-walled translucent cysts, filled with clear fluid, are usually found in the upper part of the epididymis, and lie above the testis. There are commonly multiple tiny cysts, in addition to the one that is palpable, and therefore development of further palpable cysts is likely. Excision is only recommended if a cyst is symptomatic, and should be avoided if future fertility is desired as surgery carries a risk of occlusion to sperm flow. Excision is undertaken by a scrotal incision over the cyst until its surface is reached. Dissection is then on the surface of the cysts, and an attempt should be made to shell them out intact.

Hydroceles

Hydoceles, in which an underlying testicular malignancy has been excluded, can be approached through a scrotal incision. The anterior scrotal skin is held taut over the hydrocele with one hand and an incision made through skin and dartos. An artery forceps applied to the remaining coverings and the tunica vaginalis before incising into the hydrocele will enable the sucker to be inserted more easily to drain the fluid. The opening is then enlarged to a size through which the testis can be delivered. The aim of the operation is to leave the testis so that the fluid produced by its tunica albuginea can drain into a different tissue plane. This is mostly simply achieved by several absorbable sutures which plicate the tunica vaginalis so that it lies as a cuff behind the testis (Fig. 24.12). The dartos and scrotal skin are then drawn back over the testis and closed. The scrotal incision is satisfactorily closed with a continuous absorbable haemostatic suture in the dartos, and a subcuticular absorbable suture in the skin.

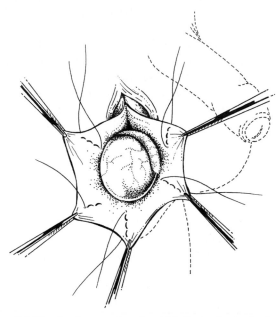

Figure 24.12 *Lord's procedure, in which the tunica vaginalis of a hydrocele is plicated to prevent recurrence.*

Aspiration of a hydrocele is usually only a very temporary solution as the fluid re-collects. Injection of a sclerosant after aspiration can obliterate the space and prevent recurrence. However, this may cause severe pain unless mixed with a short- and long-acting local anaesthetic agent. A mixture containing 2 mL of a 3 per cent solution of sodium tetradecyl sulphate mixed with 5 mL of 1 per cent lignocaine and 5 mL of 0.25 per cent bupivicaine has proved satisfactory. The procedure can be repeated if necessary.

Varicoceles

The treatment of symptomatic varicoceles – or those believed to be the cause of reduced sperm counts – has now become almost exclusively a radiological procedure in which the testicular veins are embolized endoluminally. The surgical treatment consists of ligation and division of the two to four dilated testicular venous channels at the deep inguinal ring. Excessively dilated cremasteric veins, which may be secondarily implicated, can also be ligated. Although it is tempting to undertake scrotal excision of veins, this can result in the loss of a testicle.

PREPUTIAL SURGERY

Except for some minor surgery on the prepuce, surgery of the penis is performed almost exclusively by adult or paediatric urological surgeons, or those general surgeons who have also undertaken urological training and are offering an additional relatively comprehensive urological service. However, some descriptions of purely urological operations are included for the benefit of the isolated general surgeons who find themselves forced by circumstances to undertake the occasional urological procedure.

Circumcision

This is performed for congenital and acquired phimosis, and for religious and cultural reasons. In the infant the foreskin does not retract due to physiological adhesions between foreskin and glans. In the young child, a non-retractile foreskin may be due either to a phimosis or to the persistence of these adhesions. Differentiation is important as congenital adhesions will usually separate spontaneously in the absence of infections and a circumcision is not required.

Operative procedure

A general anaesthetic is preferable in children, but in adults local infiltrative anaesthesia, or regional anaesthesia with a caudal or subpubic block is also satisfactory. The inner and the outer layer of the foreskin is removed. Sufficient skin on the penile shaft must be retained to allow an erection without skin tension, and it is helpful to mark the intended site of the circumferential skin incision before commencing the operation. Excessive suprapubic fat, especially in the young child, may carry abdominal skin onto the shaft of the penis, and before marking, this should be pushed firmly down onto the pubic symphysis so that the shaft is covered only by penile skin (Fig. 24.13a). The excision of the inner layer of foreskin should be to within a few millimetres of the coronal sulcus. Too long an inner layer, especially if associated with a long outer layer, can result in a suture line which falls forwards over the glans and may heal with a constrictive circular band which, again, prevents full retraction.

A variety of circumcision techniques will all achieve good results. The foreskin is first fully retracted, any glandular adhesions separated, the area cleaned with antiseptic and the foreskin replaced. The phimotic band must be stretched or divided to achieve this. Many paediatric surgeons favour the

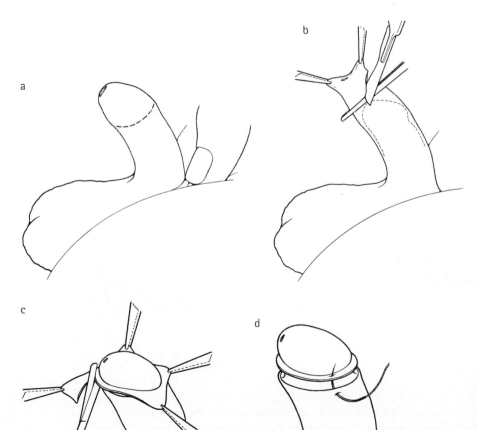

Figure 24.13 *Circumcision. (a) Adequate skin must be left on the penile shaft; it is always safer to mark the intended line of circumferential incision before commencing the operation. (b) A method of amputating the foreskin favoured by many paediatric surgeons. Great care must be taken to avoid injury to the glans. (c) The inner layer of the prepuce is then trimmed. (d) The inner and outer cut layers of prepuce are apposed with fine interrupted sutures.*

technique illustrated in Figure 24.13. The tip of the prepuce is grasped with two artery forceps and pulled forwards with light traction. A narrow clamp is placed obliquely across the prepuce distal to the glans and parallel to the corona, after which the prepuce is divided immediately distal to the clamp (Fig. 24.13b). The inner layer of the prepuce will still be excessive, and so is trimmed to leave a cuff of about 3 mm (Fig. 24.13c). As this technique is inherently dangerous with great potential for injury to the glans, including even amputation, the authors cannot recommend it.

Most adult circumcisions commence with a dorsal slit between two artery forceps placed close together on the phimotic band in the midline dorsally. Cleaning under the foreskin must usually be postponed until after this incision as any phimotic band is commonly too dense to stretch. The dorsal incision terminates at the skin mark on the outer layer (Fig. 24.14). The prepuce is then excised circumferentially along the skin mark. This incision, however, always leaves an excessive cuff of the internal layer of the prepuce which must then be trimmed.

The present author favours a modification in which the foreskin is first divided into two lateral flaps. Four artery forceps are applied to the phimotic edge of the foreskin, two dorsally and two ventrally. The initial dorsal slit is continued on the inner layer of the prepuce to within a few millimetres of the coronal sulcus. A second ventral slit is then made. This incision in the outer layer should reach the skin mark. In the inner layer, however, the incision is split into two around the frenular base and then further deviated laterally to carry the incision circumferentially round the inner layer of the foreskin until it meets the dorsal slit incision (Fig. 24.14b). As the inner layer can be divided accurately under direct vision a few millimetres outside the coronal sulcus, no further trim-ming is necessary. Connective tissue and vessels between the layers of foreskin can then often be released, and allowed to retract. Finally, the outer layers of the two preputial flaps are divided along the skin mark.

Haemostasis is important, as the most common postoperative complication is haemorrhage. Only *bipolar* diathermy is safe on the penis (see Appendix II) and is satisfactory for most of the bleeding points. A suture may be more effective for frenular bleeding, and in an adult circumcision there may be large veins which are more secure if ligated. Large divided veins, which are in spasm and not actively bleeding, are easily overlooked. They are most frequently found beneath the divided outer preputial skin and should be sought as otherwise they will bleed later when venous pressure increases as the patient stands up. Finally, fine interrupted absorbable sutures are used to appose the inner and outer cut edges of the foreskin (Fig. 24.13d).

The meatus should be inspected. When the circumcision is performed for balanitis xerotica obliterans, a meatal stenosis may already have developed necessitating a meatotomy. In children, however, there is often only a plaque adherent to the meatus which can be lifted off, exposing a raw surface. Application of a steroid cream postoperatively will reduce the incidence of a meatal stenosis developing during healing.

The *hooded foreskin* associated with a minor hypospadias is cosmetically unacceptable, and parents will often request early circumcision. It is important to defer this until it is certain that the skin is not required for reconstruction, remembering that a penis which is bowed when erect has a more major hypospadias than is superficially apparent. The circumcision of a hooded foreskin follows the same general principles, but excision is only required over about five-sixths of the circumference as the foreskin is absent ventrally.

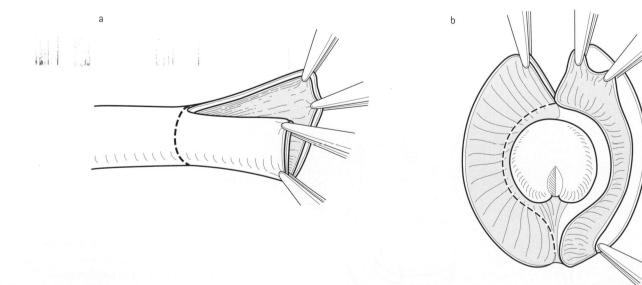

Figure 24.14 *Circumcision. (a) An initial dorsal slit is made between the forceps applied to the free edge of the prepuce. (b) A similar ventral incision has been made but, on the inner layer, it divides to skirt the frenulum. The inner layer of the foreskin can then be circumcised first under direct vision.*

DORSAL SLIT

This operation is no more than the initial dorsal incision of a circumcision followed by suturing of the wound edges. The phimosis is released and it is a satisfactory simple solution in the elderly. The cosmetic result is unacceptable to most younger men.

PREPUTIOPLASTY

This is an adaptation of the concept of the dorsal slit, but avoids the cosmetically unacceptable bifid foreskin. Small radial releasing incisions are made in the phimotic band dorsally and at each side. All three incisions are then sutured transversely. Unfortunately, re-stenosis very often occurs during healing.

FRENOPLASTY

A simple transverse release of the frenulum, which is then sutured longitudinally is indicated for a short frenulum which is tearing on intercourse.

REDUCTION OF A PARAPHIMOSIS

A paraphimosis occurs when a tight prepuce has been retracted beyond the corona and has remained there as a constricting band beyond which the inner layer of prepuce swells rapidly to form an oedematous collar. Manual replacement of the foreskin with one hand while the other is used to compress the oedematous tissue is usually successful, but a general anaesthetic may still be required, especially in a child. If reduction fails the tight band must be surgically incised, or a circumcision performed. It is therefore important that the surgical options, including circumcision, have been dis-cussed with the patient, and the necessary consent obtained, before induction of anaesthesia. A foreskin which has caused a paraphimosis will almost always finally warrant a circumcision but, if reduction can be achieved, this might be better deferred until swelling has settled.

The prepuce in reconstruction

The fine non-hair-bearing skin of the prepuce is an ideal source of full-thickness skin, whether as a local flap or as free graft. Its mobility and excellent blood supply allows it to be used as a local flap for reconstructive urethral surgery. Preputial skin acquires its blood supply both from the shaft skin and from the coronal sulcus. An incision can therefore be made along the inner layer of prepuce, close to the coronal sulcus, and the whole foreskin unfolded as a long single flap. The mobility of the penile shaft skin makes it possible to rotate this flap to the ventral aspect of the penis, or it can even be brought over the glans which is buttonholed through the flap.

Alternatively, the foreskin can be mobilized as a separate inner and outer flap with an incision along the free margin of the prepuce (Fig. 24.15a, b). The inner flap can be swung round to the ventral aspect for urethral reconstruction, either as an on-lay graft or rolled into a complete tube. It can also be folded down onto the penile shaft to cover a dorsal defect when the ventral skin cover over a urethral reconstruction has been achieved by rotation of the entire shaft skin (Fig. 24.15c). Success in all techniques depends on well-vascularized flaps without tension. The foreskin is also a valuable source of skin for free, full-thickness grafts which can be used not only for skin cover but also as a urothelial substitute in the proximal urethra (see Fig. 24.18).

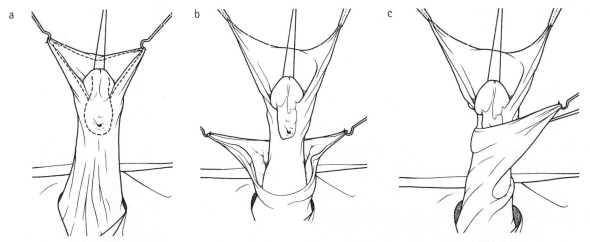

Figure 24.15 *The inner and outer layer of the foreskin can be separated along the free edge. Two flaps, each with a good blood supply, are produced and can be rotated to different areas for reconstruction. In this illustration the hooded foreskin which is often associated with hypospadias is shown. (a) The intended incisions have been marked. (b) The outer preputial flap has been mobilized with the penile shaft skin. The inner flap is still attached around five-sixths of the dorsal coronal sulcus. (c) Dorsal penile skin with the outer preputial flap has been rotated to cover a defect on the ventral aspect of the penis. If this leaves a dorsal defect it can be covered by folding down the flap from the inner layer of the prepuce.*

URETHRAL SURGERY

It is important that trauma is minimized during any intubation of the urethra. Whereas the insertion of a flexible catheter through the male urethra can be performed atraumatically with an understanding of the anatomy (Fig. 24.16), blind insertion of a rigid instrument is not recommended. Both rigid cystoscopes and flexible fibre-optic cystoscopes should be passed under direct vision, and the urethra is inspected during intubation (cystourethroscopy). Cystoscopy is discussed in Chapter 25. Many urethral procedures can be performed endoscopically. When endoscopic access will be insufficient an open surgical approach is necessary. The urethra of the penile shaft can be exposed by a subcoronal circumferential incision and proximal retraction of the penile skin. The proximal urethra is approached via a midline incision either anterior or posterior to the scrotum.

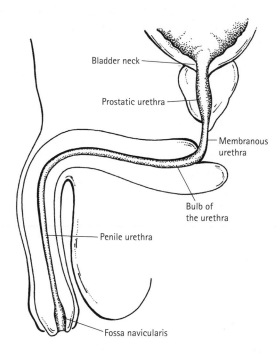

Figure 24.16   *A sagittal section of the male urethra. An appreciation of the change in direction between the bulbar and the membranous urethra is essential for any intubation.*

Urethral strictures: dilatation and urethrotomy

Strictures in the urethra should be visualized at urethroscopy, and are best treated initially by urethrotomy with an optical urethrotome. A urethrotomy is a clean releasing incision of a stricture after which re-stenosis on healing is a lesser problem than after dilatation. Subsequently, the stricture can be managed by repeat urethrotomies or sometimes by the passage of a metal sound across the stricture at regular intervals. Alternatively, the patient may be taught to pass a large-bore catheter themselves at weekly intervals to prevent re-stenosis.

Dilatation of a stricture can be accomplished with sequential passage of sounds, but nowadays this should normally only be undertaken where there are no facilities for optical urethrotomy because blind instrumentation of the urethra risks creation of false passages – a problem that has virtually vanished from those centres with optical instruments. The initial sound must be of a diameter which can traverse the stricture *without any force*. It is passed through the stricture and on into the bladder. The sound is tapered and dilates the stricture as it is advanced. Sequentially larger sounds are then passed. For narrow strictures, or strictures that are too long for optical urethrotomy, a guide wire can be threaded through the stricture under direct vision via a cystoscope and further dilators threaded over it. Healing after dilatation is commonly followed by re-stenosis and dilatation may have to be repeated every few months.

Meatotomy

A meatal stricture can be simply dilated but, as re-stenosis is common and the meatus is easily accessible, a more permanent solution is preferable. A small releasing incision is made and the urethral mucosa sutured to the skin with fine absorbable sutures (Fig. 24.17). Following circumcision a meatal stenosis may develop which is in reality only a web partially occluding an otherwise normal meatus. Simple

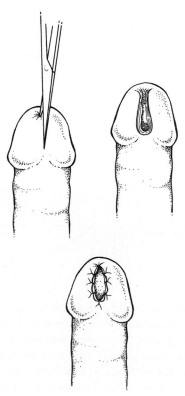

Figure 24.17   *A meatotomy.*

release of this web may be sufficient, followed by self-passage of a dilator to prevent re-stenosis during healing.

Urethroplasty

Urethral strictures which are long, dense or recurrent may be better treated by reconstruction than repeated dilatations or urethrotomies. Access to the more posterior strictures is through the perineum posterior to the scrotum. It is sometimes practical to excise a short stricture and anastomose the urethral ends, but a patch urethroplasty is usually a better solution. The buccal mucosal graft gives very good results, and is technically easy to learn. The urethra is exposed and opened along the length of the stricture (Fig. 24.18a). A full-thickness patch graft (the mucosal layer on the inside forming the urethral lumen) is then sutured to the edges of the opened urethra with fine absorbable sutures (Fig. 24.18b). Alternatively, the free graft can be taken from the inner layer of the prepuce. Pedicled skin grafts, taken from the adjoining hairy scrotal or penile skin have, in general, been superseded by buccal mucosa grafts, as hair formation in the neo-urethra can be troublesome. The skin is then closed over the reconstructed urethra, and a fine silastic urethral catheter is left *in situ* during healing.

Two-stage urethroplasty

A two-stage urethroplasty may still have a place when there are fistulae and sinuses, or excessive scar tissue from previous infection or surgery. This may well be the situation with which a general surgeon, working in an area with limited healthcare facilities, is faced. A temporary suprapubic catheter should be considered. An alternative is the creation of a perineal urethrostomy as described below to allow time for sepsis to settle, because once it has done so, a long buccal mucosal patch urethroplasty may be feasible.

An inverted U-shaped incision is made behind the scrotum (Fig. 24.19a). A vertical extension of the skin incision is then made forwards between the two halves of the scrotum and the flaps of skin and fat elevated. The urethra is incised vertically over the whole length of the stricture, and this incision must extend into healthy urethra both proximally and distally (Fig. 24.19b). The cut edges of the urethra are then sutured to the edges of the vertical skin incision, except proximally where the apex of the flap is sewn to the proximal end of the laid open urethra to form a temporary perineal urethrostomy (Fig. 24.19c). The remainder of the U-shaped flap is replaced. This first stage has on occasion been performed as an emergency when a patient presents with a para-urethral abscess associated with an impassable stricture. The external drainage of the abscess is then combined with release of the stricture and the formation of a temporary perineal urethrostomy.

The traditional second stage of this operation was to use the scrotal skin to complete the urethral tube (Fig. 24.19d, e), but a long buccal patch can be inserted at this stage, as shown in Figure 24.18b, and this provides much more satisfactory results.

Urethral injury

Urethral injury is very rare in women except as a consequence of prolonged untreated obstructed labour. Urethral

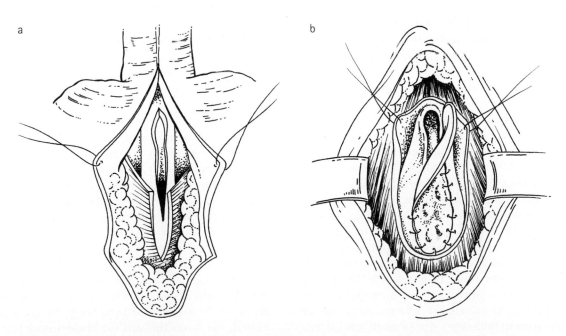

Figure 24.18 *A patch urethroplasty. (a) The whole length of the stricture and a short segment of healthy urethra proximal and distal is laid open. (b) A buccal mucosal graft is sewn to the cut edges of the urethra. The mucosal surface must face into the urethral lumen. The skin edges are closed over the mucosal patch.*

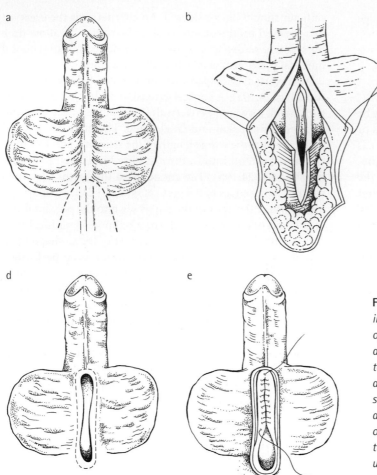

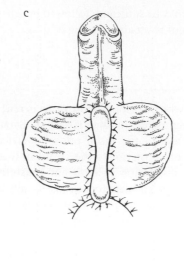

Figure 24.19   *A two-stage urethroplasty. (a) The initial inverted U-incision. (b) The whole length of the stricture is laid open, including a short segment of healthy urethra both proximal and distal to the stricture. (c) The cut edges of urethra are sewn to the skin so that the segment of stenosed urethra is exteriorized as a groove in the perineal skin. The proximal opened urethra is sewn to the skin of the apex of the flap. (d) At the second stage an incision was made a few centimetres outside the exposed part of the urethra, and the isolated skin rolled into a tube. (e) The skin tube was fashioned into a neo-urethra and the skin edges undermined and closed over it. Steps (d) and (e) are now achieved more satisfactorily using a buccal mucosal patch.*

injury must always be considered in male patients with a penile or perineal injury. Urethral injuries are also associated, particularly in the male, with displaced anterior pelvic fractures, and these patients frequently have multiple other injuries.

Early bladder catheterization may be indicated for the monitoring of a severely injured patient. Alternatively, a patient with an isolated penile or perineal injury may have developed urinary retention, and it should be remembered that this is the most frequent clinical course of a man with urethral disruption. When a urethral injury is suspected, the safe initial management is suprapubic catheterization, followed by specialist urological assessment. However, when it is thought that injury is relatively unlikely, it is reasonable to attempt urethral catheterization. A large soft catheter, when passed through a urethra distended with lubricating jelly, is least likely to compound any damage. Adequate analgesia is essential. One-and-a-half tubes of anaesthetic lubricating jelly is inserted into the urethra, but is not massaged up. The urethra is held closed to prevent the jelly escaping, and the remaining jelly used to lubricate a size 16 or 18 soft (preferably silicone) urethral catheter. If passage becomes difficult the procedure is stopped and a suprapubic catheter is placed, ideally under ultrasound control. If the catheter passes easily

into the bladder with drainage of urine, significant urethral injury is unlikely.

Penile urethral injuries may be associated with lacerations into the erectile tissue and large haematomas. Early exploration with evacuation of the haematoma and direct repair of both the urethra and the erectile tissue will give the best results.

Membranous and supra-membranous urethral injuries are often circumferential, and the continuity of the urethra is completely lost as the prostate and bladder neck dislocate upwards and backwards (see Fig. 24.20a). Rectal examination may demonstrate the displaced prostate. Suprapubic catheter drainage should be established, and arrangements made for the patient to be managed by a surgeon with experience of these injuries. Direct surgical repair of the injury is difficult, but is now believed to provide the best results in skilled hands. It must, however, be delayed for several days while bruising and oedema settles. The traditional manoeuvre of re-establishing urethral continuity without formal repair was by passing one metal bougie up the urethra, and a second one down through the bladder neck from an open cystostomy. It was then possible to manipulate the displaced tissues into position so that the two bougies touched (Fig. 24.20b). The distal bougie could then be guided up into the

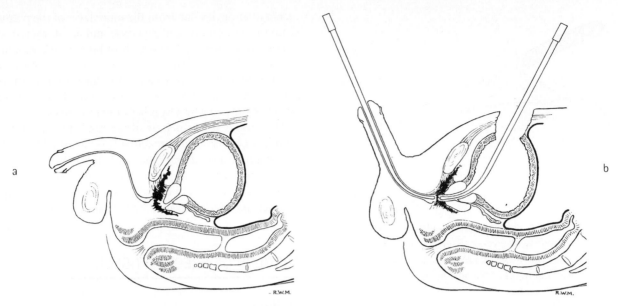

Figure 24.20 *This simple method of alignment of a disrupted membranous urethra is not now recommended as the long-term results are poor.*

bladder in contact with the upper one as it was withdrawn. The external end of a catheter was fitted over the end of the bougie and drawn retrogradely through the urethra. It was then attached to a balloon catheter which was drawn up into the bladder. After inflation of the balloon, gentle retraction held the reduction and urethral apposition. Healing with stricture formation was common and final continence was often poor. This, now historic, technique is described only as it may be the sole practical option for a general surgeon with no access to urological expertise.

Hypospadias

A hypospadiac urethra may open on the ventral aspect of the glans, the coronal sulcus or the penile shaft, or even onto the perineum. Many different reconstruction techniques have been developed.[13] The surgery of hypospadias is specialized and is carried out almost exclusively by paediatric urologists or plastic surgeons, although it is important that any surgeon undertaking circumcisions in childhood is aware of the potential value of the associated hooded foreskin for reconstruction. A general surgeon should only perform hypospadiac reconstruction if referral for expert surgery is impossible. In these circumstances, although an attempt at correction of a more major abnormality is justified, mainly cosmetic improvement of a minor glandular or coronal hypospadias is usually not.

The hypospadiac meatal opening may be stenosed and a meatotomy may be required prior to the full reconstructive operation, which is normally postponed until around 18 months of age. In many cases the hypospadias is associated with *chordee,* in which the infant's erect penis is ventrally bowed by abnormal fibrous tethering of tissue on the ventral aspect of the penile shaft. The diagnosis of chordee can be confirmed by creating an artificial erection under anaesthesia. A constricting band is placed around the base of the penis, and normal saline is injected into the erectile tissue. It is a useful test at the start of surgery, and also to check during the operation, whether surgical release has been sufficient.

The significance of the *urethral plate* has only recently been appreciated. This is the strip of urethral mucosa extending from the hypospadiac meatus to the glans and is thus ideal tissue with which to fashion the neo-urethra. However, this strip was initially thought to be the main factor tethering the short urethra to a more distal position on the penis than it could reach, and thus the cause of the chordee. It was therefore often sacrificed in the initial dissection. It has now been shown that the cause of the chordee is the abnormal fibrous attachments of this strip to the underlying erectile tissue, and not the urethral plate itself.

The first step in the repair of a hypospadias is the release of chordee by the dissection of the urethral plate off the corpora cavernosa (Fig. 24.21). Any fibrous tissue representing atretic corpus spongiosum is excised, and the urethral plate is seen to lengthen and narrow as the chordee corrects, and the meatus then lies more proximally on the penile shaft than previously. The mobilized urethral plate can now be rolled over to form a complete neo-urethra if it is sufficiently wide (Fig. 24.22). Often, it is too narrow but can still be used to form half of the circumference. In some techniques reliance is placed on the concept that a buried skin strip forms an epithelial tube by proliferation from the edges, but the formation of a tube at operation is preferable. The simplest solution to complete the tube is shown in Figure 24.23, but is not ideal as this skin may later become hairy. Alternatively, a

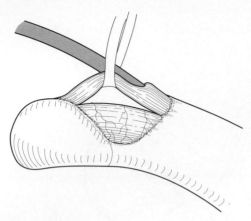

Figure 24.21   *The meatus, the distal urethra and the urethral plate are dissected off the underlying erectile tissue and held in a sling. A catheter is in situ. The distal dissection requires extensive mobilization of the lateral wings of the bifid glans.*

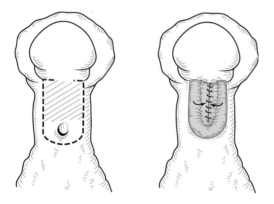

Figure 24.22   *The wide urethral plate, shown as the hatched area, has been released, rolled and sutured to form a neo-urethra. Skin cover is now required for the shaded area.*

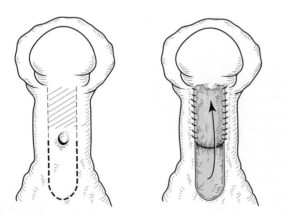

Figure 24.23   *This urethral plate is too narrow to be rolled into a complete tube. A distal skin flap has been turned over and sutured to form part of the tube of the neo-urethra, but is less satisfactory than a free graft of buccal mucosa. Skin cover is now required for the shaded area.*

rectangular on-lay flap from the inner layer of the prepuce is swung round on a vascular pedicle and anastomosed to the hypospadiac meatus. A free graft of buccal mucosa can also be used. Skin cover is then required to cover the neo-urethra. Penile skin is mobile and elastic, and the skin from the outer layer of the hooded foreskin can be brought to the ventral aspect of the penis by a number of manoeuvres.

The surgery is very delicate when carried out at around 18 months of age. Fine absorbable sutures are used (6/0 or 7/0) and magnification devices may be helpful. A tourniquet will provide control of bleeding during surgery. Broad-spectrum antibiotic cover should be used, and urethral or suprapubic catheter drainage instigated for around 10 days.

SURGERY OF ERECTILE TISSUE

Trauma

A tear of the tunica albuginea may occur from a penile laceration, or the fracture of an erect penis. A circumferential sub-coronal incision allows the loose penile skin to be retracted proximally, thus exposing the entire penile shaft. Haematoma is evacuated and the tunica repaired with strong, long-acting absorbable sutures. An associated injury to the penile urethra should be sought and repaired if present. Catheter drainage should be instituted.

Priapism

Detumescence can usually be achieved by the insertion of a 16-gauge cannula into the corpora, aspiration of blood, followed by injection with normal saline. If unsuccessful, treatment is then pharmocological, with local injection of phenylephrine. As a last resort, shunts can be created by taking a Trucut biopsy of the fascia separating the corpora spongiosum and cavernosum. The Trucut needle is introduced bilaterally through the glans and advanced in line with the penile shaft into each corpus cavernosum.

Penile amputation

Squamous cell carcinoma of the penis usually arises beneath the prepuce. Although it is perceived as an old man's cancer, UK statistics show this cancer to be occurring in men from age 40 years onwards, and survival is poor. Whenever possible, treatment should be undertaken in the context of a multidisciplinary cancer team, as the surgical and non-surgical options depend on the stage of the cancer. Surgical options include local removal and skin grafting of the glans, various levels of amputation, and complete penile removal with a perineal urethrostomy. If there is invasion of more than 2 mm in depth, then bilateral or unilateral lymph node dissection is usually indicated. In the absence of such an approach, penile amputation is often undertaken, although this will be undermanagement in some cases and overmanagement in others.

In a penile amputation the amputated corpora are oversewn and skin flaps brought over the end. It is essential to form a mucosal-skin anastomosis of the urethra to prevent stenosis. The urethra can either be brought out through the suture line or through the longer flap (Fig. 24.24). Very late presentation is common in remote hospitals, and the surgeon is faced with a fungating growth which has destroyed the penis and is invading the scrotum. A total excision of penis and scrotum with the urethral stump anastomosed to the perineal skin as a perineal urethrostomy may be the only surgical solution which will give local control. This may have to be followed by an inguinal node dissection for control of nodal metastases.

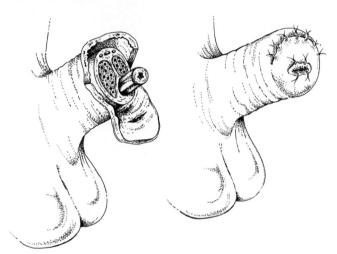

Figure 24.24 *An accurate mucosa-skin apposition is essential to prevent stenosis of the new meatus after penile amputation.*

REFERENCES

1. Cheek CM, Black NA, Devlin HB, *et al.* Groin hernia surgery; a systematic review. *Ann Roy Coll Surg Engl* 1998; **80** (Suppl. 1): S1–80.
2. MRC Laparoscopic Groin Hernia Trial Group. Laparoscopic versus open repair of groin hernia: a randomised comparison. *Lancet* 1999; **354**: 185–90.
3. Kingsnorth A. Treating inguinal hernias. Editorial. *Br Med J* 2004; **328**: 59–60.
4. Macintyre IMC. Best practice in groin hernia repair. Leading article. *Br J Surg* 2003; **90**: 131–2.
5. Ravichandran D, Kalambe BG, Pain JA. Pilot randomised controlled study of preservation or division of ilioinguinal nerve in open mesh repair of inguinal hernia. *Br J Surg* 2000; 87: 1166–7.
6. Nicholson S. Inguinal hernia repair. Leading article. *Br J Surg* 1999; **86**: 577–8.
7. Shouldice EE. The treatment of hernia. *Ontario Medical Review* 1953; 1–14.
8. Farquharson EL. Early ambulation with special reference to herniorrhaphy as an outpatient procedure. *Lancet* 1955; **11**: 517–19.
9. *Paediatric Surgery.* JD Attwell. London: Arnold, 1998.
10. Coughlin MI, Bellinger MF, La Porte RE, Lee PA. Testicular suture: a significant risk factor for infertility among formerly cryptorchid men. *J Pediatr Surg* 1998; **33**: 1790–3.
11. Swerdlow AJ, Higgins CD, Pike MC. Risk of testicular cancer in cohort of boys with cryptorchism. *Br Med J* 1997; **314**: 1507–11.
12. Frank JD, O'Brien M. Fixation of the testis. Review. *Br J Urol* 2002; **89**: 331–3.
13. *Operative Pediatric Urology*, 2nd edn. JD Frank, JP Gearhart, HM Snyder (eds). Edinburgh: Elsevier Churchill Livingstone, 2002.

25

UROLOGICAL SURGERY FOR THE GENERAL SURGEON

There is increasing specialization within all branches of surgery, and urology is now considered, in most countries, to be a separate surgical specialty from general surgery. In some parts of the world, either because of low population density or poor healthcare resources, there is a need for surgeons with a very wide remit. As the practice of these surgeons often includes both general surgery and urology, it is important that they have also received specialist training in urology. Some basic urology has been included in this chapter for the benefit of the general surgical trainee who is working in a remote unit where urology still forms part of general surgical practice. The coverage is, of necessity, limited and more comprehensive urological texts should be consulted.[1,2]

However, even the general surgeon, whose practice does not include urology, must still understand the principles underlying this branch of surgery – just as the urologist should understand general surgery. Cooperation between the specialities is often required, both for reconstructive procedures and for advanced pathology involving adjacent organs. Damage to a ureter, or to the bladder, may occur during a general surgical or gynaecological operation. In most situations, a general surgeon who unexpectedly encounters, or causes, urological trauma, or who encounters pathology which extends into urological organs, can obtain the assistance (or at least the advice) of a urological colleague. Occasionally, however, a general surgeon may be forced by circumstances to operate in 'urological territory', in the absence of any specialist expertise or equipment.

GENERAL PRINCIPLES

Renal function

No surgery should be undertaken on a kidney or ureter without knowledge of the function both of that kidney and of the other kidney. In elective urological surgery, preoperative imaging, and more sophisticated tests of differential function if indicated, will have been carried out. In the situations in which a general surgeon may be involved this information is often scant or absent. Palpation at operation can identify the anatomical presence of a second kidney, but provides no information on function. In cases of unexpected retroperitoneal or pelvic masses, beware the ectopic kidney! A preoperative intravenous urogram (IVU), or a computed tomography (CT) scan with contrast, will demonstrate where the kidneys are, and whether they are functioning. If neither investigation has been performed, an on-table IVU is recommended. A single high-dose late film, taken at 20 minutes, should provide the maximum information.

Renal vascularity

The kidneys receive one-fifth of the total cardiac output, and haemorrhage from the kidneys can be profuse. This may render any surgery *through* the renal parenchyma, and any surgery to repair renal trauma extremely difficult (see Chapter 14). Temporary vascular control of the renal vessels may be essential, and the anterior approach, in which access to the renal pedicle is superior, is recommended in these circumstances. During vascular occlusion it must be remembered that renal tissue is damaged by ischaemia faster than any other tissue, except brain.

Urinary drainage

In any functioning kidney, urine will continue to collect in the renal pelvis, and adequate drainage to the bladder, or to the exterior, is essential. An obstructed kidney eventually ceases to function, and finally this functional loss becomes irreversible. Bilateral obstruction causes post-renal failure. It should also be remembered that severe bladder outlet obstruction can finally cause bilateral upper urinary tract obstruction. Stagnant urine is also prone to infection.

- A *nephrostomy* drains the urine directly to the exterior.
- A *ureteric stent,* placed between the renal pelvis and bladder, improves drainage of urine to the bladder.
- A *urethral* or *suprapubic catheter* is employed to drain an obstructed bladder. Free catheter drainage of the bladder is also recommended for 10–14 days after the closure of a surgical or traumatic bladder incision, as normal micturition pressure can cause disruption.

Malignant ureteric obstruction: Advanced pelvic malignancies may cause unilateral, or bilateral, ureteric obstruction. Often, the diagnosis of inoperable, or recurrent, cervical, prostatic, bladder or rectal cancer is already established but the patient presents with anuria. Nephrostomy drainage, or the placement of ureteric stents (from either above or below) across the malignant stricture will prolong life. It may, however, deny the patient a relatively pain-free death from anuria and prolong the suffering from advanced pelvic malignancy.

Patients who present with ureteric obstruction before a definitive diagnosis has been reached pose combined challenges of diagnosis and initial management. Malignancy should be confirmed histologically, and benign retroperitoneal fibrosis excluded. The occasional malignancy is still amenable to curative surgery at this stage, but this is uncommon. Other malignancies may respond to radiotherapy, chemotherapy or hormone manipulation, with the potential for regression and long-term palliation. Initial nephrostomy or ureteric stents will therefore be required at least until tissue diagnosis is obtained and decisions reached on appropriate management.

Stone formation

Any foreign body in contact with urine can stimulate stone formation, and consequently all sutures must be absorbable. Stents and catheters will eventually encrust, although the materials from which long-term catheters are fashioned are designed to reduce this. A high fluid intake, with resultant dilute urine, also reduces encrustation, although stents and catheters should still be changed approximately every 3 months.

SURGICAL ANATOMY

The kidneys

The kidney is enveloped in a *fibrous capsule* and consists of the parenchyma and the collecting system. The glomeruli are within the outer parenchyma or *cortex.* The collecting tubules in the inner parenchyma, or *medulla,* open on the papillae into the *calyces* of the collecting system. The calyces unite to form the *renal pelvis.* The collecting system lies partially enclosed within the renal parenchyma, but usually some portion of the renal pelvis lies extrarenal before it tapers to the *pelvi-ureteric junction.* The *renal fascia* encloses the kidney, the adrenal gland and the perinephric fat (Fig. 25.1).

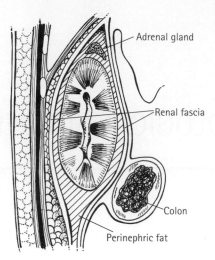

Figure 25.1 *A sagittal section of a kidney showing its relationships to perinephric fat, adrenal, renal fascia, pleura and colon.*

The *renal pedicle* consists of the renal vein which lies anterior, the ureter which is posterior, and the renal artery which lies between the two. The right renal vein is short as the right kidney lies very close to the inferior vena cava (IVC) (Fig. 25.2). Anatomical variants are common, and include variable hilar vascular anatomy, complete or partial duplex systems, horse-shoe kidneys, and crossed ectopia in which a kidney lies on the opposite side from the insertion of its ureter. All may confuse the unwary.

The kidneys lie retroperitoneally, and may be approached from the abdomen or from the loin. The abdominal approach may be retroperitoneal, but is more commonly transperitoneal. The loin approach is retroperitoneal. The abdominal and loin incisions for open surgery are described in Chapter 12. Laparoscopic renal surgery can also be performed using either approach. The duodenum and hepatic flexure lie anterior to the right kidney: the splenic flexure, pancreatic tail and spleen are closely applied to the left (see Fig. 13.2, page 219).

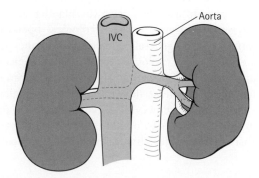

Figure 25.2 *The standard vascular anatomy of the renal pedicle. The right renal vein is short. The longer left renal vein crosses anterior to the aorta. The renal arteries, which may be multiple, are behind the veins. Nephrectomy is, in essence, an operation on the great vessels.*

The ureters

The ureters commence at the pelvi-ureteric junctions and run distally in the retroperitoneum to end at the ureteric orifices in the bladder. Their final intravesical segment runs an oblique course through the bladder wall musculature, which acts as a valve during bladder filling and micturition, preventing ureteric reflux. The ureteric wall is muscular and visible contractions, or *vermiculation*, enable the surgeon to identify the ureters at laparotomy.

X-ray position: on an IVU, classically the course of the ureters lies from the renal pelvis down the tips of the transverse processes of the lumbar vertebrae, over the sacroiliac joints, laterally towards the ischial spines and then medially to the bladder.

During intra-abdominal surgery the ureter must be identified early in any operation which might place it at risk of injury. Mobilization of the caecum or pelvic colon commences with incision of the peritoneum lateral to the bowel, which is then swung medially. Dissection proceeds with great care and the ureter is identified. It lies behind the gonadal vessels on the psoas muscle and crosses the pelvic brim approximately at the bifurcation of the common iliac vessels. It is therefore also at risk in aorto-iliac vascular surgery. In the pelvis the ureter is at greatest risk as it turns medially towards the trigone of the bladder. It crosses underneath the uterine arteries in the base of the broad ligament (hence the saying 'water under the bridge') and may be inadvertently included in the ligation of the uterine arteries during hysterectomy.

In any difficult pelvic dissection, the ureters should be identified above the pelvic brim and followed on their anterior surface into the pelvis, and towards the bladder. A tunnel is created by gently inserting an artery forceps distally along the anterior surface of the ureter from the portion which is already displayed. Tissue lying anterior to the ureters can be safely divided. This plane can be followed until the ureter enters the bladder wall. Ureteric catheters or stents make ureteric identification easier, and the general surgeon, when embarking on a pelvic dissection where difficulty is anticipated, will find the short delay while a urological colleague places the stents amply rewarded. In those patients in whom it will be most helpful, the placement of ureteric catheters may also be difficult due to distortion of the anatomy.

The bladder and prostate

The bladder lies behind the pubis and is mainly extraperitoneal, lying below the peritoneal reflexion. In the male it is separated inferiorly from the pelvic floor musculature by the prostate gland, and posteriorly it is separated from the rectum by the seminal vesicles and Denonvillier's fascia (Fig. 25.3). In the female, the bladder lies directly on the pelvic floor and is separated posteriorly from the rectum by the vagina. The ureters enter the bladder posterolaterally within a centimetre or two of the internal urethral opening.

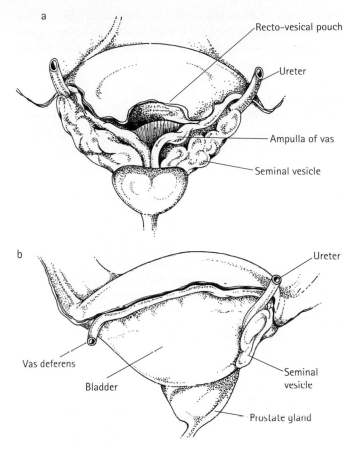

Figure 25.3   *(a) The posterior view of the bladder. (b) A lateral view of the bladder.*

RENAL TRAUMA

This is discussed in Chapter 14.

NEPHRECTOMY

The most common operation that a general surgeon will perform on the kidney will be a nephrectomy. The abdomen is often already open either for an emergency laparotomy following trauma, or rarely for the resection of a malignant mass which is found to involve a kidney. When a nephrectomy is undertaken as a planned procedure, following preoperative investigations which indicate pathology confined to the kidney, there is a choice of the abdominal or the loin approach. The transperitoneal *abdominal approach* is usually considered superior in renal malignancy for the better access it gives to the great vessels. However, for very large upper renal tumours, or for retroperitoneal sarcomas, a thoraco-abdominal approach, with or without liver mobilization, provides very extensive access. The alternative retroperitoneal *loin approach* for nephrectomy may be preferable in elective surgery for infective and other benign conditions.

Laparoscopic nephrectomy is now the method of choice when nephrectomy is required for benign disease. It is also a good approach for smaller renal tumours not suitable for partial nephrectomy.

Anterior approach

The abdomen may already have been opened through a midline incision for an emergency laparotomy or for a large bowel resection. When access is required only for a nephrectomy, a transverse-orientated incision may be preferred. The peritoneum is opened, and the small bowel is packed into the opposite side of the abdomen. The peritoneum of the posterior wall is incised along the lateral aspect of the ascending colon, hepatic flexure and second part of the duodenum on the right side, or the descending colon and splenic flexure on the left side. The colon is mobilized and displaced medially to expose the anterior surface of the kidney and its pedicle.

Mobilization and vascular control

Dissection around the kidney allows full mobilization of the organ. In benign pathology, the plane immediately outside the fibrous capsule of the kidney is followed. In renal tumours a plane should be followed *outside* the perinephric fat which is resected with the kidney (see Fig. 25.1). If there is good preoperative imaging and there is no evidence of tumour in the adrenal, it is no longer considered necessary to remove the ipsilateral adrenal gland, whereas it used to be routine to do so, especially for upper pole tumours. Adrenal vessels can be difficult to secure, particularly the right adrenal veins which may lie high in the triangle between the liver and the inferior vena cava and open directly into the inferior vena cava.

A large renal tumour may have acquired additional vascular supply and drainage from surrounding tissues, and additional vessels will have to be secured. Many accessory peripheral dilated veins should warn the surgeon that the main venous drainage may be obstructed by tumour, if not already shown on preoperative imaging. A hypernephroma may also invade the renal vein and grow within its lumen. It may, therefore, be necessary to open the IVC to remove intravascular tumour. In extreme cases this has only been possible to accomplish with the aid of circulatory arrest and cardiopulmonary bypass.

During mobilization, excessive traction on the renal pedicle must be avoided, or tears of major veins can occur. Early ligation of the renal vessels, prior to full mobilization, reduces vascularity and is one advantage of the abdominal over the loin approach. In the pedicle, the renal vein lies anteriorly, and the surgeon approaching from the front may be tempted to ligate this first to improve access. A kidney with the venous return ligated, but the arterial inflow intact, will enlarge and any haemorrhage from it will dramatically increase. It is nearly always possible to ligate the artery as the initial vascular procedure (Fig. 25.4). In situations where there is a large right renal tumour closely applied to the infe-

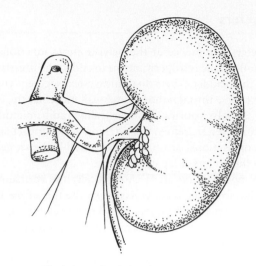

Figure 25.4 *The left renal vein has been retracted to expose the renal artery. It can be retracted cranially or caudally. Ligation of the artery before the vein prevents renal engorgement.*

rior vena cava it can help to ligate the right renal artery by approaching it between the aorta and the inferior vena cava. Change in colour of only a portion of the kidney should raise the suspicion that there is more than one renal artery. Artery, vein and ureter should be ligated separately.

The vessels should be ligated in continuity prior to division, and some surgeons prefer double ligation or transfixion ligation for additional security. The ligation should be undertaken with a thick gauge absorbable ligature, such as No. 1 Vicryl. Black silk sutures should not be used as there is an appreciable incidence of postoperative sinus formation, with discharge of suture material over many years. The exact technique is dependent upon surgeon preference, but a secure ligature is essential on these large vessels. The practice of clamping, dividing and only then ligating the vessels is not recommended as haemorrhage can be torrential if a clamp slips. The right renal vein is short and may be difficult to ligate in the way described, especially if there is tumour in its lumen. If this is so, a Satinsky clamp can be applied laterally on the vena cava where the vein enters (see Fig. 5.2, page 72). The vein is then divided distal to the clamp and the cava sutured with a continuous 5/0 vascular suture before the clamp is removed. When undertaking renal surgery it is always wise to have a Satinsky clamp immediately available.

If the kidney has been operated on before, or is infected, and there are dense adhesions, it may be impossible to identify, isolate and ligate the vessels in the way described. In such cases the pedicle can be clamped en masse and the kidney removed, leaving, beyond the clamp, sufficient tissue to allow the stumps of the main vessels to be picked up with forceps and ligated separately before removing the clamp. If even this manoeuvre is impossible, the pedicle may be ligated en masse, using a heavy absorbable transfixion suture. Where there has been prolonged severe infection, the plane between the capsule and the surrounding fat may have been obliterated. A more radical approach, similar to that employed for malignancy, may be preferable, as this will give good exposure of the vessels. However, very occasionally the inflammation is such that all planes appear obliterated, and it may be necessary to perform a subcapsular nephrectomy. Even when there is the most marked inflammatory change, the subcapsular plane remains intact. An incision is made through the renal capsule on the lateral aspect of the kidney and, by finger and gauze dissection, the plane of cleavage between it and the kidney is opened up. The separation is continued on all surfaces as far as the pedicle, where the everted capsule must be incised so that the vessels of the pedicle can be dissected out.

Finally, the ureter is ligated and divided and the kidney is lifted free from its bed.

Haemorrhage from the renal pedicle

A clamp or ligature may have slipped, or a vessel may have been injured during dissection. Profuse bleeding obscures all structures. In this situation the first rule is not to panic. No attempt should be made to secure the bleeding vessel by plunging artery forceps into a pool of blood in the hope that the vessel and nothing else will be picked up. Instead, gauze packs are pressed into the wound and the haemorrhage controlled by digital pressure. Advise the anaesthetist of the situation so that adequate venous access can be assured and blood obtained from the transfusion service. If possible, call for extra assistance. If the haemorrhage is from a divided vessel, it should be possible to remove the packs after a delay of at least 10 minutes and find that the bleeding has slowed enough for the severed vessel to be seen and secured. More frequently, especially on the right, the bleeding is from a side tear in the cava. This will not reduce spontaneously, as a partially divided vessel cannot close with spasm. Digital pressure through swabs can temporarily control the situation. The pressure is then withdrawn sequentially from above until recommencement of bleeding indicates the proximal extent of the caval tear. A continuous vascular suture is started at this point, and continued distally as the digital control is sequentially withdrawn down the cava. It is sometimes possible to apply a large Satinsky clamp to isolate the tear while it is sutured.

Open loin approach

This is an approach favoured for an elective nephrectomy for benign conditions, and is also suitable for early malignant tumours of the kidney which have not breached the renal capsule. It is therefore an approach of more limited value to the general surgeon. The loin incisions for this operation are described briefly in Chapter 12. Care is taken to sweep the peritoneum anteriorly, and the perinephric fat is opened to expose the lateral border of the kidney. The renal capsule is freed from the perinephric fat, and once the upper pole has been freed the kidney becomes much more mobile. Dissection of the pedicle, and division of the artery, vein and

ureter will then allow the kidney to be removed. The modifications which may be necessary when there are dense adhesions from chronic infection are described above.

Laparoscopic extraperitoneal approach

Those urologists who have developed laparoscopic skills are prepared to undertake an increasing range of operations on the kidney, including nephrectomy, using this technique. The recovery time is greatly reduced as both the anterior and the loin wounds required for open surgery may be a significant source of early postoperative pain and morbidity. However, if bleeding occurs during a laparoscopic nephrectomy it can be very difficult to control, and the mortality at the time of writing is between 0.5 and 1 per cent, which is higher than it is for open nephrectomy.

It must be remembered that the duodenum and colonic flexures are in close association with the anterior surface of the kidneys and are vulnerable to injury even when a retroperitoneal approach has been used, whether open or laparoscopic. A general surgeon must bear this in mind when asked by a colleague to see a postoperative urological patient who has any abdominal signs suspicious of peritonitis.

Nephro–ureterectomy

In this operation the whole length of the ureter is excised in continuity with the kidney. It is the standard treatment for *transitional cell carcinoma* in the renal pelvis, calyces or ureter. After completion of the nephrectomy, the kidney is left in the wound attached to the ureter, but nothing else. The nephrectomy wound is closed and the lower part of the ureter is approached through a separate incision in the lower abdomen. The ureterovesical junction is exposed by dividing the superior vesical vascular pedicle. Careful blunt dissection through the muscle of the bladder will liberate a delta-shaped protrusion of mucosa which will include the ureteric orifice. This is circumcised and the bladder is closed with absorbable sutures. The suture line is protected by an indwelling urethral catheter left on free drainage for 10 days. The kidney and attached ureter are removed through the lower abdominal incision.

Hemi–nephrectomy

This operation is indicated when one moiety alone of a *duplex kidney* is severely damaged by infection or trauma. There may be obstruction, or reflux, in one of the duplex ureters, with subsequent stone formation, infection, renal scarring and loss of function only in the part drained by that ureter. The associated vascular separation of the two halves makes a hemi-nephrectomy an attractive option. The hilum is dissected to identify vessels and ureters to the moiety to be removed. After ligation of these vessels, the two moieties can be separated with minimal blood loss.

Partial nephrectomy

Partial nephrectomy is a more difficult procedure than a total nephrectomy due to renal parenchymal vascularity, and in contrast to a hemi-nephrectomy in a duplex kidney, there is no natural anatomical separation to aid the surgeon. The operation should, however, be considered when only one part of the kidney is involved in pathology but the remainder of the kidney is healthy. Stone formation in a non-duplex kidney is an occasional indication for a partial nephrectomy. Although *renal tuberculosis* can be eradicated with anti-tuberculous chemotherapy, a solitary calyceal ulcer may heal with fibrosis, and a stenosed calyceal stem is common. The segment of kidney draining into this calyx is frequently also scarred but, as the remainder of the kidney is healthy, a limited resection is appropriate. Partial nephrectomy may also be indicated for a small *hypernephroma,* especially if arising in a solitary kidney. Partial nephrectomy is seldom an option in the situations with which a general surgeon is faced, but it must occasionally be attempted in trauma when there is an absent, non-functioning or poorly functioning contralateral kidney.

Access for surgery on the *in-situ* kidney is difficult in the depths of an abdominal incision, and therefore in elective situations a loin approach may be favoured. Good hilar access, however, is essential as temporary occlusion of the renal artery with a soft cross-clamp is necessary during dissection to reduce blood loss. The duration of this occlusion must however be minimized as temporary damage occurs after 15 minutes of warm ischaemia, and some permanent loss of function by 30 minutes. Cooling of the kidney increases the parenchymal tolerance of ischaemia. It is most easily accom-plished by packing sterile ice slush around the cross-clamped mobilized kidney. However, a significant reduction of temperature in the centre of the kidney is only obtained after 10–15 minutes, during which time surgery cannot proceed without partially removing the ice. Sufficient ice is then removed to enable surgery to proceed.

The arteries and veins to the portion of kidney to be excised may be ligated in the hilum, in which case a colour demarcation between perfused and non-perfused kidney will appear and form a guide to the surgeon in choosing the line of incision. The capsule is incised in the coronal plane over the pole to be removed, and is reflected back as an anterior and posterior flap (Fig. 25.5a). The kidney parenchyma is then divided along the line of demarcation, with a hilar occlusion clamp in place. Vessels in the cut surface are secured and ligated prior to release of the clamp. Opened calyces are closed with a continuous absorbable suture (Fig. 25.5b). Finally, the capsule is folded back over the raw surface and loosely sutured.

SURGERY FOR RENAL CALCULI

Renal stones may be within a calyx, or within the renal pelvis. Stones of >7 mm diameter seldom pass spontaneously, but as many are slow-growing and may remain symptomless, removal is not always indicated.

Lithotripsy: most renal calculi can be broken up by shock-waves into fragments of a size which can then pass spontaneously. A double J-stent is first passed so that the ureter dilates and fragments of stone can pass more easily.

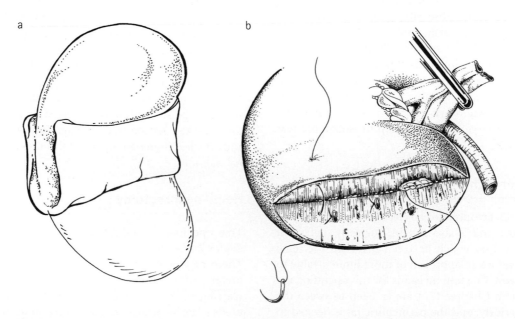

a   b

Figure 25.5 *A partial nephrectomy. The vascular pedicle is cross clamped to reduce haemorrhage. (a) The capsule is incised in the coronal plane and reflected. (b) The parenchyma has been divided as two flaps and parenchymal vessels ligated. The inner suture is closing the opened collecting system before closure of the parenchyma and the capsular flaps.*

Pyelolithotomy: the renal pelvis is opened and a stone removed from the pelvis, or from an accessible calyx (Fig. 25.6). An *extended pyelolithotomy* is a technique in which the plane is developed between the intrarenal pelvis and the overlying renal parenchyma, which is then retracted. The incision into the pelvis can then be extended into the necks of the calyces to remove a staghorn calculus. The incision is closed with absorbable sutures and a ureteric stent left *in situ* for a few weeks. This type of open surgery is very rarely undertaken by surgeons who have access to lithotripsy, or to percutaneous pyelolithotomy.

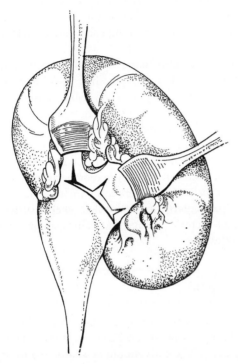

Figure 25.6 *A pyelolithotomy. Retraction to open the plane between renal parenchyma and intrarenal pelvis allows the incision to be extended into the major calyces.*

Nephrolithotomy: the incision is made directly through the renal parenchyma into a calyx. Haemorrhage may be brisk.

Total or partial nephrectomy: a total nephrectomy is the optimum treatment for a non-functioning kidney with a staghorn calculus which is the seat of recurrent urinary sepsis. A hemi-nephrectomy is a good option in a duplex kidney, and occasionally a partial nephrectomy may be justified if only part of a non-duplex kidney is affected.

Minimal access techniques: these techniques have greatly reduced the need for open surgery for renal calculi. A nephrolithotomy can be performed percutaneously, and a nephroscope is passed into the renal pelvis. Alternatively, a pyelolithotomy can be performed laparoscopically. It is also possible to reach the renal pelvis ureteroscopically at cystoscopy. Calculi can be removed from the kidney via all these approaches. A *percutaneous nephrolithotomy* has become the

treatment of choice for stones in the renal pelvis which cannot be treated solely by lithotripsy. When complete removal at percutaneous nephrolithotomy proves impossible, a staghorn calculus can be debulked and lithotripsy then used to break up remaining fragments.

SURGERY FOR HYDRONEPHROSIS

Hydronephrosis means dilatation of the pelvis and calyces of the kidney. It may be congenital, secondary to a muscular incoordination resulting in a functional obstruction, or it may be due to a mechanical obstruction from a stone, a benign stricture or a tumour. Dilatation can also occur without any evidence of obstruction, and is frequently bilateral and associated with hydroureters. This is seen in pregnancy and in ureteric reflux. Differentiation between a dilated and an obstructed collecting system is essential, as a system which is simply *dilated* often requires no intervention. The stagnant urine is, however, susceptible to infection.

An *obstructed* system requires drainage, or correction of the underlying pathology, as the increased pressure in the calyces results in a deterioration in renal function, which eventually becomes irreversible. The urgency of the situation depends on the completeness of the obstruction, whether one or both kidneys are obstructed and whether there is infection. Bilateral obstruction, or obstruction in a solitary kidney, is thus of greater urgency, and an obstructed infected kidney, *pyonephrosis*, is an emergency which should be addressed within a few hours (see Chapter 14). Delays of more than a few days should, however, be avoided even in a unilateral obstruction without infection as, especially in complete obstruction, some irreversible damage is already occurring to the kidney.

Nephrostomy

An image-guided percutaneous nephrostomy drainage tube inserted by a radiologist is usually the first choice in management of a pyonephrosis. If ultrasound-guided percutaneous drainage is not available, an attempt can be made to drain the kidney endoscopically from below by guiding a catheter up the ureter past the obstruction under image intensifier control, but this is usually not possible, and an open nephrostomy through a loin approach may be the only option.

Pyeloplasty

An *idiopathic congenital pelvi-ureteric junction (PUJ) obstruction* is secondary to a muscular incoordination at this site, and results in a hydronephrosis. Surgical correction by pyeloplasty is indicated for obstruction rather than for simple dilatation, and careful preoperative assessment of this is essential. The PUJ is divided, and reconstructed to form a wider junction with more dependent drainage. The excess renal pelvic tissue is excised. There are multiple refinements of the technique, a simple form of which is shown diagrammatically in Figure 25.7. The operation can be performed as an open, or as a laparoscopic, retroperitoneal procedure. Absorbable sutures must be used to reconstruct the junction and a ureteric stent (if used) is left *in situ* for about 3 weeks. If there is an abnormal lower pole vessel, the reconstruction is carried out anterior to this. Pelvi-calyceal dilation may be little altered at follow-up imaging, but the potentially damaging obstructive element should have been relieved.

Endoscopic balloon dilatation, with or without incision of the PUJ, is a newer technique with variable long-term results.

RENAL TRANSPLANTS

A patient with a renal transplant may present to the general surgeon with other unrelated intra-abdominal pathology. The donor kidney may cause problems with diagnosis, and with surgical access. It has most commonly been placed retroperitoneally in an iliac fossa, and it is turned so that its original posterior surface lies anteriorly. The renal pelvis and the ureter are therefore lying anteromedially and the hilar vessels posterolaterally. The donor renal artery will have been anastomosed end-to-end to the internal iliac artery or, in the case of multiple renal arteries, to the side of the external iliac artery using a donor arterial patch. The donor renal vein is anastomosed end-to-side to the external iliac vein. This anastomotic arrangement may have been contraindicated by atheroma, and alternative donor vessels, including the splenic, may have been used. In children, the transplant may have been placed intraperitoneally, with the anastomoses to the aorta and IVC in the lower abdomen.

URETERIC DAMAGE

Most ureteric trauma is iatrogenic in general and gynaecological surgery. In some instances it is inevitable when a ureter is invaded by an otherwise resectable primary tumour. In other instances, inadvertent damage occurs. A ureter may be ligated in error and unless the injury is bilateral, or in the only functioning kidney, the surgeon may remain unaware of the problem. A non-functioning kidney may then be an incidental finding some years later, but this can also occur when the ureter has not been ligated or divided. A difficult dissection close to the ureter can cause ischaemic damage with late stricturing and obstruction. Damage to a ureter can also be caused by diathermy, especially during a laparoscopic procedure.

When it is realized that a ureter has been damaged the surgeon should, if at all possible, seek assistance. It is generally true that any surgeon who causes inadvertent damage to any organ in the body is much less likely to perform a good repair than a colleague who was not involved in the original injury. In the case of accidental damage to the ureter there is often a range of surgical options and, as in all surgery, the choice of procedure may be as important as the technical aspects of the operation which is undertaken. It is therefore particularly important that when a surgeon causes inadvertent ureteric damage that help is sought from a urological colleague.

Simple repair

Simple repair with interrupted fine absorbable sutures is ideal, but it is only possible when there is minimal loss of tissue (Fig. 25.8). The ends should be spatulated to reduce the chance of an anastomotic stricture. A ureteric double **J** or pigtail stent is inserted both up and down from the point of injury, and should be left *in situ* for 3–4 weeks postoperatively. The guide wire within the stent holds the curled ends straight

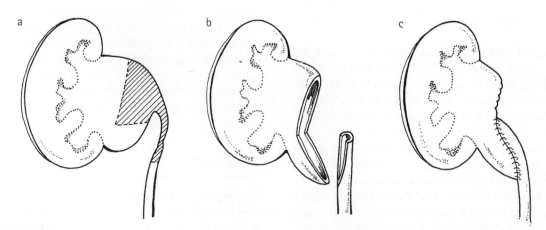

Figure 25.7   *An Anderson–Hynes pyeloplasty. This operation and all the modifications of it are designed to produce a wide dependent pelvi-ureteric junction for improved drainage.*

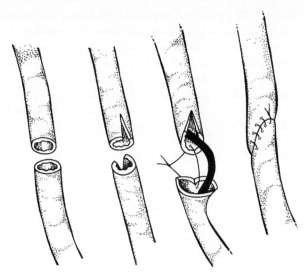

Figure 25.8   *An end-to-end anastomotic repair of a divided ureter. Each end of the ureter is spatulated. This results in a wide oblique anastomosis which is carried out with interrupted sutures over a ureteric stent.*

during insertion. The guide wire is then removed and the curl returns to the ends. It is these curled portions lying within the renal pelvis, and within the bladder, which prevent stent migration. It is particularly important with any ureteric stent that the lower end is in the bladder, and not curled in the distal ureter where it will be difficult to remove. If there is any doubt, the position of the lower end is easily checked by cystoscopy. Subsequent removal may be performed with a flexible cystoscope as a local anaesthestic procedure.

Re-implantation into the bladder

This is a reconstructive option that should be considered when simple repair is not possible. It is particularly suitable when the ureteric division is close to the bladder. The bladder is opened, and the divided ureter is spatulated to produce a wider anastomosis with less chance of a stenosis. An oblique tunnel is created through the bladder wall. The anastomosis is performed over a ureteric stent. Mucosal apposition is achieved with fine absorbable sutures, and the bladder muscle wall closed around the ureter with sutures which also tether the muscular coat of the ureter to the bladder (Fig. 25.9). Any tension on the anastomosis must be avoided and a *psoas hitch,* in which the bladder is hitched up and fixed to the psoas muscle prior to the re-implantation, is a useful manoeuvre (Fig. 25.10). It may help to make re-implantation possible when there is some loss of ureteric length. A flap of bladder (a *Boari flap*) can also be raised and formed into a tubular extension to the bladder which will reach a surprisingly high level (Fig. 25.11). An isolated ileal loop, fashioned to form a ureteric replacement, is another option when there is a long segment of proximal ureter to be replaced, but this is very much a last resort procedure.

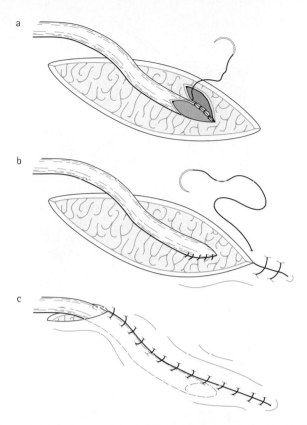

Figure 25.9   *Direct re-implantation of a ureter into the bladder is occasionally possible after a distal injury if there is sufficient length. The creation of an intramural tunnel will prevent reflux. (a) A 2 to 3 cm incision is made through the muscle coat of the bladder. At one end the incision is deepened through the mucosa. This mucosal incision should create an aperture of similar diameter to that of the spatulated ureter. An anastomosis is performed. (b) The muscle layer of the bladder wall is closed over the ureter. (c) The ureter is lying in an intramural tunnel. The final suture of the muscle layer can also be used to pick up the outer layers of the ureter to reduce any possible traction on the anastomosis.*

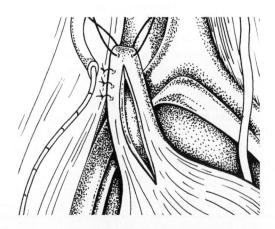

Figure 25.10   *A psoas hitch. The bladder is drawn up, out of the pelvis, and fixed to the psoas muscle. This shortens the distance over which the ureter has to reach and reduces anastomotic tension.*

a

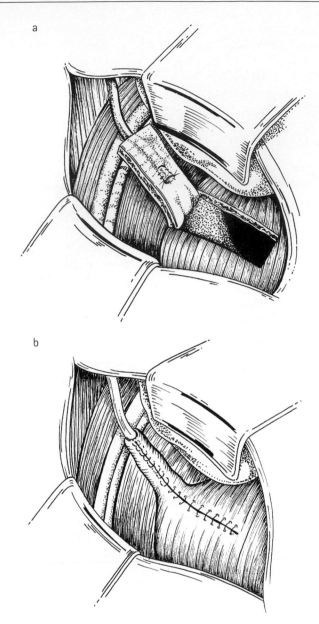

b

Figure 25.11 *A Boari flap. (a) The bladder must be drawn over to the side of the injury, and increased mobility will be obtained by mobilizing the opposite side of the bladder. A long flap, with a superolateral base, has been cut from the bladder. The ureter is anastomosed to the flap, with a submucosal tunnel. (b) The flap is tubularized and the suture line continued to close the donor defect.*

Re-implantation of a ureter into the bladder may also be needed for distal ureteric obstruction and for ureteric reflux, and re-implantation of the ureter forms part of the operation of renal transplantation.

Uretero–ureterostomy

Re-implantation of a divided ureter into the other ureter can always be considered in any situation where direct repair is impractical, and the proximal divided end does not reach to the bladder. The proximal portion of the ureter is dissected and freed so that it can be drawn across the midline. The other ureter will also need some mobilization before a tension-free anastomosis can be achieved. Ureters can be mobilized over a considerable distance without suffering ischaemia as there is an excellent anastomotic intramural blood supply. The divided end is spatulated and anastomosed end to side into the other ureter which should be stented (Fig. 25.12).

Although the advantages of re-implantation in preserving a functioning kidney are obvious, the surgery will add to the magnitude of the operation and may be an unjustifiable additional procedure in the occasional patient. It must be remembered also that, if complications develop, the future of the contralateral previously healthy kidney may also have been jeopardized.

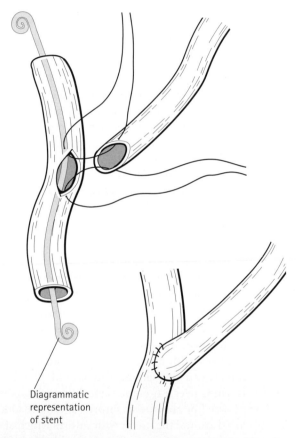

Diagrammatic representation of stent

Figure 25.12 *Implantation of a divided ureter into the other ureter is frequently the most satisfactory solution when a ureter has been damaged and length has been lost. The ureteric stent is placed in the normal ureter.*

Simple ligation

Simple ligation of the proximal ureter is an option when a segment has been excised which precludes a simple repair, and the condition of the patient contraindicates extending the surgery further. The presence of a functioning contralateral kidney must be established. The obstructed kidney atrophies and seldom produces any complications such as urine leakage from the ureteric stump with the development of a ureteric fistula, pain from the initial hydronephrosis or the development of a pyonephrosis. This is in essence little different from the situation where a non-functioning kidney is discovered incidentally some years after pelvic surgery and unsuspected inadvertent ureteric damage, or ligation, at that operation is the most likely explanation.

Nephrectomy

This may occasionally be indicated if ureteric re-implantation is not possible, or is contraindicated. It will prevent any complications which might develop in the obstructed kidney if a ureter is simply ligated, but it also increases the magnitude of the surgery.

URETERIC STONE REMOVAL

Ureteric calculi often cause renal colic and temporary partial obstruction before passing spontaneously. Stones above 5 mm in diameter are less likely to pass spontaneously, but for smaller stones, a short trial of conservative management is usually appropriate. The exceptions are complete obstruction of a solitary kidney or proximal infection. The need for urgent intervention in these situations is discussed above. Ureteric stone removal is more commonly an elective procedure when it becomes apparent that the stone will not pass spontaneously. If obstruction is only intermittent, or partial, a delay of some weeks may not be detrimental to renal function.

Open surgery to remove a ureteric calculus is seldom required in urological practice today. Calculi can usually be retrieved, or broken up, endoscopically, either under image control or with direct vision through a ureteroscope. If this is unsuccessful, it is usually possible to pass a guide wire alongside the stone up to the kidney, and a fine stent can then be introduced over the guide wire. The stent is left *in situ* while further treatment is arranged. For stones in the upper one-third of the ureter, the generally safe option is to push the stone back into the renal pelvis and then to arrange for the patient to undergo lithotripsy (the push bang procedure). Alternative techniques of endoscopic lithotripsy, and especially direct vision basketry, carry increased risks and are best not attempted outside of a stone management centre. A general surgeon practising in a remote area without access to a urologist, a lithotriptor or any image control may still need to remove a ureteric stone by open surgery.

Ureterolithotomy

An X-ray should be taken on the operating table before commencing surgery to check that the position of the stone has not altered. The site of the incision will depend on the position of the stone, and the ureter is approached retroperitoneally. Difficulty in finding the ureter can occur if the middle third becomes raised up on the under-surface of the peritoneum. The lower one-third may also be difficult to identify. It may then be easier to identify the ureter at a higher level in the pelvis, or even at the pelvic brim, and then follow it distally.

The ureter is first identified above the stone and a tape passed around it to prevent upward displacement of the stone. The ureter is then followed distally and the position of the stone is recognized by a fusiform swelling of the ureter, and is confirmed by palpation. A second tape is passed around the ureter below the stone. Two stay sutures are inserted into the ureter at the level of the stone and the stone is steadied between finger and thumb. A longitudinal incision is made through the ureter, between the stay sutures and directly over the stone. The incision begins over the thickest part of the stone and extends upwards to a level just above its upper end (Fig. 25.13). The stone is delivered out through the incision. A ureteric catheter is then passed up and down to wash out any further debris. The incision in the ureter may be repaired with fine absorbable sutures which do not penetrate the mucosa (Fig. 25.14). When the ureteric wall is traumatized and oedematous, sutures may be contraindicated and the incision can be left open. A drain should be left to the ureter as, even if it has been closed, urine leakage for a few days is common. If a ureteric stent is employed it can be removed about 4 weeks later.

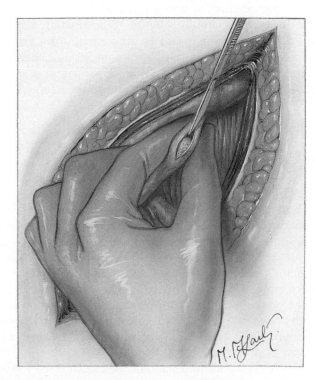

Figure 25.13 *Uretero-lithotomy. An original drawing by Margaret McLarty for the 1st edition of this book published in 1954.*

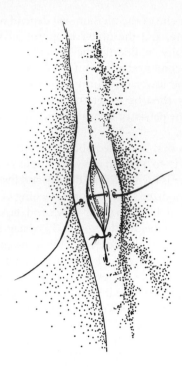

Figure 25.14   *Closure of a longitudinal incision into a ureter has the potential to cause a stricture. Sutures should be loose, well-spaced and ideally should exclude the mucosa.*

URINARY DIVERSION

When there is an intact upper urinary system, but the bladder has been excised, or does not function adequately, then some form of urinary diversion or reconstruction may be required. Diversion may also be appropriate for a grossly symptomatic bladder damaged by tumour, chronic infection or radiotherapy. It is also an alternative to a permanent indwelling catheter or intermittent self-catheterization.

Ileal conduits

This is the standard procedure for urinary diversion. The ureters are re-implanted into an isolated small bowel conduit which is brought out as a permanent urinary stoma. A loop of ileum, at least 15 cm from the ileocaecal valve, is isolated on its mesentery. The loop must be long enough to extend without tension from the midline posteriorly to some 5 cm beyond the site chosen preoperatively on the anterior abdominal wall for the stoma. The ileal mesentery is divided sufficiently to allow the necessary mobility while preserving a good blood supply (Fig. 25.15a). The loop will function as a urinary conduit ending as an ileostomy stoma. Small bowel continuity is re-established by an anastomosis in front of the isolated loop.

The ureters are identified and divided as far distally as is practical. Some mobilization of the caecum and sigmoid colon will usually be necessary at this stage, and it is recom-

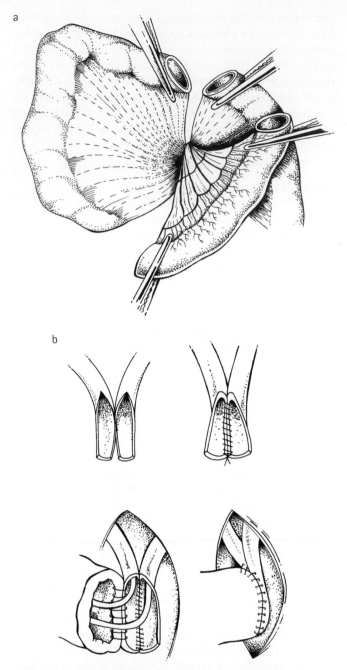

Figure 25.15   *An ileal conduit. (a) A suitable loop of ileum is isolated. The divided ends of ileum will then be brought in front of it for the anastomosis to restore continuity. (b) The ureters are implanted into the proximal end of the loop, the distal end of which is then brought through the abdominal wall as an end ileostomy.*

mended that an appendicectomy is performed as subsequent surgery for appendicitis may be difficult. The left ureter is then tunnelled medially, under the pelvic mesocolon, to lie alongside the right ureter. Both ureters are implanted into the isolated ileal loop and the distal end of this ileal conduit is then brought out, through the abdominal wall, as an ileostomy stoma (see Chapter 21). A variety of methods are employed to perform the anastomoses of the ureters into the ileum. Spatulation of the ureters, and accurate mucosal apposition, may be important in the prevention of anastomotic strictures, but as reflux is not a problem an intramural tunnel is not required (Fig. 25.15b). The anastomoses of ureters to ileum are normally stented for 2 weeks.

Ureterosigmoidostomy

This was a popular solution as it avoided a stoma and is still used in those countries where a stoma is unacceptable, or where stoma appliances are unavailable. However, there are significantly more complications than with ileal conduits. The rectal contents become fluid and if there is any impairment of sphincter function some degree of incontinence is inevitable. Ascending infection of the upper renal tract is common, even when the ureter is tunnelled obliquely though the colonic wall to minimize reflux (Fig. 25.16). Absorption of urine leads to metabolic disturbances, and urine is carcinogenic in contact with colonic mucosa. This appears to be a particular risk when there is mixing of urinary and faecal contents within the lumen, and patients who have this form of diversion should ideally, after about 10 years, have regular colonoscopy to inspect for malignant lesions near the site of the ureterocolonic anastomosis.

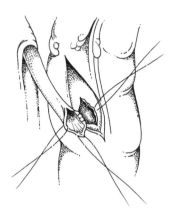

Figure 25.16 *Uterosigmoidostomy. Accurate mucosal apposition is followed by closure of the seromuscular coat of the colon over the ureter to create a submucosal tunnel. Even with this refinement to prevent reflux, ascending infections are common.*

Ureterostomy

This is the simplest diversion of the ureter, directly to the skin, as a urinary stoma. There are several disadvantages:

- two ureters require two separate stomas as ureteric length is usually insufficient to bring them out together;
- ureteric length is often still insufficient to reach the skin without tension in a fat patient; and
- the stoma is liable to stenose.

Eversion of the stoma to produce a spout similar to an ileostomy and accurate skin mucosal apposition will to some extent prevent stenosis, but this is only possible with sufficient ureteric length. Although a ureterostomy may be useful as a temporary procedure in children, it is generally impractical in adults because of insufficient ureteral length and almost universal stenosis.

CATHETERIZATION

Urethral catheterization

This is required for many non-urological surgical patients in the perioperative and early postoperative phases, and the catheter is frequently inserted after induction of anaesthesia. On other occasions, a catheter has to be inserted postoperatively for a patient in urinary retention. As with all invasive urological procedures, antibiotic cover is advisable. A small Foley type catheter (size 12–14) with a 5–10 mL self-retaining balloon is satisfactory. A wider catheter and larger balloon merely causes more urethral trauma and bladder irritation.

Difficulties in *female* patients are usually related to an invisible urethral orifice which has been drawn up the anterior vaginal wall into a stenosed vagina. The position of the urethral orifice can usually be identified digitally, as lying in the midline at the junction between the smooth vulval and the corrugated vaginal mucosa, and the catheter is then guided in, on the index finger.

Difficulties in *male* patients are often related to inadequate lubrication and a lack of appreciation of the curves of the male urethra (see Fig. 24.16, page 478). Force is inappropriate as false passages can be created. If there is difficulty, further trauma to the urethra should be avoided. Either a suprapubic catheter should be inserted, or the urethra visualized by cystoscopy. A failed urethral catheterization at the start of an abdominal operation can wait for a suprapubic catheter to be inserted once the abdomen is open.

Percutaneous suprapubic catheterization

This is an alternative to urethral catheterization, and is relatively simple when there is an enlarged palpable bladder. Local anaesthesia is injected into the midline skin and abdominal wall 5 cm above the pubis. Confirmation that the swelling is indeed bladder can be obtained by aspiration of urine through a needle prior to proceeding further. A 1- to 2-cm skin and linea alba incision is made, through which a trocar and cannula is introduced into the bladder. The trocar is withdrawn and the backflow of urine can be temporarily controlled with a finger until the self-retaining catheter is inserted down the cannula into the bladder. The proprietary suprapubic catheterization sets have a cannula which splits into two portions. This makes it easier to remove once the catheter is in place.

Extraperitoneal perforations, which may be deliberate with extensive tumour resections, will require catheter drainage for 10–14 days. Intraperitoneal perforations may require laparotomy and closure.

TRANSURETHRAL RESECTION OF THE PROSTATE

This is the standard operation for urinary retention, or severe urinary symptoms attributable to the prostate. A retropubic prostatectomy will usually be a safer option in the hands of a general surgeon without endoscopic expertise, and is a suitable alternative except for obstruction from a malignant prostate.

It may not be necessary to resect small obstructed glands as they can be treated by a bladder neck incision. This is a full-thickness cut made from below one of the ureteric orifices, through the prostatic capsule to the level of the verumontanum. After this procedure the bladder neck can be seen to 'spring open'. However, larger prostates will need to be resected.

Operative procedure

The object of the resection is to remove the central adenomatous tissue, leaving the prostatic capsule. For full operative details the reader should refer to a standard text on transurethral resection.[4] The resectoscope is passed as for the resection of a bladder tumour. Different surgeons then proceed in a variety of ways. One method is to start the resection at around the 5 o'clock position, cutting a groove from the bladder neck down to the verumontanum, and deepening the channel until the more fibrous prostatic capsule is seen. A similar groove is cut at the 7 o'clock position, and the whole of the posterior middle lobe can be resected. Haemostasis is secured with the patient slightly head-down, and a similar groove is cut anteriorly at 12 o'clock to the level of the verumontanum, again exposing the capsule. The channel is widened on one side and, by resecting at the level of the capsule, the lateral lobe can be detached from the capsule, and it will fall medially. When the majority of the lobe has been detached it can be resected piecemeal, and capsular haemostasis obtained. A similar procedure is then carried out on the opposite side. The most important point in the technique is to ensure haemostasis after each stage of the procedure. If vision is lost it may be safer to stop resecting, insert a catheter and, if necessary, repeat the resection some months later.

At the end of the operation, after haemostasis has been checked, the bladder is drained with a stiff 22/24 three-way irrigating catheter.

OPEN BLADDER AND PROSTATIC SURGERY

The bladder and prostate are usually approached through a suprapubic incision, and the dissection is in the pre-peritoneal plane. The general surgeon, however, is more likely to be involved with the bladder from within the peritoneal cavity when it is involved in trauma, or in intestinal pathology.

Trauma

Bladder trauma can be divided into intraperitoneal and extraperitoneal rupture. *Cystography* may be useful in diagnosis. Intraperitoneal rupture requires a laparotomy and closure of the bladder wall with absorbable sutures, followed by a period of at least 10 days during which the bladder undergoes continuous catheter drainage to allow healing. Extraperitoneal rupture can usually be managed by catheter drainage alone. However, it may well be associated with major pelvic trauma, and suprapubic urinary drainage may then be more appropriate. Injuries of the proximal urethra are discussed in Chapter 24. Iatrogenic trauma is most often in the form of an inadvertent entry into the bladder when opening the abdomen, or during pelvic dissection. Closure of the opening with absorbable sutures, and urethral drainage, is all that is required.

Vesicovaginal fistulae

The most common cause of these fistulae is a childbirth injury. The repair is described in more detail in Chapter 26.

Bladder calculi

The removal of calculi which are too large to be removed endoscopically is a straightforward procedure through a preperitoneal suprapubic approach. In adults, bladder calculi are usually associated with bladder outflow obstruction, or a large residual urine, and the underlying cause should be addressed. Bladder calculi in young children are common in some parts of the developing world, and this is a condition for which a general surgeon may have to operate. After removal of the calculus the bladder is closed and drained as described above.

Partial cystectomy

This is an operation which is probably performed more frequently by general surgeons than by urologists. A disc of bladder may be excised which is adherent to, and possibly invaded by, a sigmoid cancer. A diverticular mass may also be densely adherent to the bladder, but can often be 'pinched off'. However, at the time of surgery, malignancy may still be suspected and a disc of bladder is then often resected en bloc, to avoid opening potential tumour planes and compromising a curative resection. Both sigmoid malignancy and diverticular disease may be associated with a colovesical fistula. The main concern is the proximity of the involved bladder to the trigone and the ureteric orifices. A preoperative cystoscopy will often demonstrate the area of tethered or inflamed mucosa. If it is close to the trigone, or difficulty is anticipated, ureteric catheterization will make identification of the ureters easier during the dissection. After excision of a disc of bladder, the bladder wall is closed in two layers, and drained by a catheter until healing is sound. The more distal rectovesical fistulae, which is associated with locally invasive rectal or bladder cancer, will commonly involve the bladder trigone. A colorectal surgeon operating on a patient with a high rectal cancer with a fistula into the bladder should not anticipate that a partial cystectomy will be an option, as the ureteric orifices will almost certainly also be involved. The surgical options will be either a palliative colostomy to reduce the faecal contamination of the urinary tract, or a combined operation with a urologist to perform a pelvic exenteration and urinary diversion.

Total cystectomy

Total cystectomy is the best potentially curative option in some patients with locally invasive bladder cancer. However, in truly advanced bladder malignancy it has little place as distant metastases are usually present. It is also indicated in patients who present with superficial bladder cancer associated with widespread carcinoma *in situ*, who fail to respond to intravesical immunotherapy or chemotherapy. Intravesical BCG may reverse the changes in the transitional epithelium, but maintenance treatment and careful surveillance with multiple biopsies is important. If no action is taken, progression to invasive tumour is almost inevitable. The following is a summary of the operation, but a surgeon embarking on this procedure will require more operative detail.[5]

Operative procedure
At laparotomy, the extent of the disease is ascertained and, if still thought suitable for operation, the initial procedure is bilateral dissection and removal of the common iliac and obturator lymph nodes. The vasa and obliterated umbilical vessels are divided, and the ureters identified at the pelvic brim and dissected free down to the bladder, dividing the superior vesical vascular pedicles laterally. Posteriorly, the peritoneum in the rectovesical pouch is divided, and the plane between the rectum and Denonvillier's fascia posteriorly, and the bladder, seminal vesicles and prostate anteriorly, is opened. The ureters are divided as low down as is convenient.

The anterior surface of the bladder and prostate are exposed and the endopelvic fascia, attaching the prostate to the back of the pubis, is divided. The dorsal venous complex at the apex of the prostate can be divided between sutures, exposing the urethra. This (and the *in-situ* urethral catheter) is then divided, and haemostasis of the distal end, and the dorsal venous complex, can be achieved by sutures. The bladder and prostate can then be removed en bloc by division of the inferior vesical plexus. In the female, total cystectomy is combined with a hysterectomy.

The standard urinary diversion is via an ileal conduit.

Today, for younger patients, bladder reconstructive procedures are feasible.

Total cystectomy also forms part of the total pelvic exenteration which is sometimes indicated for a locally advanced rectal, cervical or uterine cancer. The urologist, general surgeon and gynaecologist may operate together in such cases. The dissection is modified so that planes between the bladder and adjacent involved organs are not breached.

Bladder reconstruction

An isolated segment of bowel can be used to replace part, or all, of the bladder. The complete replacement of the bladder with a neo-bladder fashioned from an ileal loop, is a relatively new technique which can provide good functional results when the surgery is undertaken by urologists with a special interest. The neo-bladder is created from a de-tubularized loop of ileum or colon, which is isolated from the gastrointestinal tract in a similar manner to that described for an ileal conduit. The ureters are implanted into the neo-bladder, which is then anastomosed to the proximal urethra or trigone.

A de-tubularized bowel loop can also be used to augment a small shrunken bladder. The bladder is split coronally to receive the bowel loop which augments the bladder volume.

Retropubic prostatectomy

In benign pathology, the enlarged prostate can be removed at open surgery by either a retropubic or a transvesical route. Only the retropubic approach has remained in common use, and even the indications for this method are dwindling as transurethral resection has become the standard treatment in skilled hands, for even very large prostates.

Operative procedure
A cystoscopy should be performed before a retropubic prostatectomy to exclude any associated bladder pathology. The patient is then placed supine, and the table tilted headdown. The extraperitoneal plane is entered via a lower midline or transverse suprapubic incision (Fig. 25.18a). The wound is held open with a self-retaining retractor and pressure is exerted on the bladder with a swab held in forceps. This tilts the prostate away from the pubis and exposes the fat on the surface of the prostatic capsule. The vessels within this fat must be secured with coagulation diathermy, or ligation, so that the fat can be cleared to expose the capsule and the fibres of the puboprostatic ligaments meeting in a **V** at the bladder neck. The prostatic capsule will be opened transversely a centimetre or two below the bladder neck. Deep absorbable stay sutures are placed above and below the point chosen for this incision. These sutures are tied to reduce bleeding from the capsule (Fig. 25.18b). A generous transverse incision is then made through the prostatic capsule to expose the white surface of the adenoma.

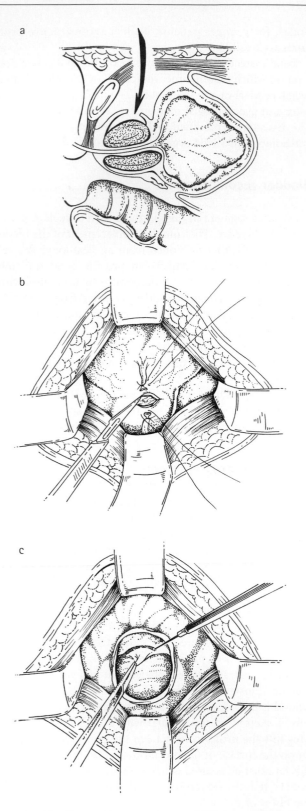

Figure 25.18 *Retropubic prostatectomy. (a) The pre-peritoneal space is entered suprapubically. (b) The anterior prostatic capsule is completely cleared of fat and veins, and is incised transversely between stay sutures. (c) The bladder neck has been grasped with tissue forceps and the middle lobe of the prostate is excised. Identification of the ureteric orifices is important at this stage to avoid damaging them when the bladder neck suture is placed.*

The anterior commissure of the prostatic lobes is then opened digitally to enable the surgeon's index finger to enter the prostatic urethra and feel the veru montanum and the prostatic adenoma from within the urethra. Digital pressure with the index finger posterolaterally just above the level of the veru will produce a split in the urethra. This split can be extended around the apex of the prostatic adenoma by further digital pressure, and the remainder of the plane between the adenoma and the prostatic capsule is then freed in a similar manner. The adenomatous lobe is then delivered out of the capsule and its remaining attachment at the bladder neck divided with scissors. The procedure is then repeated on the other side.

The prostatic cavity is then packed with swabs, and attention turned to the middle lobe. The top of the middle lobe is grasped in tissue forceps and drawn forwards, while a small swab on a stick, placed in the base of the bladder, is drawn anteriorly. This will demonstrate the interureteric bar and the ureteric orifices. The middle lobe is then resected. A diathermy incision is commenced in the midline behind the middle lobe (Fig. 25.18c). The incision is carried anterolaterally in front of each ureteric orifice to the bladder neck. The posterior prostatic urethra can then be divided with scissors just above the level of the veru montanum and the enucleation of the middle lobe completed.

Haemostasis can be improved by suturing the posterior bladder mucosa to the bladder neck with an absorbable suture. The first stitch of the capsular closure is inserted beyond each end of the capsular opening. A strong absorbable material is used and a deep bite is taken. Tying of these stitches reduces the prostatic capsular bleeding, whilst the prostatic cavity is checked for bleeding points which can be sealed with diathermy coagulation. Finally, the closure of the capsule is completed from both ends with a haemostatic continuous suture. Pressure on the bladder, similar to that used before the capsule was opened, will improve access for closure. A rigid plastic 22/24 three-way catheter is guided into the bladder before the capsular closure is completed. The tip will tend to catch on the bladder neck, and has to be lifted forwards. After capsular closure, the catheter balloon is inflated with 30 mL of water and the bladder filled to check for leakage at the closure site. Additional sutures can be placed if there is any leakage, or continuing suture-line haemorrhage. When there is excessive bleeding from the prostatic bed, it may be advisable to place an additional suprapubic catheter through the anterior wall of the bladder before the capsular closure is complete. This can be used for extra irrigation.

A retropubic drain is advisable for the first 48 hours. The urethral catheter is placed on continuous irrigation and continuous drainage. Irrigation can be stopped when bleeding reduces, and no further clots are in danger of blocking the catheter. The catheter can normally be removed after around 5–6 days. A blocked catheter requires saline irrigation with a bladder syringe. Occasionally, a patient has to be returned to theatre for excessive bleeding. A resectoscope is passed, the clot washed out and bleeding points are sought, but seldom found. Fortunately, even if no bleeding point is identified, the bleeding usually settles after such a washout.

Radical prostatectomy

The diagnosis and management of prostate cancer is a major aspect of urological practice, but is outwith the scope of a general surgical text. Biochemical screening, in conjunction with prostatic biopsy, can be used to identify men with presymptomatic early prostate cancer. In those with a life expectancy of over 10 years, radical retropubic prostatectomy is now one of the treatment options. Radical prostatectomy is only an option in early disease and, even in expert hands, carries a significant morbidity of incontinence and impotence.

Radiotherapy is another potentially curative option in localized prostate cancer. Medical castration therapy with hormone manipulation is an important treatment both for the elderly patient with a limited life expectancy, and for those with metastatic disease in whom it can abolish the pain from metastases. In those countries with limited healthcare resources, bilateral orchidectomy remains a useful alterna-

tive to medical castration. A transurethral resection of the malignant prostate may be required for outflow obstruction.

SURGERY OF THE URETHRA

For details, see Chapter 24.

REFERENCES

1. *Campbell's Urology*, 8th edn. P. Walsh, *et al.* Philadelphia: Elsevier, 2002.
2. *Smith's General Urology*, 15th edn. EA Tanagho, JW McAninch (eds). London: McGraw-Hill, 2000.
3. Perrin LC, Penfold C, McLeish A. A prospective randomized controlled trial comparing suprapubic with urethral catheterization in rectal surgery. *Aust NZ J Surg* 1997; **67**: 554–6.
4. *Transurethral Resection*, 4th edn. JP Blandy, RG Notley (eds). London: Martin Dunitz, 1998.
5. Moffat L. How I do it – radical cystectomy and ileal conduit for invasive bladder tumour. *J R Coll Surg Edinb* 1999; **44**: 379–85.

26

GYNAECOLOGICAL ENCOUNTERS IN GENERAL SURGERY

Not infrequently, the general surgeon, when performing a laparotomy, encounters an unexpected gynaecological condition, the correct management of which may cause some doubt and anxiety. The surgeon can usually call on the assistance of a gynaecological colleague, and should do so if at all possible. However, on occasion, and without access to a gynaecological opinion, the general surgeon must accept responsibility for deciding what, if any, operative procedure is indicated and for mastering the techniques required. It is mainly for such guidance that this chapter is written.

There are some general surgeons working in small remote hospitals who are offering a simple, but reasonably comprehensive, obstetric and gynaecological service. This chapter cannot cover their operative surgical needs, and further training and reading is recommended.[1-4] There are, however, other surgeons whose normal practice does not include obstetrics or gynaecology but who may be summoned unexpectedly in a small hospital as the only available surgeon to operate in a life-threatening obstetric or gynaecological emergency. These situations are covered briefly in the following text.

Many of the scenarios outlined below would ideally be treated by less invasive procedures if a preoperative diagnosis could have been established, and if the necessary equipment and expertise were available. For example, many ectopic pregnancies can be managed laparoscopically, and massive obstetric haemorrhage may sometimes be best controlled by embolization of pelvic vessels. However, on the occasions when a general surgeon has to be involved in an obstetric or gynaecological emergency, these techniques are seldom an option.

SURGICAL ANATOMY

The female genital tract, which lies between the rectum and the bladder, is confined to the pelvis except in pregnancy.

The vagina

The vagina lies in close proximity to the bladder and urethra anteriorly, and to the rectum and anus posteriorly. Below the peritoneal reflection, the vaginal and rectal walls are separated by the rectovaginal septum, and above the peritoneal reflection by the rectovaginal pouch, or 'Pouch of Douglas'. The vault of the vagina is invaginated anteriorly by the uterine cervix which divides the vault into anterior, lateral and posterior fornices. The ureters and the uterine arteries are closely related to the lateral fornices.

- The *labia majora* skin folds lie on either side of the vaginal introitus, with the smaller *labia minora* medially.
- Flanking the vaginal introitus are *Bartholin's glands* and their ducts which open into the vagina distal to the hymen.

The uterus

The uterus lies between the bladder and the rectum, as a mainly intraperitoneal organ. Anteriorly, the peritoneum is reflected onto the upper surface of the bladder from the shallow *uterovesical pouch*; posteriorly, it sweeps downwards over the posterior fornix and then is reflected onto the anterior aspect of the mid-rectum, thus forming the *rectovaginal Pouch of Douglas*. The uterine *cervix* is below the peritoneal reflection. The supravaginal portion of the cervix is related to the bladder anteriorly, to which it is connected by some loose fibrous strands.

- The *Fallopian (uterine) tube* lies along the upper free border of the broad ligament, the upper part of which is the *mesosalpinx*. Medially, the Fallopian tubes traverse the uterine wall to open into the upper angle of the uterine cavity. The lateral ends emerge from the posterior layer of the broad ligament and divide into multiple finger-like processes termed *fimbriae*. This open lateral end is in communication with the peritoneal cavity and lies close to the ovary.

- The *broad ligament* is a fold of peritoneum which stretches from the lateral wall of the uterus to the pelvic side wall (Fig. 26.1). Its upper free border contains the uterine tube in its medial four-fifths; its lateral one-fifth, containing the ovarian vessels, constitutes the *infundibulopelvic ligament*. The uterine vessels lie between the layers of the ligament, first along its base, and then close to its attachment to the side of the uterus.
- The *round ligament* raises a ridge on the anterior surface of the broad ligament as it passes from the uterus to the deep inguinal ring.

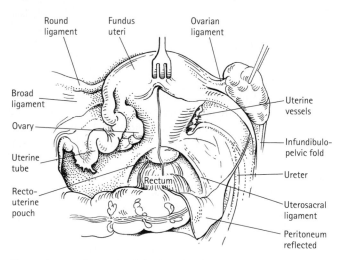

Figure 26.1 *Anatomy of the female pelvis, viewed from above at laparotomy (after Anson).*

The ovary

The ovary lies on the lateral part of the posterior surface of the broad ligament to which it is attached by a small fold of peritoneum, the *mesovarium*. Apart from its mesovarian attachment, the ovary is devoid of peritoneal covering. A normal ovary is 3–5 cm in length. It is greyish-white in colour, but its size, shape and surface can vary considerably throughout the menstrual cycle. In pre-pubertal girls it is smooth, but following puberty the surface becomes wrinkled and scarred, and it may contain several or single cysts.

- The *ovarian ligament* attaches the ovary to the uterus, and raises a small ridge on the posterior surface of the broad ligament.
- The *infundibulopelvic ligament* attaches the ovary to the pelvic side wall and carries the ovarian vessels.

Vessels

The female genital organs have a rich blood supply, and in pregnancy the uterine arteries enlarge substantially.

- The *uterine artery* arises from the anterior division of the internal iliac; it runs forward to the base of the broad ligament, and then medially within it above the lateral fornix of the vagina, where it crosses the ureter 1–2 cm lateral to the supravaginal part of the cervix; finally, it runs upwards along the lateral margin of the uterus, to which it gives numerous branches, including one to the uterine tube.
- The *ovarian artery* arises from the aorta, a little below the renal artery, and runs down the posterior abdominal wall; it then passes forwards and medially to reach the ovary via the infundibulopelvic ligament.

ANTERIOR PERINEAL PROBLEMS

Bartholin's abscess

A Bartholin's gland may distend and form a cyst if the duct becomes blocked. An infected cyst forms a painful abscess. The operation of choice is that of marsupialization of the gland, and this can be performed under local anaesthetic. Marsupialization is the preferred technique as it leads to the preservation of the gland's lubricating function, and if a stoma opening of adequate size is created there is a low risk of recurrence.

Operative procedure

An elliptical incision of 1–2 cm is made over the convexity of the abscess on the hymenal side, so that the stoma will drain into the vagina. The skin ellipse is excised, after which a similar ellipse is excised from the cyst wall and the abscess is drained. It is preferable, but not always possible, to excise these two ellipses separately. A series of fine absorbable interrupted sutures is placed around the circumference to include both layers, forming an elliptical stoma. The large size of the stoma should not alarm the surgeon, as once all inflammation has settled the final diameter is much smaller.

Vesicovaginal fistulae

These fistulae are common in areas where skilled intervention is unavailable during an obstructed labour. The pressure of the foetal head against the pubic symphysis causes ischaemic necrosis of the vaginal and bladder walls before finally, after several days of obstructed labour, a stillborn baby is delivered. Although repair should rightly be viewed as a specialized urogynaecological challenge, in practice these injuries are repaired by generalists, often in relatively remote hospitals. Expertise has been developed in the Addis Ababa Fistula Hospital and their training courses and video are recommended to surgeons wishing to undertake these repairs.[5] No specialized equipment is needed.

Operative procedure

Most repairs are performed from the perineum. A urethral catheter is passed and will be left on free drainage for 2 weeks postoperatively while the bladder heals. The fistula may be close to the ureteric orifices, which must be identified and preserved. The plane between the bladder and vagina is infiltrated with a dilute adrenaline solution and the two organs are separated by a combination of sharp and blunt dissection. Extensive mobilization of the tissues is required. The bladder and vagina are repaired as separate layers with absorbable sutures, and a Martius flap interposition (see Chapter 23, page 449) has proved valuable in bringing well-vascularized tissue between the two suture lines.

Perineal third degree tears with anal sphincter disruption

The repair of these obstetric injuries to the anal sphincters is discussed in Chapter 23.

Rectoceles

These are commonly the result of obstetric damage to the rectovaginal septum. Many require no operative intervention, but those which come to surgery may be operated on by either gynaecologists or coloproctologists. The surgical options are discussed in Chapter 23.

CONDITIONS AFFECTING THE FALLOPIAN TUBE

Salpingitis

Pelvic peritonitis from salpingitis may be indistinguishable pre-operatively from pelvic peritonitis caused by appendicitis. Even after the abdomen has been opened, the diagnosis may initially still be in doubt. Fallopian tubes lying within an appendix abscess will be inflamed, and an appendix lying within the pus of a severe salpingitis will show serosal inflammation (see Chapter 21). Once the diagnosis of salpingitis is established, only a bacteriological swab and peritoneal toilet are required before closure of the abdominal incision and the instigation of antibiotic therapy. An endocervical swab should also be taken to check for *Chlamydia*. Salpingitis in a scarred blocked tube may form a pyosalpinx; this trapped pus requires drainage either by simple incision, or preferably by a salpingectomy.

Ruptured ectopic pregnancy

Most ectopic pregnancies implant in the extrauterine portion of the Fallopian tube, and rupture occurs at around 5–7 weeks' gestation. However, an ectopic pregnancy in the interstitial portion of the tube, or in the cervix, ruptures later, at 9–16 weeks.

Rupture of an ectopic pregnancy is usually an acute emergency event. It should always be suspected in a woman of childbearing years who has collapsed with shock and lower abdominal pain. Classically, there is a history of a missed period, and signs and symptoms of early pregnancy, but frequently these clues are absent. Pregnancy tests are unreliable, and a previous sterilization operation does not preclude the diagnosis. Haemodynamically unstable patients with this acute presentation require simultaneous resuscitation and surgical exploration. Thus, a general surgeon, working in a hospital with no gynaecological service, will be unable to transfer such a patient and will have to operate.

An ectopic pregnancy can be a subacute event, however. The signs and symptoms are largely related to whether the ectopic pregnancy is intact, has aborted into the peritoneal cavity, or has ruptured through the tubal wall into the peritoneum or into the broad ligament. Pelvic peritoneal irritation may produce tenesmus and diarrhoea, or mimic appendicitis. Intraperitoneal blood can irritate the diaphragm and produce shoulder tip pain. If the diagnosis of an ectopic has not been suspected preoperatively, a general surgeon may have made an incorrect alternative surgical diagnosis, proceeded to surgery, and the ectopic pregnancy is only diagnosed at operation.

In those women who are bleeding profusely, the first priority is to control the haemorrhage. After the peritoneal cavity has been entered, it may be difficult, because of the amount of blood in the pelvis and the continuing bleeding, to identify the affected tube. A hand inserted into the blood can feel the uterus, draw it up and then palpate the tubes to identify the affected side. Digital compression of the broad ligament, proximal and distal to the mass, will effect temporary control of haemorrhage until a clamp can be applied. Autotransfusion of the intraperitoneal blood is occasionally possible (see Appendix II).

SURGICAL OPTIONS

There are a number of surgical options to treat ruptured ectopic pregnancies, and debate continues regarding the merit of tubal linear salpingotomy, mid-tube resection with a later re-anastomosis, and fimbrial evacuation. However, unilateral simple salpingectomy has the merit of controlling the haemorrhage, excising the whole pregnancy, and not leaving a damaged tube to give rise to a further ectopic. If the other tube is absent or severely damaged, and further children are wanted, a conservative operation should be considered.

Simple salpingectomy

The affected tube is clamped close to its uterine end. Whilst the tube is held up by Babcock forceps, the mesosalpinx is divided close to the tube, between a series of clamps (Fig. 26.2). The tube is removed and the pedicles are tied off with absorbable transfixion sutures. The peritoneal cavity is cleared of blood and clot, and if the pregnancy has already ruptured a search should be made for the pregnancy sac to ensure its removal.

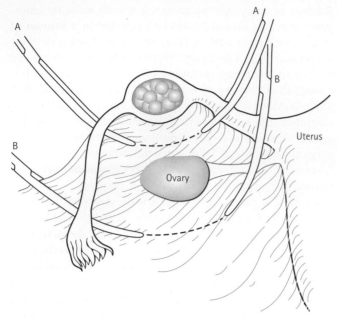

Figure 26.2 *Salpingectomy for ectopic pregnancy. Clamps are placed on the mesosalpinx and on the uterine end of the tube (**AA**). The infundibulopelvic ligament carrying the ovarian vessels is preserved. If the decision is made to remove the ovary along with the tube, then the tissue between the clamps (**BB**) is removed.*

Fimbrial evacuation

If the tubal pregnancy is about to abort from the fimbrial end, then an attempt to complete the process by gentle pressure is permissible, but care should be taken to leave no trophoblastic tissue behind.

Linear salpingotomy

The incision allows complete removal of the pregnancy sac. Haemostasis is controlled with diathermy, and the incision in the tube does not require closure.

ATYPICAL ECTOPIC PREGNANCY

These rarer forms of ectopic pregnancy present with atypical symptoms and signs, and thus there may be a delay in reaching the diagnosis.

Interstitial pregnancy

Ectopic gestation in the intramural portion of the Fallopian tube, although rare, can be the cause of rapid and profound haemorrhage. Cornual resection to remove the whole pregnancy is followed by a two-layer haemostatic repair of the uterus with deep interrupted sutures. Where haemorrhage cannot be controlled, a subtotal or total hysterectomy may be necessary.

Cervical ectopic

In this rare event, the only treatment may be a total hysterectomy. Sometimes, however, it may be possible to save the uterus if haemorrhage can be controlled either by tamponade with a Foley catheter or by embolization.

CONDITIONS AFFECTING THE OVARY

Ovarian cysts and tumours

Even with sophisticated preoperative imaging the general surgeon will still occasionally operate, without a firm diagnosis, on a pelvic or abdominal mass and discover on entering the abdomen that the mass is ovarian. Similarly, a laparotomy for suspected peritonitis may reveal that the peritoneal irritation is from a complication of an ovarian cyst. Ovarian cysts are also not infrequently encountered by general surgeons as an incidental finding during the course of a laparotomy for some unrelated pathology. Gynaecological advice should be sought, but if this is not available then the general surgeon will require some knowledge of the pathophysiology of ovarian cysts and solid tumours in order to respond appropriately.

- *Physiological cysts* include the single or multiple follicular cysts which contain straw-coloured fluid, and the corpus luteal cysts which are associated with haemorrhage of varying degree, either into the cyst or into the peritoneal cavity. Physiological cysts are seldom more than a few centimetres in diameter.
- *Endometriotic cysts* may be associated with other manifestations of endometriosis in the pelvis, and the ovary may be densely adherent to surrounding structures. Surface chocolate staining is often absent as these cysts have a thick capsule. Incision reveals single, or multiple, tense dark cysts which contain altered blood, and sometimes blood pigment stones.
- *Serous cystomas* are unilateral, benign unilocular cysts with no glandular element; they can grow to contain several litres of clear fluid.
- *Dermoid cysts*, a form of ovarian teratoma, are semi-solid. They can be single or bilateral, and may involve the whole or only part of an ovary. They contain sebaceous material and can also contain any tissue, including teeth. They are usually an incidental finding unless they have undergone torsion or rupture. When the latter happens the leaked material is irritant and may induce a chemical peritonitis.
- *Solid benign tumours* are easily misdiagnosed as malignant by a general surgeon. Ascites can occur with a benign fibroma, and when combined with a right hydrothorax, is known as Meig's syndrome, but it is comparatively rare.
- *Cystadenomas* are glandular cysts of the ovary, and have a significant potential for malignant change. The serous cystadenoma contains straw-coloured fluid, and the mucinous cystadenoma contains mucin. These cysts may be single or bilateral, unilocular or multilocular, and they may grow to a large size.
- *Cystadenocarcinomas*. Malignancy should be suspected if there are solid areas within the cyst, or if there are surface papillomatous excrescences either on the serosal

surface or the cyst lining. General metastatic seeding on peritoneal surfaces, including the greater omentum, and the presence of ascites may make the diagnosis of malignancy more certain.

COMPLICATIONS OF OVARIAN CYSTS

Any ovarian cyst can undergo a complication. These include haemorrhage, rupture, torsion and infection, and are the events which commonly bring the cyst to the attention of the surgeon. The complication is treated and the cyst is then managed on its merits.

- *Haemorrhage* may be into a cyst, with resultant tension and pain, or into the peritoneal cavity. Active bleeding from an otherwise harmless cyst may require diathermy coagulation or a haemostatic suture.
- *Rupture* of a cyst evokes a chemical peritonitis of varying severity, and the torn edges may bleed.
- *Torsion* of a normal ovary can occur, but it is more common when there is an ovarian mass. The torsion may be partial, with an engorged but viable ovary, or of several turns with complete vascular occlusion and rapid infarction. The Fallopian tube and ovary undergo torsion as a single unit and the pedicle thus formed can be simply clamped, divided and ligated if the ovary and tube are infarcted and require excision. In a partial torsion, untwisting may reveal a viable ovary which can be preserved.
- *Infection* is almost always secondary to another intraperitoneal infection. The cyst contents form an abscess which must be drained.

SURGICAL OPTIONS

When a surgeon encounters a small physiological cyst in a premenopausal woman, no treatment is required. When an apparently benign cyst is of significant size – that is more than 5 cm in diameter – it is usually in the patient's interest that it should be removed. In considering the options, the surgeon should remember that only about 13 per cent of ovarian tumours that come to surgery before the menopause are malignant, in contrast to about 45 per cent after the menopause. Ovarian function should not be sacrificed in premenopausal women without good evidence of its necessity.

- An *ovarian cystectomy* preserves the ovarian tissue, even of the affected ovary. It is an appropriate operation for small, clinically benign cysts in a premenopausal ovary.
- A *unilateral oophorectomy* preserves the function of the contralateral ovary. It may be the more appropriate treatment of a larger benign cyst, where little functioning ovarian tissue remains, and is also the recommended treatment of a benign solid tumour of a premenopausal ovary. If, however, the contralateral ovary is absent, or there is bilateral pathology, as is often the case in dermoid tumours, an ovarian cystectomy must always be considered.
- In the postmenopausal patient, a *bilateral oophorectomy* is usually recommended, even for an apparently benign cyst.

Occasionally, the surgeon strongly suspects that an ovarian tumour may be malignant. The standard surgical treatment of an ovarian primary cancer confined to the ovary is a total hysterectomy with a bilateral salpingo-oophorectomy and infracolic omentectomy. This wide excision gives the best chance of total surgical removal of any malignant spread, and provides staging information which will influence subsequent treatment. However, the general surgeon will not be operating with a preoperative diagnosis of ovarian cancer, and, although the ovary may appear malignant, there is no histological proof. There should be a reluctance to proceed with a major resection, in another surgical discipline, which will not have been indicated if the histology is finally reported as benign. The patient may be unprepared for such a major resection and feel that adequate preoperative discussion was not undertaken. For all of these reasons, a unilateral salpingo-oophorectomy is probably the best strategy for the general surgeon faced with this situation. When there is still no contamination of the peritoneal surface from tumour excrescences on the serosal surface, complete removal without spillage is extremely important. If malignancy is confirmed and further surgery indicated it can be completed at a second procedure.

More frequently in ovarian cancer, the tumour is found to have already disseminated intraperitoneally at the time of laparotomy. A total hysterectomy, bilateral salpingo-oophorectomy and infracolic omentectomy are indicated as a debulking procedure, as chemotherapy is more effective on small volume disease. In contrast to most disseminated gastrointestinal malignancies, ovarian cancer is responsive to chemotherapy and a long remission can be achieved even in advanced disease. However, general surgeons who find themselves unexpectedly in such an abdomen, without gynaecological advice, may find it best simply to take a generous biopsy of the involved omentum for histological confirmation. If ovarian cancer is confirmed, the patient can then be transferred to a gynae-oncology centre for optimal further management.

In very advanced disease, the initial laparotomy has often been performed by a general surgeon as the patient has presented with abdominal distension and an intestinal obstruction, the aetiology of which is obscure until the abdomen is opened. Disseminated malignancy and malignant adhesions are encountered and the primary lesion is thought probably to be ovarian. Small bowel obstructions can be bypassed, but a large bowel obstruction in the pelvis will usually require a proximal loop colostomy. If an omental biopsy confirms disseminated ovarian malignancy, chemotherapy may still offer some palliation.

The surgeon must remember that malignant ovarian

tumours may also be secondary deposits, which are often larger and more apparent than the primary tumour, and they may occur either with, or without, other evidence of intraperitoneal seeding. *Pseudomyxoma peritonei syndrome* and *disseminated mucous producing gastrointestinal adenocarcinoma* can produce a clinical picture identical to that of a disseminated ovarian primary. In either pathology there may be extensive intraperitoneal disease, or the pathology may appear initially to be confined to an ovary. If pseudomyxoma peritonei is confirmed histologically, the patient should be referred to a specialist centre, and subsequent surgery in the pelvis will be more hazardous if an initial hysterectomy has been performed (see Chapter 15). Secondary tumours in the ovaries from gastrointestinal or breast malignancy may be large and cause symptoms. There may be no other macroscopic metastatic spread and a bilateral oophorectomy may give very worthwhile palliation. This is also discussed further in Chapter 15.

OVARIAN SURGERY

Surgery on the ovary is generally straightforward unless an ovary is found densely adherent to adjacent structures, or is lying retroperitoneally.

Ovarian cystectomy

An incision is made through the ovarian cortex around the base of the cyst, deep enough to expose a plane of cleavage which is developed by sharp or blunt dissection so that the cyst can be enucleated (Fig. 26.3). After haemostasis, the ovary can be closed with an absorbable suture, taking care to abolish a dead space which may fill with blood.

Oophorectomy

This requires the division between clamps and subsequent ligation of the infundibular pelvic ligament to secure the ovarian vessels. Separate ligation of the ovarian ligament may also be necessary (Fig. 26.4).

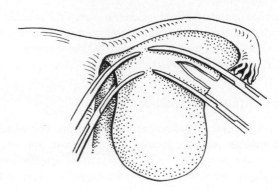

Figure 26.4   *Oophorectomy. The indundibulopelvic fold and the ovarian ligament are divided between clamps.*

Salpingo–oophorectomy

This is often the better option in a large cyst with the Fallopian tube stretched over its surface (Fig. 26.5). A large serous cystoma can be drained down to a more manageable size before removal. A needle, attached to low-pressure suction, is passed through a purse-string suture placed in the cyst wall. It is important to isolate the area with packs and to minimize any spillage during aspiration. The needle is then withdrawn, the defect closed with the purse-string, and removal of the cyst or ovary completed. This manoeuvre will enable the surgeon to remove the cyst through a smaller abdominal incision. However, the surgeon must remember that a large cyst, especially in a postmenopausal woman, may ultimately prove to be malignant. If malignancy is a possibility, aspiration is contraindicated as it is so important that there is no contamination of the peritoneal cavity with malignant cells. Instead, the abdominal wound must be enlarged to allow adequate access for gentle delivery of the cyst and identification of its pedicle.

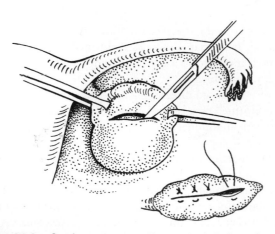

Figure 26.3   *Ovarian cystectomy. The cyst is shelled out through an incision around the base of the cyst. A sutured repair of the ovary is shown in the inset.*

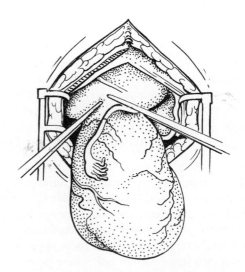

Figure 26.5   *Salpingo-oophorectomy. The lateral pedicle clamp is on the infundibulopelvic fold containing the ovarian vessels. On the uterine side the clamp is across the ovarian ligament and the proximal Fallopian tube.*

The lateral part of the pedicle is formed by the infundibulo-pelvic ligament containing the ovarian vessels which, in the case of a large cyst, are likely to be much dilated. The medial or uterine part of the pedicle contains the Fallopian tube and the ovarian ligament. Separate clamps are placed on the two parts of the pedicle. Care must be taken to avoid inclusion of the ureter in the clamps on the lateral pedicle. It is advised that two proximal clamps and a transfixion ligature should be employed on the lateral pedicle as, if a clamp or ligature slips, the cut ovarian vessels may retract behind the peritoneum. Haemorrhage may be profuse and the cut ends difficult to identify.

Excision of retroperitoneal ovarian cysts may be challenging. They tend to form when the cyst develops in the presence of surface adhesions, and are not uncommon after a previous hysterectomy. One distinguishing feature is that both Fallopian tubes and round ligaments are stretched over the surface. These cysts are rarely malignant, and seldom contain glandular tissue. The best approach is to open the peritoneum over the surface of the cyst between the round ligament and the Fallopian tube. A plane of cleavage is sought and developed digitally. The vascular pedicles should not be clamped until the ureter has been identified as it lies in close proximity to the posterior surface of the cyst.

CONDITIONS AFFECTING THE UTERUS

General surgical practice is less commonly affected by uterine pathology than tubo-ovarian pathology. However, an enlarged fibroid uterus may obscure surgical access to the pelvis, and an advanced tumour of the uterine body or cervix may invade the bowel.

Endometriosis

This gynaecological condition of ectopic endometrial tissue may have an impact on general surgical practice. The most common variety is of pelvic peritoneal nodules which cause pelvic pain, and a laparotomy may have been performed by a general surgeon for some other suspected pathology. Early lesions are dark brown or purplish nodules a few millimetres in diameter, but later puckering and scarring of the peritoneum is more prevalent. Dense adhesions may form around the Fallopian tubes, and in severe cases adhesions obliterate the rectovaginal pouch involving the anterior rectal wall in the scar tissue. When encountered unexpectedly by the general surgeon, no surgical action is required. The overall management of endometriosis is complex, and any surgery which is indicated is supported by hormone manipulation.

Rarer forms of the disease are often only diagnosed after excision. A small bowel loop may be strictured by the scarring from a nodule of endometriosis on its wall. A sigmoid or rectal wall lesion may present with a stricture or with ulcera-tion into the lumen and haemorrhage. A tender lump within a Caesarean section scar, explored as a possible incisional hernia, will sometimes prove to be ectopic endometrial tissue.

Hysterectomy

The general surgeon may have to remove the uterus en bloc with a rectal or sigmoid cancer which is invading the cervix or body of the uterus, and the hysterectomy is combined with a radical colonic or rectal resection. A similar challenge is posed by a locally advanced gynaecological cancer invading the rectum. These operations should ideally be performed as a combined procedure involving both specialists, but a colorectal surgeon will find that the additional dissection necessary for the hysterectomy is often relatively minor in this situation. In addition, the standard steps described in a hysterectomy must be modified so that the dissection does not breach the area of tumour invasion between the two organs. Occasionally, although the hysterectomy is not required for oncological reasons, pelvic access is restricted by a bulky fibroid uterus, and a hysterectomy has to be performed to allow a safe rectal dissection. Rarely, a general surgeon working in a hospital without gynaecological colleagues, may have to perform an emergency hysterectomy for obstetric haemorrhage.

Total and subtotal hysterectomy are described, but vaginal hysterectomy, and the extended Wertheim hysterectomy for carcinoma of the cervix are outwith the scope of a general surgical operative text. In the total operation the whole of the uterus, including the cervix, is removed. The subtotal operation removes the body of the uterus, but leaves the cervix. Carcinoma of the cervical stump is uncommon, but the patient should be advised to continue with cervical smears if they are available. The subtotal operation is quicker and easier to perform, with a faster recovery, and lower mortality and morbidity. It should always be considered in benign disease when there is poor access to the cervix due to obesity, fibroids or adhesions, or when the patient's condition precludes a more prolonged procedure.

In both the total and the subtotal hysterectomy, conservation of the ovaries is preferable in the premenopausal woman, if at all possible. However, a bilateral oophorectomy should be offered when planning a hysterectomy in the postmenopausal woman, as the additional morbidity is minimal, and ovarian removal almost completely prevents the development of a subsequent ovarian malignancy.

TOTAL HYSTERECTOMY

In the situations where a general surgeon is involved the abdomen will normally already have been opened through a midline incision. A Pfannenstiel incision, however, also provides good access for a hysterectomy. All pelvic surgery is easier with the patient tipped head-down and the small bowel held out of the pelvis with packs. A general surgeon will probably choose first to identify the ureters in familiar territory above the pelvic brim and to follow them distally before embarking on any pelvic dissection.

The uterus is elevated and a clamp, such as a Jessop, Oschner or Kocher, is placed across each cornu, incorporating the round ligament, the ovarian ligament and the Fallopian tube. The tip of each clamp is angled laterally into an avascular 'window' in the broad ligament. Further clamps are applied alongside and parallel to the first, and the tissue divided between them. The pedicles are transfixed and ligated. The original cornual clamps remain in place and are used to retract the uterus. If the ovaries and tubes are to be removed, the round ligament is clamped lateral to where it separates from the Fallopian tube, and the infundibulopelvic ligament containing the ovarian vessels must also be secured as already described in the section on salpingo-oophorectomy.

Digital development of the space between the leaves of the broad ligament can be helpful at this stage. The peritoneal incision in the anterior leaf of the broad ligament is then carried downwards close to the uterus towards the base of the ligament, and is then continued towards the midline across the uterovesical pouch at the junction between uterus and cervix where the peritoneum is loose (Fig. 26.6a). The anterior flap of peritoneum is raised to expose the bladder. The fascial strands between the cervix and bladder are divided to open a plane of cleavage. The bladder, with the lower half of the vesicouterine fold of peritoneum is now

a

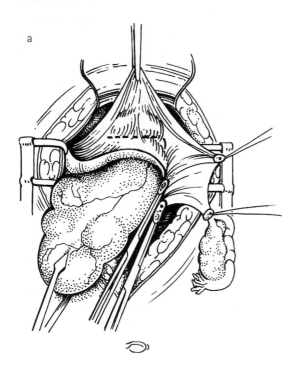

b

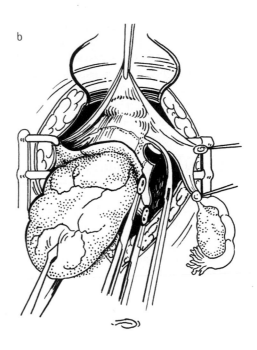

c

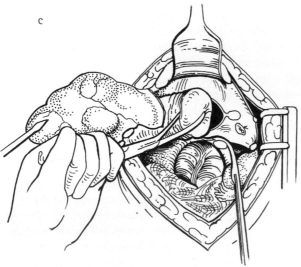

Figure 26.6 *Hysterectomy (after Shaw). (a) The right Fallopian tube and round ligament have been clamped separately in this illustration. The laterally placed clamps have been tied-off, and the medial retained as retractors. The uterovesical peritoneal fold has been elevated and the planned incision is shown. (b) The bladder has been displaced downwards off the cervix. The uterine vessels are then clamped close to the uterine wall. (c) The vagina is opened and a vulsellum retractor placed on the cervix for retraction while the vaginal division is completed.*

pushed down off the cervix and the upper part of the vagina. This carries the ureter downwards with the bladder to below the level of the uterine artery, and should safeguard it when the vessel is clamped. More laterally, stripping must be done gently as parametrial venous plexuses may be torn. When the cervix is long, or there is scarring from a previous Caesarean section, it may be necessary to leave the final dissection of the bladder off the cervix and vaginal vault until the uterine vessel pedicles have been divided.

The uterine vascular pedicle is secured with a clamp, angled at almost 90 degrees to the cervix, with the tip on the cervix itself so that when the clamp is closed the tip slips off to grip tissue as close to the cervix as possible. A second clamp is applied, parallel to the first, the uterine vessels are divided and then transfixed and ligated (Fig. 26.6b).

Any further dissection to expose the vagina is completed and the vagina is opened transversely, with scalpel or diathermy, in the midline anteriorly, until a Vulsellum retractor can be placed on the anterior lip of the cervix (Fig. 26.6c). Combined upward traction on the Vulsellum and the cornual clamps places the lateral vaginal angle on tension. An angled Kocher clamp is applied to incorporate the lateral vaginal angle, the descending cervical branch of the uterine artery and the uterosacral ligament posteriorly. The uterosacral ligaments may need to be taken separately if they are thickened due to endometriosis or chronic inflammation. Releasing the uterosacral ligaments usually results in the uterus becoming more mobile and may aid the surgery. The circumferential vaginal incision is completed posteriorly and the uterus removed.

In situations where there is a malignancy invading across the rectovaginal pouch, the posterior incision through the vaginal wall must be well below any tumour invasion, and access will have to be from the sides. The excised tumour specimen may then include a major portion of the posterior vaginal wall.

Each vaginal angle is undersewn by an over-and-over suture, starting at the tip of the clamp and working laterally. It incorporates the vagina at front and back, with the last pass being under the heel of the clamp. The clamp is removed and the suture drawn tight and tied. The vagina is then closed with a continuous haemostatic suture (no. 1 Dexon is suitable). If there is concern over haemostasis the vaginal edge should be oversewn to leave a central aperture through which a wide T-tube drain can be placed. There is no need to close the pelvic peritoneum.

SUBTOTAL HYSTERECTOMY

The operation is performed as for a total hysterectomy up to, and including, the ligation of the uterine vascular pedicles. The dissection is not then carried so deeply into the pelvis, and the bladder is not separated from the vaginal vault. The cervix is divided through its extravaginal portion and oversewn with absorbable sutures. This closure can be improved if the two halves of the cervix are cut into a V-shaped wedge.

POST-PARTUM HYSTERECTOMY

Very occasionally, a general surgeon may be required to carry out this operation for uncontrollable haemorrhage. Generally, the tissue planes are well developed and the enlarged blood vessels easy to identify. However, identifying the limits of the dilated cervix may be difficult and can lead to incomplete removal. The surgeon unfamiliar with total abdominal hysterectomy would be wise to consider the subtotal operation. A hysterectomy must occasionally be combined with a Caesarean section. Closure of the uterine Caesarean incision before embarking on the hysterectomy is recommended to reduce haemorrhage.

SURGERY IN PREGNANCY

Any surgical pathology may present in pregnancy. Surgery in the first trimester is complicated by concerns regarding the possible teratogenic effects of anaesthetic drugs, and any abortifacient effect of the condition requiring surgery or of the surgery itself. Elective surgery should therefore be avoided during this period. However, as intraperitoneal sepsis is a more powerful factor than a laparotomy in inducing a miscarriage, the surgeon should not err on the side of conservative management when, for example, appendicitis is suspected.

In mid trimester the chances of miscarriage are low, the risk of major teratogenic effects has passed, and the uterus is not yet obscuring access. This is therefore the optimum period to operate if postponement of surgery until after delivery appears unwise. Diagnosis of abdominal conditions in late pregnancy can be difficult as the uterus is in contact with most of the anterior abdominal wall masking physical signs from gastrointestinal pathology, and all the abdominal organs are displaced cranially from their normal anatomical sites. Access for surgery is difficult, and in addition the patient lying supine will often obstruct her venous return by the weight of the gravid uterus on the inferior vena cava. The surgeon will thus have to operate with the patient tilted, usually into a partial left lateral position. Close to term, a laparotomy for surgical pathology may sometimes be best combined with a Caesarean delivery.

Avoidance of radiation to the foetus is important throughout pregnancy, and surgery may be hampered by the lack of preoperative or intraoperative imaging. Ultrasound and MRI can be safely used in pregnancy.

The life-threatening emergencies associated with pregnancy itself, and which require urgent surgical intervention, will only involve a general surgeon if no gynaecologist is available. Ectopic pregnancy was discussed on page 507.

Emergency Caesarean section

Operative intervention to deliver a baby may be necessary either in late pregnancy or in labour. There may be extreme urgency when severe foetal distress indicates that the life of the baby is threatened from whatever cause. There is also urgency to deliver, even a stillbirth, when the life of the mother is threatened by eclampsia, or by haemorrhage. Neither eclampsia nor haemorrhage can be controlled until the uterus is emptied. These are probably the only situations in which a general surgeon may unexpectedly have to act as an obstetrician in an emergency. Intervention with less urgency may be required during a labour which fails to progress whether for mechanical or physiological reasons.

In the emergency situation, a Caesarean section is necessary if imminent vaginal delivery cannot be achieved. Assisted vaginal delivery by forceps, or vacuum extraction, is often preferable if the head is engaged in the pelvis and the cervix is fully dilated. A symphysiotomy (see below) should be considered, and a vaginal delivery of a dead foetus after cranioclast collapse of the cranium may also be a safer alternative to a Caesarean section in some circumstances.

Today, an emergency Caesarean section virtually always utilizes a lower-segment incision rather than the classical procedure. In a classical Caesarean section the upper segment of the uterus is opened through a vertical incision and the foetus is delivered as a breech. In the lower-segment operation, the lower uterine segment is incised transversely and the foetus is delivered head-first if the vertex is presenting. A lower midline incision in the abdominal wall can be used for both, but the transverse Pfannenstiel approach is favoured for most lower-segment operations and only takes marginally longer to perform.

LOWER-SEGMENT CAESAREAN SECTION

The operation can be performed under general, spinal, epidural or even local infiltrative anaesthesia. A general anaesthetic in labour, without adequate airway protection, carries a high risk of inhalation of gastric contents. In addition, anaesthetic drugs will cross the placenta and may depress the baby's respiratory efforts after delivery. Regional anaesthesia may therefore be safer if anaesthetic skills are limited. The mother should be catheterized and placed with a 10- to 15-degree left lateral tilt to prevent pressure of the uterus on the vena cava.

Operative procedure

Whichever incision is chosen, it must be long enough to accommodate the foetal head with a hand alongside. Care must be taken on opening the peritoneum to avoid injury to the bladder. The uterus is then checked for rotation, which is virtually always to the right. If wet packs are used to isolate the uterus from the rest of the peritoneal cavity, a pack placed first on the right side may help to correct this rotation.

The lower segment is identified as that area beneath the vesicouterine reflection of peritoneum where the peritoneum lies free of the uterine wall. This fold of peritoneum is picked up and incised transversely almost as far as the broad ligament. The lower half, with the bladder attached, is then pushed down to expose the lower segment. There may be dilated veins overlying the lower segment. These can be oversewn or merely kept compressed by an assistant whilst the lower segment is opened. A Doyen, or similar retractor, is used to hold the bladder and peritoneum down and out of the way.

A 3- to 4-cm transverse incision is made in the uterine muscle, high in the lower segment, and deepened until the membranes bulge – which they will do if amniotic fluid is still present in quantity. It does not matter if the membranes are opened at the initial incision, but there is greater control if this is done as a separate layer. Too low an incision in the lower segment must be avoided, as it may not be possible to create a long enough incision in this narrower portion to deliver the foetus, and tearing can occur either down into the cervix or laterally into the uterine vessels or ureter. The lower uterine segment may be very thinned after a prolonged labour, and care must be taken not to cut too deep and lacerate the foetus.

The incision is then extended laterally, and a finger can be inserted to protect the foetus. Before labour is established, and particularly in a pre-term pregnancy, the lower segment is poorly developed and there is a danger of entering the uterine arteries as the incision is carried laterally. A 'smile'-shaped incision with the lateral extensions curved upwards may overcome this problem and is a better solution than the classical incision. It is wise to place a stay suture at the mid-point of the lower edge of the uterine incision so that it can be found more easily when closing the uterus.

The presenting part must now be delivered up from the pelvis. In a cephalic presentation the surgeon slides the fingers of one hand down alongside the head to release the vacuum of a tight fit: there is more room over the face. The hand is then used as a 'scoop', or one forceps blade as a 'shoehorn', to draw the head up to the lower-segment opening. Fundal pressure then assists delivery. The head should be allowed to deliver slowly and flexion should be maintained to reduce the diameters.

A deeply impacted head may be difficult to deliver up, and an assistant pushing it up from the vagina is helpful. A high, free-floating head can also pose difficulty, and is easiest solved by finding the anterior ankle, doing a podalic version and delivering the baby by breech extraction.

The baby is delivered and its airway is attended to by an assistant while the surgeon completes the operation. The umbilical cord is ligated, or clamped, and divided. Ergometrine is given to speed the natural contraction of the empty uterus and the separation of the placenta. Normal physiological separation of the placenta should then be awaited but, if delay occurs, gentle cord traction can be applied if the fundus is contracted. Meanwhile, brisk bleeding from the edges of the uterine incision can be controlled with non-crushing Green–Armitage or Rampley clamps.

The placenta and membranes should be checked for completeness, and the uterine cavity is checked digitally. If a closed internal os is felt it should be gently stretched with a finger to allow free drainage of lochia.

The uterine incision is then closed. A continuous haemostatic suture is satisfactory, and should be started from both ends, as haemorrhage is not only most profuse from the lateral angles but access is most difficult. These initial lateral angle sutures can be placed before delivery of the placenta and will reduce blood loss. A heavy, long-acting absorbable material such as 0 or 1 Dexon is suitable for uterine closure. A two-layer closure is recommended. Beware of including the bladder in the stitch or of sewing the upper edge of the uterine incision to the posterior wall of the uterus. Any isolated bleeding points can be controlled by an additional interrupted suture. It used to be traditional to close the vesicouterine fold of peritoneum as a loose third layer, but this is now often omitted. The peritoneal cavity is cleared of liquor and blood, and the abdomen closed.

CLASSICAL CAESAREAN SECTION

The classical vertical incision through the uterine body leaves a scar which is more liable to rupture in future pregnancies, and should be avoided if possible. Indications for a classical incision may be absolute or relative, but include a mother who is dead though her baby is still alive, a gross foetal abnormality, a cervical cancer, an anterior placenta praevia, and a very premature pregnancy with a poorly defined lower segment.

The preparation of the patient is similar, the abdomen is opened through a lower midline incision and a midline vertical incision of at least 15 cm is made in the body of the uterus. A cephalic presentation is then delivered as a breech extraction. The management of the third stage and the uterine closure is similar to that described for a lower-segment Caesarean section.

Symphysiotomy

A symphysiotomy is a deliberate surgical separation, either full or partial, of the symphysis pubis, so as to enlarge the capacity of the pelvis and allow the passage of a living child. It is a safer procedure in unskilled hands than a Caesarean section in difficult circumstances, but the potential for long-term skeletal and urinary morbidity has made it an historic procedure in the developed world. However, a symphysiotomy avoids a uterine scar and the symphysis can separate again in a subsequent labour. This is a safer scenario for a woman who is living far from medical facilities, who has a mildly contracted pelvis, and who will probably have multiple further pregnancies.

The ligaments of the pubic symphysis are softened by pregnancy and divide easily with a scalpel. A firm urethral catheter is inserted. A finger within the vagina can then hold the urethra safely to one side during the release. Local anaesthesia is infiltrated down to the periosteum. A large scalpel, with its cutting edge facing the perineum, is passed through the skin overlying the junction of the upper and middle thirds of the symphysis pubis, and is advanced through the symphysis until the tip can just be felt by the vaginal finger. The distal two-thirds of the symphysis is then divided with a sawing movement. If the superior ligament can be left intact, the post-delivery morbidity will be reduced, but if necessary this can also be divided. A large episiotomy is performed but a forceps or vacuum extraction may still be necessary. The symphysis should open by 2–3 cm, but excessive diastasis must be prevented especially as the head is crowned. It is important that after the symphysiotomy has been performed that the patient's legs are not fixed in supports in the lithotomy position, and that two assistants are delegated to support the legs, restricting the degree of abduction and giving lateral support to the pelvis. In this way the degree of separation of the divided joint can be controlled.

The pubic symphysis heals spontaneously and no fixation is required. Urinary catheterization should be continued for several days and early mobilization encouraged with adequate analgesia.

Severe haemorrhage in the obstetric patient

In all situations, maternal blood loss will continue unabated until the baby and the placenta have been delivered and the uterus can contract and close the open sinusoids. Retained products of conception, or even blood clot, can also prevent satisfactory uterine contraction.

PRE- AND INTRA-PARTUM HAEMORRHAGE

If the foetus is still *in utero*, it must be delivered immediately and this will usually require a Caesarean section. A retained placenta is also associated with haemorrhage, and the first priority, alongside resuscitation, is delivery of the placenta. A general surgeon is unlikely to be involved until after the standard manoeuvres of oxytocin administration, fundal rubbing and controlled cord traction have failed. Manual removal of the placenta is the next step, and if this fails, due to a morbidly adherent placenta that intrudes through the uterine wall, an emergency hysterectomy may be required to control haemorrhage. Uterine inversion, sometimes associated with a placenta that is still attached, presents with haemorrhage, profound shock out of proportion to the blood loss, and a mass in or outside the vagina. The uterus should be returned to its normal position as soon as possible, before the cervix contracts necessitating a general anaesthetic for replacement. Reduction is achieved by manual manipulation within the vagina, and any attempt to remove a retained placenta is delayed until the uterus has been restored to its normal position. After reduction, and the additional manual removal of the placenta if it is still attached, the surgeon's hand should remain inside the uterine cavity until the uterus starts to contract. A uterine inversion can also be reduced by hydrostatic pressure. Saline (2 L) is run into the posterior fornix from a height of 2 metres, and both hands are used to hold the vagina closed and prevent fluid escape.

POST-PARTUM HAEMORRHAGE

Resuscitation should run parallel with the assessment of the cause of haemorrhage. The abdomen is palpated, and if the uterus is found to be well-contracted, the likely source is genital tract haemorrhage from trauma to the perineum, vagina or cervix. This should be explored and repaired. A *cervical laceration* can cause massive haemorrhage immediately after delivery, and can usually be sutured per vaginum.

If the uterus is not contracted, the standard obstetric manoeuvres of oxytocin and prostaglandin administration, fundal rubbing, and even manual exploration of the uterine cavity to remove clot and retained membranes, will almost always have been undertaken before a general surgeon is involved. Packing of the uterine cavity may have been tried but is seldom helpful. Tamponade with a Sengstaken–Blakemore tube, inflated up to 300 mL, may be a better temporary solution. (A Foley catheter balloon can be used for a similar haemorrhage in early pregnancy.) The patient can then be fully resuscitated and clotting restored to normal. With haemorrhage continuing from an atonic empty uterus, the choices are embolization, a brace suture to compress the uterus, uterine or internal artery ligation, or a hysterectomy.

Brace B–Lynch suture

This ingenious compression suture was first described in 1997.[6] The patient is anaesthetized in a semi-lithotomy position so that the rate of bleeding per vaginum can be monitored. The abdomen is opened and the uterus lifted out of the abdominal cavity and manually compressed. If this manoeuvre successfully stems the haemorrhage, the suture is worth trying. The vesicouterine peritoneal fold is divided as for a Caesarean section, and the lower segment exposed. A heavy absorbable suture (originally described with No. 2 chromic catgut) on a large round-bodied needle is required. The needle is passed from below upwards, entering the right side of the uterus 3 cm below the limit of the lower segment and 3 cm from the lateral border. The suture is brought out 3 cm above the limit of the lower segment and 4 cm from the lateral border. The stitch is then taken up and over the compressed fundus, 3–4 cm from the right cornual border. The suture is then carried down and enters the posterior wall of the uterus opposite and at the same level as the upper entry point at the front, and is carried through and around to emerge at the same level on the left posterior surface. It is then carried up the back and over the fundus 3–4 cm from the left cornual border, down the front of the uterus to enter 3 cm above the lower segment and emerges 3 cm below at the same distances as on the right side (Fig. 26.7a). The two ends are then pulled tight, an assistant compressing the uterus bimanually, and tied (Fig. 26.7b). The original report recommends that the lower segment is opened. However, those using this technique have not always found this step necessary for success. If the lower segment has been opened, it is then closed in a similar manner to that after a lower-segment Caesarean section.

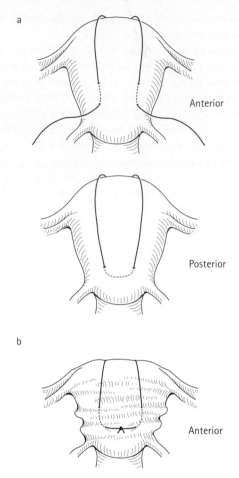

Figure 26.7 *Brace suture. (a) The position of the suture viewed from in front and behind before it is tightened. (b) The suture is tightened compressing the uterus and its arterial inflow.*

Internal iliac artery ligation

About 50 per cent of emergency hysterectomies for haemorrhage can be prevented by using this technique. However, it is not an easy operation and the surgeon must remember that the first priority is to save the life of the woman, and this must not be further jeopardized by futile attempts to save her uterus. A uterine rupture or cervical laceration which extends out into a uterine vessel can cause major haemorrhage which cannot be controlled as the torn ends of the uterine vessel cannot be safely secured. Blind sutures risk injury to the ureter. Ligation of the internal iliac artery, or its posterior division, on the side of the haemorrhage is occasionally effective. However, there is an extensive collateral blood supply to the pregnant uterus and even bilateral internal iliac artery ligation may not stem a post-partum haemorrhage, whether from an atonic uterus or from obstetric trauma. This is a similar situation to that encountered in major pelvic fractures where the haemorrhage is more satisfactorily controlled by embolization (see Chapter 4, page 55). Unfortunately, in situations where a general surgeon is involved, in the absence of a gynaecological colleague, there are often no interventional radio-logical skills available either.

REFERENCES

1. *Gynaecology*, 3rd edn. RW Shaw, WP Soutter, SL Stanton (eds). Edinburgh: Churchill Livingstone, 2003.
2. *Dewhurst's Textbook of Obstetrics and Gynaecology for Postgraduates*, 6th edn. DK Edmonds, CJ Dewhurst (eds). Oxford: Blackwell Science, 1999.
3. *Munro Kerr's Operative Obstetrics*, 10th edn. PR Myerscough (ed.). London: Macmillan, 1982.
4. *Bonney's Gynaecological Surgery*, 10th edn. JM Monaghan, R Nauk, L Tito (eds). Oxford: Blackwell Science, 2003.
5. Addis Ababa Fistula Hospital. e-mail: fistula-hospital@telecom.net.et
6. B-Lynch C, Coker A, Lawal AH, *et al*. The B-Lynch surgical technique for the control of massive postpartum haemorrhage: an alternative to hysterectomy? Five cases reported. *Br J Obstet Gynaecol* 1997; **104**(3): 372–5.

Appendix I

PREOPERATIVE PREPARATION

Successful surgery requires an understanding of surgical pathology, judgement regarding the appropriateness of an operation, and good surgical technique. Preoperative and postoperative care are also vitally important and, in general, are the responsibility of the surgeon. The preoperative period should be used for relevant investigations, and for preparation for surgery. This preparation may relate to the surgery to be undertaken; for example, mechanical bowel preparation before colonic surgery, or the control of thyrotoxicosis before thyroid surgery. The preparation also includes the specific management of certain coexistent medical conditions and optimization of the patient's general condition.

The risks of surgery and general anaesthesia are increased in the patient who has poor perfusion and oxygen delivery to vital tissue. Many patients requiring emergency surgery are in this compromised state. The underlying pathology may be hypovolaemia, cardiac failure, anaemia, sepsis or respiratory failure. Adequate delivery of nutrients to tissue is also important, as is the ability to eliminate metabolites. Hepatic or renal impairment will jeopardize these essential functions. Any hepatic or renal impairment will be compounded by poor oxygen delivery to the liver or kidneys. Sepsis is increased if the gut is underperfused. Thus, the improvement in oxygen delivery to the tissues is the most important general resuscitative goal in the ill patient prior to emergency surgery. Improved oxygen delivery has been shown to improve outcome in both elective and emergency surgery.[1] In elective surgery, preoperative treatment of concomitant cardiorespiratory pathology, and improvement in nutritional status, can also be achieved.

AVAILABLE TIME FOR PREOPERATIVE OPTIMIZATION

The time available for general preoperative preparation of a patient is highly variable and dependent on the rate of deterioration of the underlying surgical condition. The surgeon may have from a few minutes to many months in which to make improvements.

The 4-minute window

This is the situation when the patient's only chance of survival is with immediate surgery. Surgery cannot await full resuscitation which has to proceed alongside it, as attempts at further resuscitation are proving futile – for example, in the face of exsanguinating haemorrhage. The commonest scenarios are massive haemorrhage from abdominal or thoracic trauma, or from the spontaneous rupture of an aortic aneurysm. Surgical control of the bleeding, as discussed in Chapters 5, 7 and 14, is the first priority. Once bleeding has been controlled, general resuscitation may then be appropriate before definitive surgery (see *Damage limitation* in Chapter 14).

The 4-hour window

Many gastrointestinal surgical emergencies are included in this category. Patients commonly are fluid- and electrolyte-depleted. Baseline haematological and biochemical values can be obtained, and a chest X-ray and ECG performed. Preoperative resuscitation to increase oxygen delivery to all vital tissue reduces morbidity and mortality. During the delay, however, the underlying pathology will be deteriorating and timing of surgery is important (see Chapters 11 and 14).

FLUID AND ELECTROLYTE REPLACEMENT

The initial loss of fluid and electrolytes is from the intravascular compartment. Equilibration occurs rapidly within the whole extracellular compartment, and interstitial fluid is drawn into the circulation. Equilibration between the intracellular and extracellular fluid compartments follows. A standard 70-kg man has a total body water content of 40 L (60 per cent of the total body weight). Fluid and electrolyte loss which has occurred over several days will therefore have depleted all fluid compartments, and the total deficit may exceed 10 L. There is frequently relative sparing of intracellular fluid. Fluid replaced into the intravascular compartment must again equilibrate with other compartments, and a too-rapid replacement will merely overload the circulation with deterioration in perfusion and oxygen delivery. Central venous pressure measurement (ideally 3–8 mmHg) and urine output (over 30–50 mL per hour) are good guides during rehydration unless there is also renal impairment or cardiac failure, when more intensive monitoring may be required.

The sodium and potassium content of gastrointestinal secretions is shown in Table 11.1, page 191. Fluid lost from burns has a similar high sodium content. Normal saline is therefore the basic fluid for replacement of abnormal fluid losses. A fall in serum potassium is a late indicator of depletion of total body potassium which is mainly in the intracellular fluid. Therefore, if potassium is known to have been lost, it should be replaced even if the serum potassium is not below normal. Solutions of 5 per cent dextrose have no place in the replacement of abnormal losses and can only compensate for reduced oral fluid intake.

CARDIORESPIRATORY IMPAIRMENT

Improvements in cardiac output, perfusion and systolic blood pressure should occur as dehydration and hypovolaemic shock are treated. An inefficient cardiac rhythm can be corrected; for example, fast atrial fibrillation can be controlled by intravenous digoxin. Congestive cardiac failure may be improved with a fast-acting diuretic. Bronchodilators or steroids may improve bronchospasm. A decision may be taken preoperatively that a patient will require postoperative admission to an intensive care unit for a period of planned artificial ventilation and inotropic cardiac support.

Intensive preoperative maximization of oxygen delivery

This requires intensive care monitoring, including measurements of cardiac output and arterial oxygen saturation. An oxygen delivery of 600 mL/min/m^2 is sought. Fluid replacement, increased inspired oxygen concentrations and inotropes may be needed to achieve this level.[2]

CORRECTION OF ABNORMALITIES OF CLOTTING

Bleeding complications increase when surgery is performed on patients with abnormalities of clotting. A patient's brief family history, and also a personal history, will help to identify likely congenital problems. Acquired coagulation defects are more common, particularly in the context of an acutely ill patient. A drug history is also important; aspirin induces a defect in platelet function, associated with a prolonged bleeding time and 'oozing' at operation. Measurement of full blood count and a coagulation screen help in the initial assessment when a clotting abnormality is suspected. A low platelet count ($<50 \times 10^9$/L) should be corrected with platelet transfusion. A prolonged prothrombin time (PT) and activated partial thromboplastin time (APPT) due to vitamin K deficiency or liver impairment can be corrected by using fresh-frozen plasma. Patients on warfarin should receive vitamin K in addition to fresh-frozen plasma. Heparin anticoagulation can be stopped, and reversed if necessary with protamine, although low molecular-weight heparin may only be partially reversed.

ENDOCRINE ABNORMALITIES

A *diabetic* patient may be extremely unstable in an emergency situation. Commonly, they are ketoacidotic, but diabetic control will not be fully possible until the necrotic tissue or septic focus has been treated surgically. Surgery has to proceed alongside the management of their ketoacidosis. The occasional patient will be hypoglycaemic from a long-acting oral agent, or insulin, and a cessation of oral intake. Any patient on oral *steroids* requires parenteral steroid administration at increased dosages (see below).

The 4–day window

A delay of several days allows more formal preparation for surgery. A laparotomy for a non-strangulating bowel obstruction, surgery for obstructive jaundice or an amputation for irreversible ischaemia of a limb may all fall into this category. Medical treatment can be instituted for cardiac failure or hypertension. Preoperative treatment of obstructive airways disease, or a respiratory infection, with physiotherapy, bronchodilators and antibiotics may all be beneficial. Anaemia can be corrected with blood transfusion preoperatively. Perioperative diabetic management can be planned, and diabetic patients on oral agents are usually temporarily converted to insulin. Jaundiced patients are at increased risk of postoperative renal failure. This is now believed to be mainly secondary to fluid shifts with an overall fluid and electrolyte depletion, and should be corrected preoperatively. Obstructive jaundice classically causes a prolonged PT which may reverse with administration of vitamin K.

Warfarin anticoagulation can be either partially or fully reversed, dependent upon the thrombotic risk of the patient. When the thrombotic risk is extremely high, the patient is converted to intravenous heparin anticoagulation, for easier control (see below). There is time for the insertion of an IVC filter if this is indicated.

If a patient has had no effective oral intake in the week before surgery, and a gastrointestinal operation is planned after which oral intake will be further delayed, the institution of IV feeding before surgery may be beneficial. Abdominal surgery which may involve surgery of the left colon is safer if the colon is empty, and there is time for a mechanical bowel preparation if not contraindicated by intestinal obstruction.

The 4-week window

Most cancer surgery can be delayed for several weeks, without detriment. This allows better medical control of severe hypertension or other cardiorespiratory pathology. There is also time for benefit to accrue from the cessation of smoking. Occasionally, this window must be utilized for the surgical correction of other pathology which, if uncorrected, will make surgery more hazardous. For example, a carotid endarterectomy will greatly reduce the incidence of an intra-operative stroke in a patient with a severe carotid stenosis who requires another major procedure. The contraceptive pill, or aspirin therapy, can be stopped with normalization of the risk of thromboembolism or operative bleeding. There is also time to plan the management of those patients on anti-coagulants, and those who have greatly increased thrombotic risk (see below).

The over 4-month window

Truly elective surgery should be postponed if the risk of surgery is significant and can be reduced with the passage of time, or when some medical or surgical prior intervention will reduce the overall risk. During the first 6 months after a myocardial infarct the risk of a further infarct in the perioperative period is increased by 30 per cent. A delay of at least 6 months should be observed if the underlying condition will not deteriorate significantly during this period. The risk of a further stroke after a cerebral vascular accident is also increased, and a similar delay is recommended. Grossly overweight patients can sometimes manage a significant weight reduction, but more often they are unsuccessful in losing weight. It may be appropriate to delay surgery until after a carotid endarterectomy, a cardiac valvular replacement, an aortic aneurysm repair, a coronary bypass graft or angioplasty if it is felt this will reduce the overall mortality or morbidity.

PATIENT INFORMATION AND 'CONSENT'

There has been much recent interest in this issue from patient groups and medicolegal sources, and surgeons feel under increasing pressure to explain an operation and its complications, sometimes in more detail than a patient wishes to know. All patients must however understand – at least in a general way – the aims, limitations and risks of the surgery they are to undergo, and have the opportunity to ask for more information if they wish. If there is a choice of management, the patient may wish to be involved in the decision or may prefer to abdicate the choice to 'an expert'. Surgery

which alters body image (amputation of a limb, mastectomy or the formation of a stoma) can be particularly distressing. Preoperative counselling by a specialist nurse, patient information leaflets and a visit from a former patient who underwent similar surgery may all be helpful. Further reading on the legal aspects of 'consent' is essential,[3] as misconceptions are common as to who is entitled to give consent and what constitutes 'informed consent'.

GASTROINTESTINAL PREPARATION FOR SURGERY

For any general anaesthetic the stomach should ideally be empty to reduce the risk of aspiration of gastric contents, especially during induction of, and recovery from, anaesthesia. In elective surgery, a period of 6 hours without food is normally requested by anaesthetists, and traditionally clear fluids were allowed until 4 hours before induction. Many anaesthetists now allow clear fluids to be continued up to 2 hours before anaesthesia. In some emergency situations, however, surgery cannot be delayed for 6 hours. In addition, a patient with an intestinal obstruction will often not have an empty stomach, even if fasted and a nasogastric tube is in place. A patient who suffers limb trauma following a meal develops gastric stasis, and the stomach may remain full for many hours. In all of these situations the anaesthetist has to proceed with the increased risk of a full stomach, taking care to ensure that rapid intubation can be safely achieved.

An empty colon is generally considered safer than one full of faeces if colonic surgery is required. Although a right hemi-colectomy can be performed on unprepared bowel without any increased risk, most surgeons prefer an empty colon if a left-sided colonic anastomosis is planned. Mechanical clearance of the colon can be achieved in the 36 hours before surgery by a variety of means, but oral proprietary preparations of ethylene glycol or sodium picosulphate have proved the most satisfactory. Preoperative bowel preparation is not possible when there is an intestinal obstruction, and an intraoperative on-table lavage is an alternative (this is described in Chapter 22). The once-favoured oral preoperative antibiotics, given to reduce the colonic bacterial load, have been abandoned as they carry a risk of intestinal superinfection with yeasts and resistant bacteria.

DIABETES

Diabetic patients undergoing elective surgery should ideally no longer have residual long-acting insulin or oral hypoglycaemic agents affecting their blood glucose levels at the time of surgery. Conversion during the previous 24 hours to short-acting soluble insulin allows greater flexibility if blood glucose levels become labile. Most hospitals have a standard protocol for the management of diabetic surgical patients, and although there is variation, in general, the insulin is usually given as a continuous infusion (1–3–IU/hour) and adjusted according to blood glucose levels. Conversion back to the original regime should await re-establishment of a normal oral food intake. Even after minor surgery the patient must be warned that he or she may initially have increased insulin requirements relating to the stress response and increased steroid production.

Failure to recognize and treat hypoglycaemia during surgery may have disastrous consequences. Emergency surgery on diabetic patients is often complicated by failure of diabetic control, and this failure most frequently takes the form of ketoacidosis as discussed above.

STEROID THERAPY

Preoperatively, a patient may be unable to continue with their oral steroid regime due to restriction of oral intake or poor absorption. An alternative parenteral steroid must be substituted. Patients on long-term steroids, whether as replacement therapy or at therapeutic dosage, have suppressed adrenals and are unable to mount the normal steroid response to stress. Peroperatively, both groups should receive parenteral hydrocortisone which is then maintained during the postoperative period, initially parenterally and later orally. On the day of surgery, 100 mg of hydrocortisone is given an hour before surgery, and a further 100 mg 8-hourly. The dose is reduced as the stress from surgery diminishes until finally the preoperative dose is achieved. Even after relatively minor surgery, increased levels are required for several days and, after major procedures, often for over 2 weeks. Too rapid a reduction is unphysiological, and leaves the patient at best tired and depressed, and at worst with a full-blown hypotensive Addisonian crisis.

THYROTOXICOSIS, PHAECHROMOCYTOMA AND CARCINOID SYNDROME

High levels of circulating thyroxine, adrenaline, nor-adrenaline or 5-hydroxytryptamine (5-HT, serotonin) can result in a patient developing extreme cardiovascular instability during anaesthesia. The situation is compounded in surgery to remove a hormone-secreting tumour, or overactive gland, when surgical manipulation can cause sudden bolus release into the circulation of the active hormone. However, the diagnosis in these patients is usually already established, and the effects of the abnormal secretions can be blocked pharmacologically prior to surgery. The greatest surgical risk is in those in whom the diagnosis has not been made preoperatively, and who may be undergoing un-related surgery.

BLOOD CLOTTING AND SURGERY

Thromboembolic prophylaxis

Deep venous thrombosis (DVT) and pulmonary embolus (PE), following otherwise successful surgery, remains a significant cause of postoperative mortality and morbidity. Stasis, hypercoagulability and intimal damage are all implicated in the pathophysiology. The incidence can be reduced by the assessment of the risk in each patient and the institution of physical and pharmacological preventative measures appropriate to the level of risk. A scoring system, in which various risk factors carry different weighting, can divide patients into low-, moderate- and high-risk groups.

The most important general risk factors for thrombosis include a personal or family history of DVT or PE, carriage of the thrombophilic factor, immobility, increasing age, obesity, pregnancy and the combined contraceptive pill. Severe infection, inflammatory bowel disease and underlying malignancy also increase the risk of thrombosis. Major additional risk factors relate to the magnitude of the operation and the immobility associated with it. In particular, trauma and surgery to the hip, pelvis and lower limb are associated with increased risk.

Preventive strategies can be divided into physical measures which help to prevent stasis, and pharmacological measures to reduce the coagulability of the blood. Early mobilization, elevation of the legs and graduated compression stockings after surgery are important in preventing postoperative stasis, but most thromboses develop during surgery. A variety of mechanical devices which cause intermittent calf compression, either by direct external pressure or by initiating calf muscle contraction with intermittent foot impulse, are available in the operating theatre.

Low-dose heparin prophylaxis is the most widely used pharmacological measure. Low molecular-weight heparins have the advantage of a longer half-life, allowing a single daily dose. The regime is normally started an hour before surgery but, for certain procedures including epidural anaesthesia, it may be reserved until after completion of surgery if there is concern that it may increase haemorrhagic complications.

Early mobilization and graduated compression stockings is all that is recommended in low-risk patients. In patients with a moderate risk of thrombosis, either heparin or intermittent foot impulse is added to the prevention regime, whereas in high-risk patients the two strategies can be used in combination. Additional measures such as an IVC filter and extended warfarin prophylaxis should also be considered.

Abnormal clotting associated with another disease

- *Platelet production* may be depressed in any patient with a haematological malignancy, or in any patient with marrow depression from cytotoxic drug therapy or alcohol. Malignant marrow replacement can also suppress platelet production. A platelet count is important preoperatively in those patients in whom a depressed count is likely. A normal count does not always reflect normal function.

- *Platelet destruction* in idiopathic thrombocytopenia is the most common scenario in which a surgeon has to operate on a patient with a low platelet count, as a splenectomy may be required when other treatment modalities have failed. Platelet infusions may be required to cover the period of surgery, but it must be remembered that the half-life of platelets in this condition is very short. Platelets for transfusion are prepared from several donors, and have a shelf-life of 5 days. They must be ABO compatible (see Appendix II).

- *Obstructive jaundice* results in prolonged clotting from poor production of clotting factors secondary to a deficiency of vitamin K. It is reversed by administration of vitamin K a few days preoperatively.

- *Liver failure* also results in prolonged clotting from poor production of clotting factors by the failing liver. Vitamin K may not be effective. Surgery will be very high risk and clotting abnormalities have to be treated with fresh-frozen plasma transfusions.

- *Inherited defects of clotting* such as haemophilia (Factor VIII deficiency), Factor II deficiency and Von Willebrand's disease may affect up to 5 per cent of the population. Good communication with the haematologist is the key to the planning of safe surgery. Often, the presence of inhibitors in the patient's serum makes the simple replacement of clotting factors less effective than theoretically predicted.

Management of patients on anticoagulation

Management of anticoagulation during the perioperative period is dependent on the indications for therapeutic anticoagulation, the thrombotic risk of the patient, and the haemorrhagic risk associated with the surgery. Surgery on a fully anticoagulated patient is likely to be complicated by bleeding, and anticoagulation should be reversed before all elective surgery unless the risk of clotting is extremely high. For the majority of patients on warfarin, this can be safely stopped 3 or 4 days preoperatively and the clotting should have returned to near normal by the time of the operation. The International Normalized Ratio (INR) is checked immediately preoperatively, and should be less than 1.8 for surgery to proceed safely. Warfarin can be restarted once the risk of early postoperative bleeding has passed. After minor surgery the patient can return to their normal drug regime the day after surgery, and therapeutic levels will gradually be restored over several days. More urgent reversal of warfarin anticoagulation can be achieved with low-dose vitamin K, which takes around 6 hours. This is combined with fresh-frozen plasma, or a clotting factor concentrate, when there is greater urgency or when a patient is over anticoagulated.

Patients with a high risk of thrombosis – for example those with a recent personal history of thrombosis, thrombophilic factors and mechanical heart valves – should have a protocol tailored to their needs by liaison with a haematologist. The balance between thrombosis and surgical haemorrhage can be very fine, with no safe middle ground. Conversion from warfarin to heparin anticoagulation is usually instituted as the effects of heparin can be quickly reversed, enabling the patient's coagulation status to be more suppressed both during and after surgery than would be safe with warfarin. The infusion of non-fractionated, short-acting intravenous heparin is simply stopped 1 hour prior to the surgery itself. The half-life is only 1.5 hours, but if more rapid reversal becomes necessary then protamine can be given. Cooperation is essential between surgeon, anaesthetist, cardiologist and haematologist in managing these high-risk patients.

An IVC filter may be considered, but will only protect against a pulmonary embolus. It does not prevent a deep venous thrombosis, or the complication of thrombus formation on a prosthetic heart valve, within the atria or in an arterial graft. The IVC filters are usually inserted by a radiologist a few days before surgery.

An increasing number of patients are on low-dose aspirin for prevention of thromboembolic events. Aspirin and other anti-platelet agents produce an irreversible platelet dysfunction, and haemostasis can only return to normal as new platelets are formed. Therefore, if these agents are to be discontinued prior to surgery, at least a week must elapse for platelet activity to improve significantly. Aspirin is often ignored by surgeons, but it can cause major haemorrhagic problems as patient response to the drug is variable. It is, therefore, advisable to stop aspirin therapy at least 10 days before all surgery, unless it is felt that this will place the patient at significant additional thromboembolic risk.

INTRAVENOUS ACCESS

Peripheral vein access is adequate for the administration of fluid, blood or drugs. The hypertonic solutions for parenteral nutrition are irritant to endothelium, and in a narrow-calibre vein, with small volume flow, cause early phlebitis and vein occlusion with adherent thrombus. Central venous access is therefore usually established when hypertonic irritant fluid or drugs have to be administered intravenously. It is also required for the measurement of central venous pressure. Although long catheters can be threaded centrally from peripheral veins, direct cannulation of the subclavian or internal jugular vein is preferable.

Percutaneous peripheral vein cannulation

The veins on the dorsum of the hand and forearm are the most suitable. The needle, with the overlying plastic cannula, is introduced into a vein, the needle withdrawn and the plastic cannula advanced up the lumen of the vein and strapped in place. A cannula which crosses a joint may occlude when the joint is flexed and, in addition, movement results in increased trauma to the endothelium. The prominent superficial veins in the antecubital fossa, although ideal for emergency access, are therefore less suitable for longer term cannulation. The use of leg veins should be avoided as cannulation will restrict mobility and may increase the risk of DVT.

The 'lifespan' of peripheral cannula access is extremely variable. Once any phlebitis develops, occlusion is inevitable. The cannula should be replaced in another vein at the first evidence of phlebitis. To await the inevitable occlusion risks a severe local reaction and the occlusion of adjacent segments of vein which will not then be available for later cannulation. In addition, there is a significant risk of septicaemia. The lifespan of a cannula will be greater if it is inserted using an antiseptic technique and if endothelial irritation from hypertonic solutions is minimized. Mechanical trauma from movement can be reduced if the vicinity of joints is avoided, and a small cannula in a large vein causes less endothelial trauma. A small cannula is, however, inappropriate in any patient who may require rapid replacement of fluid or blood.

Peripheral vein 'cut down'

This technique can produce rapid, large-diameter, secure intravenous access. It may be appropriate in a shocked patient in whom peripheral veins are collapsed, and difficult to enter, and central catheterization skills are unavailable, or have failed. It also provides secure intravenous access for several days which can be difficult to achieve, especially in a small child, if appropriate plastic cannulae or intravenous infusion needles are unavailable.

A transverse incision is made over a vein. The subcutaneous tissue is opened by sharp or blunt dissection on either side of the vein, until an artery forceps can be passed beneath it and used to draw a ligature round under the vein. This ligature is then tied as far distally as possible, and a second ligature passed beneath the vein more proximally. The second ligature is left untied until the cannula is in place. A small incision is made between the ligatures, the plastic or metal cannula inserted, and the second ligature tied to hold the vein snugly against the outside of the cannula. In a small child the long saphenous vein at the ankle is the most suitable as the risk of DVT is not a consideration, and this vein is of large calibre and anatomically in a standard position.

Interosseous access

This was a common route for infusion of blood or fluids in the early years of the twentieth century. It fell into disuse as intravenous techniques improved, but regained popularity during the 1990s as the fastest route for circulatory access in a young child. The most suitable site is the anteromedial surface of the proximal tibia, 1–3 cm below the tibial tubercle. An 18–20-gauge needle is satisfactory in babies, but over 1 year of age a 13–16-gauge is more suitable. The needle should be stiff so that it does not break on insertion into bone, and have a stylet to prevent marrow plugging the lumen during insertion. The needle is inserted at an angle of about 15 degrees from the perpendicular, away from the tibial growth plate, and the stylet removed.

Central venous catheterization

Central lines are used with increasing frequency in surgical patients. Peripheral thrombophlebitis from mechanical and chemical irritation is reduced, and the lifespan of access greatly increased. Multi-channel lines, with two to five channels, allow monitoring of central venous pressure through one channel, continuous administration of intravenous fluids through a second, infusion pump administration of insulin, heparin or an inotrope through a third. Further channels can then be used for bolus administration of drugs and for removal of blood samples, etc.

These lines may be inserted after induction of anaesthesia as part of peroperative anaesthetic care, or they can be inserted in the conscious patient either pre- or postoperatively. Sterility is mandatory if infective complications are to be minimized. The patient is placed supine and tilted 15–30 degrees head-down to fill the veins of the neck and the superior mediastinum. There are multiple commercial kits for cannulation, but all are based on initial entry into the vein with a needle followed by manoeuvres to advance a long catheter safely into the superior vena cava (SVC). It is dangerous to advance the catheter through a needle, as in this technique the needle can cut the catheter with a resultant embolus of the catheter tip. In the *Seldinger technique* a flexible guide wire is inserted down the needle. The needle is then removed and a long catheter is advanced over the wire, which is finally removed. Intermediate dilating cannulae may be used over the wire if a large-bore catheter is required. An alternative to the Seldinger technique is to use a needle and cannula together for the initial venous insertion. The needle is withdrawn and a long catheter can be threaded safely through the cannula. An initial small skin incision is essential if any catheter is to be threaded over a wire, otherwise the catheter cannot be passed through the skin. In the conscious patient, a bleb of local anaesthesia is infiltrated in the skin followed by deeper infiltration onto the vein.

Central lines are not without complications. Insertion can be associated with a pneumothorax or, occasionally, a major haemorrhage. The tip may be advanced too far and cause arrhythmias, or may turn up into the jugular veins from a subclavian insertion. An X-ray immediately after insertion is therefore essential. Infection of a central line commonly presents with septicaemia, but thrombophlebitis and occlusion can also occur. Full sterile precautions for insertion are therefore mandatory. An infected line must be removed and important access is lost. Multi-channel, multi-purpose lines unfortunately are prone to infective complications unless all personnel using them observe similar strict precautions. Single-channel dedicated lines are therefore used when long-term access is required for prolonged intravenous feeding or the administration of cytotoxic drugs.

Internal jugular cannulation

This is favoured by anaesthetists, but the position of the cannula is awkward for the conscious patient. The head is turned to the opposite side. The surface marking of the vein is from the ear lobe to the medial end of the clavicle. The vein is overlapped by the sternocleidomastoid muscle, but is often palpable in the lower one-third where it lies between the sternal and clavicular heads of the muscle. The carotid artery lies posteromedial to the vein. The fingers of the left hand retract the carotid artery medially, and skin entry is at the apex of the triangle formed by the confluence of the two heads of sternocleidomastoid. The needle is slanted at 30 degrees to the skin and advanced caudally. Resistance is felt, then lost, as first deep fascia is encountered followed by vein wall.

Subclavian vein cannulation

This is the most satisfactory long-term central venous access. The vein runs horizontally behind the clavicle to join the internal jugular vein behind the sternoclavicular joint. It is closely related to the subclavian artery, and the dome of the pleura with the underlying lung apex. These structures may be injured during the insertion of a subclavian line. A sandbag is placed under the upper thoracic spine so that the shoulders fall back, the arm is retracted downwards to depress the shoulder girdle, and the head is turned to the opposite side. The needle is inserted 1 cm below the junction of the middle and outer thirds of the clavicle, and is angled so that it passes deep to the clavicle in the direction of the ipsilateral sternoclavicular joint. Insertion on the right side is a more natural procedure for a right-handed surgeon, but on the left side it is often easier to advance the cannula into the optimum position as the angle into the SVC is less acute.

When long-term cannulation is required, a subcutaneous tunnelled length of line, as illustrated in Figure 11.5, page 195 will reduce infective complications.

REFERENCES

1. Wilson J, Woods I, Fawcett J, *et al.* Reducing the risk of major elective surgery: randomised controlled trial of preoperative optimisation of oxygen delivery. *Br Med J* 1999; **318**: 1099–103.
2. Curran JE, Grounds RM. Ward *versus* intensive care management of high-risk surgical patients. *Br J Surg* 1998; **85**: 956–61.
3. Department of Health. *Good Practice in Consent Implementation Guide: consent to examination and treatment.* London: HMSO, 2001.

Appendix II

INTRAOPERATIVE CARE

ANAESTHESIA

For almost all surgery some form of general or regional anaesthesia is essential. Except for local infiltrative anaesthesia, this is primarily the responsibility of the anaesthetists, who also have the maintenance of all the patient's vital functions under their control during the operation. The anaesthetist will choose the most appropriate anaesthetic, but often only after discussion with the surgeon, as the planned position of an incision or the expected length of a procedure may influence the decision. In addition, the surgeon may require specific intraoperative conditions, for example, abdominal muscle relaxation or low central venous pressure.

Local infiltrative anaesthesia

This is the standard technique for all minor surgery on the skin or subcutaneous tissue. It can also be used for more major procedures such as inguinal herniorrhaphy, but care must be exercised that toxic doses are not exceeded (see Chapters 1 and 24). It is important, except when the most minor procedure is performed under local anaesthesia, that an anaesthetist is present or immediately available. This is particularly important when local anaesthesia has been chosen for an elderly patient who has cardiovascular co-morbidity. Apprehension or pain will increase both metabolic requirements and adrenaline output, and arrhythmias, angina and acute ventricular failure may be precipitated. A combination of sedation and local anaesthesia can be particularly dangerous in such patients. Over-sedation can result in confusion, but sedation then has to be increased further for the surgeon to complete the operation on a confused uncooperative patient. Finally, the surgeon can be operating on a semi-anaesthetized patient, with significant cardiac or respiratory co-morbidity, without either adequate monitoring or airway protection. When operating under local infiltrative anaesthesia, handling of the peritoneum or spermatic cord can cause bradycardia, hypotension or vomiting. It is important therefore that patients for this form of surgery are fasted, monitored and the assistance of an anaesthetist is available if required.

Peripheral nerve blocks

These can give good anaesthesia for orthopaedic, and occasionally for vascular, procedures. Lignocaine without adrenaline is infiltrated around a nerve. Direct puncture of the nerve is not only extremely painful but may cause axonal damage. A good knowledge of anatomy is essential as major vessels are often in close proximity to major nerves and are in danger of injury. Further reading is recommended for surgeons who are interested in this technique for anything other than digital or intercostal nerve blocks.[1]

Epidural and spinal regional anaesthesia

If possible, an anaesthetist should be responsible for these forms of anaesthesia. They cannot be easily instituted, monitored and adjusted by the surgeon, although the occasional isolated surgeon practising in an area with limited healthcare resources has to compromise. The surgeon establishes the epidural, or spinal anaesthetic, and then leaves the patient partially under the care of an assistant while proceeding with the surgery, but with continuing overall responsibility for the anaesthetic issues as well.

Regional intravenous anaesthesia

Also known as a Bier's block, this is a simple technique for distal limb anaesthesia and useful for the setting of a displaced wrist fracture. A cannula is inserted into a distal vein and the limb is exsanguinated either by bandaging or, if too painful, by elevation. A proximal tourniquet is inflated and a dilute solution of prilocaine is injected through the cannula into the isolated veins. A dose of 4 mg/kg should not be exceeded, but the volume must be sufficient to fill the veins, and around 40 mL will be required for an adult arm. After 5 minutes sufficient anaesthetic agent will have infiltrated out into the tissue to allow manipulation of the fracture. After 20 minutes, almost all of the anaesthetic should have diffused out of the vessels into the tissues and the cuff can be safely deflated. The simplicity of this technique encouraged surgeons to use it themselves in accident departments. Unfortunately, premature deflation of the tourniquet, for whatever reason, floods the circulation with a large bolus of local anaesthetic, with serious and even fatal cardiovascular and CNS toxicity. It is therefore considered a potentially dangerous technique, and it is now recommended that, ideally, it should only be used by anaesthetists who will be more able to deal with complications should they occur.

General anaesthesia

For most major surgery this is the ideal anaesthetic. Inhalational or intravenous drugs, or a combination of these, are used to keep the patient in a state of unconsciousness for the duration of the surgery. Patients may be breathing spontaneously, or may be paralysed and mechanically ventilated, but with either technique they are unable to protect their airway which is vulnerable to obstruction from the tongue or from inhalation of vomit or secretions. Mechanical obstruction from the tongue can be prevented by an oral 'airway', combined with skilful holding of the lower jaw forwards while the face-mask is simultaneously held in place. Most anaesthetists now favour a laryngeal mask. However, only an endotracheal tube gives reliable protection against inhalation of secretions or gastric contents.

Ketamine has proved to be an extremely safe agent where anaesthetic skills are limited. It provides a state of 'disassociative anaesthesia' – a profound analgesia with light sleep, and surgery is possible on a patient who can still protect his or her own airway. Slow recovery and unpleasant dreams have restricted its more general use.

PATIENT POSITIONING

The anaesthetized patient requires more than just protection of the airway. The eyelids must be kept closed to protect the cornea from drying and abrasions. The patient is also unable to protect joints from excessive movement which can damage both the joint and the adjacent structures. (Patients who have regional anaesthesia are equally vulnerable in the paralysed and anaesthetized areas.) An anaesthetized patient who has to be turned or moved into a different position for surgery requires particular attention to prevent excessive move-

ment of the neck. Arms may become trapped or fall unsupported and, in general, during re-positioning they should be held straight and adducted alongside the patient's trunk. Legs which have to be elevated should be moved together to prevent an uneven strain on the lumbar spine. An unstable position may be necessary to allow the surgeon satisfactory access, and the patient must be made secure in, for example, a lateral position, with the upper arm supported, and the table 'broken'. The ideal position for the surgeon may not be satisfactory for an anaesthetized patient. For example, abduction of the arm should be kept to less than 90 degrees and, if legs have to be elevated for a long procedure, extreme flexion of knees and hips should be avoided (see Fig. 23.3a and b, page 438). Even a Lloyd–Davis position can compromise the perfusion of the legs in a very long operation, and a postoperative calf compartment syndrome is a well-recognized, but fortunately rare, complication. Consideration must be given to mechanical prophylaxis of deep venous thrombosis (see Appendix I).

The most vulnerable area of skin is that on which the patient is lying. The initial ischaemic insult in a postoperative sacral, or heel, pressure sore has most often occurred during the surgery itself. Pressure damage can be reduced by the use of a soft surface, a 'jelly mat' or a sheepskin, and heel pressure can be further reduced by spreading the area of weight-bearing skin with a soft support under the Achilles tendon. It is also important during long operations to tip the table in different directions to alter the pressure points. Localized pressure from restraining straps, armrests and lithotomy poles can also cause pressure damage to skin, or to a superficial nerve. The ulnar and the lateral popliteal nerve are the most vulnerable. No skin should be in contact with any metal part of the operating table, or its attachments, or there is a danger of a diathermy burn.

MONITORING DURING SURGERY

In all surgery under general anaesthesia the surgeon is only marginally involved in the monitoring of the patient's overall homeostasis. The anaesthetist may however need to know whether measurements of urine output or blood loss are realistic. Ascitic fluid, mixed with blood and weighed in swabs, may be erroneously recorded as blood, and in open genitourinary surgery urine output may significantly exceed the urine collected by catheter. A surgical observation that the blood pooling in the pelvis is no longer clotting often predates confirmation of a clotting abnormality on laboratory tests.

In minor surgery under local infiltrative anaesthesia, no monitoring may be necessary but, when a surgeon is operating on an elderly unfit patient for a more major procedure, monitoring is desirable. An ECG, pulse oximetry and blood pressure monitoring are straightforward to set up and may alert the surgeon to a deteriorating situation. The patient should also have an intravenous cannula in place in case emergency intravenous access is required.

Intraoperative imaging

X-ray monitoring is routine in many urological, orthopaedic, vascular and biliary procedures. A single exposure can demonstrate the position of a fracture after reduction or can confirm the free flow of contrast along a vessel, a duct or a ureter on which surgery has been performed. An image intensifier allows surgery to be performed with continuous radiological screening to guide the passage of the tip of an instrument which is not visible or palpable by the surgeon. Inappropriate or excessive X-ray exposure of both patient and staff must be avoided. The guidelines for safe practice are strict, but must be observed.[2] Intraoperative ultrasound has an increasing role in surgery and does not pose the safety hazards of X-ray monitoring.

PREVENTION OF INFECTION

Sterilization of instruments and the use of antiseptic skin preparations, sterile drapes and towels does not ensure total sterility. Bacteria are released into the operating theatre air from the skin and respiratory tract of everyone present in the theatre. Masks prevent droplet contamination of the wound if a surgeon sneezes, but are largely ineffective in reducing the general contamination of the air with organisms. Decontamination of the surgeon's hands and forearms by an antiseptic wash, followed by the wearing of a sterile surgical gown and gloves, is no longer an effective barrier if a non-permeable gown becomes soaked with body fluids, or gloves are torn. Preparation of the patient's skin in the operation field with antiseptic does not destroy the bacteria in the hair follicles or sweat glands. These bacteria may come to the surface with secretions during surgery. Sterile drapes over unprepared skin are not an effective barrier if they are permeable and soaked with body fluids. Surgery which opens into the gastrointestinal tract is always contaminated.

Surgery should be undertaken in as clean an environment as is possible. Floors and surfaces should be washed, and shoes and outer clothing changed. Controlled air flow can also reduce the bacterial counts in the air. Sterile instruments, sutures and surgical gloves are used, and any skin not treated with antiseptic is isolated from the operative field by sterile drapes.

'Scrub' procedure is the antiseptic wash of the hands and forearms of those involved in the surgery. The traditional abrasive scrub is no longer recommended as it damages skin, and increases infection. Hands are simply washed in a detergent solution containing added chlorhexidine or an iodine-based antiseptic. Alternatively, an alcohol rub of already clean hands can be employed.

Skin preparation of the operation site with an antiseptic solution is standard. Suitable solutions again include iodine-based antiseptic solutions, and chlorhexidine in water or spirit. Spirit-based solutions should be avoided, or used with great care, if diathermy is to be employed as ignition of spirit-soaked drapes, and of puddles of spirit in the vagina or umbilicus, has been reported. Hairs obscure the surgeon's view, and shaving of hair-bearing skin is standard. It does not, as originally believed, reduce infection, and may, if carried out more than a few hours before surgery, increase the bacterial colonization of hair follicles.

Sterilization of instruments

Initial sterility of instruments is mandatory to prevent patient-to-patient spread of virulent organisms. (Instruments open to the theatre air will no longer be totally sterile at the end of a long operation.) Sterility can be achieved by the destruction of bacteria and viruses by thermal, chemical or irradiation damage. The resistance of some organisms to all methods of sterilization is greater than others, and it is on the properties of these organisms that sterilization schedules have to be based. The choice of method employed is most often dictated by the properties of the material or instrument to be sterilized. Heat-tolerant materials and instruments can be sterilized by pressurized steam. The higher the temperature, the shorter the time that the temperature must be held for sterilization, and several alternative cycles are available in standard autoclaves. The cycle commences with vacuum extraction of air, except in the small, portable steam sterilizers. The latter may therefore fail to sterilize an instrument with a lumen in which air is trapped and steam fails to enter. Heat without steam is less effective, and temperatures of 180°C for 60 minutes are required. Commercially, ethylene oxide gas and irradiation are used to sterilize single-use instruments and equipment. Instruments, such as fibre-optic telescopes, are damaged by the temperatures necessary for steam sterilization. Formaldehyde, or glutaraldehyde in an aqueous solution, is the most common alternative used in hospitals for multi-use heat-intolerant equipment. Unfortunately, this will not kill all spores and viruses, and must be regarded as a disinfection rather than a sterilization procedure.

Antibiotic prophylaxis

Despite all the above measures, infective complications remain a significant source of postoperative morbidity in some procedures unless prophylactic antibiotic therapy is employed. It is based on the concept that bacterial contamination occurs during surgery, and that the administration of the antibiotic used for prevention must be timed for optimum blood levels during the operation.

Bacterial contamination of the blood may progress to bacteraemic shock, or to infective vegetations, either on damaged heart valves or on the vascular anastomoses between native vessel and a prosthetic arterial graft.

Bacterial contamination of collections of blood or body fluid introduces organisms to an excellent culture medium, and abscess formation frequently follows. The administration of antibiotics once an abscess has formed is seldom sufficient definitive treatment. However, the complication can be prevented if there are high concentrations of antibiotic in these collections, making them an unfavourable culture medium. Antibiotic prophylaxis should therefore be administered immediately before, or during, surgery. Further prophylaxis for 48 hours postoperatively is justified if oozing of blood or tissue fluid from internal raw surfaces is expected to continue during this period. The choice of antibiotic is dictated by the likely pathogenic contaminants.

Anti-staphylococcal prophylaxis

This is most often considered in 'clean' surgery. The source of infection may be the patient's own skin or upper respiratory tract, or that of the personnel in theatre. The incidence of infection is low in clean surgery, but antibiotic prophylaxis is recommended if foreign material is used as infection of a joint prosthesis, an arterial graft or the mesh in a hernia repair can all have disastrous consequences. The emergence of methicillin-resistant *Staphylococcus aureus* (MRSA) is posing increasing difficulty in offering effective anti-staphylococcal prophylaxis without the inappropriate use of antibiotics which should be reserved for the treatment of severe infections with resistant organisms.

Intestinal organisms

These include a wide range of potential pathogens many of which are anaerobic. Antibiotic prophylaxis is recommended for all surgery in which the gastrointestinal tract is opened and is of particular importance in colonic surgery. A combination of a broad-spectrum antibiotic, such as a cephalosporin with metronidazole, which is effective against anaerobes, is commonly employed. The anaerobic clostridial organisms are commensals of the colon and encountered in the soil. Penicillin provides effective prophylaxis against gas gangrene and tetanus, and the risk should be remembered in contaminated wounds, especially if there is muscle ischaemia. Penicillin prophylaxis is recommended for all lower-limb amputations for ischaemia.

Urology

A transient bacteraemia is common in urethral instrumentation, even of an apparently non-infected urinary tract, and occasionally progresses to bacteraemic shock. This serious complication can be almost eliminated by a single dose of gentamicin.

Endocarditis

The risk is greatest in those patients with cardiac valvular lesions or a cardiac valve replacement, but prosthetic vascular grafts are also vulnerable. At-risk patients require antibiotic prophylaxis against possible pathogens. Anaerobic streptococci, which are sensitive to amoxycillin, are the most common pathogens although other organisms can be implicated. Dental surgery therefore carries the highest risk, but any general anaesthetic can result in a bacteraemia with oral organisms including *Streptococcus viridans*. In gastrointestinal or urinary tract surgery, antibiotic prophylaxis should also cover Gram-negative and anaerobic organisms, and gentamicin is given in addition to amoxycillin.

Viruses and prions

These agents now pose an increasing threat to the safety of all surgery. The long latent period before clinical symptoms, and the serious and frequently fatal consequences of infection, are major concerns. Hepatitis and HIV can be spread by small quantities of infected blood or tissue fluid, and it is mainly needle-stick injuries which are responsible for infection between the operating personnel and the patient. Additional precautions, such as double-gloves and the use of impermeable gowns, are commonly practised in a high-risk patient, but many carriers of these viruses are not identified. Great care should therefore be taken in the handling of needles and scalpels during every operation, and eye protection is also recommended. Diathermy for skin incision and dissection, the use of blunt needles for fascial closure, and clips for skin closure, can significantly reduce the risk, by eliminating sharp instruments from the operation. All surgeons should be immunized against hepatitis B. Immunization against hepatitis C and HIV is not currently available, but HIV prophylaxis should be instituted after a needle-stick injury involving contamination from a known HIV carrier. Conversely, any surgeon who is a carrier of any of these viruses is a risk to patients and should not continue operating. The prion responsible for new variant Creutzfeldt-Jakob disease (CJD) is not destroyed by normal sterilization techniques and, although it is a rare disease, this knowledge has led to calls for single-use instruments for surgery. The financial implications of this for all surgery would be prohibitive, however.

Surgery for infective pathology

Antibiotics in this situation are given to treat, rather than merely to prevent, infection, and therefore must be given for an adequate period of time. A 5-day course is usually the minimum, but in certain situations relapse is common unless antibiotics are continued for 2 weeks or more. Broad-spectrum antibacterial activity is necessary until bacteriological results are available, and adequate blood levels can often only be assured with parenteral administration. In gastrointestinal infective pathology, prophylactic regimens of cephalosporin and metronidazole are inadequate. Either gentamicin must be added to the regime, or treatment with a broad-spectrum antibiotic such as Tazocin (a piperacillin/tazobactam combination) substituted.

DIATHERMY

Haemostasis by diathermy coagulation has been available for over 50 years. Refinements in technology have led to increased use of diathermy for dissection with the advantage of greater precision in an almost bloodless operative field.

Monopolar diathermy

A high-frequency alternating electric current is passed through the patient. Heat is produced wherever the current is locally concentrated. A large plate electrode is held in contact with the patient's skin. The other point of patient contact is concentrated in a small area of tissue with a fine point or forceps with resultant thermal damage. A *pulsed electrical output* has a coagulation effect. A *continuous output,* used to create an arc between the diathermy tip and the tissue, vaporizes cell water and cuts tissue with minimal charring. A 'blend' of the two forms of current can provide the surgeon with a haemostatic cutting tip which combines minimal charring with effective coagulation of small vessels.

In all monopolar diathermy there is a danger of burns from the wide plate if it is mal-positioned and in contact with only a small area of skin. Burns may also occur if any part of the patient is in contact with earthed metal such as a drip stand. Current passes through the patient and, although normally harmless, there is a risk in certain circumstances. Metal jewellery which a patient cannot remove may result in a local burn. Monopolar diathermy on an extremity with a narrow pedicle can result in a high concentration of energy in the tissue of the pedicle and thermal damage. The spermatic cord is thus at risk if diathermy is used on a testis which has been mobilized out of the scrotum, and urethral burns have been reported when monopolar diathermy was used during a circumcision. Diathermy current passing through a cardiac pacemaker can disrupt its function, and current can also be channelled along the wires and cause myocardial burns. The diathermy pad can sometimes be positioned to minimize the current through the pacemaker, but bipolar diathermy will be a safer alternative.

Bipolar diathermy

This is a less versatile, but safer, form of electric current haemostasis. There is no pad attached to the patient and the current only passes between the two tips of the diathermy forceps, coagulating the tissue held between them. Current will not pass from the tips along another instrument to the patient, and it therefore cannot be used to coagulate a vessel already held by ordinary forceps. Neither can it be used as a 'bloodless scalpel' for dissection as no spark or arc can be created between the diathermy tips and the tissue.

LASERS

These have a wide range of application in the controlled destruction of tissue by a beam of electromagnetic radiation. In addition to their use endoscopically for the control of inoperable malignancies, the general surgeon is most likely to use a laser for coagulation.

Argon beamers

A jet of argon, combined with a laser beam of electromagnetic energy, produces a 'spray' of coagulation to tissue a few millimetres from the tip of the instrument. The coagulation is very superficial with minimal deeper thermal damage, and is a useful technique for large oozing surfaces such as a liver laceration, or the remaining part of the spleen after avulsion of one pole.

BLOOD TRANSFUSION

Blood has been used in the treatment of haemorrhage since the early twentieth century. The crucial development in safe transfusion was Landsteiner's discovery in 1901 of the major human ABO groups. Blood can now be separated into its components for individual use: red cells, platelet concentrates, fresh-frozen plasma, cryoprecipitate, albumin, high-purity Factor VIII, and combination factors are also available. This allows more targeted therapy. Preselection, and screening of donors and donated blood, for blood-borne pathogens is crucial. However, infection remains a hazard. Provision of safe blood requires a high level of organization and strict protocol. If an accredited blood transfusion service is not available, avoidance of blood products, unless absolutely necessary, is extremely important. Deaths also occur due to basic administrative errors in labelling blood samples from patients, and incorrect patient identification techniques. Although a basic understanding of the red cell antigen system is necessary, probably more important for the surgeon is the appreciation of the risks of blood transfusion.

Blood banks
A blood bank transfusion service is the system within which most blood transfusions are given and the surgeon does not need a detailed knowledge of the collection, storage and compatibility testing of blood. It must be remembered that the most common cause of a serious transfusion reaction is either incorrect labelling of the blood sample sent from a patient for cross-matching, or failure to ensure that the blood from the blood bank is administered to the correct patient. The importance of following all checking procedures in the ward or operating theatre cannot be overstated. Blood must also be ordered from the blood bank in time for all tests on antibodies and compatibility to be performed. The possibility that a blood transfusion may be

needed during an operation should therefore be addressed preoperatively. If transfusion is unlikely, the patient's blood should be sent for grouping and antibody testing. If the patient then does need a transfusion, blood can be issued from the blood bank within 30 minutes with a high degree of safety. It is rare to transfuse blood without some form of emergency compatibility test, but it is justified to transfuse uncrossmatched Group O Rhesus negative blood in situations of massive blood loss. Transfusion of uncrossmatched Group O blood carries a risk of a reaction to other antigens, especially in patients who have had previous transfusions.

Infection and blood

Blood collection must be performed using a sterile technique. A citrate anticoagulant solution is added, and the blood stored at 4°C. The shelf-life of blood is 35 days. Blood transfusion may transmit viral and protozoal infections in addition to bacterial infections. Protozoal infections which can be transmitted by blood include malaria, babesiosis, leishmaniasis, toxoplasmosis and trypanosomiasis. Viral infections potentially transmitted by blood include hepatitis A, B and C, cytomegalovirus, Epstein–Barr virus, human T-lymphocytotrophic virus, parvovirus B19, HIV and new-variant CJD. As the red cell component of blood is not subject to sterilization or virucidal treatment, donor selection and screening is crucial.

Transfusion reactions

A reaction during a blood transfusion may be one of pyrexia, shock, urticaria, or of headache and backache. It is often not clear initially whether it is a haemolytic transfusion reaction, a more minor allergic or febrile reaction, a bacteraemia from contamination, or an unrelated deterioration in the patient's condition. The initial management of all suspected reactions is the discontinuation of the blood transfusion, followed by assessment. The blood bank should be informed immediately. During anaesthesia and surgery a transfusion reaction is more difficult to diagnose as there are multiple other potential causes for a pyrexia, cardiovascular instability or allergic reaction.

- An *allergic reaction* is only rarely of a severe anaphylactic type requiring adrenaline and steroids. A minor reaction can be managed with antihistamines and continuation of the transfusion.
- A *febrile reaction* used to occur commonly, particularly with patients who had had multiple transfusions, due to sensitization to platelet or leukocyte antigens. In the UK, leukocyte-depleted blood is now supplied, making this reaction uncommon. A red cell mismatch must be excluded.
- A *haemolytic transfusion reaction* to an ABO

incompatibility is associated with a high mortality. It may commence after only a small amount of blood has been transfused. Shock, rigors and back pain are characteristic. The immediate dangers are of shock, hyperkalaemia and renal failure. Treatment is supportive resuscitation, and includes intravenous hydrocortisone and the maintenance of a good urine output. Dialysis may prove necessary.

- A *delayed haemolytic transfusion reaction* can result from minor blood group incompatibilities. Within a few days of the transfusion, the patient becomes jaundiced and anaemic with a low-grade fever. Treatment is supportive.

Autologous transfusions

Many of the hazards of blood transfusion can be avoided by transfusion of the patient's own blood. There are three ways in which this can be achieved, but each has inherent limitations. Bacterial contamination and infection remain a risk.

- *Preoperative donation*, over a period of 5–6 weeks, can accumulate 2–4 units of the patient's own blood, which is available for transfusion at the time of surgery. The operation must be reliably scheduled, and the patient must be fit to withstand repeated venesection without detriment. Oral iron and additional erythropoeitin will help the patient recover a normal haemoglobin level more quickly.
- *Normovolaemic haemodilution* immediately before surgery consists of the withdrawal of 2 units of blood, and replacement with three times the volume of crystalloid. The blood then available for transfusion is fresh with active platelets and clotting factors. It is seldom possible, however, to withdraw more than 2 units in this way.
- *Intraoperative blood salvage* with re-infusion into the patient can be an excellent technique for conserving blood. It is sometimes used in an elective setting in knee surgery. In the emergency situation, massive haemorrhage into the peritoneal or pleural cavity is usually the only circumstance in which it is practical. It is not suitable if the blood is contaminated with gastrointestinal bacteria, or with malignant cells. In its simplest form the blood is drawn into an evacuated container, containing citrate anticoagulant, and returned to the patient through a blood filter. The disadvantages of the technique in an emergency are the difficulties in setting up the collection of the blood on an occasional basis in a situation with exsanguinating haemorrhage. There are also the dangers associated with the infusion of activated clotting factors and of bacterial contamination. More sophisticated systems can wash and filter before re-infusion. This may either be a *cell*

washer in the theatre or the blood can be collected and taken to a central site for processing. The delays involved make these refinements less suitable in an emergency.

REFERENCES

1. *Atlas of Regional Anaesthesia*, 2nd edn. DL Brown, A Ross. Philadelphia: WB Saunders, 1998.
2. The Ionising Radiation (Medical Exposure) Regulations 2000. www.legislation.hmso.gov.uk/si/si2000/20001059.htm

Appendix III

POSTOPERATIVE CARE

The main responsibility for postoperative care rests with the surgeon. The advantages of good surgery can be lost if such care is sub-optimal.

LEVEL OF CARE

The appropriate level should be considered preoperatively, and the decision reviewed at the completion of surgery if unexpected problems have been encountered.

Day surgery

This is appropriate in those patients who are ambulant and who can resume normal oral intake within a few hours. There should be no metabolic or cardiovascular instability, and no respiratory compromise anticipated, either as the result of the procedure or from co-morbidity. Satisfactory pain relief must be possible with agents which are suitable for use at home. After a general anaesthetic patients must have a responsible adult who can care for them for the first 24 hours, and a similar arrangement is also essential after more major operations under local anaesthesia. The patient should be aware of the emergency management of any complication which might occur at home. However, if a complication would still be significantly more serious out of the hospital environment, the advisability of discharge home should be reconsidered.

Surgical ward

A surgical ward is an appropriate environment for those patients who require nursing care, basic monitoring of vital functions, and pain relief or other treatment which can not be managed at home.

- *Nursing care* may include the dressing of open wounds, fistulae and stomas, or the management of urinary catheters, nasogastric tubes and chest, abdominal or superficial drains. Alternatively, it may be simply the basic nursing care of an immobile patient.

- *Monitoring* of blood pressure, pulse, temperature, urine output and fluid balance are all standard ward procedures. Blood glucose can be monitored in diabetic patients and measurement of oxygen saturation and central venous pressure (CVP) are also practical. More advanced monitoring will require a more intensive environment.
- *Pain relief* with patient controlled intravenous opiate or with an epidural infusion are impractical at home, but both can be managed in an appropriate surgical ward environment.
- *Other treatment* may be necessary which, although not practical at home, can be managed safely on an ordinary ward. Intravenous fluid replacement or parenteral feeding is straightforward, unless the patient is cardiovascularly or metabolically unstable. Minor respiratory compromise can be treated with oxygen therapy and chest physiotherapy.

Intensive care or high–dependency environments

These are necessary when a patient is cardiovascularly unstable, or has incipient, or established, respiratory or renal failure. The definition of these units varies in different localities, as does the balance of medical supervision. The surgeon, the anaesthetist or the medical intensivist may be the lead clinician, but the surgical input remains of paramount importance. Patients who require mechanical ventilation, inotrope support or dialysis are obviously candidates for this environment, but those in incipient cardiac, respiratory or renal failure will often have an improved prognosis if they can be transferred early to an environment where intensive monitoring and intervention are possible.

PAIN CONTROL

Pain after surgery is feared by patients, and control is important if only to avoid the distress it causes. In addition, uncontrolled pain delays recovery and increases postoperative complications. Pain from chest and upper abdominal incisions inhibits both adequate respiratory effort and the clearance of secretions. Control of pain reduces the incidence of postoperative chest infections. Pain after abdominal incisions is a potent factor in postoperative ileus, and the reduction of this complication in laparoscopic surgery is probably in part related to a reduction in abdominal wall wound pain. Pain is also associated with many of the troublesome postoperative nausea and hypotensive episodes which prevent satisfactory discharge after day surgery.

Oral analgesia

This is the mainstay for day surgery pain relief. A combination of a non-steroidal anti-inflammatory drug (NSAID) with a preparation of paracetamol and codeine proves satisfactory in most patients. Pain control can be improved by commencing analgesic drugs immediately prior to surgery. Patients in whom a NSAID is contraindicated will require an increased dosage of codeine. This may cause nausea and should be anticipated with an oral anti-emetic. Postoperative nausea and vomiting also prevents the satisfactory administration of oral pain relief.

Local anaesthetic infiltration

Local infiltration of bupivicaine into the wound provides excellent pain relief in the critical first 6 hours after surgery, and may be more effective if given at the start rather than the end of the operation. This technique is used extensively in day surgery, but is less effective in a long abdominal or thoracic wound where both superficial and deep anaesthesia is required. Further bupivicaine can be administered to prolong the anaesthesia if a wound catheter is left *in situ*.

Intramuscular opiates

These are administered as bolus injections when required every 4–6 hours, and were for many years the mainstay of postoperative inpatient pain relief. The patient frequently requires intramuscular or intravenous pain relief in the recovery area, and this is followed by further injections as necessary. This is still a satisfactory method in those patients in whom only a few boluses are anticipated, and who are expected to be ambulant and able to take oral medication within 24–48 hours. However, if severe prolonged pain is anticipated this method is unsatisfactory as it produces widely fluctuating levels of pain relief, even with 4-hourly boluses. Hourly boluses are safe if the patient is still in pain, but the situation must be carefully monitored to prevent overdosage.

Intravenous opiates

This is the fastest method of bringing severe pain under control. A 2.5 mg dose of intravenous morphine is safe for an adult in severe pain, and can be repeated at 5-minute intervals, if necessary up to a total of 10 mg. Once the pain is under control, a longer term plan for adequate pain relief can be instituted.

Patient-controlled analgesia (PCA)

This is a system of delivery of intravenous opiate, the dose of which is controlled by the patient. The patient can administer a bolus (usually of 1 mg in adults) by pressing the control button. It should be possible for a patient to control pain without the risk of overdosage, as an oversedated patient will be too sleepy to press the button. Various safety 'lock-out' devices have had to be built into the system, however, to prevent a rapid delivery of repeated boluses. A 5-minute period during which the system will not respond to a second request for a bolus is usually satisfactory. A further hazard can be button pressure by child visitors!

Epidural analgesia

This is an extremely satisfactory method of ensuring a pain-free early postoperative period after major abdominal or thoracic surgery, without the sedation of systemic opiates. An epidural catheter is placed *in situ* by the anaesthetist and analgesia is maintained by continuous infusion of local anaesthetic agents or opiates into the epidural space. The excellent pain control can reduce postoperative respiratory complications and enables the patient to turn and move more freely. Analgesia can be maintained without distal paralysis, and although the legs are frequently too weak for weight-bearing, leg movement should still be possible. Epidural pain relief is, however, not without complications. Overdosage can be responsible for hypotension, and failure of delivery from a blocked or misplaced catheter can result in severe breakthrough pain which is sometimes difficult to get under control. Infection in the epidural space is a potential disaster. Catheters must be sited under sterile conditions and precautions taken to prevent subsequent introduction of infection. An epidural catheter should be removed as soon as it is no longer in use, and its retention for over 3 days should generally be avoided. A haematoma at insertion is a rare, but potentially catastrophic, complication. The signs of cord compression from an expanding haematoma may be mistaken for the effects of the epidural infusion until cord damage is irreversible. Management consists of early awareness of the possibility, confirmatory imaging and urgent neurosurgical transfer for decompression of the cord. Prevention includes good insertion technique and the avoidance of epidural anaesthesia, or analgesia, in patients with an underlying clotting abnormality. Prophylactic heparin should also be withheld during the period of epidural catheter insertion and removal.

INTRAVENOUS FLUID REQUIREMENTS

Many postoperative patients, especially those who have had intra-abdominal surgery, will be unable to take oral fluids for several days. Maintenance fluid and electrolytes are given intravenously. The daily maintenance requirements for adults and children are given in Table AIII.1. To this must be added fluid and electrolytes to correct pre-existing dehydration and

Table AIII.1 *Daily maintenance requirements.*

	Water	Sodium	Potassium
Adult and older child	100 mL/kg for the 1st 10 kg +50 mL/kg for the 2nd 10 kg +25 mL/kg for each subsequent 10 kg	1.5–2 mmol/kg	1 mmol/kg
Children weighing <10 kg	150 mL/kg	1.5–2 mmol/kg	1 mmol / kg

to replace continuing abnormal fluid losses (see Appendix I). In the early postoperative phase the correct volumes can be difficult to calculate. In addition, fluid shifts may result in an imbalance with hypovolaemia in association with increased interstitial fluid. An adequate circulatory volume, CVP and urine output can then only be maintained by a positive fluid balance. Conversely, increased output of antidiuretic hormone postoperatively inhibits the excretion of excess intravascular fluid, and subsequently fluid overload, particularly in the elderly, can precipitate congestive cardiac failure.

In adult practice the maintenance fluid and electrolyte requirements are seldom calculated accurately according to weight. Instead, a standard regime of 2–3 L of fluid is given of which one-third to one-quarter is normal saline and the remainder is 5 per cent dextrose. These solutions are available with potassium included (usually 40 mmol/L) but alternatively potassium can be added in aliquots of 27 mmol. A small elderly patient would therefore receive as maintenance 500 mL of saline and 1.5 L of 5 per cent dextrose, and a large younger patient 1 L of saline and 2 L of 5 per cent dextrose (Table AIII.2).

PARENTERAL FEEDING

Cardiac, respiratory and renal failure are all well recognized by clinicians as life-threatening conditions for which medical intervention is indicated to reduce mortality. Nutritional failure presents more assiduously, and although eventually equally serious is often ignored. Starvation or nutritional failure is a contributory cause of death in many patients who die in hospital of complications some weeks after surgery. This was discussed in Chapter 11, as it is of particular relevance in gastrointestinal surgery. The simpler and more satisfactory option of enteral feeding should always be considered, and this is also discussed in Chapter 11. However, it

may not be practical in the presence of gastrointestinal complications, and parenteral feeding has to be instituted.

Although oral intake of food comprises ingestion of large molecules of protein or starch, intravenous feeding is with the molecules to which these foodstuffs are reduced in the gut before absorption into the circulation. Solutions of amino acids and glucose, and emulsions of lipids form the basis of intravenous feeding. It is now standard practice to combine the lipids, glucose and amino acids in a single bag to which is added a customized amount of additional electrolytes, vitamins and trace elements. These bags (2.5 or 3 L in adult practice) are prepared in the pharmacy under sterile conditions which minimize the septic complications from bedside additions to what is an excellent culture medium. The solutions used for parenteral nutrition are hypertonic and irritant to peripheral veins. A central venous line is therefore usually established (see Appendix I). Sterility is paramount, as infection causes septicaemia and central vein thrombosis. A feeding line should, therefore, be a dedicated line and not used for intravenous access for other purposes. For long-term feeding a length of line tunnelled subcutaneously can reduce septic complications and prolong the life of the line (see Fig. 11.5, page 195).

Energy

Food is the fuel for the body. Carbohydrate supplies approximately 4 kcal/g and fat 9 kcal/g. Fat, although apparently a more valuable fuel source, cannot be metabolized efficiently on its own. It is therefore still important to provide nutritional support to the obese patient. Protein is a fuel source which is sometimes neglected in calculations; it supplies approximately 4 kcal/g when broken down, with the release of nitrogen to be excreted as urea. Skeletal muscle is therefore an important source of fuel in the starved patient. However, some of the amino acids given intravenously dur-

Table AIII.2 *Maintenance regimes.*

Body weight/Status	Total intake	Fluid	Sodium
40-kg elderly woman	1.5 L dextrose 500 mL saline 54 mmol K^+	2 L	70 mmol (1.5–2 mmol/kg)
80-kg young man	2 L dextrose 1 L saline 81 mmol K^+	3 L	140 mmol (1.5–2 mmol/kg)

ing well-balanced parenteral nutrition should be destined for the replacement of enzymes and for structural repair. Fuel is required by every cell of the body for the maintenance of its cell membrane function, and also for essential mechanical and enzymatic functions within the cell. Proportionally more is required by cells which are performing vital metabolic functions for the whole body; for example, in the resting state the liver accounts for 26 per cent of the total basal metabolic requirements.

Specific nutrients

Food is essential for the provision of specific nutrients for chemical reactions, and for structural intra- and extracellular materials. Amino acids are the most important building blocks of tissue, but lipids and carbohydrates are also required for structural mucopolysaccharides, glycoproteins and glycolipids. The balance of amino acids is important, in particular when feeding a very sick patient with an already compromised metabolism. Although an imbalance can to some extent be overcome by metabolic pathways which convert one amino acid to another, there are still problems. Some 'essential' amino acids cannot be manufactured by normal human metabolic pathways. Others, 'conditionally essential', can only be made in ideal metabolic circumstances. In addition, a poorly balanced combination places an additional strain on the patient's already compromised metabolic pathways. Much of an excess amino acid is then often simply broken down, lost to the amino acid pool, and although some protein calories are extracted, the nitrogen must be excreted, placing further demand on suboptimal hepatic and renal function.

Daily requirements

The daily requirements of energy and specific nutrients are normally calculated according to body weight, although a calculation by lean body mass is probably more appropriate.

Basic energy requirements
These are of the order of 25–30 kcal/kg body weight per day (1800–2100 kcal/day for a 70-kg man):

- 1.5 L of 20 per cent dextrose contains 300 g of glucose and will provide 1200 kcal
- 0.5 L of 20 per cent lipid emulsion contains 100 g of lipid and will provide 900 kcal
- Thus, a combination will provide 2100 kcal in 2 L of fluid.

Protein requirement
This is estimated as approximately 1 g/kg/day (70 g/day for a 70-kg man), although 0.8 g/kg/day is usually sufficient (56 g/day for a 70-kg man).

- As nitrogen accounts for 16 per cent of protein, the requirement for nitrogen is approximately 8.9 g nitrogen per day for a 70-kg man (16% of 56 g = 8.9 g).

- 0.5 L of amino acid solution can thus complete the usual nutritional requirements within the daily fluid allowance. Commonly, one of the standard compound 24-hour preparations is used.

Different concentrations of nutrients are available. For example:

- 9 g nitrogen/2200 calories; or
- 14 g nitrogen/2400 calories.

Many postoperative patients in whom oral feeding is delayed due to a prolonged ileus only require a simple basic maintenance regime, as outlined above, for a period of 1–2 weeks. The temptation to over-feed a severely malnourished patient must be resisted. Initially, their daily requirements are *less* and not more than the standard requirements. A process of 'reductive adaptation' will have occurred. Enzyme reserves are reduced with increased cellular efficiency. A sudden increase in nutrients is beyond the metabolic capacity of the cells, and damage occurs from toxic metabolites which the cells are unable to clear. Re-feeding must be introduced very gradually.

Hypercatabolic states

Some patients have greatly increased energy requirements, and also an increased need for essential nutrients for extensive tissue repair after injury. However, many of these patients initially are in the 'flow' stage of the general metabolic mobilization triggered by the cytokines of the systemic inflammatory response syndrome (SIRS). Skeletal muscle is broken down and amino acids are released into the circulation. Additional amino acids also enter the circulation from tissue destroyed by bacterial, chemical or thermal insults.

- The basal metabolic rate (BMR) rises 13 per cent for each 1° Centigrade rise in temperature.
- Severe sepsis can double the energy requirements.
- A 40 per cent burn increases the BMR by 60 per cent.

Attempts to match the energy requirements from external sources during this early catabolic phase are misguided, as it will not stop the mobilization of structural protein. The mobilization is usually in excess of that needed for the repair and replacement which the body can undertake at this stage. As there is therefore already a major source of fuel, feeding with excessive additional intravenous glucose results only in hyperglycaemia. Excessive administration of amino acids is also counterproductive in this early phase, as they place additional strain on the already stressed metabolic pathways and merely require to be broken down and the nitrogen excreted. A positive nitrogen balance cannot be achieved until the anabolic recovery phase has been reached. The monitoring of nitrogen losses in the urine may give an indication of the severity of the insult suffered or the time it will take for full convalescence, but does not provide any guide as to the requirements of nitrogen in the ensuing 24–48 hours.

In those patients in whom a high-calorie, high-protein regime is desirable, simply increasing the intravenous feeding regime to increase calories and nutrients has problems. Fluid overload and nutrient overload can occur. Lipid is poorly cleared from the circulation, and poorly metabolized, in severe infections. Glucose oxidation and storage is also impaired by sepsis and other causes of SIRS, although utilization can be restored to near-normal by insulin administration on a sliding scale to keep blood glucose concentrations within the normal range. There is, however, a metabolic ceiling for glucose oxidation, even in a patient who is not metabolically compromised.

Although rates of 4.1 mg glucose per kg fat free body mass per minute have been reported, the upper safe limit is usually taken as:

- 3 mg of glucose/kg of total body weight per minute; or
- 12 600 mg of glucose per hour for a 70-kg man; which equates to
- 750 g of glucose per day for a 70-kg man.

Therefore, a total of 3000 carbohydrate calories a day can seldom be exceeded in an adult.

The nitrogen content in a regimen can be increased, and this is important in those patients who have large external losses from burns or fistulae. Increased urinary nitrogen loss as explained above is seldom an indication for increasing parenteral delivery of nitrogen. Low serum albumin levels are more often an indication of a severe underlying illness, or ongoing sepsis, and are not specific or sensitive markers of severe malnutrition.

Amino acids should not be given without a simultaneous energy supply.

- 100–200 carbohydrate kcal/g of nitrogen is recommended.

Long-term parenteral feeding

Long-term parenteral feeding for established intestinal failure was discussed in Chapter 11. The requirements of micronutrients, trace elements and vitamins become of increasing importance, and the general surgeon may wish the involvement of a clinician with a nutritional and metabolic interest.

Children

The principles of intravenous feeding in children are similar to those in adults. However, in the neonate or baby, growth and development is rapid and the nutritional requirements higher. These very small patients with intestinal failure should be under the care of paediatric surgeons and physicians rather than a general surgeon.

POSTOPERATIVE COMPLICATIONS

Respiratory

Many patients already have some degree of respiratory compromise preoperatively, but respiratory function is further challenged by a general anaesthetic and surgery. In general, management consists of the correction of mechanical problems, adequate pain relief, intensive physiotherapy, antibiotics and additional oxygen in the inspired air. If despite these measures the P_aO falls below 8 kPa, or the P_aCO rises above 7 kPa, then mechanical ventilation should be considered.

Atelectasis
Anaesthetic gases are irritant to the respiratory epithelium, and an increase in bronchial secretions is to be expected. Impaired clearance of secretions is common postoperatively. This not only predisposes the patient to a postoperative respiratory infection, but a plug of mucus can occlude a segmental, or even a main bronchus, with atelectic collapse distally. Coughing may be too painful, and once analgesia is sufficient the patient may be too sedated to wish to cough unless encouraged to do so. Adequate analgesia and regular well-timed chest physiotherapy is therefore essential. An established atelectasis may be treated by dislodgement of the mucus plug by intensive physiotherapy, but bronchoscopy is still sometimes indicated.

Mechanical failure
Mechanical failure of adequate ventilation due to a pleural space filled with air, fluid or blood must be excluded. Tidal volume can also be reduced by a diaphragm which is splinted from raised intra-abdominal pressure and, when gastric dilatation is partly the cause, the situation can be improved by gastric aspiration.

Adult respiratory distress syndrome (ARDS)
This is a diffuse lung injury which occurs 24–72 hours after a range of initial insults (see 'Multi-organ failure' below). General opacification of the lung fields on X-ray is obvious, and the deterioration of respiratory function will often require mechanical ventilation.

Chest infections
These are a common postoperative complication. The normal commensals of the upper respiratory tract become opportunist pathogens in the increased stagnant secretions of the lower tract. A respiratory tract infection is the most common cause of a pyrexia during the first 3 days after surgery. A pulmonary embolus may also present with dyspnoea and pleuritic chest pain. Differentiation from an infective problem can be difficult when symptoms, signs and X-rays suggest an area of pneumonia.

Cardiovascular

Strokes and myocardial infarctions

Cardiovascular instability, and especially periods of hypotension, are potentially serious to any patient with a stenosis of an artery supplying the myocardium or brain. A perioperative myocardial infarction or cerebrovascular accident can follow an episode of poor perfusion prior to, during or immediately after an operation. Later, the increased coagulability of the blood during the postoperative period predisposes to arterial thrombosis on stenosed arteries, and may again be precipitated by a fall in perfusion. This fall may be associated with a secondary postoperative haemorrhage or with sepsis from an anastomotic leak.[1] The surgeon must be aware of this combination of pathologies, or only the secondary medical problem may be diagnosed and the underlying surgically amenable complication may be missed.

Cardiac failure and inotrope support

Cardiac output and arterial blood pressure may both be depressed in an ill patient. When perfusion of vital organs becomes threatened, inotropic support with adrenaline, noradrenaline or other pressor agent becomes necessary. Such patients require intensive monitoring, and frequently also mechanical ventilation, and will have to be transferred to an intensive care unit.

Venous thrombosis and embolus

The prophylaxis of venous thrombosis and pulmonary embolus was discussed in Appendix I, and should continue during the postoperative period until the patient is fully mobile, which in practice is often the time of discharge home. The treatment of an established thrombosis or embolus is anticoagulation.

A clinical diagnosis of deep vein thrombosis is difficult as signs are unreliable. However, recently developed algorithms may help in decisions over management. Unfortunately, D-dimer levels are not helpful during the perioperative period. Doppler ultrasound by an experienced operator is a sensitive investigation, although venography remains the 'gold standard'.

Accurate clinical diagnosis of pulmonary embolism is also difficult. Treatment must often be started on a presumptive diagnosis, based on clinical suspicion, combined with an analysis of ECG or blood gas results. Subsequently, radiological investigations are important to establish the diagnosis, as if excluded, treatment can be discontinued, and several months of further prophylactic anticoagulation therapy will be avoided. Investigations will depend on the facilities available. CT pulmonary angiography is the current gold standard, but ventilation–perfusion (VQ) scanning and conventional invasive pulmonary angiography are also in common use.

The initial treatment is classically with a loading dose of 10 000 units of non-fractionated heparin (100–200 units/kg) intravenously. A heparin infusion is then established at a rate of 30 000 units per 24 hours. Adjustment of dose is influenced by monitoring of the activated partial thromboplastin time (APTT), which should be maintained at twice the normal range. Once the diagnosis is confirmed, warfarin anticoagulation is commenced unless there is still a risk of postoperative bleeding. The heparin is stopped once the patient is fully anticoagulated, and the warfarin should be continued for 3–6 months. A large pulmonary embolus with right-heart failure may require more active treatment with thrombolysis through a pulmonary artery catheter placed by a radiologist. The surgical alternative of a pulmonary embolectomy (see Chapter 7) is almost never undertaken. An IVC filter should be considered in patients at high risk of further emboli – those with free-floating IVC clot, with repeat emboli after commencement of heparin and in those in whom anticoagulation is contraindicated.

Renal complications

Oliguria

Oliguria, usually defined as a urinary output of <20 mL per hour, requires action. Urine retention or a blocked catheter must first be excluded. If the patient is hypotensive or shocked, volume replacement of the extracellular fluid compartment is the first priority. Similarly, if the oliguria is secondary to poor perfusion due to cardiac failure this should be treated. If neither hypovolaemia nor cardiac failure are the apparent cause, a fluid bolus of 200 mL should then be given. If this fails to produce a diuresis, a CVP measurement will be helpful. (Further fluid boluses will be detrimental if the CVP is high, and a diuretic challenge contraindicated if the patient is hypovolaemic.) Diuretics, in conjunction with generous fluid replacement, can protect against renal failure by maintaining a good urine flow and preventing sludging in the collecting system. A frusemide challenge will often improve urine output in oliguria, but in high dosage it can be nephrotoxic.

Established renal failure

This requires intensive fluid and electrolyte monitoring. Transfer of the patient to an intensive care or high-dependency environment becomes necessary and the management of their renal failure passes to the intensivists. Fluid overload, hyperkalaemia and acidosis are the main threats. The risk of upper gastrointestinal bleeding is increased and prophylactic H_2 antagonists or sucralfate should be given. Nephrotoxic drugs must be avoided. Hyperkalaemia of over 6.5 mmol must be reduced urgently. Conservative measures to reduce potassium levels include correction of the acidosis, glucose and insulin infusions, oral exchange resins, intravenous calcium administration and high-dose frusemide. Renal replacement therapy is indicated for hypervolaemia, and for a hyperkalaemia or acidosis which does not respond to conservative treatment (a persistent potassium over 6.5 or a pH below 7.2). A variety of renal replacement techniques are available, but the most commonly used in the acute postoperative patient is continuous venovenous haemofiltration

(CVVH) with a pump providing the flow through the system. In the postoperative patient, renal failure is most commonly part of a multi-system failure, and often the patient also requires cardiac inotropes and mechanical ventilatory support.

Intestinal complications

Temporary intestinal failure after abdominal – and particularly gastrointestinal – surgery is common. An ileus usually resolves spontaneously and is seldom life-threatening, but more severe manifestations are discussed in Chapter 11. Prolonged intestinal failure results in severe malnutrition. This often goes unrecognized, but is an important cause of increased mortality and morbidity in the surgical patient.

Infective complications

The diagnosis of sepsis during the postoperative period is not always straightforward. A pyrexia and rise in white blood cell count (WBC) may also occur as part of a systemic inflammatory reaction to sterile tissue damage. An overwhelming sepsis may result in a fall in WBCs, and, particularly in the elderly, the most obvious clinical features may be of cardiovascular decompensation, which is easily misdiagnosed as a primary cardiac complication.

During the first 48 hours after surgery any infection is most likely to be related to the original septic pathology for which surgery was undertaken, or to be a respiratory infection. A central line sepsis must also be considered. Dead tissue, whether gut or the soft tissue of an amputation stump, may also present as 'sepsis'. Evidence of sepsis at 7–14 days after any intra-abdominal anastomosis must raise the possibility of an anastomotic leak. This must be excluded as urgent re-laparotomy will often be indicated. Intra-abdominal, pelvic and wound abscesses may also present at this time, and respiratory, central line and urinary infections are all further possibilities. Antibiotic therapy alone is insufficient if there is necrotic tissue or extensive contamination with infected gastrointestinal contents. Dead tissue must be excised, and any pus drained.

Multi-organ failure

Direct tissue injury, whether from a traumatic, surgical, thermal or infective cause, releases into the circulation chemicals from damaged cells which incite a systemic inflammatory response. The effects include endothelial damage in capillaries throughout the body and subsequent damage in all organs. In addition, these damaged capillaries allow excessive fluid out of the circulation, and even if there is no bleeding wound or weeping burn there can be a profound hypovolaemia. If aggressive fluid replacement is not initiated early there is inadequate tissue perfusion and further damage to vital tissue. The mainstay of management is intensive support including inotropes, mechanical ventilation and haemofiltration. The surgeon, however, must be alert to the possibility that there might be an underlying surgically amenable pathology which requires action. An abdominal abscess, dead gut or an intraperitoneal or mediastinal leak from a gastrointestinal anastomosis are the most common scenarios.

REHABILITATION

Healing of tissue at the site of operation continues after a patient has been discharged home. Generalized weakness and tiredness following major surgery may take several months to settle, especially if the surgery or the underlying pathology was associated with sepsis or a profound weight loss. Patients require some guidance on return to normal activities, as some unrealistically expect an immediate return to peak physical fitness, while others will delay their full recovery by restricting their activities. Some patients may require specific dietary advice or a course of physiotherapy.

For some patients, a return to their preoperative level of health and lifestyle is not possible. The physical and psychological adjustments to a prosthetic limb, a breast prosthesis or a stoma should not be underestimated. Other patients have to adjust to a shortened life expectancy or a life with major restrictions. A surgeon who decides that they do not need to see a patient after discharge from hospital must be assured that the patient has sufficient other professional or social support for their further recovery from surgery.

REFERENCE

1. Sutton CD, Marshall LJ, Williams N, *et al.* Colo-rectal anastomotic leakage often masquerades as a cardiac complication. *Colorectal Dis* 2004; **6**: 21–2.

Index